Handbook of
Veterinary Drugs

SECOND EDITION

Handbook of Veterinary Drugs

SECOND EDITION

Dana G. Allen
DVM, MSc, Diplomate ACVIM (Internal Medicine)
Professor
Department of Clinical Studies
Ontario Veterinary College; University of Guelph
Guelph, Ontario

John K. Pringle
DVM, DVSc, PhD, Diplomate ACVIM (Internal Medicine)
Associate Professor of Large Animal Medicine
Department of Health Management
Atlantic Veterinary College;
University of Prince Edward Island
Charlottetown, Prince Edward Island

Dale A. Smith
DVM, DVSc
Associate Professor
Department of Pathobiology
Ontario Veterinary College; University of Guelph
Guelph, Ontario

with

Associate Editor
Kirby Pasloske
BSc, DVM, DVSc (Clinical Pharmacology)
Veterinary Researcher
Merck and Company, Incorporated
Branchburg Farm
Somerville, New Jersey

Assistant Editor
Kendra Day
BSc (Pharm)
Director of Pharmacy
Atlantic Veterinary College;
University of Prince Edward Island
Charlottetown, Prince Edward Island

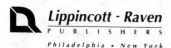

Lippincott - Raven
PUBLISHERS
Philadelphia • New York

Acquisitions Editor: Paula Callaghan
Developmental Editor: Lesa Ramsey
Indexer: Barbara Littlewood
Cover Designer: Karen Quigley
Supervising Editor: Kimberly Swan
Production Service: P. M. Gordon Associates
Compositor: Circle Graphics
Printer/Binder: R. R. Donnelley & Sons

Printed in the United States of America

9 8 7 6 5 4 3 2 1

Library of Congress Cataloging-in-Publication Data

Allen, Dana G. (Dana Gray)
    Handbook of veterinary drugs / Dana G. Allen, John K. Pringle, Dale A. Smith
with Kirby Pasloske and Kendra Day. — 2nd ed.
        p.   cm.
    Includes index.
    ISBN 0-397-58435-0
    1. Veterinary drugs—Handbooks, manuals, etc.   I. Pringle, John K.   II. Smith,
Dale A.   III. Title.
SF917.A44 1998
636.089'51—dc21   98-9454
                                                                                                                CIP

Care has been taken to confirm the accuracy of the information presented and to
describe generally accepted practices. However, the authors, editors, and publisher are
not responsible for errors or omissions or for any consequences from application of the
information in this book and make no warranty, express or implied, with respect to
the contents of the publication.

The authors, editors and publisher have exerted every effort to ensure that drug
selection and dosage set forth in this text are in accordance with current
recommendations and practice at the time of publication. However, in view of
ongoing research, changes in government regulations, and the constant flow of
information relating to drug therapy and drug reactions, the reader is urged to check
the package insert for each drug for any change in indications and dosage and for
added warnings and precautions. This is particularly important when the
recommended agent is a new or infrequently employed drug.

Some new drugs and medical devices presented in this publication have Food and
Drug Administration (FDA) clearance for limited use in restricted research settings. It
is the responsibility of the health care provider to ascertain the FDA status of each
drug or device planned for use in their clinical practice.

CONTENTS

Part III: Exotics 597

PREFACE

In undertaking the revision of *Handbook of Veterinary Drugs*, we endeavored to provide readers with the same useful and practical data, dosing information, and user-friendly format that made the first edition a success. *Handbook of Veterinary Drugs* serves as a useful reference for commonly used drugs in veterinary medicine.

We designed *Handbook of Veterinary Drugs* to be a practical aid to both veterinary students and busy practitioners. To provide readers with rapid access, the book is divided into three sections: Small Animals (dogs and cats); Large Animals (horses, ruminant species, and pigs); and Exotic Species (avian species, ferrets, reptiles, rodents, and rabbits). Each section begins by listing common drug dosages and routes of administration. The reader then finds tables listing parasites and useful anthelmintics (Large Animals) and bacteria and useful antibiotics (Small and Large Animal sections). The second part of each section describes those drugs listed in drug doses under the following headings.

INDICATIONS: A description of the drug and its use(s) is listed. Where available, serum drug levels are given. Common trade names in Canada ♣ and the United States ★ are included to facilitate acquisition of the drug.

ADVERSE AND COMMON SIDE EFFECTS: Emphasis is placed on information as it pertains to veterinary medicine. When these data are not available, reference to human experience with the drug is given. Management of drug toxicity is discussed in cases where appropriate data are available.

DRUG INTERACTIONS: Where such information is available for animals, it is provided. However, some of the data are derived from experience in human medicine.

SUPPLIED AS: This section provides common drug formulations. As in other sections, veterinary-specific information is listed where available, with human medicine filling in some of the gaps. Note that available formulations may change over the course of this publication, and they may differ in Canada versus the United States.

OTHER USES: This segment discusses off-label uses, including drug dose(s), where available. Although we generally do not condone off-label use, such uses may be necessary in practice, especially when treating exotic species. Much of the information contained herein has been derived from empirical use and not from scientifically controlled studies. In those cases in which conventional therapy has been unsuccessful or has not been established for the condition present, alternative drug therapy is supplied for the reader's information. Informed consent must be obtained from owners or agents before such use of the drug is employed.

Additional features of *Handbook of Veterinary Drugs* include a body weight-to-body surface area conversion chart located at the front of the Small Animals section. We have added a description of the idiosyncrasies of drug use in the various exotic species. A list of abbreviations is provided to clarify areas of possible confusion. Along with drugs licensed for use in the stated species, some drugs that are not licensed for specific use are listed. This book makes no attempt to validate reports of drugs for off-label use. Practitioners are urged to follow manufacturers' recommendations concerning the use of any drug. In the Large Animal section, dosage regimens for aerosol medications also are included, and withdrawal times for meat and milk for Canada and the United States are given. In the Exotic Animal section, drug dosages derived from scientific studies are distinguished from dosages derived from empirical use alone. Readers will not find data pertaining to pharmacokinetic studies unless that information is important to the practitioner's use of the drug. To keep the book practical and portable, references have been omitted. References are available on request to the editor(s).

We also have created an electronic version of the *Handbook*, providing users with multimedia links between dosing tables and specific drug entries. The electronic version also allows practitioners to print side and adverse effects for clients. The CD-ROM adds to the book's practicality by providing the speed and flexibility of a computer. We hope that both media will be as popular as the first edition with veterinarians in training and in practice.

LIST OF ABBREVIATIONS

bid—twice daily
tid—three times daily
q—every
qid—four times daily
qod—every other day

IC—intracardiac
IM—intramuscular
IP—intraperitoneal
IV—intravenous
PO—per os
PRN—as required
SC—subcutaneous

BUN—blood urea nitrogen
D_5W—5% dextrose in water
g—gram
gr—grain
IU—international unit
L—liter
lb—pound
m^2—square meter (body surface area)
μg—microgram
mEq—milliequivalent
OD—right eye
OS—left eye
OU—both eyes
w/v—weight (of solute) per volume (of solvent)

♣—Canadian usage
★—U.S. usage

Part I

Small Animals

Conversion of Body Weight to Body Surface Area in Dogs

Body Weight (kg)	Body Surface Area (m²)	Body Weight (kg)	Body Surface Area (m²)
0.5	0.06	29.0	0.94
1.0	0.10	30.0	0.96
2.0	0.15	31.0	0.99
3.0	0.20	32.0	1.01
4.0	0.25	33.0	1.03
5.0	0.29	34.0	1.05
6.0	0.33	35.0	1.07
7.0	0.36	36.0	1.09
8.0	0.40	37.0	1.11
9.0	0.43	38.0	1.13
10.0	0.46	39.0	1.15
11.0	0.49	40.0	1.17
12.0	0.52	41.0	1.19
13.0	0.55	42.0	1.21
14.0	0.58	43.0	1.23
15.0	0.60	44.0	1.25
16.0	0.63	45.0	1.26
17.0	0.66	46.0	1.28
18.0	0.69	47.0	1.30
19.0	0.71	48.0	1.32
20.0	0.74	49.0	1.34
21.0	0.76	50.0	1.36
22.0	0.78	51.0	1.38
23.0	0.81	52.0	1.40
24.0	0.83	53.0	1.41
25.0	0.85	54.0	1.43
26.0	0.88	55.0	1.45
27.0	0.90	56.0	1.47
28.0	0.92	57.0	1.48

From Ettinger SJ. *Textbook of veterinary internal medicine.* Vol. I. Philadelphia: WB Saunders, 1975:146.

Conversion of Body Weight to Body Surface Area in Cats

Body Weight (kg)	Body Surface Area (m²)
2.3	0.165
2.8	0.187
3.2	0.207
3.6	0.222
4.1	0.244
4.6	0.261
5.1	0.278
5.5	0.294
6.0	0.311
6.4	0.326
6.9	0.342
7.4	0.356
7.8	0.371
8.2	0.385
8.7	0.399
9.2	0.413

Handbook of Veterinary Drugs, Second Edition, edited by Dana Allen,
Lippincott–Raven Publishers, Philadelphia. © 1998

Section 1

Common Dosages for Dogs and Cats

*Drugs listed in boldface indicate that additional dosing information (uses) is available in Section 3: Description of Drugs for Small Animals.

Drug*	Dog	Cat
Acemannan	1 mg/kg weekly, IP for up to 6 wks, followed by monthly injections for 1 year plus 2 mg intratumor before surgery for up to 6 wks; surgical excision of tumor at 4th to 7th wk then radiation treatment started (fibrosarcoma)	Same **OR** FeLV or FIV-induced syndromes; 2 mg/kg once weekly; IV, SC, IP for 6 wks (FeLV) or 12 wks (FIV), followed by 2 mg/kg once monthly (FIV)
Acepromazine	0.55 to 2.2 mg/kg; PO 0.025 to 0.200 mg/kg; IV (max 3 mg) **OR** 0.10 to 0.25 mg/kg; IM, PO (restraint, sedation)	1.1 to 2.2 mg/kg; PO 0.05 to 0.10 mg/kg; IV, IM, SC (max 1 mg) (restraint, sedation)
Acetaminophen	10 mg/kg bid; PO	None
Acetazolamide	10 mg/kg qid; PO (metabolic acidosis) 2 to 5 mg/kg tid; PO (glaucoma)	Same 50 mg/kg once; IV 7 mg/kg tid; PO (glaucoma)

Drug*	Dog	Cat
Acetylcysteine (10% and 20% solutions available)	50 mL/hr for 30 to 60 min bid; by nebulization (respiratory disease)	140 mg/kg; PO, then 70 mg/kg qid; PO for 7 treatments (acetaminophen toxicosis)
Albendazole	25 mg/kg bid; PO for 10 days (Paragonimus)	Same
	Giardia: 4 doses at 25 mg/kg	Giardia: 10 doses at 25 mg/kg
Albuterol	0.02 to 0.04 mg/kg 1 to 3 times daily; PO	Unknown
Aldactazide	2 mg/kg once to twice daily; PO	Same
Allopurinol	10 mg/kg bid–tid for 1 mo, then reduce to 10 mg/kg daily **OR** 15 mg/kg bid; PO; if poor response, increase dose by 10–25% (urate calculi)	None
Alpha-keri	1 capful to 1 to 2 quarts of water for final rinse, or spray aerosol onto wet coat and rub well	Same
Aluminum hydroxide	30 to 90 mg/kg once to 3 times daily; PO (hyperphosphatemia) **OR** 2 to 10 mL every 2 to 4 hrs; PO (antacid)	30 to 90 mg/kg/day; PO (hyperphosphatemia)
Amikacin	5 mg/kg tid; IM, IV, SC	Same
Aminopentamide	0.1 mg to 0.4 mg bid–tid; SC, IM (antiemetic, decrease tenesmus) **OR** up to 10 lbs, 0.1 mg bid–tid; IM, SC, PO	0.1 to 0.4 mg bid–tid; IM, SC (antiemetic)

Drug*	Dog	Cat
Aminopentamide (continued)	11 to 20 lbs, 0.2 mg as above 21 to 50 lbs, 0.3 mg as above 51 to 100 lbs, 0.4 mg as above >100 lbs, 0.5 mg as above	
Aminophylline	10 mg/kg tid; PO, IM, IV	5 mg/kg bid–tid; PO **OR** 4 mg/kg bid; PO, IM
Amitraz	10.6 mL in 2 gallons of water; dip every 2 wks for 3 to 6 treatments; let dry on coat **OR** 0.125% applied half-body daily; topically	0.0125% applied weekly; topically (demodex)
Amitriptyline	2.2 to 4.4 mg/kg once daily; PO **OR** 2.2 mg/kg once to twice daily; PO (separation anxiety) **OR** 1 to 6 mg/kg once to twice daily; PO 1 mg/ kg bid; PO (pruritus)	5 to 10 mg once daily; PO **OR** 0.5 to 1 mg/kg/day; PO
Ammonium chloride	200 mg/kg div. tid; PO	20 mg/kg bid; PO
Amoxicillin	10 to 20 mg/kg bid; PO, SC, IV **OR** 11 to 22 mg/kg bid–tid; PO	Same
Amphotericin B	0.15 to 1 mg/kg dissolved in 5 to 20 mL D$_5$W; rapidly IV 3 times weekly for 2 to 4 mos (not to exceed 2 mL/kg) **OR**	Same

Drug*	Dog	Cat
Amphotericin B (continued)	0.25 to 0.5 mg/kg in 0.5 to 1 L D$_5$W; IV over 6 to 8 hrs; qod to total dose of 8 to 10 mg/kg or BUN and creatinine increase	
Ampicillin	22 mg/kg tid; PO **OR** 11 to 22 mg/kg tid–qid; SC, IV, IM	Same
Amprolium	100 to 200 mg/kg once daily; PO in food or water for 7 to 10 days	Unknown
Amrinone	1 to 3 mg/kg; IV bolus followed by 30 to 100 µg/kg/min	Unknown
Apomorphine	0.04 mg/kg; IV 0.08 mg/kg; IM, SC	Same
Ascorbic acid	100 to 500 mg/day; PO (maintenance) 100 to 500 mg 1 to 3 times daily; PO (urine acidification)	100 mg/day; PO (maintenance) 100 mg 1 to 3 times daily; PO (urine acidification) 30 mg/kg qid; PO for 7 treatments (acetaminophen toxicosis)
Asparaginase	10,000 to 30,000 IU/m^2; IM weekly (lymphosarcoma) **OR** 400 U/kg; IM once (thrombocytopenia)	10,000 IU/m^2; IM, SC every 1 to 3 wks (neoplastic disease)
Aspirin	10 mg/kg bid; PO (antipyretic) 25 to 35 mg/kg tid; PO (musculoskeletal pain)10 mg/kg once daily; PO **OR** 0.5 mg/kg bid (antithrombotic therapy)	6 mg/kg every 48 to 72 hrs; PO (antipyretic) 40 mg/kg every 72 hrs (antirheumatic) 25 mg/kg twice weekly; PO (antithrombotic therapy)

Drug*	Dog	Cat
Aspirin (continued)	5 to 10 mg/kg once daily; PO (heartworm therapy)	10 mg/kg every 48 to 72 hrs; PO **OR**
	10 to 25 mg/kg bid–tid; PO (analgesia)	10 to 20 mg/kg every 48 hrs; PO (analgesia)
Atenolol	6.25 to 12.5 mg bid; PO **OR**	6.25 to 12.5 mg once daily; PO **OR**
	0.25 to 1 mg/kg once to twice daily; PO	5 mg once to twice daily; PO **OR**
		3 mg/kg bid; PO
Atracurium	0.22 mg/kg; IV; give ¹⁄₁₀ to ¹⁄₆ initially as a priming dose, then 4 to 6 min later, the remainder with a sedative or hypnotic agent (induction dose)	Same
	0.11 mg/kg; IV (intraoperative dose)	
Atropine	0.022 to 0.044 mg/kg PRN; IM, IV, SC or 0.04 mg/kg tid–qid; PO (sinus bradycardia, sinus block, AV block)	Same
	0.02 to 0.04 mg/kg; SC, IM (preanesthetic)	Same
	0.2 to 2 mg/kg; ¹⁄₄ dose IV, rest SC, IM (cholinergic toxicity)	
Auranofin	0.05 to 0.2 mg/kg bid; PO	Unknown
Aurothioglucose	1st wk: 5 mg; IM 2nd wk: 10 mg; IM, then 1 mg/kg once weekly; IM, decreasing to once monthly	1st wk: 1 mg; IM 2nd wk: 2 mg; IM, then 1 mg/kg once weekly; IM, decreasing to once monthly
Azathioprine	2 mg/kg once daily; PO	1.1 mg/kg qid; PO (with caution)

Drug*	Dog	Cat
BAL: Dimercaprol	4 mg/kg every 4 to 6 hrs until recovered; IM	Same
Benazepril	0.25 mg/kg once daily; PO (dose may be doubled as indicated)	Unknown
Benzoyl peroxide	Bathe every 3 to 4 days to once every 1 to 2 wks; leave on skin for 10 min and rinse	Same
Betamethasone	0.15 mg/kg once; IM	Unknown
Bethanechol	5 to 25 mg tid; PO 2.5 to 10 mg tid; SC	2.5 to 5 mg tid; PO
Bisacodyl	5 to 20 mg once daily; PO	5 mg once daily; PO
Bismuth subsalicylate	10 to 30 mL every 4 to 6 hrs; PO **OR** 2 mL/kg tid–qid; PO	1 to 2 mL/kg every 4 to 6 hrs; PO
Bleomycin	0.2 to 0.6 mg/m²; SC or IV, daily for 5 days, then twice a week for 5 wks	Same
Bromide; Potassium	Initially 70 to 80 mg/kg once daily; PO (used as a single agent) 22 to 30 mg/kg once daily; PO (those also on phenobarbital) 22 to 40 mg/kg/day; PO **OR** 10 mg/kg bid; PO as a 100-mg/mL soln diluted in water with food	Same
Buprenorphine	0.005 to 0.02 mg/kg every 4 to 8 hrs; IV, IM	0.005 to 0.01 mg/kg every 4 to 8 hrs; IV, IM

Drug*	Dog	Cat
Buspirone	2.5 to 10 mg bid–tid; PO **OR** 1 to 2 mg/kg 1 to 3 times daily; PO (behavioral problems)	2.5 to 5 mg bid–tid; PO 5 mg bid; PO; if no response, increase to 7.5 mg bid; PO (urine spraying) 0.5 to 1 mg/kg 1 to 3 times daily; PO (behavioral problems)
Butorphanol	0.55 mg/kg bid–qid; PO to a max of 5 mg/4.5 kg **OR** 0.5 to 1 mg/kg bid–qid; PO **OR** 0.05 to 0.12 mg/kg bid–tid; PO (antitussive) 0.2 to 0.4 mg/kg every 2 to 5 hrs; IM, IV **OR** 0.4 mg/kg; SC, IM **OR** 0.2 to 0.8 mg/kg every 1 to 3 hrs; IM, IV, SC (analgesia)	0.5 to 1 mg/kg bid–qid; PO (antitussive) 0.1 to 0.4 mg/kg; IV, IM, SC (lasts 2–5 hrs) **OR** 0.8 mg/kg; IV (lasts 2 hrs) **OR** 0.2 to 1.0 mg/kg every 4 to 6 hrs; PO (analgesia)
Calcitonin-salmon	4 to 7 U/kg tid–qid; SC **OR** 4 to 6 IU/kg every 2 to 3 hrs; SC, IM until serum calcium stabilizes **OR** 4 U/kg; IV initially followed by 4 to 8 U/kg once to twice daily; SC	Unknown
Calcitriol	0.03 to 0.06 µg/kg once daily; PO 2.5 ng/kg once daily; PO (chronic renal failure)	Same
Calcium carbonate	1 to 4 g/day; PO **OR** 100 to 150 mg/kg div. bid–tid; PO	Same

Drug*	Dog	Cat
Calcium chloride (10% solution)	1 mL per 10 kg; IV (ventricular asystole) 0.1 mL/kg (100- mg/mL soln); IV (hyper-kalemia or hypocal-cemia)	Same
Calcium EDTA	100 mg/kg/day for 5 days; make soln of 1 g versenate per 100 mL D₅W, div. total quantity into 20 aliquots at 1 dose; SC qid for 5 days (lead poisoning)	Same
Calcium gluconate (10% solution)	0.5 to 1.5 mL/kg over 20 to 30 min; IV; may repeat tid–qid **OR** 10 to 15 mg/kg/hr; IV inf	Same **OR** 5 to 10 mL/cat; IV
Calcium lactate	0.5 to 2 g; PO **OR** 130 to 200 mg/kg tid; PO	0.2 to 0.5 g; PO **OR** Same
Captopril	0.5 to 2 mg/kg bid–tid; PO	2 mg bid–tid; PO
Carbenicillin	15 mg/kg tid; PO, IV	Same
Carboplatin	300 mg/m² every 21 days; IV	Unknown
Carnitine	2 g bid–tid; PO **OR** 100 mg/kg bid; PO **OR** 220 mg/kg/day; IV, or div. daily; PO (cardiomyopathy)	250 to 500 mg once daily; PO **OR** 50 to 100 mg/kg; PO (hepatic lipidosis)
Carprofen	2.2 mg/kg bid; PO 4 mg/kg; IV initially (surgical pain) 4 mg/kg; IV (chronic pain)	Unknown Same Same
Cefaclor	4 to 20 mg/kg tid; PO	Same
Cefadroxil	22 mg/kg bid; PO	Same

Drug*	Dog	Cat
Cefamandole	6 to 40 mg/kg tid–qid; IM, IV	Same
Cefazolin	5 to 15 mg/kg tid–qid; IM, IV	Same
Cefixime	5 mg/kg once daily; PO	Unknown
Cefotaxime	20 to 80 mg/kg tid; IM, IV, SC	20 to 80 mg/kg qid; IM, IV, SC
	25 to 50 mg/kg tid; IM, IV, SC	Same
Cefoxitin	6 to 20 mg/kg tid; IM, IV, SC **OR** 6 to 40 mg/kg tid–qid; IV **OR** 30 mg/kg every 5 hrs; IV and 30 mg/kg tid; SC	22 to 30 mg/kg tid; IM, IV, SC
Ceftazidime	25 mg/kg bid–tid; IM, SC	Same
Cephalexin	20 to 40 mg/kg bid–tid; PO	Same
Cephalothin	20 to 35 mg/kg tid–qid; IM, IV, SC	Same
Cephapirin	20 to 30 mg/kg tid; IM, IV, SC	Same
Cephradine	20 to 40 mg/kg tid; PO, IV, IM	Same
Charcoal (activated)	1 g/5 mL water; give 10 mL slurry/kg; PO	Same
Chlorambucil	2 to 8 mg/m^2 once daily; PO for 3 wks beyond remission, then 1.5 mg/m^2 once daily; PO for 15 days, then every 3rd day	1.5 mg/m^2 once daily; PO then as for dog 0.2 mg/kg/day; PO (immune-mediated anemia)
Chloramphenicol	50 mg/kg tid; PO, IM, IV, SC	50 mg/kg bid; PO, IM, IV, SC
Chlorhexidine (1%)	Apply ointment after cleansing area; repeat PRN	Same

Drug*	Dog	Cat
Chlorothiazide	20 to 40 mg/kg bid; PO	Same
Chlorpheniramine	0.5 to 1 mg/kg bid–tid; PO	1 to 2 mg bid–tid; PO
	0.22 mg/kg tid; PO (pruritus)	2 to 4 mg bid; PO (pruritus)
Chlorpromazine	3.3 mg/kg 1 to 4 times daily; PO **OR** 1.1 to 6.6 mg/kg 1 to 4 times daily; IM **OR** 0.55 to 4.4 mg/kg 1 to 4 times daily; IV	Same
	0.5 mg/kg tid; IM (antiemetic)	Same
	3 mg/kg bid; PO **OR** 0.5 mg/kg bid; IM, IV (sedative, restraint)	Same **OR** 0.5 mg/kg once daily; IM, IV
	up to 1.1 mg/kg; IM 1 to 1.5 hrs before surgery (preanesthetic)	Same
	0.5 to 3.3 mg/kg 1 to 4 times daily; PO (behavioral problems)	Same
Chlorpropamide	10 to 40 mg/kg once daily; PO	Unknown
Cimetidine	5 to 10 mg/kg tid–qid; PO, IV, IM (chronic gastritis, GI ulcer)	5 mg/kg tid–qid; PO, IV **OR** 10 mg/kg bid; PO, IM, IV **OR** 2.5 to 5 mg/kg bid; PO, IV
Ciprofloxacin	10 to 15 mg/kg bid; PO **OR** 5 to 11 mg/kg bid; PO	Unknown Same
Cisapride	0.1 to 0.5 mg/kg bid–tid; PO	Same **OR** 2.5 mg tid; PO <4 kg 5 mg tid; PO >4 kg **OR** 1 mg/kg tid; PO **OR** 1.5 mg/kg bid; PO

Drug*	Dog	Cat
Cisplatin	60 mg/m²; slowly IV over 20 min every 3 wks; pretreat with IV fluids 4 hrs before (20 mL/kg/hr) and 2 hrs after **OR** 70 mg/m² every 21 days; IV over 20 min; saline given for 3 hrs before cisplatin at 25 mL/kg/hr and after at same rate for 1 hr	None
Clavamox	13.75 mg/kg bid; PO	62.5 mg bid; PO
Clemastine	0.05 to 0.1 mg/kg bid; PO	0.68 mg bid; PO
Clindamycin	5.5 mg/kg bid; PO (wounds, abscesses, dental infection) 11 mg/kg bid; PO (osteomyelitis)	5.5 to 11 mg/kg bid; PO (susceptible infections)
	5 to 11 mg/kg tid; PO, IM, IV (infections)	Same
	3 to 13 mg/kg tid; PO, IM **OR** 10 to 20 mg/kg bid; PO, IM (for 2 wks for toxoplasmosis and *Neospora caninum*)	10 to 20 mg/kg bid; PO, IM for 3 to 6 wks **OR** 25 to 50 mg/kg/day div. for 2 to 3 wks (toxoplasmosis)
Clonazepam	1 to 10 mg once to 4 times daily; PO **OR** 1.5 mg/kg div. tid; PO 0.1 to 0.5 mg/kg bid–tid; PO (behavioral problems)	0.016 mg/kg 1 to 4 times daily; PO (behavioral problems)
Clorazepate	2 mg/kg bid; PO 0.55 to 2.2 mg/kg once to twice daily; PO or PRN (behavioral problems)	Same (behavioral problems)

Drug*	Dog	Cat
Clotrimazole	Apply to lesions bid for 2 to 4 wks; continue treatment 1 wk beyond clinical cure	Same
Cloxacillin	10 to 15 mg/kg qid; PO, IM, IV	Same
Coal tar shampoos	May be used daily or less often; leave in contact with skin for 10 min, then rinse	None
Codeine	0.1 to 0.3 mg/kg tid–qid; PO **OR** 1 to 2 mg/kg tid; PO (cough) 0.5 to 1 mg/kg tid–qid; PO **OR** 1 to 4 mg/kg every 1 to 6 hrs; PO (pain) 0.25 to 0.5 mg/kg tid–qid; PO (diarrhea)	1 to 2 mg/kg bid; PO (with caution) 1 to 2 mg/kg tid; PO (cough)
Colchicine	0.03 mg/kg tid; PO, SC **OR** 0.025 to 0.03 mg/kg/day; PO	None
Cyclophosphamide	50 mg/m² once daily; PO for 4 days a wk for 3 to 4 wks (immune thrombocytopenia) 2 mg/kg/day 4 days of each wk; PO (immune hemolytic anemia) 1 mg/kg/day for 4 days of each wk; PO (polymyositis)	10 mg/kg weekly; IV 100 mg/m²; PO every 3 wks [with doxorubicin] (mammary cancer) 1.5 mg/kg/day **OR** 10 mg/kg once weekly; PO (immune-mediated anemia)
Cyclosporine	20 mg/kg once daily; PO 10 mg/kg once to twice daily; PO (AIHA) **OR**	10 mg/kg bid; PO **OR** 8 to 10 mg/kg/day; PO (immune-mediated anemia)

Drug*	Dog	Cat
Cyclosporine (continued)	10 to 20 mg/kg/day; IM, PO for 5 days, stop for 2 days, resume at 5 mg/kg/day on a 5-days-on, 2-days-off regimen as clinical signs warrant	
Cyproheptadine	1.1 mg/kg bid–tid; PO (antihistamine) 5 to 20 mg once to twice daily; PO (appetite stimulant)	2 to 4 mg once to twice daily; PO (appetite stimulant) **OR** 8 mg 1 to 3 times daily; PO
Cytarabine	5 to 10 mg/kg once daily for 2 wks **OR** 30 to 50 mg/kg once a wk; IV, IM, SC **OR** 100 mg/m^2 once daily; IV, IM for 4 days, then 150 mg/m^2	Same
Cythioate	3.3 mg/kg every 3rd day or twice weekly; PO (tablets) 0.22 mL/kg every 3rd day or twice weekly; PO (liquid)	Same
Dacarbazine	200 mg/m^2 once daily; IV for 5 days; repeat every 3 wks	Same
Dactinomycin	0.015 mg/kg once daily for 3 to 5 days; IV; wait 3 wks for marrow recovery 1.5 mg/m^2 once weekly **OR** 0.5 to 1.1 mg/m^2 every 2 to 3 wks; IV **OR** 0.6 to 0.7 mg/m^2 every 3 wks; IV	Same Same

Drug*	Dog	Cat
Danazol	5 mg/kg bid; PO **OR** 5 mg/kg tid; PO **OR** 10 to 20 mg/kg/day div. bid–tid; PO (AIHA)	5 mg/kg bid; PO for 2 to 4 wks (immune-mediated anemia)
Dantrolene	3 to 15 mg div. bid–tid; PO **OR** 1 to 5 mg/kg bid; PO (urethral obstruction)	Same **OR** 0.5 to 2.0 mg/kg tid; PO (urethral obstruction)
Dapsone	1.1 mg/kg tid–qid; PO **OR** 1 mg/kg tid; PO (subcorneal pustular dermatosis)	Same **OR** 50 mg bid; PO (mycobacteriosis)
Dehydrocholic acid	10 to 15 mg/kg tid; PO until urine negative for bilirubin	Same
Demeclocycline	6 to 12 mg/kg bid–qid; PO (human dose)	Unknown
Derm Caps	1 capsule per 9 kg once daily; PO	Same
Derm Caps (liquid)	To 4.5 kg, give 0.35 mL; to 9 kg, give 0.7 mL; to 13.6 kg, give 1.05 mL	Same
Derm Caps ES	1 capsule per 31.5 to 40 kg	Same
Derm Caps ES (liquid)	To 13.6 kg, give 0.5 mL; to 27.2 kg, give 1 mL; to 40.8 kg, give 1.5 mL	Same
Desmopressin acetate [DDAVP 100 µg/mL] (1 drop = 1.5–4.0 µg; 1 spray = 10 µg)	1 to 4 drops intranasally or in conjunctival sac once to twice daily **OR** 2 µg once to twice daily; SC (central DI) 1 µg/kg; IV, SC **OR** 0.3 µg/kg; IV (diluted in 50 mL saline and infused over 15 to	Same

Unknown |

Drug*	Dog	Cat
Desmopressin acetate (continued)	30 min), repeat PRN (von Wille-brand's disease)	
Desoxycorticosterone pivalate (DOCP)	2.2 mg/kg; every 25 days; IM	Unknown
Dexamethasone	2 mg/kg; IV, then 1 mg/kg tid–qid; SC in decreasing doses **OR** 1 to 4 mg/kg; IV followed by gradually tapering doses every 6 to 8 hrs (cerebral edema) 2 to 3 mg/kg; IV, then 1 mg/kg bid–tid; SC, IV for 24 hrs, then 0.2 mg/kg bid–tid; SC in decreasing doses for 5 to 8 days (spinal cord trauma) 2 to 8 mg/kg; slowly IV (shock) 0.25 to 0.30 mg/kg once; SC, then 0.10 to 0.15 mg/kg bid for 5 to 7 days; SC, switch to oral and taper (immune thrombo-cytopenia) 0.1 to 0.5 mg/kg every 4 to 8 hrs; SC, IV (allergic reactions) 0.11 mg/kg every 48 hrs (pruritus)	Same 0.2 mg/kg every 48 hrs (pruritus)
Dextran 40 and 70	10 to 20 mL/kg/day; IV then 10 mL/kg/day thereafter **OR** 2 to 5 mL/kg/hr; IV inf	Same

Drug*	Dog	Cat
Dextroamphetamine	5 to 10 mg tid; PO (narcolepsy) 0.2 to 1.3 mg/kg PRN; PO (hyperkinesis)	None
Dextromethorphan	2 mg/kg tid–qid; PO	2 mg/kg qid; PO, SC, IV
Diazepam	0.5 to 1 mg/kg; IV in increments of 5 to 10 mg to effect (status epilepticus) 1 to 4 mg/kg div. tid–qid; PO (seizures) 0.5 to 2 mg/kg of injectable soln per rectum (cluster seizures) 2 to 10 mg tid; PO (relax urinary sphincter)	2 to 5 mg tid; PO, IV (seizures) 0.05 to 0.15 mg/kg once to every other day; IV or 1 mg once daily; PO (appetite stimulant) 2.5 mg tid–qid; PO (relax urinary sphincter)
Diazoxide	10 to 40 mg/kg/day div.; PO **OR** 5 to 13 mg/kg bid; PO	None
Dichlorphenamide	2 to 4 mg/kg bid–tid; PO	1 mg/kg bid–tid; PO
Dichlorvos	11 to 22 mg/kg; PO, repeat in 3 wks	Same
Dicloxacillin	10 to 20 mg/kg tid; PO **OR** 50 mg/kg tid; PO	Same
Diethylcarbamazine	6.6 mg/kg once daily; PO (heartworm prevention)	None
Diethylstilbestrol	0.1 to 0.4 mg/kg/day for 3 to 5 days; PO, then once to twice weekly for maintenance (urinary incontinence)	0.05 to 0.1 mg/day; PO (urinary incontinence)
Digitoxin	0.04 to 0.1 mg/kg div. tid; PO	0.005 to 0.015 mg/kg once daily; PO

Drug*	Dog	Cat
Digoxin	0.005 to 0.008 mg/kg bid; PO (elixir) 0.005 to 0.010 mg/kg bid; PO (tablet) 0.22 mg/m² bid; PO	0.003 to 0.004 mg/kg bid; PO (elixir)
Dihydrostreptomycin	5 to 10 mg/kg bid; IM, SC **OR** 12.5 mg/kg bid–tid; IM, SC	Same
Dihydrotachysterol	0.03 mg/kg once daily for 2 days then 0.01 to 0.02 mg/kg/day; PO	Same **OR** 1 to 2 drops once to twice daily; PO
Diltiazem	0.5 to 1.5 mg/kg tid; PO **OR** 0.75 to 1.5 mg/kg tid; PO	1.75 to 2.5 mg/kg bid–tid; PO **OR** 1 mg/kg tid; PO **OR** 3.5 to 7 mg/kg tid; PO 0.2 mg/kg; IV **OR** 10 mg/kg/day; PO (long-acting form)
Dimethyl sulfoxide	Apply topically tid–qid; 1 g/kg; slowly (over 45 min) IV (increased CSF pressure from head trauma)	None
Diphenhydramine	2 to 4 mg/kg tid–qid; PO, IM, IV 2.2 mg/kg tid (pruritus)	Same Unknown
Diphenoxylate	2.5 to 10 mg qid; PO **OR** 2.5 mg bid–qid; PO	0.6 to 1.2 mg bid–tid; PO
Dipyrone	28 mg/kg tid; IM, IV, SC	Same
Disopyramide	dog >18 kg 100 mg tid–qid; PO	None
Dobutamine	250 mg in 1 L of 5% dextrose at 2.5 µg/kg/min; IV **OR** 10 to 20 µg/kg/min const rate inf	2.5 to 10 µg/kg/min const rate inf; IV

Drug*	Dog	Cat
Docusate calcium	50 to 100 mg once to twice daily; PO	50 mg once to twice daily; PO
Docusate sodium	50 to 200 mg bid–tid; PO	50 mg once to twice daily; PO
Dopamine	2 to 15 µg/kg/min; IV inf (inotrope) 2 to 4 µg/kg/min; IV inf in D_5W (renal vasodilator; acute renal failure)	Same
Doxapram	5 to 10 mg/kg once; IV; may be repeated in 15 to 20 min	Same
Doxorubicin	30 mg/m² in 150 mL D_5W once every 3 to 9 wks; IV (not to exceed total dose of 250 mg/m²)	Same (not to exceed 90 mg/m²)
Doxycycline	5 mg/kg; PO as a loading dose followed in 12 hrs by 2.5 mg/kg, then 2.5 mg/kg every 24 hrs thereafter **OR** 5 to 10 mg/kg bid; PO, IV **OR** 15 to 20 mg/kg bid; PO	Same **OR** 2.5 to 5 mg/kg bid; PO (hemobartonella)
Econazole	Apply topically bid for 2 to 4 wks	Unknown
Edrophonium chloride	0.1 to 0.2 mg/kg; IV (max 5 mg) **OR** 0.1 to 0.5 mg; IV (puppies)	2.5 mg/cat; IV
Enalapril	0.5 mg/kg once to twice daily; PO	0.25 to 0.5 mg/kg once to twice daily; PO
Enilconazole	Apply 10 to 20 mg/kg bid topically for 10 to 14 days (10% soln div. 50:50 with water) [aspergillosis]	Unknown

Drug*	Dog	Cat
Enilconazole (continued)	Wash 4 times at 3- to 4-day intervals (0.2% soln) [dermatophytes]	
Enrofloxacin	2.5 to 5 mg/kg bid; PO **OR** 5 to 20 mg/kg/day div. bid; PO (max 30 days) **OR** 5 to 15 mg/kg bid; PO 2.5 mg/kg bid; IM for 3 days	Same
Ephedrine	5 to 15 mg bid–tid; PO (bronchodilator) 5 to 15 mg tid; PO (urethral sphincter incompetence) 0.05 to 0.2 mg/kg; IV **OR** 0.1 to 0.25 mg/kg; IV; may be repeated up to 3 times (hypotension)	2 to 5 mg bid–tid; PO (bronchodilator) 2 to 4 mg tid; PO (urethral sphincter incompetence) Same
Epinephrine (1:10,000 solution)	0.1 mL/kg; IC (cardiac arrest) 0.5 to 1.5 mL; IV, repeat in 30 min (anaphylaxis)	Same Same 0.1 mg every 4 to 6 hrs; SC (feline asthma)
Epsiprantel	5.5 mg/kg once; PO	2.75 mg/kg once; PO
Erythromycin	10 to 20 mg/kg tid; PO	Same
Erythropoietin	100 U/kg 3 times weekly; SC until PCV in low normal range then dose interval decreased to twice weekly; if adequate control not achieved with this regimen, increase	Same

Drug*	Dog	Cat
Erythropoietin (continued)	dose by 25 to 50 U/kg maintaining dose interval between once and 3 times weekly	
Estradiol cypionate	44 µg/kg; IM 3 to 5 days after onset of estrus (pregnancy termination)	250 µg 40 hrs postcoitum; IM (pregnancy termination)
Ethacrynic acid	0.2 to 0.4 mg/kg every 4 to 12 hrs; IM, IV	Same
Etidronate	5 mg/kg/day **OR** 15 mg/kg bid; PO	10 mg/kg/day; PO
Etretinate	1 mg/kg once daily; PO	Unknown
Famotidine	0.5 to 1 mg/kg once to twice daily; PO, IV **OR** 5 mg/kg once daily; IM, SC, PO	Unknown
Fenbendazole	50 mg/kg once daily for 3 days; repeat in 3 wks; PO	30 mg/kg once daily for 3 to 6 days; PO
Fentanyl	0.04 to 0.08 mg/kg; IM, IV, SC (provides 2 hrs of analgesia)	Topical patch—see Drug Descriptions
Ferrous sulfate	100 to 300 mg once daily; PO	50 to 100 mg once daily; PO
Fluconazole	2.5 to 5 mg/kg div. bid with food for 8 wks; PO **OR** 50 mg/day; PO	50 mg/kg bid; PO (cryptococcosis)
Flucytosine	30 to 50 mg/kg tid–qid; PO **OR** 50 to 75 mg/kg tid; PO	Same
Fludrocortisone	0.1 to 0.8 mg daily; PO **OR** 0.02 mg/kg/day; PO	0.1 to 0.2 mg daily; PO
Flumethasone	0.06 to 0.25 mg once daily; PO, IM, IV, SC	0.03 to 0.125 mg once daily; PO, IM, IV, SC

Drug*	Dog	Cat
Flunixin meglumine	0.5 mg/kg bid; IV for 1 to 2 treatments (ocular disease) 1 mg/kg once; IV (acute gastric dilatation) 0.5 mg/kg once to twice daily for 3 treatments; IV (GIT obstruction) 0.5 to 1 mg/kg/day; IV (not to exceed 5 days) 0.25 to 1 mg/kg; IV, SC, IM; can be repeated in 1 to 2 treatments (ocular disease) 0.25 mg/kg; IV, SC, IM; once, can be repeated in 12 to 24 hrs if needed (pyrexia) 1 mg/kg; IM, IV, SC daily (surgical pain)	0.25 mg/kg once; SC; can be repeated in 12 to 24 hrs (surgical pain)
Fluorouracil	150 mg/m^2 once weekly; IV	None
Folic acid	5 mg/day; PO (dietary supplement) 1 mg/day; PO (supplement to pyrimethamine)	2.5 mg/day; PO Same
Fomepizole	20 mg/kg; IV loading dose; then 15 mg/kg (12 hrs), 15 mg/kg (24 hrs), and 5 mg/kg (36 hrs); then 5 mg/kg bid PRN	None
Furosemide	2 to 4 mg/kg bid–tid; PO, IM, IV (diuresis—heart failure) 1 to 2 mg/kg once to twice daily; PO,	1 to 4 mg/kg bid–tid; PO, IM, IV, SC Same

Drug*	Dog	Cat
Furosemide (continued)	SC (ascites from liver failure) 1 to 2 mg/kg bid–tid; IV, IM (diuresis—hypercalcemia) 5 to 20 mg PRN; IV (initiate diuresis in acute renal failure) 2 to 4 mg/kg every 4 to 12 hrs; PO, IM, IV (pulmonary edema) 1 to 2 mg/kg bid; PO (hypertension)	
Gentamicin	2 mg/kg tid; IM, SC	Same
Glipizide	0.25 to 0.5 mg/kg bid; PO	Same **OR** 2.5 to 5 mg bid–tid; PO
Glyburide	0.2 mg/kg once daily; PO	0.2 mg/kg once daily; PO (nonmicronized product)
Glycopyrrolate	0.005 to 0.010 mg/kg; IV, **OR** 0.01 to 0.02 mg/kg; SC, IM (sinus bradycardia, SA block, AV block)	Same
Gonadorelin	50 to 100 µg; SC, IV; if no response, repeat in 4 to 6 days (undescended testes)	25 µg; IM after mating (stimulate ovulation)
Granulocyte colony-stimulating factor (human)	5 µg/kg once daily; SC	Same
Griseofulvin	20 to 50 mg/kg once daily for 3 to 6 wks; PO	Same
Guaifenesin	44 to 88 mg/kg; IV **OR** 33 to 88 mg/kg; IV with 1.1 mg/kg ketamine (restraint)	None

Drug*	Dog	Cat
Guaifenesin (continued)	110 mg/kg; IV (to cause muscle relaxation with strychnine or tetanus)	
Halothane	Induction: 3% Maintenance: 0.5% to 1.5%	Same
Heparin	200 IU/kg; IV, then 50 to 100 IU/kg tid–qid; SC (arterial thromboembolism) 75 to 100 IU/kg qid; IV (DIC) 100 IU/kg bid; SC (acute pancreatitis) 100 to 200 IU/kg for 1 to 4 treatments; IV (burns)	Same
Hetastarch	20 mL/kg/day; IV, then 10 mL/kg/day; IV **OR** 25 to 30 mL/kg over 6 to 8 hrs; 2nd dose immediately after 1st (severe hypoproteinemia with volume depletion, pulmonary edema, or effusion) In severe cases give concurrent crystalloids at ⅔ daily dosing requirements	Same
Hydralazine	1 to 3 mg/kg bid; PO (arterial vasodilator) 0.5 to 2 mg/kg bid–tid; PO (systemic hypertension)	2.5 mg bid; PO (arterial vasodilator and systemic hypertension)
Hydrochlorothiazide	2 to 4 mg/kg bid; PO	Same
Hydrocodone	0.22 mg/kg bid–tid; PO	2.5 to 5 mg bid–tid; PO (with caution)

Drug*	Dog	Cat
Hydrocortisone sodium succinate	8 to 20 mg/kg; IV **OR** 50 to 150 mg/kg; IV (shock)	Same
	5 to 20 mg/kg every 2 to 6 hrs; IV (hypo-adrenocortical crisis)	1 to 3 mg/kg; IV (asthma)
Hydroxyurea	50 mg/kg once daily, 3 days/wk; PO	25 mg/kg once daily, 3 days/wk; PO **OR** 12.2 mg/kg once daily for 16 days fol-lowed by mainte-nance dose every other day; PO
Hydroxyzine	2 mg/kg tid–qid; PO, IM 2.2 mg/kg tid (pruritus)	10 mg bid; PO Unknown
	2.2 mg/kg bid–tid; PO (behavioral prob-lems)	Same
Imipenem-Cilastatin	2 to 5 mg/kg tid; IV	Same
Imipramine	0.5 to 1 mg/kg tid; PO **OR** 1 mg/kg div. bid; PO (max 3 mg/kg/day)	2.5 to 5 mg bid; PO
Immunoglobulin G	0.4 to 0.5 mg/kg/day for 5 days; IV (re-peat PRN) **OR** 0.5 to 1.5 g/kg; IV as a 12-hr inf	Unknown
Innovar-Vet (fentanyl-droperidol)	0.3 to 0.5 mL/55 kg; IV (tranquillization) 1 mL/20 kg; IM (preanesthetic)	None
Insulin Regular	Initially 0.2 U/kg; IM, then 0.1 U/kg hourly until glucose is less than 250 mg/dL [13.8 mmol/L] **OR**	Same
	2.2 U/kg/day; slow IV inf (ketoacidosis)	Unknown

Drug*	Dog	Cat
Intermediate-acting [NPH, Lente]	<15 kg, 1 U/kg once to twice daily; SC >25 kg, 0.5 U/kg once to twice daily; SC	0.25 to 0.5 U/kg bid; SC [NPH]
Long-acting [Ultralente]	0.5 U/kg once daily; SC	1 to 3 U once to twice daily; SC
Interferon	Unknown	30 IU once daily for 7 days; PO on a 1-wk-on/1-wk-off basis
Ipecac (syrup)	5 to 15 mL; PO **OR** 3 to 6 mL; PO	Same **OR** 2 to 6 mL; PO
Iron dextran injection	10 to 20 mg/kg once; IM, followed by oral ferrous sulfate	50 mg; IM at 18 days of age (to prevent transient neonatal iron deficiency anemia)
Isoflurane	Induction: 5% Maintenance: 1.5% to 2.5%	Same
Isoproterenol	15 to 30 mg every 4 hrs; PO	Same
	0.1 to 0.2 mg qid; IM, SC	Same
	1 mg in 250 mL D_5W at 0.01 µg/kg/min; IV **OR** 0.04 to 0.08 µg/kg/min; IV	0.5 mg in 250 mL D_5W; IV to effect
Isotretinoin	1 to 3 mg/kg/day; PO	Same
Itraconazole	2.5 mg/kg bid to 5 mg/kg once daily; PO **OR** 5 mg/kg bid; PO for 60 days (blastomycosis) **OR** 5 to 10 mg/kg bid; **OR** 10 mg/kg once daily; PO	10 mg/kg/day; PO **OR** 50 mg/day cats <3.2 kg and 100 mg/day cats >3.2 kg min 2 mos beyond clinical remission (cryptococcus) and 10 mg/kg once daily; PO for 4 to 6 mos (pulmonary mycoses)

Drug*	Dog	Cat
Ivermectin	50 to 200 µg/kg once; PO (microfilaricide) 6 to 12 µg/kg once monthly; PO (heartworm prevention)	200 µg/kg; SC (*Otodectes cynotis*) 400 µg/kg; SC (*Notoedres cati* and cheyletiella)
Kanamycin	10 to 12 mg/kg qid; PO 5 to 7.5 mg/kg bid; IM, SC 4 to 6 mg/kg qid; IM, SC	Same Same Same
Kaolin-pectin	1 to 2 mL/kg every 2 to 6 hrs; PO	Same
Ketamine hydrochloride	5.5 to 22 mg/kg; IV, IM with adjunctive sedative or tranquilizer	11 mg/kg; IM (restraint) 22 to 33 mg/kg; IM **OR** 2.2 to 4.4 mg/kg; IV (anesthesia) 0.5 to 1.0 mg/kg; IM 1.0 to 4.0 mg/kg; IV (analgesia; lasts 30 min)
Ketoconazole	10 to 40 mg/kg/day or div. bid; PO (fungal disease) 5 to 10 mg/kg once to twice daily (dermatophytes)	10 mg/kg once to twice daily; PO
Ketoprofen	2 mg/kg; IM, IV, SC on day 1, then continue 1 mg/kg once daily; PO for 4 days For more severe cases, give 2 mg/kg; IM, IV, SC once daily for 3 days 2 mg/kg initially; PO, then 1 mg/kg/day (chronic pain)	Same Same

Drug*	Dog	Cat
Ketorolac	0.5 mg/kg tid up to 48 hrs; IM or slowly IV; dose can be increased to 0.75 mg/kg if pain persists. If pain relief persists beyond 8 to 12 hrs, decrease dose by 50% 0.5 mg/kg tid; PO 0.3 to 0.5 mg/kg bid–tid for 1 to 2 treatments, IV, IM (surgical pain) Dogs 20 to 30 kg, 5 mg bid; PO for 6 treatments Dogs >30 kg, 10 mg bid; PO for 6 treatments (panosteitis)	0.25 mg/kg bid; IM; dose can be increased to 0.5 mg/kg in cases of severe pain 0.25 mg/kg bid–tid; IM for 1 to 2 treatments
Lactulose	0.5 mL/kg tid; PO (hepatic encephalopathy) 1 mL per 4.5 kg tid; PO (constipation)	2.5 to 5 mL/cat tid; PO (hepatic encephalopathy) Same
Levamisole	10 mg/kg once daily for 6 to 10 days; PO (microfilaricide) 0.5 to 2 mg/kg 3 times weekly; PO (immunostimulant)	20 to 40 mg/kg qod for 5 to 6 treatments; PO (lungworm) 25 mg qod for 3 treatments; PO (plasma cell gingivitis)
Levothyroxine (T₄)	22 µg/kg bid; PO **OR** 0.02 mg/kg bid; PO **OR** 0.5 mg/m² daily; PO	20 to 30 µg/kg/day; PO once daily or div. bid **OR** 0.1 to 0.2 mg/day; PO
Lidocaine	2 to 4 mg/kg over 1 to 2 min; IV **OR** 25 to 80 µg/kg/min; IV inf	0.25 to 0.75 mg/kg; slowly IV (with caution) **OR** 10 to 40 µg/kg/min; IV inf

Drug*	Dog	Cat
Lincomycin	15 mg/kg tid; PO 10 mg/kg bid; IM, IV	Same
Liothyroxine (T_3)	4 to 6 µg/kg tid; PO	4.4 µg/kg bid–tid; PO
Loperamide	0.08 mg/kg tid; PO	0.1 to 0.3 mg/kg once to twice daily; PO (with caution)
Magnesium hydroxide	5 to 30 mL once to twice daily; PO (antacid) 3 to 5 times antacid dose (cathartic)	5 to 15 mL once to twice daily; PO (antacid) Same
Magnesium sulfate	2 g (in 250–500 mL) over 1 to 2 hrs; IV **OR** 300 mg qid for 7 to 10 days; PO (mild deficiency) 2 to 4 g (in 250–500 mL) over 4 to 6 hrs; IV (moderate) 2 g (in 20 mL) over 2 min, then 2 g (in 100 mL) over 20 min, then 2 to 4 g (in 250 mL) over 2 to 4 hrs; IV (severe)	Unknown
Mannitol	1 to 2 g/kg every 6 hrs; IV (20% soln) 0.25 to 2 g/kg; IV over 20 min; repeat every 3 to 8 hrs for a maximum of 3 doses over 24 hrs (25% soln) [head trauma]	Same Same
Mebendazole	22 mg/kg once daily for 3 days; PO (with food)	None

Drug*	Dog	Cat
Meclofenamic acid	1.1 mg/kg daily for 5 to 7 days; PO; maintain dose if effective; if signs worsen, give 1.1 mg/kg every 3rd day for 7 days; if still effective, give every 4th day, then every 5th day, etc., until signs recur	None
Medetomidine	750 µg; IV **OR** 100 µg; IM/m² **OR** 30 to 40 µg/kg; IM (max 50 µg/kg)	80 to 110 µg/kg; IM (max 120 µg/kg)
Medium-chain triglyceride (MCT) oil	1 to 2 mL/kg/day; PO (in food)	Same
Medroxy-progesterone acetate	20 mg/kg once; IM; repeat in 3 to 6 mos if needed (skin conditions) 10 mg/kg PRN; IM, SC (behavioral conditions)	50 to 100 mg once; IM repeat in 3 to 6 mos if needed (skin conditions) 10 to 20 mg/kg PRN; SC (behavioral conditions)
Megestrol acetate	1 mg/kg/day; PO (skin conditions) 0.5 mg/kg/day for 8 days; PO (pseudocyesis) 2 to 4 mg/kg once daily; PO; reduce to half dose at 8 days (behavioral conditions)	5 to 10 mg qod; PO for 10 to 14 treatments, then every 2nd wk (eosinophilic ulcers) 2.5 mg once daily for 10 days, then qod for 5 treatments, then PRN; PO (plasma cell gingivitis)
Melarsomine	2.5 mg/kg; IM twice; 24 hrs apart via deep lumbar injection (L_3–L_5 only)	None
Melphalan	1.5 mg/m² once daily for 7 to 10 days, then no treatment	Same

Drug*	Dog	Cat
Melphalan (continued)	for 2 to 3 wks **OR** 0.05 to 0.1 mg/kg once daily; PO	Same
Meperidine	5 to 10 mg/kg PRN; IM	1 to 4 mg/kg; IM (with caution)
Mercaptopurine	50 mg/m^2 once daily; PO **OR** 2 mg/kg once daily; PO	None
Metamucil	2 to 10 g once to twice daily (in moistened food)	2 to 4 g once to twice daily (in moistened food)
Methenamine mandelate	10 mg/kg qid; PO	None
Methimazole	None	5 mg once to 3 times daily; PO
Methionine	0.2 to 1 g tid; PO	0.2 to 1 g once daily; PO
Methocarbamol	Injectable; for relief of moderate conditions, 44 mg/kg; IV. For controlling severe effects of strychnine and tetanus, 55 to 220 mg/kg; IV; give half dose rapidly, wait until relaxation occurs, and continue [not to exceed 330 mg/kg/day]	Same
	Initially 132 mg/kg/day div. bid–tid; PO, then 61 to 132 mg/kg div. bid–tid; PO; if no response in 5 days, discontinue	Same
	15 to 20 mg/kg tid; PO (for muscle relaxation of intervertebral disc disease)	Unknown

Drug*	Dog	Cat
Methotrexate	2.5 mg/m^2 daily; PO (neoplasia) 5 mg/m^2 on days 1 and 5 of a weekly maintenance schedule (lymphoma)	2.5 mg/m^2 2 to 3 times weekly; PO **OR** 0.3 to 0.8 mg/m^2 every 7 days; IV (neoplasia) 2.5 to 5 mg/m^2 2 to 3 times per wk; PO (lymphoma)
Methoxyflurane	Induction: 3% Maintenance: 0.5 to 1.5%	Same
Methylene blue	8.8 mg/kg (1% soln); slowly IV; repeat PRN 100 to 300 mg daily; PO (methemoglobinemia)	Same
Methylphenidate hydrochloride	5 to 10 mg bid–tid; PO (narcolepsy) 2 to 4 mg/kg PRN; PO (hyperkinesis)	None
Methylprednisolone sodium succinate	30 to 35 mg/kg; IV (shock)	Unknown
	30 mg/kg; IV, then 15 mg/kg; IV 2 hrs later, then 10 mg/kg; IV, SC for 2 days, then taper dose over 5 to 7 days (spinal trauma)	Same
	Initially 30 mg/kg; IV, then 15 mg/kg; IV at 2 and 6 hrs, then 2.5 mg/kg/hr for 42 hrs (head trauma) **OR** 30 mg/kg; IV bolus followed by 5.4 mg/kg/hr infusion for 23 hrs (spinal trauma)	Same

Drug*	Dog	Cat
Metoclopramide	0.2 to 0.5 mg/kg tid; PO, SC **OR** 1 to 2 mg/kg/day; IV inf (antiemetic)	0.2 to 0.5 mg/kg tid; PO, SC (GIT motility disorders, esophageal reflux)
Metoprolol	5 to 50 mg tid; PO	2.5 to 5 mg tid; PO
Metronidazole	25 to 65 mg/kg once daily for 5 days; PO **OR** 25 mg/kg bid; PO for 5 days (giardiasis)	10 to 25 mg/kg once daily for 5 days; PO **OR** 12 to 25 mg/kg bid; PO for 5 days (giardiasis)
Mexiletine	4 to 10 mg/kg tid; PO	Unknown
Mibolerone	1 to 11 kg, 30 µg/day; PO 12 to 22 kg, 60 µg/day; PO 23 to 45 kg, 120 µg/day; PO >45 kg, 180 µg/day; PO (estrus prevention)	None
Midazolam	0.066 to 0.22 mg/kg; IM, IV (preoperative agent) **OR** 0.1 mg/kg; IV	Same Unknown
Milbemycin	Up to 4.5 kg, 2.3 mg 5 to 11 kg, 5.75 mg 12 to 22 kg, 11.5 mg 23 to 45 kg, 23 mg	None
Mineral oil	5 to 30 mL; PO **OR** 1 to 2 mL/kg per rectum	5 to 20 mL bid; PO **OR** per rectum
Minocycline	5 to 15 mg/kg bid; PO	Same
Misoprostol	2 to 5 µg/kg bid–tid; PO	Unknown
Mitotane	40 to 50 mg/kg/day for 7 to 10 days, then once weekly; PO	None
Mitoxantrone	5 mg/m^2 once every 3 wks; IV	2.5 to 6.5 mg/m^2 every 3 wks; IV

Drug*	Dog	Cat
Morphine sulfate	0.5 to 1 mg/kg PRN; IM, SC 0.05 to 0.4 mg/kg every 1 to 4 hrs; IV **OR** 0.2 to 1 mg/kg every 2 to 6 hrs; IM, SC 0.3 to 3 mg/kg every 4 to 8 hrs; PO **OR** 0.3 to 3 mg/kg bid–tid; PO (slow-release)	0.05 to 0.1 mg/kg PRN; IM, SC (with caution) **OR** 0.05 to 0.2 mg/kg every 2 to 6 hrs; IM, SC
Nafcillin	10 mg/kg qid; PO, IM	Same
Naloxone	0.04 mg/kg; IM, IV, SC (opioid reversal)	0.05 to 0.1 mg/kg; IV (opioid reversal)
Nandrolone decanoate	1 to 5 mg/kg/wk; IM (max 200 mg/wk); anabolic effect	Same (anabolic effect) 10 to 20 mg/wk; IM (marrow stimulant)
Neomycin	2.5 to 10 mg/kg bid–qid; PO **OR** 20 mg/kg bid–tid; PO 3.5 mg/kg tid; IM, IV, SC	Same Same Same
Neostigmine	0.5 mg/kg bid–tid; PO (myasthenia gravis) 1 to 2 mg PRN; IM 5 to 15 mg PRN; PO	None
Nitrofurantoin	4 mg/kg tid–qid; PO	Same
Nitroglycerin ointment	¼ to 1 inch tid–qid; topically	⅛ to ¼ inch tid–qid; topically
Nitroprusside	1 to 10 µg/kg/min; IV inf	Same
Nitroscanate	50 mg/kg; PO	Same
Norfloxacin	22 mg/kg bid; PO	Same **OR** 5 mg/kg bid; PO (urinary tract infection)
Novobiocin	10 mg/kg tid; PO	Unknown
Nystatin	100,000 U qid; PO	Same
Omeprazole	0.7 mg/kg once daily; PO **OR**	Same

Drug*	Dog	Cat
Omeprazole (continued)	>20 kg, 1 capsule (20 mg) daily; PO <20 kg, ½ capsule (10 mg) daily; PO <5 kg, ¼ capsule (5 mg) daily; PO	
Ondansteron	0.1 mg/kg bid–tid; IV **OR** 0.5 to 1 mg/kg; PO **OR** 0.5 mg/kg loading dose; IV followed by 0.5 mg/kg/hr infusion for 6 hrs	Unknown
Orbifloxacin	2.5 mg/kg once daily; PO **NB:** dose may be increased to 7.5 mg/kg once daily; PO if required	Same
Oxacillin	15 to 25 mg/kg tid–qid; PO 8.8 to 20 mg/kg every 4 to 6 hrs; IM, IV	Same
Oxazepam	0.2 to 1 mg/kg once to twice daily; PO (behavioral problems)	0.2 to 0.5 mg/kg once to twice daily; PO (appetite stimulant)
Oxtriphylline	14 mg/kg tid–qid; PO **OR** 30 mg/kg bid; PO (sustained-release)	6 mg/kg bid–tid; PO
Oxybutynin	5 mg bid–tid; PO	0.5 mg bid; PO
Oxymetholone	1 mg/kg once to twice daily; PO	Same
Oxymorphone	0.05 to 0.1 mg/kg; IM, IV **OR** 0.1 to 0.2 mg/kg; IM, SC (sedation) 0.02 to 0.1 mg/kg every 2 to 4 hrs; IV (analgesia)	0.02 mg/kg; IV (with caution) **OR** 0.05 to 0.2 mg/kg; IV, IM (analgesia; lasts 2–5 hrs)

Drug*	Dog	Cat
Oxymorphone (continued)	0.05 to 0.2 mg/kg every 2 to 6 hrs; IM, SC (analgesia)	
Oxytetracycline	22 mg/kg tid; PO	Same **OR** 25 mg/kg tid; PO (hemobartonella)
	7 to 12 mg bid; IM, IV	Same
Oxytocin	5 to 20 U; IM once (uterine prolapse)	5 U; IM once (uterine prolapse)
	5 to 20 U; IM or IV inf; may repeat in 30 to 60 min (uterine inertia)	2.5 to 5 U; IM or IV inf (uterine inertia)
	Spray intranasally 5 to 10 min before nursing (stimulate milk letdown)	
Pancuronium	0.1 mg/kg; IV **OR** 0.03 mg/kg; IV with methoxyflurane 0.06 mg/kg; IV with halothane	0.044 to 0.11 mg/kg; IV (higher dose used initially; lower doses if drug repeated)
Penicillamine	15 mg/kg bid; PO (cystine urolithiasis) 10 to 15 mg/kg bid; PO (copper hepatopathy) 33 to 100 mg/kg/day div. qid for 7 days, wait 7 days, repeat; PO (lead poisoning)	None
Penicillin G (aqueous) Potassium	20,000 U/kg every 4 hrs; IM, IV, SC 40,000 U/kg qid; PO	Same
Sodium	20,000 U/kg every 4 hrs; IM, IV, SC 40,000 U/kg qid; PO	Same
Penicillin G (procaine)	20,000 U/kg once to twice daily; IM, SC	Same

Drug*	Dog	Cat
Penicillin V	10 mg/kg tid; PO	Same
Pentastarch (10%)	10 to 20 mL/kg/day over 1 to 24 hrs as indicated for up to 3 days	5 to 10 mL/kg/day over 1 to 24 hrs as indicated for up to 3 days
Pentazocine	0.2 to 0.5 mg/kg PRN; IM **OR** 1 to 3 mg/kg every 30 min to 3 hrs; IM, IV (analgesia)	2.2 to 3.3 mg/kg; IM, IV, SC (with caution) 2 to 3 mg/kg; IM, IV, SC (analgesia; lasts 2–4 hrs)
Pentobarbital	2 to 4 mg/kg; IV (sedation) 10 to 30 mg/kg; IV (anesthesia)	Same 25 mg/kg; IV (anesthesia)
Pentosan polysulfate	3 mg/kg (1 mL/33 kg) every 5 to 7 days for 4 treatments; SC	None
Phenobarbital grain = 65 mg	1 to 2 mg/kg bid; PO [may require up to 16 mg/kg/day] (seizures) 3 to 30 mg/kg; IV to effect (status epilepticus) 2.2 mg/kg bid; PO (irritable colon)	1/8 to 1/4 grain once to twice daily; PO (seizures) 6 mg/kg bid–qid; IM, IV (status epilepticus) 1 mg/kg bid; PO (sedation)
Phenoxybenzamine	5 to 15 mg once daily; PO **OR** 2.5 to 30 mg tid; PO (urinary incontinence)	0.5 mg/kg once daily; PO **OR** 0.25 mg/kg tid; PO (urinary incontinence)
Phenylbutazone	15 to 22 mg/kg bid–tid; PO (max 800 mg/day)	None
Phenylpropanolamine	12.5 to 50 mg tid; PO (urinary incontinence) 1 to 2 mg/kg bid; PO (decongestant)	12.5 mg tid; PO (urinary incontinence) Same (decongestant)
Phenytoin	15 to 40 mg/kg tid; PO (seizure)	None

Drug*	Dog	Cat
Phenytoin (continued)	2 to 4 mg/kg in increments, up to 10 mg/kg total dose; IV (arrhythmias) 6 mg/kg bid–tid; PO (tumor-induced hypoglycemia)	
Phosphate enemas (Fleet)	1 to 2 mL/kg (medium to large dogs)	None
Piperazine	100 mg/kg; PO; repeat in 3 wks	Same
Piroxicam	0.3 mg/kg every 48 hrs; PO (degenerative joint disease/pain)	None
Plicamycin	25 µg/kg; IV (hypercalcemia)	Unknown
Polymyxin B	2 mg/kg bid; IM	Same
Polysulfated glycosaminoglycans [Adequan]	4.4 mg/kg twice weekly; IM (maximum of 8 injections) **OR** 5 mg/kg every 3 to 5 days; IM (repeated 5–10 times)	Unknown
Potassium chloride	0.5 mEq/kg/day; not to exceed 0.5 mEq/kg/hr	Same
	1 to 3 g/day; PO, IV **OR** 0.1 to 0.25 mL/kg tid; PO (dilute with water 1:1) 1.5 to 2 mEq/kg; IV (chemical defibrillation)	0.2 g/day; PO
Potassium citrate	100 to 150 mg/kg/day; PO (calcium oxalate urolithiasis)	Unknown
Potassium gluconate	2.2 mEq/100 kcal of energy/day; PO **OR** 5 mEq bid–tid; PO (Kaon® elixir)	Same **OR** 5 to 10 mEq div. bid–tid; PO (severe cases); decrease to

Drug*	Dog	Cat
Potassium gluconate (continued)		4 to 6 mEq/day with clinical improvement; 2 to 4 mEq/day; PO (maintenance) (Kaon® elixir) 5 to 8 mEq once to twice daily; PO (Tumil-K®)
Potassium iodide	40 mg/kg tid; PO	20 mg/kg bid; PO (with food) **OR** 30 to 100 mg/cat daily for 10 to 14 days
Potassium phosphate	0.01 to 0.03 mmol/kg/hr; IV for 6 hrs	Same **OR** 0.011 to 0.017 mmol/kg/hr for 6 to 12 hrs; IV
Praziquantel	½ tab per 2.5 kg; PO (max 5 tabs)	Up to 1.8 kg, ½ tab; PO 2.3 to 5 kg, 1 tab; PO >5 kg, 1½ tabs; PO
Prazosin	1 mg/15 kg tid; PO	0.03 mg/kg; IV in combination with dantrolene (1 mg/kg) (urethral obstruction)
Prednisolone and Prednisone	0.2 to 0.4 mg/kg once daily to qod; PO (hypoadrenocortical maintenance)	Same
	0.5 mg/kg bid; PO, IM (allergy)	1 mg/kg bid; PO, IM (allergy)
	2 to 4 mg/kg/day; PO, IM (immunosuppression)	3 mg/kg bid; PO, IM (immunosuppression)
	0.5 mg/kg bid–tid; PO, IM (allergic bronchitis)	Same
	0.5 to 1 mg/kg/day; PO (pulmonary eosinophilic infiltrates)	Same

Drug*	Dog	Cat
Prednisolone and Prednisone (continued)	0.5 to 1.5 mg/kg/day div. bid; PO, taper over 3 mos (eosinophilic gastritis)	Same
	1 to 3 mg/kg once daily; PO, taper to qod (eosinophilic enteritis, colitis)	Same
	1 mg/kg bid; PO (plasmacytic/ lymphocytic enteritis)	Same
		2.5 to 5 mg once daily to every other day; PO (urethritis, hematuria)
	1 to 4 mg/kg/day div. bid; PO (immune hemolytic anemia)	Same
	2 to 3 mg/kg bid; PO (hypercalcemia)	Same
	Initially 10 to 30 mg/kg followed by gradually tapering doses every 6 to 8 hrs (head trauma)	Same
	1.1 mg/kg every 48 hrs (pruritus)	2.2 mg/kg every 48 hrs (pruritus)
Prednisolone sodium succinate	11 to 25 mg/kg; IV (shock)	Same
	2 to 4 mg/kg; IV, IM (allergic bronchitis, asthma)	1 to 3 mg/kg; IV, IM (allergic bronchitis, asthma)
Primidone	11 to 22 mg/kg tid; PO	Same
Procainamide	6 to 8 mg/kg over 5 min; IV, then 25 to 40 µg/kg/min **OR** 6 to 20 mg/kg every 4 to 6 hrs; IM 8 to 20 mg/kg qid; PO (regular tabs or caps)	7.5 to 15 mg/kg; IM 62.5 mg/cat tid; PO (sustained-release)

Drug*	Dog	Cat
Procainamide (continued)	25 to 50 mg/kg tid; PO **OR** 8 to 20 mg/kg tid–qid; PO (sustained-release)	
Prochlorperazine	0.13 mg/kg qid; IM **OR** 0.1 to 0.5 mg/kg tid–qid; IM, SC 1 mg/kg bid; PO	0.13 mg/kg bid; IM Same 0.5 mg/kg tid–qid; PO
Propantheline bromide	Small dogs: 7.5 mg tid; PO Medium dogs: 15 mg tid; PO Large dogs: 30 mg tid; PO	7.5 mg tid to every 3rd day; PO
Propionibacterium acnes	<7 kg, 0.25 to 0.5 mL; IV 6.8 to 20 kg, 0.5 to 1 mL; IV 20 to 34 kg, 1 to 1.5 mL; IV >34 kg, 1.5 to 2 mL; IV given 4 times in first 2 wks at 3- to 4-day intervals, followed by 1 injection/wk until signs abate or stabilize; maintenance dose once/month	2 injections (0.5 mL) weekly; IV for 2 wks; followed by 1 injection/wk for 20 wks or until cat tests negative by IFA and ELISA (FeLV-associated disease)
Propofol	6 mg/kg; slowly IV (induction without premed) 10 mg (1 mL)/10 to 25 kg to maintain anesthesia **OR** 0.4 to 0.8 mg/kg/min if anesthesia >15 min	Same
Propranolol	0.02 to 0.06 mg/kg over 2 to 3 min; IV 0.2 mg/kg tid; PO (arrhythmias)	0.25 to 0.5 mg; slowly IV followed by 2.5 to 5 mg tid; PO (arrhythmias)

Drug*	Dog	Cat
Propranolol (continued)	2.5 to 10 mg bid–tid; PO (systemic hypertension)	2.5 to 5 mg bid–tid; PO (systemic hypertension)
Prostaglandin F$_{2\alpha}$	0.25 mg/kg once daily; SC for 5 days (pyometra)	0.1 to 0.25 mg/kg once to twice daily; SC for 3 to 5 days (pyometra)
Protamine sulfate	1 mg for every 100 IU heparin used; given over 60 min as IV infusion	Same
Pseudoephedrine	15 to 30 mg bid–tid; PO (urinary incontinence) 15 to 50 mg tid; PO (decongestant)	Unknown 2 to 4 mg/kg bid–tid; PO (decongestant)
Pyrantel pamoate	5 mg/kg orally after a meal; repeat in 7 to 10 days	20 mg/kg orally; repeat in 7 to 10 days
Pyridostigmine bromide	0.2 to 2 mg/kg bid–tid; PO	1 to 5 mg; IV (administer anticholinergic first)
Pyrimethamine	1 mg/kg/day for 14 to 28 days; PO (5 days only for *Neosporum caninum*) **OR** 0.25 to 0.5 mg/kg bid for 2 wks; PO (toxoplasmosis and *Neospora caninum*)	0.5 to 1 mg/kg/day for 14 to 28 days; PO
Quinacrine	100 mg tid; PO **OR** 6.6 mg/kg bid; PO for 5 days (giardia)	10 mg/kg once daily; PO **OR** 2.3 mg/kg/day; PO for 12 days (giardia)
Quinidine	6 to 16 mg/kg tid–qid; PO, IM	4 to 8 mg/kg tid; IM
Ranitidine	1 to 2 mg/kg bid; PO **OR** 0.5 mg/kg bid; PO, IV, SC	3.5 mg/kg bid; PO 2.5 mg/kg bid; IV

Drug*	Dog	Cat
Rifampin	10 to 20 mg/kg bid; PO	Same
Selegiline	1 to 2 mg/kg/day; PO (pituitary-dependent hyperadrenocorticism)	Unknown
	0.5 mg/kg once daily; PO (age-related behavior disorders)	
Sodium bicarbonate	10 to 15 mg/kg tid; PO (renal failure)	Same
	0.5 to 1 mEq/kg; IV (acidosis)	Same
Sodium chloride (0.9% solution)	40 to 50 mL/kg/day; IV, SC, IP	Same
Sodium iodide	20 to 40 mg/kg bid–tid; PO for 4 to 6 wks	20 mg/kg/day; PO for 4 to 6 wks
Sodium polystyrene sulfonate	8 to 15 g tid; PO	Unknown
Spectinomycin	5 to 12 mg/kg bid; IM	Same
	20 mg/kg bid; PO	
Spironolactone	1 to 2 mg/kg bid; PO	Same
Stanozolol	2 to 10 mg bid; PO, IM	1 to 2 mg bid; PO
Sucralfate	0.5 to 1 g bid–tid; PO **OR**	0.25 g bid–tid; PO **OR**
	1 g/30 kg qid; PO	0.25 to 0.5 g bid–tid; PO
Sulfadimethoxine	25 mg/kg once to twice daily; PO, IM, IV, SC	Same
Sulfadimethoxine ormetoprim	Day 1, 55 mg/kg, then 27.5 mg/kg once daily for a maximum of 21 days; PO	None
Sulfasalazine	10 to 30 mg/kg bid–tid; PO	20 mg/kg bid; PO (pediatric suspension)
Taurine	See Drug Descriptions	250 to 500 mg bid; PO
Terbutaline	2.5 mg/dog tid; PO, SC	1.25 mg bid; PO **OR** 0.625 mg bid; PO, SC

Drug*	Dog	Cat
Testosterone Methyl	1 to 2 mg/kg once daily; PO (max 30 mg/day) [anabolic effects]	Same
Cypionate	2.2 mg/kg once every 30 days; IM	Unknown
Propionate	2 mg/kg 3 times/wk; IM, SC (urinary incontinence)	5 to 10 mg; IM (urinary incontinence)
Tetracycline	25 to 50 mg/kg tid–qid; PO **OR** 22 mg/kg tid; PO 7 mg/kg bid; IM, IV	Same
Thenium closylate	2.3 to 4.5 kg; 250 mg bid for 2 treat- ments; PO **OR** >4.5 kg, 500 mg once; PO; repeat in 3 wks (max 110 mg/kg)	None
Theophylline	6 to 11 mg/kg tid–qid; PO, IM, IV 9 mg/kg tid–qid; PO 20 mg/kg bid; PO (Theo-Dur) **OR** 25 to 30 mg/kg bid; PO (Slo-bid)	4 mg/kg bid–tid; PO 0.1 mg/kg tid; IM, IV 25 mg/kg once daily (in p.m.); PO (Theo- Dur) **OR** 25 mg/kg once daily (in p.m.); PO (Slo-bid)
Thiabendazole	50 mg/kg once daily for 3 days; PO; re- peat in 1 mo	None
Thiacetarsamide	2.2 mg/kg bid for 2 days; IV (heart- worm)	Same (with caution)
Thiamine (vitamin B₁)	1 to 2 mg/kg; IM 2 mg/kg once daily; PO	Same 4 mg/kg once daily; PO
Thiamylal sodium	18 mg/kg to effect; IV 9 mg/kg to effect; IV after premedication	Same

Drug*	Dog	Cat
Thiopental sodium	25 to 30 mg/kg; IV (to effect) 22 mg/kg; IV (after tranquilization) 11 mg/kg; IV (after narcotic premedication)	Same
Ticarcillin	40 to 75 mg/kg tid–qid; IM, IV	Same
Ticarcillin/clavulanate	30 to 50 mg/kg tid–qid; IV	Same
Tiletamine-zolazepam	9.9 to 13.2 mg/kg; IM (minor procedures) 6.6 to 9.9 mg/kg; IM (diagnostic procedures) 6 to 13 mg/kg; IM (surgery lasting 30–60 min)	9.7 to 11.9 mg/kg; IM (minor procedures) 10.6 to 12.5 mg/kg; IM (castration, lacerations) Same 14.3 to 15.8 mg/kg; IM (spay, declaw)
Tobramycin	1 mg/kg tid; IM, IV, SC	2 mg/kg tid; SC
Tocainide	10 to 20 mg/kg tid; PO	None
Triamcinolone	0.05 mg/kg bid–tid; PO (anti-inflammatory) 0.88 mg/kg every 48 hrs; PO (pruritus)	0.25 to 0.5 mg/kg once daily for 7 days; PO
Triamterene	1 to 2 mg/kg bid; PO	Unknown
Trimeprazine	1.1 to 4.4 mg/kg qid; PO	Same
Trimethoprim-sulfadiazine	15 to 30 mg/kg bid; PO, SC, IV	Same
Tylosin	5 to 15 mg/kg tid–qid; IM, IV 5 to 10 mg/kg bid–tid; PO	Same Same
Ursodiol	4 to 15 mg/kg/day; PO	Same **OR** 10 to 15 mg/kg once daily; PO

Drug*	Dog	Cat
Valproic acid	60 mg/kg tid; PO **OR** 75 to 200 mg/kg tid; PO **OR** 25 to 105 mg/kg/day; PO if used with phenobarbital	Unknown
Vasopressin (aqueous)	10 U PRN; IV, IM	Same
Verapamil	10 to 15 mg/kg/day div. bid–tid; PO 0.05 to 0.15 mg/kg; slow IV 2 to 10 µg/kg/min; IV inf	None
Vinblastine	2 mg/m² every 7 to 14 days; IV	Same
Vincristine	0.5 to 0.75 mg/m² every 7 to 14 days; IV (neoplasia) 0.02 mg/kg once weekly; IV (immune thrombocytopenia)	0.5 to 0.75 mg/m² once weekly; IV
Vitamin E	100 to 400 IU bid; PO	Same
Vitamin K$_1$	2 to 5 mg/kg/day div. bid; SC **OR** 2 to 3 mg/kg/day div. tid for 5 to 7 days; PO, then 1 mg/kg div. tid for 4 to 6 wks; PO	Same
Warfarin	0.1 mg/kg once daily; PO	0.1 to 0.2 mg/kg once daily; PO
Xylazine	1.1 mg/kg; IV 1.1 to 2.2 mg/kg; IM, SC 0.6 mg/kg; IV, IM (sedative)	Same 0.05 to 0.2 mg/kg; IV, IM (analgesia; lasts 15–30 min) 0.44 mg/kg; IM (emetic)
Zinc acetate	5 to 10 mg/kg bid; PO **OR**	Unknown

Drug*	Dog	Cat
Zinc acetate (continued)	100 mg bid; PO for 3 mos, then 50 mg bid; PO	
Zinc sulfate	220 mg once to twice daily; PO (zinc responsive dermatoses) 5 to 10 mg/kg bid; PO **OR** 2 mg/kg/day; PO (hepatic copper toxicosis)	None

AIHA, autoimmune hemolytic anemia; AV, atrioventricular; DIC, disseminated intravascular coagulation; FeLV, feline leukemia virus; FIV, feline immunodeficiency virus; GI, gastrointestinal; GIT, gastrointestinal tract; inf, infusion; soln, solution.

Note: Many of the drug doses listed are empirical. In some cases, the literature cites two or more dose scedules. The dose, efficacy, and side effects have not been determined for all drugs listed. Many of the drugs have not been approved for use in small animals. Read the product information before using the drug.

Handbook of Veterinary Drugs, Second Edition, edited by Dana Allen,
Lippincott–Raven Publishers, Philadelphia. © 1998

Section 2

Antimicrobial Agents in Dogs and Cats

TABLE 1. **Antimicrobial Agents in Dogs and Cats**

Organism	Drug(s) of Choice	Alternative Drug(s)
Anaerobic organisms		
Actinomyces sp.	Chloramphenicol Clindamycin Penicillin	Cefoxitin
Anaerobic cocci	Penicillin	Cephalosporin (1st generation) Chloramphenicol Clindamycin
Bacteroides fragilis	Cefoxitin Chloramphenicol Clavamox Metronidazole	Ampicillin Clindamycin
Bacteroides sp.	Chloramphenicol Clavamox Metronidazole Penicillin G	Ampicillin Cefoxitin Clindamycin
Clostridium perfringens	Cephalosporins Chloramphenicol Penicillin	Clindamycin Erythromycin Metronidazole
Clostridium sp.	Ampicillin Chloramphenicol Metronidazole Clavamox	Clindamycin

TABLE 1.   **(Continued)**

Organism	Drug(s) of Choice	Alternative Drug(s)
Fusobacterium sp.	Chloramphenicol Clavamox Clindamycin Ampicillin Metronidazole	
Bacillus anthracis	Ampicillin Penicillin G	Cephalothin Chlortetracycline Erythromycin Oxytetracycline
Bordetella bronchiseptica	Trimethoprim- sulfamethoxazole Enrofloxacin Doxycycline	Amikacin Chloramphenicol Gentamicin Tetracycline Tobramycin
Brucella canis	Minocycline- streptomycin	Trimethoprim- sulfamethoxazole
Campylobacter	Erythromycin	Chloramphenicol Gentamicin Neomycin Clindamycin
Chlamydia psittaci	Tetracyclines	Chloramphenicol Erythromycin Rifampin
Coccidia	Sulfonamides	Amprolium
Corynebacterium sp.	Penicillin G	Erythromycin Tetracycline

Dermatophytosis
  Microsporum
  Trichophyton
	Griseofulvin	Ketoconazole

Escherichia coli
  Urinary tract
    infections (UTIs)
	Ampicillin
	Trimethoprim-sulfa
	Enrofloxacin
	Nitrofurantoin
		Cephalosporins
		Chloramphenicol
		Nitrofurantoin
		Sulfonamides
		Tetracyclines
		Tribrissen®

Other infections	Ampicillin Chloramphenicol Tetracyclines	Aminoglycosides Polymyxin Fluoroquinolones Cephalosporin (3rd generation)

TABLE 1.   **(Continued)**

Organism	Drug(s) of Choice	Alternative Drug(s)
Giardia	Albendazole Fenbendazole	Metronidazole Quinicrine
Hemobartonella	Tetracyclines Doxycycline Oxytetracycline	Chloramphenicol Amoxicillin
Klebsiella/Enterobacter	Gentamicin Kanamycin Cephalosporin (1st generation) Enrofloxacin	Cephalosporins Chloramphenicol
Leptospira	Penicillin G with streptomycin	Tetracyclines
Lyme Borreliosis	Ampicillin Tetracycline	Doxycycline Cephalexin Chloramphenicol
Malassezia canis	Cuprimyxin 2% "tame" iodine or 25% glyceryl tri- acetate topically	—
Mycobacterium	Isoniazid with streptomycin or p-aminosalicylic acid	—
Atypical Mycobacteria *M. fortuitum* and *M. chelonei*	Aminoglycosides Doxycycline Enrofloxacin Clofazimine Chloramphenicol	—
Mycoplasma	Chloramphenicol Erythromycin Tetracycline Enrofloxacin	—
Mycotic disease Aspergillus Blastomyces *Candida* Coccidioides *Cryptococcus* Sporotrichosis	Amphotericin B +/– Ketoconazole Enilconazole (Aspergillus) Sodium or potassium iodide (sporotri- chosis)	Flucytosine (*Candida, Cryptococcus*) Ketoconazole Thiabendazole (Aspergillus)
Neorickettsia	Chloramphenicol Chlortetracycline Oxytetracycline	Ampicillin with erythromycin

TABLE 1.   **(Continued)**

Organism	Drug(s) of Choice	Alternative Drug(s)
Neorickettsia (continued)	Penicillin Sulfonamides	
Neospora caninum	Clindamycin	Pyrimethamine with a sulfonamide
Nocardia	Sulfonamides with ampicillin or Tribrissen®	Ampicillin with erythromycin Amikacin Minocycline
Pasteurella multocida	Penicillin G	Ampicillin Tetracyclines Trimethoprim-sulfamethoxazole
Pentatrichomonas	Metronidazole	—
Proteus mirabilis	Ampicillin Cephalexin Nitrofurantoin (UTI only) Enrofloxacin	Chloramphenicol Trimethoprim-sulfamethoxazole
Pseudomonas	Gentamicin + Ticarcillin or carbenicillin Ceftazidime Enrofloxacin Tetracycline Tobramycin	Chloramphenicol Fluoroquinolones Carbenicillin Ticarcillin Trimethoprim
Salmonella sp.	Trimethoprim-sulfamethoxazole	Ampicillin Cephalosporin (3rd generation) Chloramphenicol Fluoroquinolones
Staphylococcus aureus	Penicillin G sensitive Penicillin G Penicillin G resistant Cephalosporin (1st generation) Cloxacillin	Ampicillin Cephalosporin (1st generation) Cephalosporins Chloramphenicol
Staphylococcus intermedius	Clavamox Trimethoprim-sulfa	Aminoglycoside Vancomycin

TABLE 1. **(Continued)**

Organism	Drug(s) of Choice	Alternative Drug(s)
Staphylococcus intermedius (continued)	Ormetoprim-sulfa Chloramphenicol Lincomycin Erythromycin Cephalosporins Enrofloxacin	
Streptococcus	Penicillin G Ampicillin Amoxicillin	Amp (amox) icillin Cephalosporins Erythromycin Chloramphenicol Trimethoprim
Toxoplasmosis	Clindamycin	Pyrimethamine with sulfonamide
Yersinia enterocolitica	Trimethoprim-sulfamethoxazole	Ampicillin Tetracycline

TABLE 2. **Suggested Antimicrobial Treatment Pending Culture**

Condition	Bacteria	Antibiotic Choices

Bacteremia
Septicemia
Endotoxemia
	AEROBIC BACTERIA
	Staphylococcus
	Streptococcus
	E. coli
	Klebsiella
	Enterobacter
	Pseudomonas
		AEROBIC BACTERIA
		Aminoglycoside with
		  a penicillin or
		  cephalosporin

	ANAEROBIC BACTERIA Clostridium Bacteriodes	ANAEROBIC BACTERIA Penicillin Chloramphenicol Clindamycin Metronidazole Cefoxitin Moxalactam
		EMPIRIC CHOICES Cefazolin/Amikacin Cefazolin/Gentamicin Ampicillin/Amikacin Ampicillin/Gentamicin Enroflox/Clindamycin Enroflox/Ampicillin 3rd-generation cephalosporin

Bacterial endocarditis	Staphylococcus
	E. coli
	β-hemolytic
	  streptococci
		Ampicillin and
		  gentamicin,
		Cephalosporins or
		  flouroquinolones

Dentistry; in those
  with preexisting
  valvular heart
  disease
	Staphylococcus
	Streptococcus
	Facultative bacteria
	Anaerobes
		Ampicillin
		Amoxicillin
		Penicillin G
		Clindamycin

Soft tissue infection	Dogs: Staphylococcus Cats: Pasteurella	Staph: Cefazolin Cefadroxil Ormetroprim-sulfa Pasteurella: Penicillin G Ampicillin Tetracycline Trimethoprim-sulfa Bacteroides: Clavamox®

TABLE 2.   **(Continued)**

Condition	Bacteria	Antibiotic Choices
Contaminated wounds, including bite wounds	Streptococcus *Pasteurella* Penicillinase-producing staph	Clavamox® Oxacillin Dicloxacillin Cephalosporins Tetracyclines Trimethoprim-sulfa Enrofloxacin Polymicrobial aerobic and anaerobic infection: Enrofloxacin with metronidazole
Burns	*Pseudomonas* Staphylococcus Proteus *Klebsiella* *Candida* spp.	Systemic drugs: Aminoglycosides Oxacillin Dicloxacillin Clavamox® Flouroquinolones Topical creams: Silver sulfadiazine Polymyxin-Neomycin-Bacitracin Gentamicin
Gingivitis-Stomatitis	Anaerobes	Clindamycin Metronidazole Tetracycline Clavamox®
GIT bacterial overgrowth	Mixed population	Tetracyclines Trimethoprim-sulfa
	Anaerobes	Tylosin and/or Metronidazole
Severe gastroenteritis	Aerobic and anaerobic bacteria	Ampicillin or Cephalothin +/– Aminoglycoside Penicillin G (HGE) Metronidazole Flouroquinolones Trimethoprim-sulfa
Gastroduodenal surgery	Gram-positive cocci Enteric Gram-negative bacilli	Cefazolin Ampicillin

TABLE 2. **(Continued)**

Condition	Bacteria	Antibiotic Choices
Colorectal surgery	Enteric Gram-negative bacilli Anaerobes	Metronidazole plus Enro- or Ciprofloxacin Oral Neomycin plus Erythromycin
Hepatobiliary infections	*E. coli* *Clostridium* spp. Staphylococcus *Pasteurella*	Chloramphenicol Cefoxitin Cephalothin Metronidazole Kanamycin Gentamicin Ampicillin Amoxicillin Tetracyclines (dog)
Upper respiratory infections	Difficult to interpret because of abundant normal flora	Ampicillin Clavamox® Cephalosporin Chloramphenicol Chlamydia: Tetracycline
Lower respiratory infections	Dog: *E. coli* *Klebsiella* *Pasteurella* *Pseudomonas* *Bordetella* *Strep. zooepidemicus* Cat: *Bordetella* *Pasteurella*	General: Amikacin Ceftizoxime Enrofloxacin Gentamicin Gram-positives: Cephalexin Trimethoprim-sulfa Clavamox® Amoxicillin Ampicillin Anaerobes: Ampicillin Clavamox Chloramphenicol Clindamycin Metronidazole Mycoplasma: Erythromycin Tylosin Chloramphenicol Tetracycline Fluoroquinolones

TABLE 2. **(Continued)**

Condition	Bacteria	Antibiotic Choices
Lower respiratory infections (continued)		*Bordetella:* Enrofloxacin Chloramphenicol Doxycycline Trimethoprim-sulfa Aminoglycosides Cephalexin Clavamox®
		Pyothorax: Ampicillin Cephalothin Chloramphenicol Trimethoprim-sulfa
Urinary tract infection	*E. coli* Proteus *Klebsiella Pseudomonas Enterobacter Staph. aureus* β-Strep.	Ampicillin Clavamox Cephalosporins Trimethoprim-sulfa Sulfa-ormetoprim Flouroquinolones
		Recurrent gram-negative infection: Trimethoprim-sulfa Enrofloxacin Cephalexin
		Recurrent gram-positive infection: Ampicillin
		Pyelonephritis: Chloramphenicol Trimethoprim-sulfa Enrofloxacin Norfloxacin
		Fungal and yeast: Fluconazole Ketoconazole Amphotericin B
Prostatitis	*E. coli Proteus* sp. Staphylococcus Streptococcus	Gram-positive: Erythromycin Clindamycin Chloramphenicol

TABLE 2. **(Continued)**

Condition	Bacteria	Antibiotic Choices
Prostatatis (continued)		Trimethoprim-sulfa
		Fluoroquinolones
		Gram-negative:
		Trimethoprim-sulfa
		Chloramphenicol
		Enrofloxacin
		Norfloxacin
Vaginitis	*E. coli*	Chloramphenicol
	Proteus	Amoxicillin
	Staphylococcus	Lincomycin
	Streptococcus	
Pyometra and Metritis	*E. coli*	Chloramphenicol
	Proteus	Trimethoprim-sulfa
	Streptococcus	Fluoroquinolones
Intraocular infection	Chlamydia	Chloramphenicol
	Mycoplasma	
	Gram positive	Sulfacetamide
		Neomycin-
		Polymyxin-
		Bacitracin
	Gram negative	Gentamicin
		Polymyxin
Central nervous system (CNS) infection		Chloramphenicol
		Trimethoprim-sulfa
		Metronidazole
		Fluoroquinolones
		Cefotaxime
		Ceftazidime
		Inflammation allows entry into CNS by:
		Minocycline
		Doxycycline
		Erythromycin
Dermatologic infections	Staphylococcus	Trimethoprim-sulfa
		Ormetoprim-sulfa
		Chloramphenicol
		Dicloxacillin
		Oxacillin
		Clavamox®
		Cephalosporins

TABLE 2. **(Continued)**

Condition	Bacteria	Antibiotic Choices
		Erythromycin Lincomycin Fluoroquinolones
Osteomyelitis	Staphylococcus Streptococcus E. coli Proteus Pseudomonas	Gram-positive: Cephalosporins Clavamox® Imipenem
		Gram-negative: Gentamicin Amikacin Fluoroquinolones
		Penicillinase-producing Staph: Oxacillin Cloxacillin Clavamox®
		Acute infection: Oxacillin with Gentamicin
		Anaerobes: Penicillins or 3rd-generation Cephalosporins with Clindamycin
Orthopedic surgery	Staphylococus	Cefazolin
Mixed or unknown infection	Mixed/Unknown	Clinadamycin and Enrofloxacin or Imipenem

GIT, gastrointestinal tract; HGE, hemorrhagic gastroenteritis.

Handbook of Veterinary Drugs, Second Edition, edited by Dana Allen,
Lippincott–Raven Publishers, Philadelphia. © 1998

Section 3

Description of Drugs for Small Animals

ACEMANNAN

INDICATIONS: Acemannan Immunostimulant ★ (Carrisyn ★-human product) enhances macrophage release of interleukin-1, interleukin-6, tumor necrosis factor-α, prostaglandin E_2, and interferon-γ. It increases natural killer cell activity and enhances T-cell function. This agent may be beneficial in dogs and cats with fibrosarcoma when used in conjunction with surgery and radiation treatment. It also has been used in cats with feline leukemia virus (FeLV)-induced diseases. Appetite improved. Hematocrit, hemoglobin, and leukocyte numbers also improved.

ADVERSE AND COMMON SIDE EFFECTS: None reported. Anaphylaxis has been reported after bolus IV administration; this can be eliminated by diluting acemannan in 100 to 150 mL saline and by infusing the IV solution over 15 to 30 minutes. The drug has not been studied in pregnant animals.

DRUG INTERACTIONS: None reported.

SUPPLIED AS: VETERINARY PRODUCT
For injection in 10-mg vials

ACEPROMAZINE

INDICATIONS: Acepromazine [formerly Acetylpromazine] (AC Promazine ★, Atravet ✦ ★, PromAce ★) is a phenothiazine drug used as a sedative and a preanesthetic agent. Acepromazine is used to facilitate restraint of patients. It also has antiemetic, antispasmodic, and hypothermic properties. The drug significantly decreases intraurethral pressures and may be useful in the management of feline urinary tract disease. It also may have a protective effect on barbiturate-, halothane-, and epinephrine-induced cardiac arrhythmias.

ADVERSE AND COMMON SIDE EFFECTS: The following side effects have been noted with the use of acepromazine: constipation, paradoxical aggression, sinus bradycardia, depression of myocardial contractility, hypotension, collapse, and prolongation of pseudocyesis.

Acepromazine lowers the seizure threshold and should not be used in animals with the potential for seizure activity, including those patients that have undergone procedures that may precipitate seizure activity, e.g., myelography. In addition, acepromazine should not be given to animals with tetanus.

Prolonged effects of the drug (even at low doses) may be seen in older animals. Giant breeds, as well as greyhounds, appear quite sensitive to the clinical effects of the drug, yet terrier breeds appear more resistant. Conversely, boxer dogs are predisposed to the hypotensive and bradycardic effects of the drug. Concurrent administration of atropine often is recommended to counter the bradycardia.

DRUG INTERACTIONS: Acepromazine is contraindicated in animals with strychnine or organophosphate poisoning and should not be given to animals treated with succinylcholine or other cholinesterase inhibitors. Concurrent anesthetic or narcotic preparations may exacerbate central nervous system (CNS) depression associated with the use of acepromazine. Kaolin-pectin and bismuth subsalicylate compounds and antacids decrease the absorption of oral acepromazine. Concurrent administration of propranolol and acepromazine may lead to serum elevations of both drugs. Phenytoin activity may be decreased if given along with acepromazine, and concurrent use of quinidine may cause additional cardiac depression. Finally, phenothiazines are α-adrenergic blocking agents and, if used with epinephrine, may lead to profound vasodilation and tachycardia. Other CNS depressants enhance hypotension and respiratory depression if used concurrently. Atropine and other anticholinergics have additive anticholinergic potential and reduce the antipsychotic effect of phenothiazines. Barbiturate drugs increase the metabolism of phenothiazines and may reduce their effects. Barbiturate anesthetics may increase excitation (tremor, involuntary muscle movements) and hypotension. Phenothiazines may mask the ototoxic effects of aminoglycoside antibiotics. Phenothiazines inhibit phenytoin metabolism and increase its potential for toxicity. In humans, there is the unexplained possibility of sudden death if phenothiazines are used concurrently with phenylpropanolamine. Tricyclic antidepressants, e.g., amitriptyline, may intensify the sedative and anticholinergic effects of phenothiazines.

SUPPLIED AS: VETERINARY PRODUCTS
Tablets containing 10 and 25 mg
For injection containing 10 mg/mL

OTHER USES
Dogs
AMPHETAMINE TOXICOSIS
0.05 to 1 mg/kg; IM, IV, SC

PREANESTHETIC DOSE
0.1 to 0.2 mg/kg; IV, IM (maximum 3 mg)

Dogs and Cats
ARTERIAL THROMBOEMBOLIC DISEASE
i)   0.05 to 0.11 mg/kg bid–tid; SC (to promote arterial vasodilation)
ii) 0.15 to 0.30 mg/kg bid–tid; IM, SC

ACETAMINOPHEN

INDICATIONS: Acetaminophen (Atasol ★, Tempra ♣ ★, Tylenol ♣ ★) is an antipyretic, analgesic agent useful for the treatment of mild to moderate pain in dogs. The drug is reported to be as effective as aspirin in the reduction of pain and fever. It is a weak anti-inflammatory agent and is not useful in the management of rheumatoid arthritis.

ADVERSE AND COMMON SIDE EFFECTS: A dosage of 150 mg/kg in dogs and 50 to 60 mg/kg in cats may cause toxicity. The incidence of gastric ulceration is less than that reported with aspirin. Vomiting and depression are the most common clinical signs of toxicosis noted in dogs. Anorexia and abdominal pain also are reported. The drug is extremely toxic to cats. Methemoglobinemia, Heinz-body anemia, hepatic necrosis, hematuria, cyanosis, depression, anorexia, vomiting, salivation, edema of the face and paws, and death have been reported in this species. Supportive treatment includes parenteral fluids and electrolytes, cimetidine (to reduce acetaminophen hepatic metabolism), and N-acetylcysteine (loading dose of 140 mg/kg, followed by 70 mg/kg every 4 hours; PO or IV for 3 to 5 treatments).

DRUG INTERACTIONS: None of significance in small animal medicine.

SUPPLIED AS: HUMAN PRODUCTS
Tablets containing 325 and 500 mg

Syrup containing 80 mg per 5 mL solution
Drops containing 80 mg/mL

ACETAZOLAMIDE

INDICATIONS: Acetazolamide (Acetazolam ✦ ★, Diamox ✦ ★) is a carbonic anhydrase inhibitor used in the treatment of glaucoma. The drug promotes renal bicarbonate and potassium excretion accompanied by water. These properties have made it useful as a diuretic and for the management of metabolic alkalosis. Acetazolamide reduces cerebrospinal fluid (CSF) production and may be of use in the management of hydrocephalus.

ADVERSE AND COMMON SIDE EFFECTS: In dogs, carbonic anhydrase inhibitors have been associated with causing drowsiness, behavioral changes, disorientation, vomiting (oral acetazolamide causes vomiting more often than other carbonic anhydrase inhibitors, e.g., methazolamide), diarrhea, hyperventilation, polydipsia (which usually decreases after a few weeks of use), and pruritus of the paws. Other potential adverse effects include bone marrow depression (anemia, leukopenia, thrombocytopenia) and hypercalciuria. Acetazolamide is contraindicated in animals with known hypersensitivity to the sulfonamides and derivatives, e.g., thiazides.
Acetazolamide should not be used in patients with marked renal or hepatic dysfunction, hypoadrenocorticism, hyponatremia, hypokalemia, or hyperchloremic acidosis. Long-term use is contraindicated in patients with hyphema or chronic, noncongestive angleclosure glaucoma. Long-term use may cause metabolic acidosis. Caution is recommended if the drug is used in patients with diabetes mellitus or obstructive pulmonary disease, or for those receiving digitalis.

DRUG INTERACTIONS: Oral use of acetazolamide may inhibit the absorption of primidone. Concurrent use of acetazolamide with primidone or phenytoin may cause osteomalacia. Concurrent use with corticosteroids, amphotericin B, or other diuretics may predispose to hypokalemia.

SUPPLIED AS: HUMAN PRODUCTS
Capsules (extended release) containing 500 mg
Tablets containing 125 and 250 mg
For injection in 500-mg vials

OTHER USES
Dogs
HYDROCEPHALUS
10 mg/kg every 6 to 8 hours

ACETYLCYSTEINE

INDICATIONS: Acetylcysteine (Mucomyst ✚ ★) is used as a mucolytic agent to help liquefy abnormal viscous or inspissated mucous secretions of the respiratory tract and eye. The drug also is used as antidotal therapy in the management of acetaminophen toxicity.

ADVERSE AND COMMON SIDE EFFECTS: Nebulization of the drug may cause bronchospasm, especially in patients with asthma. When given orally, nausea and vomiting may occur. Because the drug has a bad taste, stomach intubation may be required for oral administration.

DRUG INTERACTIONS: Acetylcysteine is incompatible with (based on the possible formation of a precipitate or a change in the color or clarity): tetracycline, oxytetracycline, chlortetracycline, and hydrogen peroxide.

SUPPLIED AS: HUMAN PRODUCT
For oral inhalation, oral solution, or intratracheal instillation containing a 10% or a 20% sterile solution

ALBENDAZOLE

INDICATIONS: Albendazole (Valbazen ✚ ★) is an anthelmintic marketed for use in cattle. However, it has been used in small animals in the treatment of filaroidiasis, capillariasis, giardiasis, and paragonimiasis infections. The drug is safer and more effective than metronidazole or quinacrine for the treatment of giardiasis. Efficacy against *Metametorchis intermedius* in cats also is likely.

ADVERSE AND COMMON SIDE EFFECTS: Adverse drug effects have not been seen in dogs at dosages of 25 mg/kg bid, for 2 days, or at dosages of 30 mg/kg once daily for 13 weeks, but dosages of 30 to 60 mg/kg once daily for 26 weeks have resulted in leukopenia, blood dyscrasia, and reduced bone marrow cellularity. Idiosyncratic or dose-dependent pancytopenia has been reported in a dog given the drug at a dosage of 100 mg/kg once daily. The pancytopenia may resolve after drug withdrawal. Anorexia may develop in dogs receiving 50 mg/kg twice daily. In cats, lethargy, depression, and anorexia sometimes develop. Drug dosages of 100 mg/kg once daily for 14 to 21 days have caused leukopenia in cats.

DRUG INTERACTIONS: None reported.

SUPPLIED AS: VETERINARY PRODUCT
Suspension containing 113.6 mg/mL (11.36%)

OTHER USES
Dogs
FILAROIDES HIRTHI
50 mg/kg bid; PO for 5 days, repeat in 21 days
Note: Symptoms may worsen with therapy because of the reaction to
dying worms.
FILAROIDES OSLERI
25 mg/kg bid; PO for 5 days, repeat in 2 weeks
CAPILLARIA PLICA
50 mg/kg bid; PO for 10 to 14 days
GIARDIA CANIS
25 mg/kg bid; PO for 2 consecutive days

Cats
PARAGONIMUS KELLICOTTI
25 mg/kg bid; PO for 10 to 21 days
METAMETORCHIS INTERMEDIUS
50 mg/kg div. bid; PO for 10 to 14 days
GIARDIA
25 mg/kg bid; PO for 5 days

ALBUTEROL

INDICATIONS: Albuterol or Salbutamol (Ventolin ❋ ★) is a synthetic sympathomimetic amine and moderately selective β_2-adrener-
gic agonist. It has more prominent effects on β_2-receptors—particularly smooth muscles in bronchi, uteri, and vascular supply to
skeletal muscles—than on β_1-receptors in the heart. Some peripheral
vasodilation may occur. The drug produces bronchodilation and inhibits histamine release. It is used to relieve bronchospasm and alleviate cough.

ADVERSE AND COMMON SIDE EFFECTS: Caution is advised
with use of the drug in patients with cardiovascular disease, hypertension, hyperthyroid disease, or diabetes mellitus. In dogs, muscle
tremors and nervousness may be noted with initiation of therapy.
Side effects disappear within 5 to 7 days of therapy. Additional side
effects often include tachycardia, premature ventricular contractions, vomiting, tachypnea and panting, and depression. In humans,
other reported side effects have included increased or decreased
blood pressure, nausea, paradoxical bronchospasm, difficulty in
voiding, muscle cramps, and aggravation of diabetes mellitus. A
β-blocking agent such as propranolol or metoprolol may be of benefit in cases of albuterol toxicosis.

DRUG INTERACTIONS: The concurrent use of epinephrine and other sympathomimetic (adrenergic) agents and antihistamines may have additive effects and is not recommended. Monoamine inhibitors, possibly amitraz, may potentiate the action of the drug on the vascular system. Propranolol and other β-adrenergic blocking agents may inhibit the effect of the drug. Theophyllines may potentiate the bronchodilatory effects of albuterol.

SUPPLIED AS: HUMAN PRODUCTS
Tablets containing 2 or 4 mg
Oral liquid containing 0.4 mg/mL

ALDACTAZIDE

INDICATIONS: Hydrochlorothiazide-spironolactone (Aldactazide ✚ ★) acts at Henle's loop and the proximal and distal convoluted tubules, exerting a synergistic diuretic effect. The principal advantage of this combination is its potassium-sparing effect. The onset of action is slower, and its effect is longer lasting. In humans, this drug combination is recommended in patients with congestive heart failure unresponsive or poorly tolerant to other diuretics, diuretic-induced hypokalemia in those requiring diuretic therapy, cirrhosis of the liver accompanied by edema and/or ascites, essential hypertension, and nephrotic syndrome unresponsive to glucocorticoids or other diuretics.

ADVERSE AND COMMON SIDE EFFECTS: Aldactazide should not be used in patients with anuria, acute renal insufficiency, or hyperkalemia, or those sensitive to spironolactone or thiazide agents. In humans, adverse effects may include nausea, anorexia, vomiting, cramping, diarrhea or constipation, jaundice, acute pancreatitis, leukopenia, thrombocytopenia, agranulocytosis, aplastic anemia, impotence, abnormal sperm motility or counts, and irregularities of the menstrual cycle.

DRUG INTERACTIONS: Spironolactone has been shown to increase the half-life of digoxin and may result in digitalis toxicity. The drug may alter insulin requirements in diabetic patients.

SUPPLIED AS: HUMAN PRODUCT
Tablets containing 25 and 50 mg

ALLOPURINOL

INDICATIONS: Allopurinol (Zyloprim ✚ ★) is indicated in the treatment of urate urolithiasis in dogs. It inhibits the enzyme xanthine oxidase and blocks the formation and urinary excretion of uric acid. Urine urate/creatinine ratio decreases with drug administration. Urine urate/creatinine ratio in Dalmatian dogs ranges from 0.5 to 0.6 in one study to 0.6 to 1.5 in another study, versus 0.2 to 0.4 in non-Dalmatian dogs. A 50% reduction in the urine urate/creatinine ratio (reduced to 0.25 to 0.3) is recommended to decrease the recurrence of urate urolithiasis. The drug also has been used to treat leishmaniasis in a dog.

ADVERSE AND COMMON SIDE EFFECTS: Although adverse effects in dogs are uncommon, in humans the drug has been associated with nausea, vomiting, diarrhea, pancreatitis, and a reversible hepatopathy associated with transient increases in serum alkaline phosphatase, alanine aminotransferase, and aspartate aminotransferase. Rare cases of bone marrow suppression with leukopenia and thrombocytopenia also have been documented. The drug should be used with caution in patients with renal disease. In these cases, the dose should be decreased and the patient closely monitored for further deterioration in renal function. Chronic use of the drug at doses of 30 mg/kg/day may predispose the patient to xanthine urolith formation. If long-term use of the drug is required, drug dose probably should be decreased.

DRUG INTERACTIONS: Allopurinol potentiates the effects of cyclophosphamide, increasing the risk for bone marrow suppression. Because azathioprine metabolism depends on xanthine oxidase, concurrent use of this drug with allopurinol may lead to toxic levels of azathioprine. Urinary acidifiers, e.g., methionine and ammonium chloride, may reduce the solubility of uric acid and promote urolithiasis. Thiazides and possibly other diuretics increase the risk of allopurinol toxicity and hypersensitivity, especially in those with impaired renal function. Rarely, when used with trimethoprim/sulfamethoxazole, allopurinol has been associated with thrombocytopenia in humans. Large doses of allopurinol may decrease the metabolism of aminophylline and theophylline and increase their serum levels.

SUPPLIED AS: HUMAN PRODUCT
Tablets containing 100, 200, and 300 mg

OTHER USES
Dogs
LEISHMANIA SPP.
11 mg/kg/day for 4 months; PO, dose then was increased to 15 mg/kg/day for an additional 9 months

ALPHA-KERI

INDICATIONS: Alpha-keri ♣ ★ is a ,water-dispersible, antipruritic oil. It contains a dewaxed, oil-soluble, keratin-moisturizing fraction of lanolin, mineral oil, and nonionic emulsifiers. It is indicated for dry, pruritic skin conditions, including seborrhea, to relieve itching and to lubricate and soften the skin.

ADVERSE AND COMMON SIDE EFFECTS: This product should not be used on acutely inflamed skin.

DRUG INTERACTIONS: None.

SUPPLIED AS: HUMAN PRODUCTS
Bath oil available in 200- and 480-mL plastic bottles
Bar soap containing 110 g

ALUMINUM HYDROXIDE

INDICATIONS: Aluminum hydroxide (Amphojel ♣ ★, Dialume ★) is an antacid, antiflatulent medication useful in the treatment of gastric ulcers and hyperphosphatemia associated with renal failure. The aluminum component has a cytoprotective effect on the gastrointestinal tract (GIT) mucosa because of prostaglandin synthesis, which is in addition to its buffering activity. The drug may have a protective effect on the GIT when administered with poorly tolerated drugs, e.g., aminophylline and nonsteroidal anti-inflammatory agents. Aluminum hydroxide may be combined with magnesium hydroxide. The advantage of combining aluminum with magnesium hydroxide (Amphojel 500 ★, Maalox ♣ ★) is to optimize the extent and rate of acid neutralization. See also **ANTACIDS**.

ADVERSE AND COMMON SIDE EFFECTS: The drug is contraindicated in animals with alkalosis. It is poorly palatable, and the aluminum component may predispose to constipation. Aluminum-containing antacids may delay gastric emptying and should be used with caution in patients with gastric outlet obstruction. Also, aluminum hydroxide supposedly may lead to phosphate depletion, muscle weakness, bone resorption, and hypercalcemia.

DRUG INTERACTIONS: Antacid products may interfere with the absorption of oral iron preparations, digoxin, phenothiazines, glucocorticoids, captopril, ketoconazole, nitrofurantoin, penicillamine, phenothiazines, phenytoin, ranitidine, cimetidine, and the tetracyclines. Increased absorption and serum levels of the following drugs may be seen if given concurrently with antacid compounds: aspirin, quinidine, and sympathomimetic agents.

SUPPLIED AS: HUMAN PRODUCTS
Liquid containing 320 mg/5 mL [Amphojel]
400 mg/5 mL [Aluminum Hydroxide Gel ★]
600 mg/5 mL [Alternagel ★, Aluminum Hydroxide Concentrated ★]
Capsules containing 475 mg [Alu-Cap ★] and 500 mg [Dialume]
Tablets containing 600 mg [Amphojel] [each tablet has an antacid effect = 10 mL of Amphojel liquid (320 mg/5 mL)]
Liquid containing 500 mg aluminum hydroxide and magnesium hydroxide per 5 mL [Amphojel 500]

AMIKACIN

INDICATIONS: Amikacin (Amiglyde-V ♣ ★, Amikin ♣ ★) is an aminoglycoside antibiotic indicated in the treatment of genitourinary tract infections in the dog caused by susceptible strains of *Escherichia coli* and *Proteus* sp., and skin and soft tissue infections caused by *Pseudomonas* sp., *E. coli,* and *Staphylococcus* sp. Amikacin is especially useful in those infections caused by *E. coli, Pseudomonas* sp., *Klebsiella* sp., *Proteus* spp., and *Staphylococcus* spp. resistant to gentamicin, kanamycin, or other aminoglycoside antibiotics. See also **AMINOGLYCOSIDE ANTIBIOTICS.**

ADVERSE AND COMMON SIDE EFFECTS: The LD$_{50}$ of amikacin is in excess of 250 mg/kg in dogs. Like other aminoglycosides, amikacin has nephrotoxic, neurotoxic, and ototoxic potential, but usually only at exaggerated parenteral doses over a prolonged period of time. Amikacin serum concentrations should be monitored in all patients because of the large interanimal variation in pharmacokinetics. Peak serum concentrations (determined 1 hour after injection) should be four to five times the minimum inhibitory concentration (MIC) of the offending organism, but no higher than 25 µg/mL. Trough concentrations (taken just before the next dose) should be less than 5 µg/mL. In cats, amikacin has less ototoxic potential than gentamicin. Transient pain may be noted on injection.

DRUG INTERACTIONS: See **AMINOGLYCOSIDE ANTIBIOTICS.**

SUPPLIED AS: VETERINARY PRODUCT
For injection containing 50 mg/mL [Amiglyde-V]

HUMAN PRODUCT
For injection containing 50 and 250 mg/mL [Amikin]

AMINOGLYCOSIDE ANTIBIOTICS

INDICATIONS: The aminoglycoside antibiotics, which include amikacin, dihydrostreptomycin, gentamicin, kanamycin, neomycin, streptomycin, and tobramycin, are indicated in the treatment of certain gram-negative, gram-positive, and mycobacterial infections. They primarily are effective against aerobic gram-negative bacteria such as *E. coli, Klebsiella, Proteus,* and *Enterobacter*; some also are effective against *Pseudomonas* infections. Gentamicin is more effective than kanamycin but less effective than tobramycin against *Pseudomonas aeruginosa*. Amikacin sulfate injection is especially useful against *Pseudomonas* and *Klebsiella* spp. resistant to gentamicin. Steady-state drug levels of gentamicin are established in 6.5 hours in the dog. Serum concentrations are measured 1 to 2 hours after dosing (peak levels) or just before the next dose (trough levels). To establish optimum dosing levels, it is desirable to take samples at peak and trough times.

ADVERSE AND COMMON SIDE EFFECTS: Nephrotoxicity, deafness, vestibular toxicity, respiratory paralysis, and cardiovascular depression have been reported with the use of these drugs, although otic preparations of gentamicin sulfate do not adversely affect vestibular or cochlear function in healthy dogs. Endotoxemia predisposes to cardiovascular-induced depression. These drugs should be avoided in puppies and kittens because they are more likely to develop renal failure. Neomycin is the most nephrotoxic aminoglycoside, followed in decreasing order of nephrotoxicity by gentamicin, tobramycin, kanamycin, amikacin, and streptomycin. Monitoring the urine for the appearance of casts, which in this case is a more sensitive indicator of impending renal dysfunction than serum urea or creatinine, is recommended if blood levels are not measured. Hypokalemia, hypocalcemia, hypomagnesemia, metabolic acidosis, and low sodium diets may enhance gentamicin nephrotoxicity. Topical administration of gentamicin (i.e., wound lavage) also has caused nephrotoxicity in a cat.

DRUG INTERACTIONS: Aminoglycoside antibiotics can potentiate the action of neuromuscular blocking agents, leading to respiratory depression, apnea, or muscle weakness, especially in animals with renal insufficiency. The neuromuscular blocking activity can be reversed with neostigmine. Furosemide may enhance the ototoxicity and nephrotoxicity of the aminoglycosides. Gentamicin, dihydrostreptomycin, kanamycin, neomycin, and streptomycin may decrease cardiac output and produce hypotension and bradycardia and should be avoided in animals in shock or with serious cardiac insufficiency. Intravenous calcium gluconate should be used to reverse myocardial depression and restore blood pressure. Prolonged high oral doses of neomycin may cause diarrhea and malabsorption because of selective overgrowth of resistant indigenous intestinal flora. Aminoglycosides may cross the placental barrier and produce fetal intoxication and should not be given to pregnant animals. Penicillins should not be mixed with aminoglycosides before injection because inactivation of the aminoglycoside may occur.

SUPPLIED AS: See individual drug.

AMINOPENTAMIDE SULFATE

INDICATIONS: Aminopentamide (Centrine ★) is an antiemetic drug. It has antispasmodic and anticholinergic properties and is recommended for the treatment of acute abdominal visceral spasm, tenesmus, pylorospasm or hypertrophic gastritis, and associated nausea, vomiting, and/or diarrhea in dogs and cats.

ADVERSE AND COMMON SIDE EFFECTS: Adverse effects may include dry mouth, dry eyes, blurred vision, and urinary hesitancy, the latter of which usually is the result of excessive dosing. The drug is contraindicated in patients with glaucoma, and it should be given cautiously, if at all, to those with pyloric obstruction. Aminopentamide should not be used in animals with a history of sensitivity to anticholinergic drugs, tachycardia, cardiac disease, obstructive gastrointestinal (GI) disease, paralytic ileus, ulcerative colitis, urinary obstruction, or myasthenia gravis. The drug also should not be used in those with GI infections because the antimuscarinic effects decrease GI motility, contributing to retention of the infection within the GIT. In addition, antimuscarinic agents should be used with caution in patients with liver or renal disease, hyperthyroid disease, congestive heart failure, esophageal reflux, or prostatic hypertrophy, and in geriatric or pediatric patients. Although no specific information is given concerning treatment of overdose, therapy for atropine overdose may be applicable here. If oral ingestion is recent, the GIT should be emptied and the patient given activated charcoal and a saline cathartic. The animal then is treated symptomatically. Avoid the use of phenothiazines because they are likely to contribute to the anticholinergic effects. Physostigmine should only be considered in those exhibiting severe supraventricular tachyarrhythmias or extreme agitation to the point of possibly inflicting injury to themselves. The human pediatric dose that may be applicable to small animals is 0.02 mg/kg slowly IV. If clinical response is not seen, the drug is repeated every 10 minutes until cholinergic or muscarinic signs have disappeared. Adverse effects of physostigmine (bronchoconstriction, bradycardia, seizure) are treated with small doses of IV atropine.

DRUG INTERACTIONS: Although none are listed for this product, those drugs that interact with atropine may react similarly with aminopentamide. Antihistamines, procainamide, quinidine, meperidine, benzodiazepines, and phenothiazines may enhance the activity of aminopentamide. The following drugs may potentiate the adverse effects of aminopentamide: primidone, disopyramide, nitrates, and long-term corticosteroid use. Atropine (and possibly aminopentamide) may enhance the activity of nitrofurantoin, the thiazide diuretics, and sympathomimetic agents. Atropine (and possibly aminopentamide) may antagonize the action of metoclopramide.

SUPPLIED AS: VETERINARY PRODUCTS
Tablets containing 0.2 mg
For injection containing 0.5 mg/mL

AMINOPHYLLINE

INDICATIONS: Aminophylline (Phylloconton ♣ ★ and generics) is a bronchodilator principally used for the management of cough due to bronchospasm. It has mild inotropic properties and mild, transient diuretic activity.

ADVERSE AND COMMON SIDE EFFECTS: Side effects may include vomiting, anorexia or polyphagia, diarrhea, polydipsia, polyuria, restlessness, muscle twitching, cardiac arrhythmias, tachycardia, hyperglycemia, and nervousness. The drug should be used with caution in patients with cardiac disease, systemic hypertension, cardiac arrhythmias, GIT ulcers, impaired renal or hepatic function, diabetes mellitus, hyperthyroid disease, and glaucoma. Serum or plasma concentrations of theophylline should be measured after steady-state concentrations have been attained (approximately 30 hours after initiation of therapy in dogs and 40 hours in cats) and just before the next dose. Therapeutic serum concentrations are 10 to 20 µg/mL (55 to 110 µmol/L). See also **THEOPHYLLINE.**

DRUG INTERACTIONS: Serum levels may be increased by the concurrent use of thiabendazole, cimetidine, allopurinol, clindamycin, and erythromycin. Phenobarbital decreases the therapeutic effect of the drug. Concurrent use of aluminum or magnesium antacid preparations slows the absorption of theophylline. Propranolol has direct antagonistic effects because propranolol is a β-adrenergic blocking agent and aminophylline is a β-adrenergic stimulant. Phenytoin increases theophylline clearance, requiring larger doses of the drug for effect. Aminophylline should not be mixed in a syringe with other drugs. Because aminophylline solutions are alkaline, they are incompatible with epinephrine, isoproterenol, or penicillin G potassium. Aminophylline contains approximately 80% theophylline. Concurrent use of this drug with allopurinol, cimetidine, furosemide, or epinephrine may cause excessive CNS stimulation. See also **THEOPHYLLINE.**

SUPPLIED AS: HUMAN PRODUCTS
Tablets containing 100 mg aminophylline (78.9 mg theophylline)
and 200 mg aminophylline (157.8 mg theophylline)
Theophylline timed-release capsules and tablets are available in 50-,
100-, 125-, 130-, 200-, 225-, 250-, 260-, 300-, and 350-mg strengths.
For injection containing 25 mg/mL (19.7 mg/mL theophylline) and
50 mg/mL (39.4 mg/mL theophylline)

AMITRAZ

INDICATIONS: Amitraz (Mitaban ✣ ★) is indicated for the eradication of demodicosis and sarcoptic mange in dogs. The drug is
classified as a monoamine oxidase (MAO) inhibitor (causes a
build-up of norepinephrine in the CNS), although the exact mechanism of its action is unknown. It also inhibits prostaglandin synthesis and is an α-adrenergic agonist. Although not specifically
indicated for use in cats, the drug has been used safely as outlined
below.

ADVERSE AND COMMON SIDE EFFECTS: The most common
side effects of mild toxicosis are ataxia and depression. Other side effects may include transient sedation, mydriasis, hypersalivation,
transient pruritus (due to effect of dead mites), hypothermia or hyperthermia, vomiting, diarrhea, and occasionally bradycardia. Clinical signs of severe toxicosis may include hypotension, hyperglycemia, mydriasis, and hypothermia. Puppies are especially
sensitive, and cats may become toxic even when treated aurally. Safe
use of the drug in pregnant bitches and puppies less than 4 months
of age has not been established and is not recommended.

DRUG INTERACTIONS: Atropine potentiates the pressor effects
of amitraz and may cause hypertension and cardiac arrhythmias.
It also may potentiate ileus and gastric distention. Yohimbine
(0.1 mg/kg; IV) is a safe and effective antidote. The half-life of yohimbine is 1.5 to 2 hours. Therefore, it may need to be repeated.
Atipamezole (50 μg/kg; IM), a potent α$_2$-antagonist, also is an effective antagonist. Reversal of clinical signs of toxicosis are apparent
within 10 minutes after injection. In cases of ingestion, and before the
onset of clinical signs of toxicosis, vomiting should be induced.

When drug interactions to MAO inhibitors are reported throughout this text, amitraz is given as a possible example, even though
studies directly implicating it may not be available.

SUPPLIED AS: VETERINARY PRODUCT
Available in 10.6-mL units

OTHER USES
Cats
NOTOEDRES CATI
Single application of 0.025% solution applied with a toothbrush to affected skin and repeated in 2 weeks

LOCALIZED DEMODECTIC MANGE
Topical application of 0.025% solution to affected lesions twice weekly for 3 weeks

AMITRIPTYLINE HYDROCHLORIDE

INDICATIONS: Amitriptyline (Apo-amitriptyline ✦, Elavil ✦ ★, Levate ✦) is a tricyclic antidepressant drug with antihistaminic, anticholinergic, and local anesthetic properties. It is recommended for the management of anxiety-related behavioral disorders, including depression, separation anxiety in dogs, aggression, narcolepsy, compulsive behaviors and anxiety, urine spraying, and excessive grooming in cats. The drug also may have antipruritic properties in dogs. The drug also appears to ameliorate clinical signs of lower urinary tract inflammation in cats with recurrent idiopathic cystitis for at least 6 months.

ADVERSE AND COMMON SIDE EFFECTS: Sedation may be marked initially. Anticholinergic effects may include dry mouth, urine retention, constipation, tachycardia, and vomiting. Other side effects may include hallucinations, disorientation, and hyperactivity. Amitriptyline is contraindicated in animals with cardiac disease, urinary retention, or a history of seizure activity because the drug lowers the seizure threshold. Adverse effects noted in small animals may include vomiting, hyperexcitability, ataxia, lethargy, tremors, seizures, and cardiac arrhythmias. Diazepam (2.5 to 5 mg/kg; PO or IV) may be used to control the hyperexcitability. Caution is recommended if the drug is used in patients with diabetes mellitus, hyperthyroid disease, and hepatic or renal disease. After long-term use, withdrawal should be gradual.

DRUG INTERACTIONS: Amitriptyline should not be given within 14 days of an animal receiving an MAO inhibitor, e.g., amitraz (Mitaban) and selegiline. Tachycardia, hyperpyrexia, seizures, and cardiovascular instability may result. Potentiation of CNS depression may occur if the drug is given with barbiturates or sedatives. Concurrent use of epinephrine or norepinephrine and amitriptyline may cause hypertension and hyperpyrexia. Concurrent use with thyroid drugs may accelerate the onset of therapeutic effects, but also may increase the likelihood of cardiac arrhythmias.

SUPPLIED AS: HUMAN PRODUCTS
Syrup containing 10 mg/5 mL
Tablets containing 10, 25, 50, 75, 100 and 150 mg

OTHER USES
Cats
IDIOPATHIC CYSTITIS
10 mg per cat daily; PO (at bedtime)

AMMONIUM CHLORIDE

INDICATIONS: Ammonium chloride is used in the treatment of metabolic alkalosis and has a mild expectorant action. The drug also is used to acidify urine, as adjunctive therapy in the treatment of urinary tract infection, feline lower urinary tract inflammation, and struvite urolithiasis. Ammonium chloride may enhance the antibacterial properties of penicillin G, nitrofurantoin, methenamine mandelate, chlortetracycline, and oxytetracycline. It also is used to enhance the renal excretion of quinidine and the amphetamines in cases of drug intoxication.

ADVERSE AND COMMON SIDE EFFECTS: Nausea and vomiting may occur with oral use of the drug. Intoxication may follow IV use of the drug, demonstrated by metabolic acidosis, hyperventilation, arrhythmias, depression, stupor, coma, and seizure. Ammonium chloride is contraindicated in animals with severe hepatic disease and in those with renal failure. The drug may cause fetal acidosis and should not be given to pregnant animals.

DRUG INTERACTIONS: Acidification of urine may decrease the efficacy of the aminoglycosides and erythromycin.

SUPPLIED AS: HUMAN PRODUCTS (United States only)
Tablets containing 500 mg
For injection; 26.75% (5 mEq/mL) [dilute 1 or 2 vials (100–200 mEq) in 500 or 1,000 mL of sodium chloride 0.9% for injection—do not exceed 5 mL/minute] (adult human)

VETERINARY PRODUCTS
MEQ-AC ★
Granules containing 535 mg/teaspoonful
Tablets containing 357 mg

There are no products containing ammonium chloride alone in Canada. It also is available in combination with methionine as Uroeze ★ and in Canada in combination with atropine, hyoscyamine, scopolamine, and sulphisoxazole as Renazone for treatment of renal bacterial infections and renal spasm in small animals.

OTHER USES: Ammonium chloride sometimes is used in cough mixtures for its expectorant activity.

AMOXICILLIN

INDICATIONS: Amoxicillin (Amoxi-Tabs ★, Amoxi-Drop ★, Amoxi-Inject ★, Amoxil ♣ ★, Moxilean ♣, Robamox-V ★) is indicated for the treatment of genitourinary, GI, respiratory, and skin/soft tissue infections in dogs and cats sensitive to the drug. Amoxicillin has the same antibacterial spectrum as ampicillin but is better absorbed from the GIT and has a more rapid bactericidal activity and a longer duration of action. For more information, see **PENICILLIN ANTIBIOTICS.**

ADVERSE AND COMMON SIDE EFFECTS: See PENICILLIN ANTIBIOTICS.

DRUG INTERACTIONS: See PENICILLIN ANTIBIOTICS.

SUPPLIED AS: VETERINARY PRODUCTS
Tablets containing 50, 100, 200 and 400 mg
Oral suspension containing 50 mg/mL [Amoxi-Drop, Moxilean, Robamox-V]
For injection containing 3 g/vial [Amoxi-Inject]

OTHER USES
Dogs
LYME BORRELIOSIS
5 mg/kg bid; PO for 10 to 14 days

AMPHOTERICIN B

INDICATIONS: Amphotericin B (Fungizone ♣ ★) is an effective antifungal agent. The drug has been used to treat the following infections: blastomycosis, histoplasmosis, cryptococcosis, coccidioidomycosis, and candidiasis. The lipid complex form is less toxic and has been found to be as effective as amphotericin B in the treatment of blastomycosis in dogs. Mucoraceae is variably susceptible, and aspergillosis usually is resistant.

ADVERSE AND COMMON SIDE EFFECTS: The most important side effect is renal dysfunction. Serum urea and creatinine levels and urinalysis should be monitored frequently throughout the treatment regimen. Administration of the drug is discontinued, at least temporarily, when the blood urea nitrogen (BUN) exceeds 30 to 40 mg/dL (10.7–14.3 mmol/L) or serum creatinine exceeds 3 mg/dL (265 µmol/L). Two regimens have been recommended to decrease the nephrotoxicity of amphotericin B (AMB). Mannitol (12.5 g or 0.5–1 g/kg) is given concurrently with AMB by slow infusion. However, this technique may decrease the efficacy of AMB, especially in patients with blastomycosis. With the second method, sodium chloride (0.9%) is administered at a rate of 5 mL/kg, half of which is given before injection of AMB and half after AMB injection. Anorexia, nausea, vomiting, fever, phlebitis, normocytic normochromic anemia, hemolytic anemia, and cardiac arrhythmias also have been documented with use of the drug. Cats appear to be more sensitive to the drug than dogs, and lower doses are recommended by some authors. Potassium loss has not been a problem in dogs and cats as it is in humans treated with the drug.

DRUG INTERACTIONS: The concurrent use of aminoglycosides, polymyxin B, cisplatin, methoxyflurane, or vancomycin may potentiate the nephrotoxicity of AMB. When AMB is combined with minocycline and flucytosine, serum concentrations of AMB needed to inhibit growth of *Candida* or *Cryptococcus neoformans* are reduced. Rifampin enhances the effect of AMB on *Aspergillus, Candida,* and *Histoplasma capsulatum.* Similarly, ketoconazole appears to potentiate the efficacy of AMB against blastomycosis and histoplasmosis.

SUPPLIED AS: HUMAN PRODUCT
For injection containing 50 mg lyophilized AMB per vial
For detailed regimens on the preparation and administration of AMB, the reader is directed to Kirk's Current Veterinary Therapy IX: 1102

OTHER USES
Dogs
BLASTOMYCOSIS
1 mg/kg; IV every Monday, Wednesday, and Friday, and administered at a rate of 4 mg/kg/hour; (cumulative dose of 12 mg/kg; AMB lipid complex)

AMPICILLIN

INDICATIONS: Ampicillin (Omnipen ★, Penbriton ♣, Polyflex ♣ ★) is indicated in the treatment of urinary tract, GI, and respiratory tract infections susceptible to the antibiotic. Ampicillin has increased antibacterial activity against many gram-negative bacteria not affected by the natural penicillins or penicillinase-resistant penicillins, including some strains of *E. coli* and *Klebsiella*. Ampicillin also has activity against anaerobic bacteria, including clostridial organisms. Ampicillin is susceptible to β-lactamase bacteria, e.g., *Staph aureus.* For information concerning adverse and common side effects, see **PENICILLIN ANTIBIOTICS.**

DRUG INTERACTIONS: If ampicillin is given concurrently with an aminoglycoside, the efficacy of the aminoglycoside may be impaired in patients with reduced renal function. Do not administer ampicillin with bacteriostatic drugs, e.g., chloramphenicol, erythromycin, or tetracyclines, because the combination may reduce the bactericidal activity of the ampicillin.

SUPPLIED AS: VETERINARY PRODUCT
For injection in 10- and 25-g vials [Polyflex]
HUMAN PRODUCTS
Capsules containing 250 and 500 mg
Oral suspension containing 100, 125, 250, and 500 mg/mL
For injection containing 125-, 250-, and 500-mg and 1-, 2- and 10-g vials

AMPROLIUM

INDICATIONS: Amprolium (Amprol ♣, Corid ★) is an antiprotozoal agent (coccidiosis). The drug is a thiamine inhibitor.

ADVERSE AND COMMON SIDE EFFECTS: Vomiting, diarrhea, anorexia, depression, and nervous symptoms may develop. In such cases, the drug should be discontinued and the animal treated with thiamine (1–10 mg/day; IM, IV). The drug should not be used for more than 12 days in puppies.

DRUG INTERACTIONS: None reported.

SUPPLIED AS: VETERINARY PRODUCTS
Oral solution containing 96 mg/mL (9.6%) [Amprol, Corid] approved for use in calves
Soluble powder containing 20% [Corid] approved for use in calves

AMRINONE

INDICATIONS: Amrinone (Inocor ♣ ★) is a positive inotropic agent with mild arteriolar dilating properties. It is of potential benefit in increasing cardiac output and decreasing pulmonary capillary pressures in animals with congestive heart failure and cardiomyopathy.

ADVERSE AND COMMON SIDE EFFECTS: Although side effects are rare, anorexia, nausea, vomiting, diarrhea, tachycardia, arrhythmias, and hypotension may be seen. The drug should be used with caution in patients with compromised renal or hepatic function or aortic stenosis.

DRUG INTERACTIONS: If used with disopyramide, excessive hypotension may occur.

SUPPLIED AS: HUMAN PRODUCT
For injection containing 5 mg/mL

ANABOLIC STEROIDS

INDICATIONS: Anabolic androgenic steroids have been used in the treatment of aplastic anemia, myeloproliferative disease, and lymphoma accompanied by nonregenerative anemia. In addition to increasing erythrocyte mass, androgens stimulate myelopoiesis, and thrombopoiesis to a lesser degree. These drugs stimulate the production of erythropoietin, potentiate its effects, and increase the production of erythrocytes. Because of the lack of an extrarenal source of erythropoietin, dogs with anemia secondary to renal failure are less likely to respond, and the expected response essentially is proportional to the amount of functional renal tissue remaining. Several weeks to months may be required for a positive response to be seen, and reportedly, only one third of dogs and cats show a positive erythropoietic response to these drugs. These agents also are hypothesized to stimulate appetite, promote a positive nitrogen balance, enhance skeletal calcium deposition, and promote intestinal absorption of calcium. In dogs with acute uremia, however, boldenone undecylenate failed to enhance appetite or promote an anabolic effect. Danazol, a modified androgen, also has been used with corticosteroids in the management of autoimmune hemolytic anemia and immune-mediated thrombocytopenia. These agents are classified into two groups: alkylated agents (methyltestosterone, fluoxymesterone, oxymetholone, methandrostenolone, stanozolol, norethandrolone) and nonalkylated agents (testosterone, methenolone, nandrolone).

ADVERSE AND COMMON SIDE EFFECTS: Animals with compromised cardiac or renal function should be monitored closely because of the potential for sodium and water retention. Interference with normal female reproductive cycling, masculinization of fetuses during pregnancy, and a reduction in spermatogenesis may occur. Early closure of bony epiphyses in young animals and pain at injection sites have been reported. Additional adverse effects of androgens may include sodium and water retention, hepatotoxicity, recurrence and exacerbation of perianal adenoma, perineal hernia, and prostatomegaly. The nonalkylating drugs are less hepatotoxic but appear to be less effective in stimulating erythrocyte production. In addition, hepatotoxicity occurs primarily with the oral androgens. Parenteral forms essentially are considered nonhepatotoxic. Anabolic steroids also have been implicated in the etiology of hepatic carcinoma.

DRUG INTERACTIONS: See specific drug.

SUPPLIED AS: See specific drug.

ANTACIDS

INDICATIONS: Orally administered antacids contain aluminum hydroxide (Amphojel, Dialume), calcium carbonate (Titralac, Tums), magnesium compounds (Phillips' Milk of Magnesia), combinations of aluminum and magnesium hydroxide (Amphojel Plus, DiGel, Gelusil, Maalox), or aluminum and magnesium hydroxide with calcium carbonate (Camolox). The use of sodium bicarbonate (baking soda) is not recommended because this drug can lead to systemic alkalosis with repeated use. These drugs are useful in the management of gastric and duodenal bleeding or ulceration and reflux esophagitis. Aluminum-containing products bind intestinal phosphorous and also are used in the management of hyperphosphatemia associated with renal failure. Antacids reduce the amount of gastric acid and decrease the proteolytic effects of pepsin by inactivating the enzyme when the gastric pH is 6 or higher. They have a cytoprotective function through their ability to stimulate the release of prostaglandins and bind bile salts. Astringent properties enhance gastric mucus production. For optimal effect, these drugs should be given every 3 to 4 hours.

ADVERSE AND COMMON SIDE EFFECTS: The use of calcium- and aluminum-containing preparations may be associated with constipation; the use of magnesium-containing preparations may be associated with diarrhea. Calcium-containing preparations also may cause hypercalcemia, stimulation of gastric secretion, and impairment of renal function. Aluminum hydroxide also may lead to phosphate depletion, muscle weakness, bone resorption, and hypercalcemia.

DRUG INTERACTIONS: Antacid products may interfere with the absorption of oral iron preparations, digoxin, phenothiazines, glucocorticoids, captopril, ketoconazole, nitrofurantoin, penicillamine, phenothiazines, phenytoin, ranitidine, cimetidine, and the tetracyclines. Increased absorption and serum levels of the following drugs may be seen if given concurrently with antacid compounds: aspirin, quinidine, and sympathomimetic agents.

SUPPLIED AS: See specific product.

ANTIHISTAMINES

INDICATIONS: Antihistamines, including chlorpheniramine, clemastine, cyproheptadine, diphenhydramine, hydroxyzine, trimeprazine, and terfenadine, have been used to help alleviate pruritus in dogs. The percentage of dogs with atopic dermatitis that respond to antihistamines varies from 5% to 30%. Chlorpheniramine and clemastine has been used successfully to control pruritus in some cats. These drugs are histamine (H_1) antagonists with anticholinergic, local anesthetic properties and with some of those listed, sedative properties. At low doses, they block the release of histamine from mast cells and basophils. At higher doses, they may stimulate histamine release. An animal may respond to one form of antihistamine drug and not another. These drugs also have been used as antiemetics (by depressing the chemoreceptor trigger zone and inhibiting input from the vestibular apparatus), although they are less effective than the phenothiazines in this regard. Antihistamines also may relieve neuromuscular blockade associated with organophosphate toxicity.

ADVERSE AND COMMON SIDE EFFECTS: Sedation may be seen with the use of chlorpheniramine, cyproheptadine, diphenhydramine, and trimeprazine; sedative effects are mild with hydroxyzine and minimal or nonexistent with the use of terfenadine. Nausea, vomiting, diarrhea, and an increase in pruritus may occur. With drug overdose, hyperexcitability, seizure, and death may occur. Dogs receiving 100 mg/kg/day of terfenadine developed ataxia, trembling, rigidity or weakness, disorientation, or convulsions. Dosages of 150 mg/kg induced vomiting. These drugs should be avoided in patients with glaucoma, urinary retention, CNS disorders, and gastric and duodenal disorders. Some antihistamines are teratogenic and should be avoided during pregnancy.

DRUG INTERACTIONS: In humans, antihistamines should be discontinued for 4 days before skin testing for allergies. Anxiolytic agents, sedatives, narcotics, and barbiturates may enhance CNS depression, and MAO inhibitors, possibly amitraz and selegiline, may prolong and intensify the anticholinergic (drying) effects of antihistamines. Concurrent use of chlorpheniramine with phenytoin may increase the pharmacologic effects of phenytoin. In humans, normal doses of terfenadine when used in conjunction with ketoconazole or erythromycin, or in patients with severe liver disease, may cause severe and life-threatening cardiac arrhythmias. In addition, conditions that increase the risk of cardiac arrhythmias, e.g., electrolyte imbalance or the use of drugs that prolong the QT interval on an electrocardiogram, also may be associated with increased risk.

SUPPLIED AS: See the specific drug.

APOMORPHINE HYDROCHLORIDE

INDICATIONS: Apomorphine ★, Britaject ♣, is a useful and effective centrally acting emetic agent for dogs. Use of the drug in cats is controversial. Xylazine or ipecac is safer and more effective in this species. Apomorphine produces vomiting by directly stimulating the chemoreceptor trigger zone and possibly by excitation of the vestibular apparatus. Gastric emptying may be induced readily in cases of recent (less than 4 hours) oral intoxication.

ADVERSE AND COMMON SIDE EFFECTS: Respiratory depression, sedation, bradycardia, hypotension, salivation, and protracted vomiting have been reported. These signs may be controlled with the IV use of a narcotic antagonist (e.g., naloxone 0.04 mg/kg, levallorphan 0.02 mg/kg, or nalorphine 0.1 mg/kg). Where indicated, the bradycardia may be treated with atropine. The drug is contraindicated in patients with respiratory or CNS depression. Induction of vomiting is contraindicated in unconscious animals and in those that have ingested strong acids, bases, petroleum products, tranquilizers, or other antiemetics. Local induration has been reported in people at SC sites of injection. Safe use of the drug during pregnancy has not been determined.

DRUG INTERACTIONS: Phenothiazine drugs may counter the antiemetic effects of apomorphine. The drug is contraindicated in those with strychnine poisoning and in those with narcosis due to barbiturate, opiate, or other CNS depressant drug use.

SUPPLIED AS: HUMAN PRODUCT
Note: Apomorphine is difficult to obtain. In Canada, it only can be obtained on an emergency drug-release basis.
Tablets containing 6 mg ★
Ampules containing 10 mg/mL [Britaject]

ASCORBIC ACID

INDICATIONS: Ascorbic acid or vitamin C (Apo-C ♣, Redoxon ♣) is essential for the synthesis and maintenance of collagen and intercellular ground substance of body tissue cells, blood vessels, bone, cartilage, tendons, and teeth. It also is important in wound healing and resistance to infection. It may influence the immune response. Ascorbic acid is used for the treatment of methemoglobinemia due to acetaminophen toxicosis. However, acetylcysteine is the drug of choice in the treatment of acetaminophen toxicosis. Vitamin C has been recommended as adjunctive therapy in the treatment of copper-induced hepatopathy and as a urinary acidifier. Some authors also have supported its use in cases of hypertrophic osteodystrophy. However, the use of vitamin C in these cases actually may accelerate dystrophic calcification and decrease the rate of bone remodelling.

ADVERSE AND COMMON SIDE EFFECTS: Use of the vitamin is very safe. With high doses, nausea, vomiting, diarrhea, abdominal cramping, dysuria, crystalluria (calcium oxalate, cystine, or urate stones), pain at injection sites, and deep venous thrombosis with IV use have been reported in humans.

DRUG INTERACTIONS: Large doses of ascorbic acid may reduce the hypoprothrombinemic effect of oral anticoagulants in some patients.

SUPPLIED AS: HUMAN PRODUCT
Tablets containing 100, 250, 500, or 1,000 mg

OTHER USES
Dogs
COPPER-INDUCED HEPATOPATHY
500 to 1,000 mg once daily; PO

Vitamin C also is used to prevent and treat cancer. The role of vitamin C in reducing established malignancies remains controversial.

ASPARAGINASE

INDICATIONS: Asparaginase (Elspar ★, Kidrolase ♣) is a chemotherapeutic agent used in the treatment of lymphoma, lymphoblastic leukemia, mast cell tumors, and idiopathic thrombocytopenia. The drug inhibits asparaginase synthetase and depletes asparagine in tumor cells.

ADVERSE AND COMMON SIDE EFFECTS: Because this drug is a foreign protein, repeated use can lead to immediate hypersensitivity and urticaria, vomiting, diarrhea, dyspnea, hypotension, pruritus, and collapse. Anaphylaxis was reported in up to 30% of dogs given the drug intraperitoneally. Administration of the drug intramuscularly eliminated the occurrence of anaphylaxis. Hemorrhagic pancreatitis also has been observed in the dog. Prior administration of an antihistamine, e.g., diphenhydramine, may decrease the risk of hypersensitivity. If a hypersensitivity reaction does occur, diphenhydramine (0.2–0.5 mg/kg; slowly IV), dexamethasone sodium phosphate (1–2 mg/kg; IV), and fluid support is recommended. If the reaction is severe, epinephrine (0.1–0.3 mL of a 1:1,000 solution; IV) is suggested. The drug should be used with caution in patients with liver disease, diabetes mellitus, infection, or a history of urate calculi.

DRUG INTERACTIONS: Asparaginase inhibits the activity of methotrexate. These drugs should not be given concurrently. Asparaginase may reduce the hypoglycemic effect of insulin. In humans, increased toxicity may occur if the drug is used concurrently with or before prednisone or vincristine.

SUPPLIED AS: HUMAN PRODUCT
For injection containing 10,000 IU powder in 10-mL vials

OTHER USES: Asparaginase has been reported to be of some benefit to patients with hypoglycemia associated with islet cell tumors. However, the efficacy remains to be determined.

ASPIRIN

INDICATIONS: Aspirin (ASA) or acetylsalicylic acid (Ecotrin ♣, Entrophen ♣, and many others) is an effective analgesic for the management of mild to moderate pain. Therapeutic serum concentrations are in the range of 50 to 100 μg/mL. This agent is not effective for the treatment of visceral pain. ASA is an antipyretic and anti-inflammatory agent. Effective anti-inflammatory serum concentrations range from 150 to 300 μg/mL. Aspirin often is used in the therapy of degenerative joint disease. Its antiplatelet activity makes it useful in the prevention of arterial thromboembolic disease as occurs with feline cardiomyopathy (although many cats still form emboli—warfarin may be more effective), heartworm disease, and membranoproliferative glomerulonephritis. A dose that effectively and consistently inhibits thromboembolic formation in cats with cardiomyopathy or in dogs undergoing adulticide therapy for heartworm disease has not yet been established.

As a topical agent, salicylic acid (2%) has keratolytic, keratoplastic, mildly antipruritic, and bacteriostatic properties. It often is used in conjunction with captan and sulfur as a shampoo for seborrhea, pyoderma, and dermatophytosis. When combined with sulfur, a synergistic effect occurs, and the keratolytic effect is enhanced.

ADVERSE AND COMMON SIDE EFFECTS: Side effects of ASA are dose dependent. Anorexia, vomiting, gastrointestinal ulceration, seizure, and coma have been reported. The presence of food within the GIT may decrease gastric irritation. Chronic high doses of the drug have been associated with an increased incidence of gastric carcinoma in the dog. Buffered aspirin also is associated with gastric irritation, and although enteric-coated aspirin produces fewer gastric side effects, absorption of the drug is less consistent.

Aspirin has a much longer half-life in cats (44.6 hours) than in dogs (7.5 hours). It is the only nonsteroidal anti-inflammatory drug (NSAID) that can be used safely in cats. The toxic dose reported in cats is greater than 25 mg/kg/day and is greater than 50 mg/kg 3 times daily in dogs (serum concentrations greater than 500 μg/mL).

Consequently, more than 7 mL/kg of Pepto-Bismol contains enough aspirin to cause toxicity. Severe toxicity is characterized by vomiting, fever, metabolic acidosis, increased respiratory rate, GIT ulceration and bleeding, depression, seizure, and coma. In cases of toxicity, vomiting should be induced and activated charcoal given. Serum concentrations are increased in hypoalbuminemia, and drug dosages should be decreased in these animals. Serum salicylate concentrations of 50 to 100 µg/mL are in the analgesic range, and concentrations of 150 to 300 µg/mL are anti-inflammatory. Concentrations greater than 500 µg/mL usually are toxic. Serum samples are taken just before the next dose and after steady-state levels have been attained (40 hours in dogs and 8 days in cats). In cases of toxicity, treatment should include the induction of vomiting or gastric lavage with 3% to 5% sodium bicarbonate to delay salicylate absorption. Activated charcoal (2 g/kg) should be given orally to bind any unabsorbed drug. Alkalinization of the urine with sodium bicarbonate (1 to 4 mEq/kg; IV) will increase urinary excretion of the salicylate, and diuretic use (5 mg/kg IV; furosemide) will further augment urinary excretion.

Aspirin is contraindicated in animals with GIT ulceration, renal insufficiency, von Willebrand's disease, or asthma and should be discontinued approximately 1 week before elective surgery. ASA may exacerbate clinical signs associated with Scotty cramp. The drug should not be used in pregnant animals. Reproductive abnormalities, including fetal resorption and stillbirth, have been reported.

Topically applied solutions containing salicylic acid may be irritating to the skin.

DRUG INTERACTIONS: Aspirin may decrease the vasodilatory activity of captopril and enalapril and decrease the efficacy of spironolactone. Concurrent administration with digoxin may lead to increased serum digoxin levels. Its antiplatelet activity in cats may be impaired when used concurrently with propranolol. Simultaneous administration with acidifying agents, e.g., ammonium chloride, may increase the risk of ASA toxicity. Sodium bicarbonate increases the ionization of ASA in urine, promotes its excretion, and is of potential use in cases of aspirin toxicity. Increased hypoglycemic activity of insulin preparations may be seen if ASA (in moderate to large doses) and insulin preparations are given to the same animal. Concurrent use with carbonic anhydrase inhibitors, e.g., acetazolamide, may induce metabolic acidosis and enhance ASA intoxication. Concurrent use of ASA with glucocorticoids increases the risk of GI ulceration and decreases serum levels of ASA by increasing renal excretion of the drug. ASA may increase toxic methotrexate levels. Salicylates in large doses antagonize spironolactone-induced urinary excretion of sodium.

SUPPLIED AS: VETERINARY PRODUCT
Tablets containing 60 gr (3.89 g)
Note: 1 gr = 1 grain = 65 mg.

HUMAN PRODUCTS
Tablets containing 65 mg (1 gr) and 81 mg (1.25 gr)
Tablets (uncoated) containing 325 mg (5 gr) and 500 mg (7.8 gr)
Tablets (buffered uncoated) containing 325 mg (5 gr) and 500 mg (7.8 gr)

OTHER USES
Dogs
DISSEMINATED INTRAVASCULAR COAGULATION
150 to 300 mg/20 kg once daily to once every other day for 10 days; PO

ATENOLOL

INDICATIONS: Atenolol (Tenormin ♣ ★) is a selective β_1-blocking agent equal in potency to propranolol. It is the preferred drug in patients with pulmonary disease, e.g., asthma. Atenolol is useful in the management of supraventricular tachyarrhythmias, ventricular premature contractions, systemic hypertension, and hypertrophic cardiomyopathy in cats.

ADVERSE AND COMMON SIDE EFFECTS: The drug is excreted through the kidneys and should be used with caution in animals with compromised renal function. Nausea, vomiting, and diarrhea are less common in small animals than they are in people. Diarrhea, depression, lethargy, hypoglycemia (in diabetics), bradycardia, impaired atrioventricular conduction, syncope, and congestive heart failure have been documented with the use of β-blockers. The acute onset of congestive heart failure should respond to dobutamine (1–5 µg/kg/minute; IV), furosemide (1 mg/kg; IM) and oxygen therapy. Glycopyrrolate (0.01 mg/kg; IM) and dopamine hydrochloride (1–5 µg/kg/minute; IV) can be used to counter the bradycardia, and 5% dextrose in water can be used to manage the hypoglycemia.

DRUG INTERACTIONS: The simultaneous administration of negative inotropic agents, e.g., calcium channel-blocking drugs such as verapamil and diltiazem, or hypoglycemic agents, e.g., insulin, may exacerbate the adverse effects of β-blockers. Atropine and other anticholinergic agents enhance GIT absorption of atenolol. Serum lidocaine levels may be increased, predisposing to lidocaine toxicity if both drugs are used concurrently. The first dose of prazosin (Minipress) may be more severe and of a longer duration, and a dose reduction and close patient monitoring are advised if both drugs are used together.

SUPPLIED AS: HUMAN PRODUCT
Tablets containing 25, 50, and 100 mg

ATIPAMEZOLE

INDICATIONS: Atipamezole (Antisedan ♣ ★) is a synthetic α-adrenergic antagonist marketed for the reversal of the sedative and analgesic effects of medetomidine hydrochloride in dogs. Atipamezole is given on a volume-per-volume basis (mL for mL) of medetomidine administered.

ADVERSE AND COMMON SIDE EFFECTS: Occasionally, vomiting is seen. Transient excitement or apprehension may be noted, and hypersalivation, diarrhea, and tremors may occur. The drug can cause a rapid reversal of sedation and analgesia predisposing to apprehension and aggression. Patients should be monitored for persistent hypothermia, bradycardia, and depression of respiration until recovery is complete. Safety of the drug in pregnant or lactating bitches has not been established.

DRUG INTERACTIONS: Unknown.

SUPPLIED AS: VETERINARY PRODUCT
For injection containing 5 mg/mL

ATRACURIUM

INDICATIONS: Atracurium (Tracrium ♣ ★) is a nondepolarizing neuromuscular blocking agent used in conjunction with general anesthesia to produce muscle relaxation during surgery or mechanical ventilation and endotracheal intubation.

ADVERSE AND COMMON SIDE EFFECTS: The drug should not be used in patients with myasthenia gravis. Although rare, it may cause histamine release and should be used with caution in susceptible patients, e.g., asthmatics. Adverse reactions are rare and primarily related to histamine release. Side effects may include allergic reactions, prolonged or inadequate block, hypotension, bradycardia, tachycardia, dyspnea, bronchospasm, laryngospasm, rash, urticaria, and reaction at the site of injection. Reversal of blockade can be achieved by the use of an anticholinesterase, e.g., edrophonium, physostigmine, or neostigmine, in conjunction with an anticholinergic, e.g., atropine or glycopyrrolate. Reversal usually is complete within 8 to 10 minutes.

DRUG INTERACTIONS: Neuromuscular blockade may be potentiated by procainamide, quinidine, verapamil, aminoglycoside antibiotics, lincomycin, clindamycin, bacitracin, polymyxin B, magnesium sulfate, thiazide diuretics, enflurane, isoflurane, and halothane. Furosemide may increase or decrease the efficacy of atracurium. Theophylline and phenytoin may inhibit or reverse the blocking action of atracurium. Succinylcholine may hasten the onset of action and enhance the blockade of atracurium.

SUPPLIED AS: HUMAN PRODUCT
For injection containing 10 mg/mL

ATROPINE

INDICATIONS: Atropine ✤ ★ is an anticholinergic, antispasmodic, and mydriatic drug. It is indicated in the treatment of sinus bradycardia, sinus block or arrest, and incomplete atrioventricular block. It is a parasympatholytic agent that causes relaxation of the GIT, biliary, and genitourinary tract and suppresses salivary, gastric, and respiratory tract secretions (given preoperatively). Atropine is a mydriatic and cycloplegic agent, making it useful in the management of ocular inflammation. It also is used in the treatment of organophosphate and carbamate poisoning.

ADVERSE AND COMMON SIDE EFFECTS: Sinus tachycardia (at higher doses), bradycardia (at low doses or seen with initial injection), and second-degree heart block may occur. Atropine also decreases the threshold at which premature ventricular contractions are likely to occur. Dry mouth, dysphagia, constipation, vomiting, thirst, urinary hesitancy, CNS stimulation, drowsiness, ataxia, seizures, and respiratory depression may occur. With drug overdose, respiratory depression and hypotension are likely to occur. Atropine should not be used in patients with asthma because it will have a drying effect on mucous plugs in bronchi, making them difficult to mobilize. The drug should not be given to patients with glaucoma or paralytic ileus or adhesions between the iris and lens. Use of the drug also has been associated with keratoconjunctivitis sicca. Atropine should be used with caution in those with GIT infections because impaired GIT motility will prolong retention of the offending organism(s). In cases of oral drug overdose, cleanse the stomach by inducing vomiting or performing gastric lavage; follow with installation of activated charcoal. Physostigmine (0.1–0.6 mg/kg; slowly IV, repeated every 10 minutes until toxicity reversed) may be used as an antidote and diazepam may be used to control CNS stimulation. Additional supportive care includes oxygen therapy and fluid support.

DRUG INTERACTIONS: Atropine may decrease GIT absorption of oral phenothiazine drugs. Antihistamines, procainamide, quinidine, meperidine, benzodiazepines, and the phenothiazines may enhance the activity of atropine. Primidone, disopyramide, nitrates, and long-term corticosteroid use may potentiate adverse effects of atropine. Atropine may enhance the activity of nitrofurantoin, thiazide diuretics, and sympathomimetic agents. Atropine may antagonize the actions of metoclopramide.

SUPPLIED AS: VETERINARY PRODUCT
For injection containing 0.5 mg/mL, 2 mg/mL, and 15 mg/mL (organophosphate toxicity)
HUMAN PRODUCTS
Ophthalmic ointment (0.5% and 1% atropine sulfate)
Ophthalmic solution (0.5%, 1%, and 2% atropine sulfate)
For injection containing 0.05 and 0.1 mg/mL (in syringes)
For injection containing 0.3, 0.4, 0.5, 0.6, 1.0, and 1.2 mg/mL
Tablets containing 0.4 mg (regular and soluble) and 0.3, 0.4, and 0.6 mg (soluble)

AURANOFIN

INDICATIONS: Auranofin (Ridaura ✦ ★) is an oral gold salt (triethylphosphine) that has been used in dogs to treat idiopathic polyarthritis and pemphigus foliaceus. Gold compounds stabilize lysosomal membranes, decrease migration and phagocytic activity of macrophages and neutrophils, inhibit prostaglandin synthesis, and suppress immunoglobulin synthesis. Furthermore, oral gold therapy inhibits helper T-cell responses without affecting the suppressor T-cell population. A beneficial response in humans may take 3 to 4 months to be seen.

ADVERSE AND COMMON SIDE EFFECTS: An immune-mediated thrombocytopenia may develop. High doses (2.4–3.6 mg/kg/day) result in thrombocytopenia and moderate to severe hemolytic anemia. Rapid reversal of these side effects can be expected after cessation of therapy and the administration of corticosteroids. Dose-dependent diarrhea has been reported in some dogs. It resolves with discontinuation of the drug or lowering of the dose. Proteinuria has been documented in people, the incidence of which is low. A complete blood count, platelet count, serum creatinine, and urinalysis should be completed every 2 weeks for the first month, monthly until the third month, and every 3 to 4 months thereafter. Serum biochemistry should be monitored every 6 months or sooner if warranted. In humans, the drug should be used with caution in inflammatory bowel disease, liver disease, bone marrow suppression, diabetes mellitus, and congestive heart failure. The drug has been shown to be embryotoxic in rats and should not be used during pregnancy.

DRUG INTERACTIONS: None.

SUPPLIED AS: HUMAN PRODUCT
Capsules containing 3 mg

AUROTHIOGLUCOSE

INDICATIONS: Aurothioglucose suspension (Solganal ♣ ★) is used in the treatment of pemphigus foliaceus in cats, feline plasma cell stomatitis, plasma cell pododermatitis, canine bullous pemphigoid and pemphigus complex, and rheumatoid arthritis. Gold compounds stabilize lysosomal membranes, decrease migration and phagocytic activity of macrophages and neutrophils, inhibit prostaglandin synthesis, and suppress immunoglobulin synthesis. Positive clinical response should not be expected before 6 to 12 weeks of therapy. If a positive response is not noted after 16 weeks, the dose can be increased to 1.5 mg/kg/week. Once a positive response is seen, the drug can be given as needed; i.e., every 2 to 8 weeks. Aurothioglucose is the preferred parenteral form of gold therapy.

ADVERSE AND COMMON SIDE EFFECTS: Although rare, oral ulcerations, leukopenia, thrombocytopenia, anemia, nephrotic syndrome, hepatitis, miliary dermatitis, stomatitis, and anaphylaxis have been reported. There also has been a possible relationship between the use of aurothioglucose and death associated with toxic epidermal necrolysis in dogs. A complete blood count, serum biochemistry, and urinalysis should be completed every 2 weeks during the first 2 months of therapy and then monthly to quarterly as the dose is reduced. It is recommended to use a test dose for the first and second weeks (as outlined in Section 1: Common Dosages for Dogs and Cats) to rule out potential idiosyncratic reactions. Gold-containing drugs are contraindicated in patients with renal or hepatic disease, systemic lupus erythematosus, uncontrolled diabetes mellitus, or preexisting hematologic disorders. In humans, overdose is treated with BAL (dimercaprol) [to chelate the gold] at a dose of 3 mg/kg IM every 4 hours for the first 2 days, 4 injections on the third day, and 2 injections daily thereafter for 10 days until complete recovery. In milder cases, the dose may be reduced to 2.5 mg/kg.

DRUG INTERACTIONS: The concurrent use of gold salt compounds and immunosuppressant drugs (other than corticosteroids), penicillamine, or phenylbutazone increases the risk of blood dyscrasias.

SUPPLIED AS: HUMAN PRODUCT
For injection containing 50 mg/mL

AZATHIOPRINE

INDICATIONS: Azathioprine (Imuran ♣ ★) is a thiopurine antimetabolite immunosuppressive agent used primarily in the treatment of autoimmune disease. It suppresses primary and secondary antibody responses and has significant anti-inflammatory activity. More specifically, the drug has been used in the treatment of immune-mediated skin disease, autoimmune hemolytic anemia, thrombocytopenia, rheumatoid arthritis, polyarthritis, polymyositis, eosinophilic enteritis, lymphocytic–plasmacytic enteritis, myasthenia gravis, atrophic gastritis, ulcerative colitis, autoimmune uveitis with dermal depigmentation, systemic lupus erythematosus, ocular histiocytoma, and chronic active hepatitis. Azathioprine also has been used to prevent organ transplant rejection (although it is not effective in reversing ongoing rejection), and as a last resort, to control pruritus in intractable atopic dogs. The drug often is used in combination with glucocorticoids or cyclophosphamide in the management of these disorders. According to some researchers, the onset of action is slow, taking 4 to 6 weeks to produce beneficial clinical effects. However, there is no evidence that azathioprine has a slower onset of action than cyclophosphamide. In fact, it has been shown that T-cell suppression is evident within 1 week of initiation of drug use. Azathioprine is less immunosuppressive than cyclophosphamide, and it has fewer deleterious side effects.

ADVERSE AND COMMON SIDE EFFECTS: Leukopenia, anemia, and thrombocytopenia may occur. Cats are especially sensitive to bone marrow toxicity, and for this reason, it generally is not recommended in this species. If used, it is given at a reduced dose. Leukocyte counts should be monitored biweekly during the first 8 weeks of therapy, then monthly. If leukocyte counts decrease to less than 4,000 per microliter, the drug should be discontinued until the leukopenia has resolved. Other potential adverse effects associated with azathioprine may include pancreatitis, jaundice, skin eruptions, and poor hair growth. Teratogenicity also is a concern, and the drug should not be used in pregnant animals.

DRUG INTERACTIONS: Azathioprine may potentiate the neuromuscular blockade induced by succinylcholine chloride. It may inhibit the neuromuscular blocking activity of pancuronium and tubocurarine. The concurrent use of azathioprine and allopurinol increases the pharmacologic effects and toxicity of the former drug. In humans, it is recommended that the dose of azathioprine should be reduced by one third to one quarter if the two agents are used together.

SUPPLIED AS: HUMAN PRODUCTS
For injection containing 100 mg
Tablets containing 50 mg

OTHER USES
Dogs
INTRACTABLE PRURITUS
2.2 mg/kg/day until pruritus controlled (usually 2–3 weeks); then reduced to lowest effective dose

CHRONIC INFLAMMATORY BOWEL DISEASE
i)   1 to 2 mg/kg every 24 to 48 hours; PO
ii) 2 mg/kg/day for 1 week, then every 48 hours; PO

Cats
CHRONIC INFLAMMATORY BOWEL DISEASE
i)   0.3 to 0.5 mg/kg every 24 to 48 hours; PO
ii) 0.3 mg/kg every 48 hours; PO

BAL: DIMERCAPROL

INDICATIONS: BAL ✿ ★, or dimercaprol, is a sulfhydryl-containing compound that chelates arsenic. It is used principally for the treatment of arsenical toxicity and occasionally for toxicity caused by lead, mercury, and gold. BAL is not very effective in advanced cases. Therefore, it is best to administer the drug shortly after exposure.

ADVERSE AND COMMON SIDE EFFECTS: The drug is contraindicated in patients with hepatic insufficiency unless caused by the offending toxin. It should be used with caution in patients with renal impairment. To offset possible renal toxicosis, the urine should be alkalinized. Intramuscular injection is painful. Administer the drug deep into muscle. Signs of BAL toxicity include vomiting, tremors, seizures, coma, and death. Tachycardia and a transient increase in blood pressure sometimes are reported. Toxic effects at therapeutic doses generally are not severe and tend to wear off as the drug is excreted over a 3- to 4-hour period.

DRUG INTERACTIONS: Do not administer dimercaprol within 24 hours of iron or selenium compounds. Dimercaprol can form toxic complexes with iron, selenium, uranium, and cadmium.

SUPPLIED AS: HUMAN PRODUCT
For injection containing 100 mg/mL

BARBITURATES

INDICATIONS: The barbiturate drugs are used for sedation and general anesthesia and for control of seizure disorders. The barbiturates are classified as ultrashort-acting agents, including thiopental and methohexital, with a rapid onset of action (15–30 seconds) and short duration of action (5–20 minutes) primarily used as induction agents and as the primary anesthetic for short procedures. The short-acting agents include pentobarbital, hexobarbital, and secobarbital. These drugs have a rapid onset of action (30–60 seconds) after IV injection and a duration of action of 1 to 2 hours. Pentobarbital is the principal agent used in veterinary medicine in this group as a sedative and general anesthetic. Barbiturates provide little analgesia, thus necessitating high doses in painful procedures. The long-acting barbiturates include barbital and phenobarbital. These drugs have a slow onset of action after IV administration (12 minutes for phenobarbital, 22 minutes for barbital) and a duration of action of 6 to 12 hours after IV injection. This group of drugs is used mainly as sedatives and hypnotics and to control seizure activity.

ADVERSE AND COMMON SIDE EFFECTS: If given perivascularly, the alkaline pH of barbiturates irritates tissues. Apnea and respiratory depression are common after bolus administration. Other side effects may include myocardial depression, arrhythmogenesis (especially thiopental), hypotension, and hypothermia. At sedative doses, barbiturates have a wide margin of safety with few side effects. These drugs should be used with caution in animals with pre-existing arrhythmias, renal or hepatic disease, and hypoalbuminemia or acidosis (increased response and possible toxicity to barbiturates). Lack of body fat can predispose to prolonged recovery because recovery is determined by redistribution from the CNS to other organs, including body fat. Greyhounds and other sight hounds metabolize thiobarbiturates more slowly than methohexital, an oxybarbiturate, making the latter the preferred barbiturate in these breeds. The obese animal is at risk for relative drug overdose. The very young and very old patient also are at increased risk for barbiturate effects because of immature development of hepatic enzyme systems (the young) and impaired liver function (the old), leading to delayed detoxification. Hypothyroidism may predispose to increased sensitivity to anesthetic drugs. Treatment of drug overdose includes doxapram (2% solution: 3–5 mg/kg; IV, repeat as necessary), oxygen, and fluid support. See specific drug for more details. Repeated doses of barbiturates can result in excessive anesthetic times and prolonged recovery. Thiobarbiturates may induce anaphylactoid reactions mediated by histamine release via a nonimmunologic mechanism that can occur without prior drug exposure.

DRUG INTERACTIONS: Metabolic acidosis, hypoalbuminemia, renal or hepatic disease, the administration of nonsteroidal anti-inflammatory agents, certain sulfonamides, glucose, and atropine augment the anesthetic effect of barbiturates and potentiate toxicity. Any CNS depressant enhances the response to barbiturates.

SUPPLIED AS: See specific product.

BENAZEPRIL HYDROCHLORIDE

INDICATIONS: Benazepril hydrochloride (Fortekor ♣) is a second-generation angiotensin-converting enzyme (ACE) inhibitor. Like other ACE inhibitors, captopril and enalapril, it is used to manage patients with congestive heart failure caused by mitral valvular regurgitation or dilated cardiomyopathy.

ADVERSE AND COMMON SIDE EFFECTS: Although overdosage of up to 200 times was not accompanied by deleterious effects, transient reversible hypotension signalled by fatigue and dizziness may occur with overdosage. If this occurs, the dose of diuretic used should be decreased. The drug is eliminated by biliary excretion. It is recommended that plasma urea and creatinine be monitored in patients with renal insufficiency. The safety of the drug in breeding or lactating animals has not been studied.

DRUG INTERACTIONS: Benazepril may be used safely in conjunction with digoxin, diuretics and antiarrhythmic agents.

SUPPLIED AS: VETERINARY PRODUCT
Tablets containing 5 and 20 mg

BENZOYL PEROXIDE

INDICATIONS: Benzoyl peroxide (Ben-A-Derm ♣, Oxydex ★, Pyoben ♣ ★) is a degreasing, astringent, keratolytic, keratoplastic, antipruritic, topical anesthetic, wound-healing, follicular-flushing, and anti-inflammatory agent useful in the treatment of Schnauzer comedo syndrome, canine and feline acne, seborrhea, superficial pyoderma, pruritus, crusts, and scales.

ADVERSE AND COMMON SIDE EFFECTS: The 5% solution can be irritating to animals, causing dryness and local irritation. The gel often is too irritating for use in cats. Avoid contact with the eyes and mucous membranes. If irritation develops, discontinue use. Benzoyl peroxide may discolor fabrics.

DRUG INTERACTIONS: None.

SUPPLIED AS: VETERINARY PRODUCTS
Shampoos 2.5% [Ben-A-Derm; Oxydex]
Shampoo 3% [Pyoben]

BETAMETHASONE

INDICATIONS: Betamethasone (Betasone ♣ ★, Betavet soluspan ★) is a long-acting injectable glucocorticoid used for the control of pruritus in dogs. Betamethasone valerate (Valisone cream) is the cream. For more information on Indications, Adverse and Common Side Effects, and Drug Interactions, see **GLUCOCORTICOID AGENTS.**

ADVERSE AND COMMON SIDE EFFECTS: Betamethasone should be used with caution in dogs with congestive heart failure, diabetes mellitus, and renal disease. Injections of betamethasone have resulted in decreased sperm output, increased percentages of abnormal sperm, and decreased concentrations of serum testosterone. This drug, therefore, should be used with caution in stud dogs. Potent topical corticosteroid agents may be associated with the induction of steroid acne, aggravation of folliculitis, atrophy of epidermal, dermal, and SC tissues, telangiectasia, purpura, poor healing, exacerbation of ulceration, hypopigmentation, hypertrichosis, and aggravation of preexisting disease.

DRUG INTERACTIONS: The concurrent use of barbiturate agents, phenytoin, or rifampin reduces the pharmacologic effects of betamethasone by increasing its metabolism through the induction of liver enzymes. Betamethasone reduces the pharmacologic effects of other corticosteroids and aspirin, requiring higher doses of these drugs if they are given concurrently with betamethasone.

SUPPLIED AS: VETERINARY PRODUCT
For injection containing betamethasone dipropionate equivalent to 5 mg/mL betamethasone and betamethasone sodium phosphate equivalent to 2 mg/mL betamethasone
  For intraarticular injection containing betamethasone acetate equivalent to 10.8 mg/mL betamethasone and betamethasone sodium phosphate equivalent to 3 mg/mL betamethasone

BETHANECHOL CHLORIDE

INDICATIONS: Bethanechol (Duvoid ♣ ★, Urecholine ♣ ★) is a cholinergic agent used to stimulate muscular contraction of the bladder in cases of detrusor atony. Although the efficacy of the drug has been questioned in humans, in cats unable to urinate because of dysautonomia, bethanechol stimulated urination 30 to 60 minutes after an oral dose of 0.125 or 0.25 mg.

ADVERSE AND COMMON SIDE EFFECTS: Mild vomiting, diarrhea, anorexia, abdominal cramping, bradycardia, increased salivation, and lacrimation may occur with oral doses. Arrhythmias, hy-

potension, and bronchospasm generally are seen only with overdosage. The drug is contraindicated if urethral obstruction is present. Drugs used to decrease urethral outflow resistance, e.g., diazepam or phenoxybenzamine, may be used concurrently in cases of
reflex dyssynergia. The drug is contraindicated in patients with obstructive pulmonary disease, bronchial asthma, hyperthyroidism,
cystitis, bactiuria, peptic ulcer, peritonitis, atrioventricular conduction defects, severe bradycardia, hypotension, hypertension, and
epilepsy. Overdosage is treated with atropine. Epinephrine may be
used to treat symptoms of bronchospasm.

DRUG INTERACTIONS: Bethanechol should not be used concurrently with neostigmine because additive cholinergic effects and
possible toxicity may occur. Procainamide and quinidine may antagonize the cholinergic effects of the drug, and this combination
should be used with caution.

SUPPLIED AS: HUMAN PRODUCT
For injection containing 5 mg/mL
Tablets containing 5, 10, 25, and 50 mg

BISACODYL

INDICATIONS: Bisacodyl (Bisacolax ★, Dulcolax ✦ ★) is a laxative
used to help alleviate constipation and to help cleanse the colon for
colonoscopy. After rehydration to soften feces, it is a useful drug for
the treatment of severe impaction. The drug induces contractions by
direct stimulation of sensory nerve endings in the colonic wall and
expands intestinal fluid volume by increasing epithelial permeability. The drug generally acts within 6 to 12 hours.

ADVERSE AND COMMON SIDE EFFECTS: Rarely, mild cramping, nausea, and diarrhea have been observed in some patients.

DRUG INTERACTIONS: It is advised not to give oral medication
within 2 hours of administering a laxative.

SUPPLIED AS: HUMAN PRODUCTS
Microenema containing 10 mg [Dulcolax]
Suppositories containing 5 and 10 mg
Tablets containing 5 mg

BISMUTH SUBSALICYLATE

INDICATIONS: Bismuth subsalicylate (Pepto-Bismol ✦ ★) is used in
the treatment of diarrhea. It inhibits the synthesis of prostaglandins
responsible for GIT hypermotility and inflammation. The drug also

may have antibacterial and antisecretory properties. Bismuth sub-salicylate relieves indigestion by forming insoluble complexes with offending noxious agents and by forming a protective coating.

ADVERSE AND COMMON SIDE EFFECTS: The drug is contraindicated in those sensitive to salicylate drugs. Cats may be especially sensitive to the salicylate content especially in the presence of an inflamed bowel. See also **ASPIRIN.** Stool color may darken with its use. With high doses, fecal impaction may occur. Bismuth subsalicylate is radiopaque and may interfere with radiographic GIT studies.

DRUG INTERACTIONS: The antimicrobial action of tetracyclines may be reduced if these drugs are used concurrently. It is advised that tetracycline be given at least 2 hours before or after bismuth administration.

SUPPLIED AS: HUMAN PRODUCTS
Suspension containing 17.47 mg/mL
Tablets (chewable) containing 262 mg

BLEOMYCIN

INDICATIONS: Bleomycin (Blenoxane ♣ ★) is an antineoplastic glycopeptide antibiotic. In small animals, it may be useful in the treatment of nonfunctional thyroid tumors, malignant teratoma, lymphoma, and squamous cell carcinoma.

ADVERSE AND COMMON SIDE EFFECTS: Clinical signs of acute toxicity may include nausea, vomiting, fever, anaphylaxis, and other allergic reactions. Signs of delayed toxicity may include pneumonitis and pulmonary fibrosis, rash, stomatitis, and alopecia.

DRUG INTERACTIONS: Other antineoplastic agents used in conjunction with bleomycin predispose to bleomycin toxicity, including bone marrow suppression. Bleomycin decreases the GIT absorption, and pharmacologic effects of digoxin and phenytoin are reduced if used concurrently.

SUPPLIED AS: HUMAN PRODUCT
For injection containing 15 units/vial

BROMIDE SALTS

INDICATIONS: Bromide salts (potassium, sodium, and ammonium) have been used effectively in the management of seizure disorders in people.

Potassium bromide has been used in dogs unresponsive to therapeutic serum concentrations of phenobarbital (as adjunctive therapy with phenobarbital), epileptic patients with suspected anticonvulsant-induced hepatotoxicity, and in epileptics with preexisting liver dysfunction. The drug penetrates the CNS, raises the seizure threshold, and prevents the spread of epileptic discharge. Steady-state drug levels are achieved after 4 to 6 months in the dog (serum levels are measured 1 and 4 to 6 months after initiation of therapy and are taken before the next dose, preferably in the morning). Reported therapeutic serum concentrations of potassium bromide range from 0.5 to 1.6 mg/mL or 0.7 to 1.9 mg/mL and 0.7 to 2.3 mg/mL or 100 to 200 mg/dL and 7 to 17 mmol/L. Toxic levels are in excess of 20 mmol/L.

ADVERSE AND COMMON SIDE EFFECTS: Bromide sensitivity may be affected by diets high in chloride content (e.g., Hill's S/D and I/D), dehydration, vomiting, diarrhea, and impaired renal function. High chloride-containing diets decrease bromide levels necessitating an increase in drug dose. In dogs, reported side effects include polydipsia, polyphagia, excessive sedation, ataxia, depression, anisocoria, muscle pain, and stupor. Pancreatitis also has been reported from use of the combination of bromide and phenobarbital. Occasional nausea may be resolved by dividing the daily dose or switching to sodium bromide. Twenty milligrams per kilogram of potassium bromide is equal to 17.3 mg/kg of sodium bromide, i.e., if changing from potassium to sodium bromide, decrease the dose by 15%. Discontinuation of the drug and supportive therapy, including IV isotonic saline, hastens recovery from drug toxicity. Diuretic therapy, e.g., loop diuretics, also may be beneficial. In humans, neonatal bromide intoxication causing growth retardation has been associated with maternal use of the drug during pregnancy. Clinical signs of intoxication also have been reported in human infants nursing from mothers taking the drug. Experience with use of the drug in cats is limited.

The most common laboratory abnormality noted in dogs given potassium bromide is an artifactual hyperchloremia (DACOS colorimetric methodology). However, flame photometric analysis will correctly determine serum chloride levels.

DRUG INTERACTIONS: Bromide may enhance the effects of other anticonvulsants on the CNS. The use of potassium bromide alone or in combination with primidone and diphenylhydantoin predisposes to hepatotoxicity. The toxicity of bromide may be reduced by a reduction in the drug dose or frequency when it is used in conjunction with other anticonvulsants. Bromide levels increase after halothane anesthesia and remain elevated for days to weeks thereafter, although the increase is reportedly small (40–88 mg/L). Loop diuretics (ethacrynic acid, furosemide) may enhance bromide elimination.

SUPPLIED AS: HUMAN PRODUCT

Potassium bromide [Fischer Scientific, Pittsburgh, PA; ICN Biomedicals, Costa Mesa, CA; Sigma Chemical Co., St. Louis, MO; Aldrich, Milwaukee, WI; VWR Scientific, Bridgeport, NJ]]

In Canada, the drug is available only through a limited number of pharmacies. To locate a pharmacy near you, call the Ontario Veterinary College Pharmacy, Guelph, Ontario, Canada, at 519-823-8830.

BUPRENORPHINE HYDROCHLORIDE

INDICATIONS: Buprenorphine hydrochloride (Buprenex ★) is a partial opiate agonist with analgesic properties. In dogs and cats, analgesia lasts 4 to 8 hours and longer after epidural administration. Experience with the drug in small animals is limited.

ADVERSE AND COMMON SIDE EFFECTS: Respiratory depression may occur. In humans, sedation also may be noted. Opiates should be used with caution in animals with hypothyroid disease, severe renal insufficiency, hypoadrenocorticism, debilitated patients, those with head trauma or CNS dysfunction, and geriatrics. The drug is resistant to antagonism by naloxone.

DRUG INTERACTIONS: The concurrent use of other CNS depressants (anesthetics, antihistamines, tranquilizers) may potentiate CNS and respiratory depression. This drug may inhibit the analgesic effects of opiate agonists, e.g., morphine.

SUPPLIED AS: HUMAN PRODUCT

For injection containing 0.324 mg/mL in 1-mL ampules

BUSPIRONE

INDICATIONS: Buspirone (BuSpar ✚ ★) is a nonbenzodiazepine antianxiety drug. It is used to treat various behavioral disorders in dogs and cats, e.g., chronic fears/anxiety, phobias, aggression, and stereotypy-obsessive disease. It does not promote sedation or behavioral dependence. The drug is considered by some to be the drug of choice in the management of urine spraying and inappropriate urination in cats. Generally, only 1 week of therapy will determine if the drug is going to be successful in the management of urine spraying. If successful, the drug is continued for 8 weeks, after which the dose is reduced gradually. If urine spraying resumes, buspirone is continued for 6 to 12 months, and then the dose is reduced gradually. Cats from multicat households favorably respond more often than cats from single-cat households. Only half of the cats treated with buspirone resumed spraying when the drug was discontinued after 2 months of treatment versus those treated with diazepam, more than 90% of which resumed spraying.

ADVERSE AND COMMON SIDE EFFECTS: Rarely sedation may occur. Agitation after administration of the drug is similarly rare. An increase in affection toward owners and aggression toward other cats also is reported. In humans, the drug may cause an increase in liver enzymes [alanine transaminase (ALT), aspartate transaminase (AST)].

DRUG INTERACTIONS: None of significance to small animals.

SUPPLIED AS: HUMAN PRODUCT
Tablets containing 10 mg

BUTORPHANOL

INDICATIONS: Butorphanol (Torbugesic ✿ ★, Torbutrol ✿ ★) is a narcotic agonist/antagonist analgesic with potent antitussive activity in dogs. It has minimal cardiovascular effects and causes only slight respiratory depression. Alone, it causes little sedation. Analgesia occurs 30 minutes after IM injection and reaches peak activity in 1 hour. With IV injection, the analgesic effect is immediate, with peak activity in 30 minutes. Pain relief lasts 2 to 3 hours. The drug is 5 times more potent in pain relief than morphine, 15 to 30 times more potent than pentazocine, and 30 to 50 times more potent than meperidine. It provides effective visceral analgesia at low doses for up to 6 hours in cats; however, somatic analgesia is only attained at higher IV doses (0.8 mg/kg) and is only of short duration (1 to 2 hours). Butorphanol tartrate is 15 to 20 times more effective in the management of cough than codeine or dextromethorphan.

ADVERSE AND COMMON SIDE EFFECTS: Although rare, side effects after oral use may include slight sedation, anorexia, nausea, and diarrhea. Because the drug suppresses the cough reflex, it should not be used in dogs with a productive cough. Moderate to marked cardiopulmonary depression has been reported only with IV infusions given at rapid rates (0.2 mg/kg/minute). Panting may occur with doses of 0.4 mg/kg IV. In conscious dogs, the drug produces minimal cardiovascular or respiratory effects. Mydriasis lasting as long as 3 hours after an IV dose of 0.2 mg/kg may be seen in cats. Until further studies are complete, the drug should not be used in pregnant animals or male stud dogs. Butorphanol should not be given to animals with liver disease. The safety of butorphanol use in heartworm-positive dogs has not been established. The drug should not be given with other analgesic agents as the effects are additive. All opiates should be used with caution in debilitated animals and those with head trauma, increased CSF pressure, hypothyroidism, severe renal disease, or adrenocortical insufficiency.

DRUG INTERACTIONS: Butorphanol can be used as an antagonist to narcotic agonists, such as meperidine, morphine, and oxymorphone. As an antagonist, butorphanol is approximately equivalent to nalorphine and 30 times more potent than pentazocine. Marked sedation occurs when butorphanol is combined with acepromazine, more so in medium to large breed dogs. When used with other CNS depressants, such as the barbiturates and phenothiazine tranquilizers, additive respiratory depression may occur. Use these combinations with caution. Concurrent use of pancuronium may lead to conjunctival changes.

SUPPLIED AS: VETERINARY PRODUCTS
Tablets containing 1-, 5-, and 10-mg base activity
For injection containing 10 mg/mL

OTHER USES
Dogs
ANTITUSSIVE
i)   0.05 to 0.12 mg/kg bid–tid; PO

ii) 0.05 to 0.1 mg/kg bid–qid; SC, PO

ANALGESIA
0.2 to 0.4 mg/kg; IM, IV

ANTIEMETIC IN CISPLATIN-INDUCED EMESIS
0.4 mg/kg; IM at the beginning and end of a 3-hour cisplatin infusion

PREANESTHETIC
i)   0.05 mg/kg; IV or 0.4 mg/kg; SC, IM

ii) 0.1 to 0.2 mg/kg; IM

iii) 0.2 to 0.4 mg/kg; IM (with acepromazine 0.02–0.04 mg/kg; IM)

NEUROLEPTANALGESIA DOSE
Butorphanol 0.2 mg/kg; IV
Acepromazine 0.05 mg/kg; IV
Atropine 0.02 mg/kg; IV
All three agents can be mixed in one syringe. Sedation can be reversed with naloxone.

Cats
PREANESTHETIC
i)   0.1 to 0.2 mg/kg; IM

ii) 0.2 to 0.4 mg/kg; IM (with glycopyrrolate 0.01 mg/kg; IM and ketamine 4–10 mg/kg; IM)

ANALGESIA
i)   0.1 to 0.2 mg/kg; IM, IV

ii) 0.4 mg/kg; SC

CALCITONIN SALMON

INDICATIONS: Calcitonin salmon (Calcimar ♣ ★) may be an effective adjunct (in addition to fluid therapy, diuretics, and corticosteroids) to the management of hypercalcemia. The drug inhibits bone resorption. Efficacy usually is noted 4 to 12 hours after injection.

ADVERSE AND COMMON SIDE EFFECTS: Little data are available in small animals. In humans, transient nausea, anorexia, and vomiting are encountered most frequently. Local inflammatory reactions at the injection site develop in a few patients. In a few cases, administration of calcitonin has resulted in allergic reactions, e.g., bronchospasm, swelling of the tongue, and anaphylactic shock. Some hypercalcemic dogs become refractory to treatment with the drug after several days and hypercalcemia recurs. The drug may result in decreased fetal birth weights and is not advised for use in pregnancy. Calcitonin also inhibits lactation and should not be given to nursing animals.

DRUG INTERACTIONS: None.

SUPPLIED AS: HUMAN PRODUCT
For injection containing 200 IU/mL in 400-IU vials

OTHER USES: In humans, the drug also has been shown to decrease increased serum calcium levels in patients with carcinoma, multiple myeloma, and primary hyperparathyroidism.

CALCITRIOL

INDICATIONS: Calcitriol (Calcijex ♣ ★, Rocaltrol ♣ ★), a vitamin D_3 metabolite, is used in the management of hypocalcemia. It also may be used to prevent or reverse renal secondary hyperparathyroidism in dogs and cats with chronic renal failure. It has a rapid onset of action (1–4 days) and a short half-life (4–6 hours). Oral calcitriol is administered to patients after initial stabilization with fluid therapy, dietary protein, and phosphorous restriction, the use of intestinal phosphate binders and H-2 blockers as needed. Serum phosphorous should be less than 6 mg/dL (1.9 mmol/L) before initiating calcitriol.

ADVERSE AND COMMON SIDE EFFECTS: Hypercalcemia leading to polyuria, polydipsia, listlessness, depression, anorexia, vomiting, nephrocalcinosis, muscle weakness, and trembling or muscle twitching may occur. If hypercalcemia results from drug overdosage, it generally will resolve within 4 days of discontinuing the drug. Hypercalcemia usually only occurs if calcitriol is used in conjunction with intestinal phosphate binders, especially calcium carbonate. Safety of the use of this product in pregnant or lactating animals has not been established.

DRUG INTERACTIONS: Hypercalcemia may precipitate cardiac arrhythmias in patients on digitalis. Intestinal absorption may be impaired by cholestyramine and by mineral oil (when used as a laxative). Long-term use of phenytoin and the barbiturates may interfere with the action of the drug, necessitating higher doses of calcitriol. Thiazide diuretics may enhance the effects of calcitriol predisposing to hypercalcemia. Calcitriol-induced hypercalcemia may antagonize the antiarrhythmic effects of calcium channel-blocking agents.

SUPPLIED AS: HUMAN PRODUCTS
Capsules containing 0.25 and 0.50 µg
Oral solution containing 1.0 µg/mL
For injection containing 1 and 2 µg/mL

CALCIUM CARBONATE

INDICATIONS: Calcium carbonate (Apo-Cal ★, Calsan ✦ ★, Os-Cal ✦ ★) is a rapid-acting antacid drug with high neutralizing properties and relatively prolonged duration of action. It also increases lower esophageal sphincter tone. The drug also is used for the management of hyperphosphatemia associated with renal failure. Calcium carbonate is not as potent a phosphorus binder as the aluminum salts.

ADVERSE AND COMMON SIDE EFFECTS: The use of calcium-containing antacid preparations may be associated with constipation or diarrhea. Calcium-containing preparations also may cause hypercalcemia, stimulation of gastric secretion, and impairment of renal function. A slight alkalosis may develop with prolonged use of the drug. Gastric acid rebound may be caused by the release of gastrin triggered by the action of calcium in the small intestines. Liberation of carbon dioxide in the stomach causes belching in some patients. The drug is contraindicated in patients with hypercalcemia, hypercalciuria, severe renal disease, renal calculi, gastrointestinal hemorrhage or obstruction, dehydration, hypochloremic alkalosis, ventricular fibrillation, cardiac disease, and pregnancy. Cautious use of the drug is recommended in patients with decreased bowel motility, e.g., those receiving anticholinergics, antidiarrheals, or antispasmodics. Also see **ANTACIDS.**

DRUG INTERACTIONS: Calcium carbonate may decrease oral iron absorption. The absorption of oral tetracyclines and phenytoin may be decreased. Administer the tetracycline up to 3 hours before or after calcium carbonate. Calcium carbonate may antagonize the effects of calcium channel-blocking agents, e.g., verapamil, diltiazem, nifedipine. Thiazide diuretics used concurrently with large doses of calcium may cause hypercalcemia.

SUPPLIED AS: HUMAN PRODUCTS
Tablets containing 250, 500, and 750 mg
Capsules containing 500 mg

OTHER USES
Dogs

HYPOCALCEMIA   ASSOCIATED   WITH   HYPOPARATHYROIDISM
100 to 200 mg/kg bid–tid; PO

HYPERPHOSPHATEMIA ASSOCIATED WITH RENAL FAILURE
100 mg/kg/day div. bid or tid; PO

CALCIUM CHLORIDE

INDICATIONS: Calcium chloride ✤ ★ is used in the treatment of cardiac arrest (ventricular asystole and electromechanical dissociation) to stimulate cardiac excitation when epinephrine fails to improve myocardial contractions and hyperkalemic myocardial toxicity. It also may be used in the acute treatment of hypocalcemia.

ADVERSE AND COMMON SIDE EFFECTS: Hypercalcemia may occur. With rapid IV injection, hypotension, bradycardia, syncope, cardiac arrhythmias, and cardiac arrest may occur. Extravascular injection causes inflammation, tissue necrosis, and sloughing. If perivascular injection occurs, recommendations include injection of the area with normal saline, corticosteroids, 1% procaine, and hyaluronidase. In addition, heat should be applied to the affected area and the limb should be kept elevated. Calcium chloride should be used with caution in animals with nephrocalcinosis. The safety of its use during pregnancy has not been established.

DRUG INTERACTIONS: Calcium chloride may increase the risk of digitalis toxicity in patients receiving digitalis drugs. Calcium chloride-induced hypercalcemia may negate the efficacy of calcium channel-blocking agents, e.g., verapamil, diltiazem, and nifedipine. Calcium chloride for injection is incompatible with amphotericin B, bicarbonates, carbonates, cephalothin sodium, chlorpheniramine, phosphates, sulfates, and tartrate admixtures. Thiazide diuretics used concurrently with large doses of calcium may cause hypercalcemia.

SUPPLIED AS: HUMAN PRODUCT
For injection containing 100 mg/mL providing a 10% solution

CALCIUM EDTA

INDICATIONS: Calcium disodium EDTA (Calcium Disodium Versenate ✚ ★) is a favored chelating agent for the treatment of lead toxicity in the dog and cat. Before administration, calcium EDTA is diluted to a 1% solution using 5% dextrose in water.

ADVERSE AND COMMON SIDE EFFECTS: The drug is contraindicated in patients with anuria, and drug dosage should be decreased in those with renal failure. Intravenous administration may cause an increase in CSF pressure and the potential for fatal lead-induced cerebral edema. Therefore, the SC route of administration is recommended. High concentrations can cause pain at the injection site. Lidocaine can be mixed with the solution to prevent pain. Depression, vomiting, and diarrhea may occur but may be alleviated by concurrent zinc supplementation (2 mg/kg/day). The most serious potential side effect of calcium EDTA is reversible renal tubular necrosis. Dosages greater than 12 g/kg are fatal in dogs. During the first 72 hours of chelation, blood lead concentrations rapidly decrease and clinical improvement is noted, but then they become constant or even increase during the remainder of the treatment schedule. Therefore, blood lead levels should be submitted only 10 to 14 days after treatment to evaluate the efficacy of therapy.

DRUG INTERACTIONS: Concurrent administration with zinc insulin preparations will decrease the sustained action of the insulin. Renal toxicity of calcium EDTA may be potentiated by the use of corticosteroids. Calcium EDTA should be used with caution with other potentially nephrotoxic agents, e.g., aminoglycosides and amphotericin B.

SUPPLIED AS: HUMAN PRODUCT
For injection containing 200 mg/mL

CALCIUM GLUCONATE

INDICATIONS: Calcium gluconate ✚ ★ is indicated for the treatment of hypocalcemia, ventricular asystole, severe bradycardia, hyperkalemic cardiotoxicity, and eclampsia (puerperal tetany). Although calcium gluconate rapidly corrects hyperkalemic cardiotoxicity, its beneficial effects usually last only 10 to 15 minutes (it does not lower serum potassium levels). The oral form of calcium gluconate also is used to manage hypocalcemia associated with chronic renal failure.

ADVERSE AND COMMON SIDE EFFECTS: The drug is relatively contraindicated in patients with ventricular fibrillation, renal calculi, and hypercalcemia. It should be used with caution in those concurrently receiving digitalis therapy or those with renal or cardiac insufficiency. Intravenous injections must be given slowly to avoid hypercalcemia (vomiting, abdominal pain, ileus, decreased excitability of nerves and muscles, azotemia, acute pancreatitis, and potential cardiotoxicity). If the heart rate decreases significantly, infusion should be discontinued until the rate returns to normal, at which time reinfusion can begin. Extravascular injection causes inflammation, tissue necrosis, and sloughing. Oral preparations predispose to constipation and increased gastric acid secretion. Also see **CALCIUM CHLORIDE.**

DRUG INTERACTIONS: Calcium gluconate may potentiate the inotropic and toxic effects of digitalis and can precipitate arrhythmias in patients receiving these drugs. Oral calcium complexes with and decreases the effect of oral tetracyclines. Do not administer these drugs within 3 hours of each other. Calcium gluconate-induced hypercalcemia may antagonize the effectiveness of the calcium channel-blocking agents, e.g., verapamil, diltiazem, and nifedipine. Calcium gluconate reportedly is incompatible with IV fat emulsions, amphotericin B, cefamandole, cephalothin, dobutamine, methylprednisolone sodium succinate, and metoclopramide. Thiazide diuretics used concurrently with large doses of calcium may cause hypercalcemia.

SUPPLIED AS: VETERINARY PRODUCT
For injection containing 23% w/v as calcium borogluconate

HUMAN PRODUCTS
1-g tabs contain 90 mg elemental calcium
975-mg tabs contain 87.75 mg elemental calcium
650-mg tabs contain 58.5 mg elemental calcium
500-mg tabs contain 45 mg elemental calcium
For injection as a 10% solution

OTHER USES: Calcium gluconate also has been used to antagonize aminoglycoside-induced neuromuscular blockade and as a calcium challenge to diagnose Zollinger-Ellison syndrome (causes increased plasma gastrin levels in affected dogs).

CALCIUM LACTATE

INDICATIONS: The INDICATIONS, ADVERSE AND COMMON SIDE EFFECTS, AND DRUG INTERACTIONS of calcium lactate ✤ ★ are similar to those of calcium gluconate. Calcium lactate generally is used to treat mild hypocalcemia and for maintenance calcium therapy.

SUPPLIED AS: HUMAN PRODUCT
Tablets containing 325 mg (contain 42.25 mg elemental calcium) and
650 mg (contain 84.5 mg elemental calcium)

CAPTOPRIL

INDICATIONS: Captopril (Capoten ♣ ★) is an angiotensin-converting
enzyme (ACE) inhibitor. It significantly increases cardiac output
while reducing systemic vascular resistance, pulmonary capillary
wedge pressure, and right atrial pressure. Heart rate usually is unaffected. The drug has been shown to be more efficacious in improving cardiac function in people than prazosin. It is useful in conditions of congestive heart failure and in the management of systemic
hypertension. Angiotensin-converting enzyme inhibitors often improve even mild cases of congestive heart failure. Experimentally,
ACE inhibitors may slow the progression of renal disease via decreasing glomerular pressures (which contribute to the progression
of renal disease) and possibly by limiting the growth/proliferation
of glomerular cells, although clinical improvement has yet to be
proven.

ADVERSE AND COMMON SIDE EFFECTS: Hypotension causing
lethargy, anorexia, weakness, and difficulty rising—possibly in association with dehydration or azotemia—has been reported. Consequently, low initial doses are recommended, titrating the drug to effect. Anorexia, vomiting, and diarrhea (sometimes with blood) have
been observed in some dogs. Discontinuation of the drug results in
prompt resolution of these signs, and therapy usually can be resumed
at lower doses. Hyperkalemia may occur, especially if the drug is used
with potassium-sparing diuretics. Renal insufficiency has been observed in small animals (usually at doses greater than 2 mg/kg tid).
Proteinuria may occur. The drug should be used cautiously in animals
with renal disease. Captopril does not require hepatic conversion and
consequently is a better choice for patients with liver disease than
enalapril. Drug overdose may be treated with a β-agonist, e.g., dobutamine (2.5–10 μg/kg/minute; IV). Bradyarrhythmias may respond to
atropine or glycopyrrolate. A case of pancytopenia in a dog has been
reported. Pancytopenia resolved after discontinuation of the drug and
the institution of erythropoietin and recombinant human granulocyte
colony-stimulating factor (Filgrastim neupogen).

DRUG INTERACTIONS: Hypotension may be enhanced if captopril
is used in conjunction with other vasodilators, e.g., nitroglycerin.
Low-salt diets and accelerated salt loss induced by loop diuretics
may predispose to renal insufficiency and azotemia associated with
ACE inhibitor use. Treatment includes a reduction of diuretic dose

and liberalization of dietary salt intake. The antihypertensive effects of captopril may be decreased when captopril is used in conjunction with aspirin or other NSAID drugs. Hyperkalemia is a concern if captopril is used with potassium-sparing diuretics (e.g., spironolactone) or potassium supplements. Serum digoxin levels may increase if the two drugs are used simultaneously. Absorption from the GIT may be decreased if captopril is given at the same time as antacid preparations. Separate dosing of these drugs by at least 2 hours is recommended.

SUPPLIED AS: HUMAN PRODUCT
Tablets containing 12.5, 25, 50, and 100 mg

OTHER USES: Captopril may be useful in hemorrhagic or endotoxic shock by helping maintain peripheral tissue perfusion.

CARBAMATE INSECTICIDES

INDICATIONS: The carbamate insecticides are cholinesterase inhibitors used to eradicate mites, lice, fleas, and ticks. Included in this group are propoxur (Baygon, Sendran, Vet-Kem), carbaril (Sevin, Vet-Kem), methomyl (Lannate), bendiocarb (Ficam), aldicarb (Temik), and carbofuran (Furadan).

ADVERSE AND COMMON SIDE EFFECTS: Toxicity results in miosis, salivation, frequent urination and defecation, vomiting, bronchoconstriction, ataxia, incoordination, muscle tremors, convulsions, respiratory depression, paralysis, and possibly death. Carbamate products should not be used on puppies or kittens younger than 12 weeks of age or on pregnant or nursing animals. In some animals, skin irritation may develop with use of the collars, especially if the collars are applied too tightly. In case of accidental poisoning, exposed skin should be cleansed. If the drug has been ingested, gastric lavage is indicated. After lavage, activated charcoal should be given by way of stomach intubation. In all cases, atropine (0.2 mg/kg) is given to effect. One fourth of the total dose is given intravenously, and the balance is given intramuscularly or subcutaneously. Diazepam has been used to augment the effects of atropine, hastening recovery. The use of pralidoxime chloride (2-PAM) is discouraged in carbamate toxicity because it may predispose to increased toxicity.

DRUG INTERACTIONS: Phenothiazine tranquilizers may potentiate the adverse effects of carbamate products. Concurrent use of physostigmine, pyridostigmine, neostigmine, morphine, or succinylcholine also should be avoided.

CARBENICILLIN

INDICATIONS: Carbenicillin (Geopen ✚ ★, Pyopen ✚ ★) is an extended spectrum, penicillinase-sensitive, semisynthetic penicillin. It is bactericidal against a variety of gram-negative and gram-positive organisms and some anaerobes. Among susceptible bacteria are *Pseudomonas aeruginosa*, *Proteus*, susceptible strains of *E. coli*, *Enterobacter*, and *Streptococcus*.

ADVERSE AND COMMON SIDE EFFECTS: See PENICILLIN ANTIBIOTICS.

DRUG INTERACTIONS: A synergistic action occurs when carbenicillin is combined with aminoglycoside antibiotics. If, however, carbenicillin is given concurrently with a tetracycline, the bactericidal activity of the former compound may be reduced.

SUPPLIED AS: HUMAN PRODUCTS
For injection containing 1-, 2-, 5-, 10-, and 30-g vials [Geopen, Pyopen]
Tablets containing 382 mg [Geocillin ★, Geopen Oral ✚]

CARBOPLATIN

INDICATIONS: Carboplatin (Paraplatin ✚ ★) is a second-generation platinum compound that differs from cisplatin because it is less nephrotoxic and does not require saline diuresis. It also may be useful for dogs that cannot receive cisplatin because of preexisting congestive heart failure. The drug has been used in the management of canine osteosarcoma. Treatment with amputation and four doses of the drug given every 21 days resulted in a median survival time of 321 days with 35% of dogs alive at 1 year, which is longer than that reported for amputation alone and similar to that noted with two to four doses of cisplatin.

ADVERSE AND COMMON SIDE EFFECTS: The dose-limiting toxicity in dogs is neutropenia and thrombocytopenia. Transient vomiting and elevations in serum urea and creatinine may occur. Dose-limiting neutropenia and thrombocytopenia also have been documented in the cat at dosages of 200 and 250 mg/m^2. The neutrophil nadir is seen on day 17 (at 200 mg/m^2) and lasts from day 14 through 25 after drug administration.

DRUG INTERACTIONS: In people, concomitant use with aminoglycoside antibiotics may predispose to renal and auditory toxicity. Carboplatin should not be used in conjunction with other potentially nephrotoxic drugs.

SUPPLIED AS: HUMAN PRODUCTS
For injection containing 50, 150, and 450 mg
For injection containing 10 mg/mL [Paraplatin-AQ]

CARNITINE

INDICATIONS: Carnitine (Carnitor ★, VitaCarn ★, L-Carnitine ✿ ★) supplementation may be useful adjunctive therapy in the management of some dogs with dilated cardiomyopathy. It has been reported that myocardial-free carnitine deficiency occurs in approximately 50% to 90% of dogs with dilated cardiomyopathy. It has been concluded that American cocker spaniels with dilated cardiomyopathy are taurine deficient and are responsive to taurine and carnitine supplementation. Although myocardial function did not return to normal, it improved sufficiently enough to allow discontinuation of cardiovascular drug therapy. Survival of Dobermans with myocardial carnitine deficiency treated with carnitine in addition to conventional pharmacotherapy reportedly has been significantly improved. Although conventional pharmacotherapy for heart failure occasionally can be withdrawn from patients responding to carnitine, it is not considered a reasonable expectation. The drug also may have a protective effect against myocardial infarction and doxorubicin-induced cardiomyopathy. It also has been recommended as adjunct therapy in feline hepatic lipidosis, for which it is believed the drug may facilitate hepatic lipid metabolism, although other investigators suggest that carnitine deficiency has no role in the pathogenesis of this disease.

ADVERSE AND COMMON SIDE EFFECTS: The drug is very safe. Excessive drug doses have not been associated with adverse effects, although mild diarrhea has been reported in one dog. D, L-carnitine has been associated with a myasthenia-like syndrome. Therefore, it is recommended that the L-isomer (L-carnitine) formulation be used.

DRUG INTERACTIONS: D, L-carnitine sold in health food stores as vitamin B_T inhibits L-carnitine and may cause a deficiency.

SUPPLIED AS: Powder [L-carnitine; Ward Robertson Chemicals; Scarborough, Ontario]
Tablets containing 330 mg ★
Capsules containing 250 mg ★
Oral solution containing 100 mg/mL ★

OTHER USES
Dogs
AMERICAN COCKER SPANIEL DILATED CARDIOMYOPATHY
500 mg taurine bid–tid; PO with 1 g carnitine bid–tid; PO

CARPROFEN

INDICATIONS: Carprofen (Rimadyl ★) is a carboxylic acid non-steroidal anti-inflammatory agent with analgesic, anti-inflammatory and antipyretic properties. Its potency is comparable to that of indomethacin and greater than that of aspirin or phenylbutazone. The drug has been shown to be clinically effective in the management of osteoarthritis in dogs.

ADVERSE AND COMMON SIDE EFFECTS: Clinically significant adverse side effects did not develop in dogs receiving up to 5 times the recommended dosage for 42 days or 10 times the recommended dosage for 14 days. Use of the drug may be associated with vomiting, diarrhea, changes in appetite, lethargy, constipation, or aggression. Serum alanine transferase activity may be increased. Carprofen has not been reported to cause GI ulceration or renal damage. Safe use of the drug in pregnant, breeding, or lactating dogs has not been established.

DRUG INTERACTIONS: Carprofen should not be used concurrently with glucocorticoids because the possibility of adverse GI effects may be increased.

SUPPLIED AS: Caplets containing 25, 75, and 100 mg

CEFACLOR

INDICATIONS: Cefaclor (Ceclor ♣ ★) is a second-generation cephalosporin antibiotic. It has a similar spectrum of activity as other oral cephalosporins but is more active. For more information, see **CEPHALOSPORIN ANTIBIOTICS.**

ADVERSE AND COMMON SIDE EFFECTS AND DRUG INTERACTIONS: See **CEPHALOSPORIN ANTIBIOTICS.**

SUPPLIED AS: HUMAN PRODUCTS
Capsules containing 250 and 500 mg
Oral suspension containing 125 mg/5 mL, 250 mg/5 mL, and 375 mg/5 mL

CEFADROXIL

INDICATIONS: Cefadroxil (Cefa-Tabs ♣ ★, Cefa-Drops ♣ ★) is a first-generation cephalosporin. The drug is used in dogs and cats to treat infections caused by susceptible organisms of the skin, soft tissue, and genitourinary tract, including *E. coli, Proteus mirabilis, Pasteurella multocida, Staphylococcus aureus,* and *S. epidermidis,* as well as *Streptococcus* spp. For more information, see **CEPHALOSPORIN ANTIBIOTICS.**

ADVERSE AND COMMON SIDE EFFECTS: Occasional nausea and vomiting have been reported with the use of Cefa-Tabs. Administration with food appears to decrease nausea. Diarrhea and lethargy also may occur. See also **CEPHALOSPORIN ANTIBIOTICS.**

DRUG INTERACTIONS: See CEPHALOSPORIN ANTIBIOTICS.

SUPPLIED AS: VETERINARY PRODUCTS
Tablets in 50-mg, 100-g, 200-mg, and 1-g strengths [Cefa-Tabs]
For oral suspension as 750 mg/15-mL bottle and 2,500 mg/50-mL bottle

CEFAMANDOLE

INDICATIONS: Cefamandole (Mandol ✦ ⋆) is a second-generation cephalosporin with wide tissue distribution, including bile and synovia. The drug exerts high activity against *E. coli, Klebsiella, Enterobacter, Proteus, Salmonella, Hemophilus,* and *Shigella* species. For additional information, see **CEPHALOSPORIN ANTIBIOTICS.**

ADVERSE AND COMMON SIDE EFFECTS and **DRUG INTERACTIONS:** See CEPHALOSPORIN ANTIBIOTICS.

SUPPLIED AS: HUMAN PRODUCTS
For injection containing 1- and 2-g vials [Mandol]
For injection containing 1 g [ADD-Vantage; Abbott ✦]

CEFAZOLIN

INDICATIONS: Cefazolin (Ancef ✦ ⋆, Kefzol ✦ ⋆) is a short-acting, first-generation cephalosporin that achieves the greatest serum concentration and has the longest half-life. It is more active against *E. coli, Klebsiella,* and *Enterobacter* species. For additional information, see **CEPHALOSPORIN ANTIBIOTICS.**

ADVERSE AND COMMON SIDE EFFECTS and **DRUG INTERACTIONS:** See CEPHALOSPORIN ANTIBIOTICS.

SUPPLIED AS: HUMAN PRODUCTS
For injection as a powder containing 500 mg and 1, 5, 10, and 20 g
For injection (IV infusion) 500 mg and 1 g in vials and in 5% dextrose [in water] (D_5W) 50-mL bags

CEFIXIME

INDICATIONS: Cefixime (Suprax ✤ ★) is a third-generation cephalosporin antibiotic. Experience with use of the drug in small animals at this time is limited. As with other third-generation cephalosporins, cefixime has an expanded range of activity against gram-negative bacteria.

ADVERSE AND COMMON SIDE EFFECTS and **DRUG INTER-ACTIONS:** See CEPHALOSPORIN ANTIBIOTICS.

SUPPLIED AS: HUMAN PRODUCTS
Capsules containing 200 and 400 mg
Oral suspension containing 100 mg/5 mL

CEFOTAXIME

INDICATIONS: Cefotaxime (Claforan ✤ ★) is a third-generation cephalosporin. It readily penetrates into the CSF. Unlike other cephalosporins, the third-generation drugs, including cefotaxime, are somewhat effective against *Pseudomonas aeruginosa*. For more information, see **CEPHALOSPORIN ANTIBIOTICS.**

ADVERSE AND COMMON SIDE EFFECTS and **DRUG INTER-ACTIONS:** See CEPHALOSPORIN ANTIBIOTICS.

SUPPLIED AS: HUMAN PRODUCTS
For injection as a powder containing 500 mg and 1, 2, or 10 g
For injection in 50 mL, 5% dextrose bags containing 1 and 2 g cefotaxime

CEFOXITIN

INDICATIONS: Cefoxitin (Mefoxin ✤ ★) is a semisynthetic, broad-spectrum, second-generation cephalosporin antibiotic. For more information, see **CEPHALOSPORIN ANTIBIOTICS.** Cefoxitin has activity against gram-positive cocci, although less so than first-generation cephalosporins. It does, however, have good activity against many strains of *E. coli, Klebsiella,* and *Proteus* organisms that may be resistant to the first-generation drugs. Cefoxitin is one of the most effective cephalosporins for treating anaerobic infections, including those caused by Enterobacteriaceae and *B. fragilis*.

ADVERSE AND COMMON SIDE EFFECTS: See CEPHALO-SPORIN ANTIBIOTICS.

DRUG INTERACTIONS: An additive or synergistic effect is gained against some organisms when cefoxitin is used in conjunction with the penicillins, chloramphenicol, or the aminoglycoside antibiotics. However, the manufacturer advises that cefoxitin should not be administered with aminoglycoside antibiotics because of possible incompatibility. The concurrent use of cefoxitin and aminoglycosides, vancomycin, polymyxin B, or a diuretic increases the potential for nephrotoxicity, thus dictating close monitoring of renal function. Pain may occur on intramuscular injection.

SUPPLIED AS: HUMAN PRODUCTS
For injection containing 1, 2, and 10 g
For injection containing 1 and 2 g in 5% dextrose (frozen) as 1 g (20 mg/mL) and 2 g (40 mg/mL)

CEFTAZIDIME

INDICATIONS: Ceftazidime (Fortaz ✦ ★) is a third-generation, broad-spectrum cephalosporin similar to cefotaxime, with activity against gram-negative bacteria but with greater activity against *Pseudomonas aeruginosa*. The drug is used to treat infections of the lower respiratory tract, skin, urinary tract, bones, and joints, CNS infections (including meningitis), and bacteremia.

ADVERSE AND COMMON SIDE EFFECTS: The drug is contraindicated in patients with known hypersensitivity to cephalosporins and related β-lactam antibiotics. Drug dose should be decreased in patients with renal impairment. Safe use in pregnancy has not been established. Experience with use of the drug in small animals is limited. The most common adverse effects in humans include local reactions after injection (phlebitis, thrombophlebitis, pain), fever, pruritus, diarrhea, nausea, transient elevations in serum urea and creatinine, and hepatic enzymes. See also **CEPHALOSPORIN ANTIBIOTICS.**

DRUG INTERACTIONS: Concurrent use with aminoglycosides may cause an additive nephrotoxic effect. Concomitant use of furosemide and ethacrynic acid may increase the risk of renal toxicity. Chloramphenicol is antagonistic in vitro with ceftazidime. Ampicillin may produce antagonism against group B streptococci and *Listeria monocytogenes*. See also **CEPHALOSPORIN ANTIBIOTICS.**

SUPPLIED AS: HUMAN PRODUCTS
For IM or direct IV injection vials containing 500 mg or 1 g
For IV injection or infusion vials containing 1, 2, or 6 g
For injection containing 1 g in 4.4% dextrose (20 mg/mL) and 2 g in 3.2% dextrose (40 mg/mL)

CEPHALEXIN

INDICATIONS: Cephalexin (Keflex ✤ ★) is a broad-spectrum, first-generation cephalosporin. For more information, see **CEPHALOSPORIN ANTIBIOTICS.**

ADVERSE AND COMMON SIDE EFFECTS: In addition to the side effects noted for the **CEPHALOSPORIN ANTIBIOTICS,** cephalexin has been reported to cause salivation, tachypnea, and excitability in dogs, and vomiting and fever in cats. See **CEPHALOSPORIN ANTIBIOTICS.**

DRUG INTERACTIONS: See CEPHALOSPORIN ANTIBIOTICS.

SUPPLIED AS: HUMAN PRODUCTS
Capsules containing 250 and 500 mg
Tablets containing 250 and 500 mg
Oral suspension containing 25 mg/mL and 50 mg/mL

CEPHALOSPORIN ANTIBIOTICS

INDICATIONS: The cephalosporin antibiotics are bactericidal to gram-positive and several gram-negative strains. They are used in the treatment of respiratory, skeletal, genitourinary, skin, and soft tissue infections. In addition, these drugs are recommended for prophylactic use in biliary tract surgery and for treating biliary tract disease. All are effective against anaerobic infections except *Bacteroides fragilis* (cefoxitin excepted). Cephalosporins may be more effective than penicillin antibiotics in the treatment of β-lactamase–producing staphylococci. The cephalosporins usually are not effective against resistant strains of *Pseudomonas aeruginosa* (ceftazidime excepted). The first- and second-generation cephalosporin antibiotics do not readily cross the blood–brain barrier.

First-generation cephalosporins (cefadroxil, cephalexin, cephradine, cephalothin, cefazolin, cephapirin) are active against gram-positive bacteria, including penicillin-resistant staphylococci, and against some gram-negative bacteria, including *E. coli, Proteus,* and *Klebsiella* spp. First-generation drugs are relatively ineffective against *Bacteroides*. They enter the CSF only in the presence of inflammation. In vitro antimicrobial activity and serum concentrations after oral administration of cephalexin, cefadroxil, and cephradine are similar; however, serum and urine concentrations of cefadroxil are more sustained than those seen with cephalexin. These drugs are less expensive than the second- and third-generation cephalosporins.

Second-generation cephalosporins (cefamandole, cefaclor, cefoxitin) have a broader spectrum of activity and greater efficacy against gram-negative bacteria and anaerobes than the first-generation cephalosporins, but their activity against gram-positive organisms is less than that of the first-generation drugs. Cefoxitin also is effective against *Serratia* and *B. fragilis*. Cefamandole is active against *Salmonella* and *Shigella*.

Third-generation cephalosporins (cefixime, cefotaxime, cefoperazone, ceftazidime, moxalactam) have increased antibacterial activity against gram-negative bacteria and anaerobes, but activity against gram-positive organisms is minimal. The third-generation drugs have increased resistance to β-lactamase–producing bacteria and increased activity against gram-negative bacteria, including *Pseudomonas, Proteus, Enterobacter,* and *Citrobacter* spp. Moxalactam and cefotaxime readily penetrate into the CSF in healthy and inflamed meninges.

A fourth-generation cephalosporin (cefepime) is an injectable drug that has similar gram-negative activity as third-generation agents but maintains good gram-positive activity.

ADVERSE AND COMMON SIDE EFFECTS: As a group, the cephalosporin antibiotics are quite safe. Vomiting and diarrhea may occur with oral administration. Administration with food decreases nausea. Because most cephalosporins are eliminated by the kidney, their concentration is increased and their half-life is extended in cases of renal failure. All parenteral forms may cause phlebitis and myositis after IV or IM injection, respectively. Reversible blood dyscrasias, including anemia, thrombocytopenia, and neutropenia, have been induced with high-dose, long-term use of these drugs in some dogs as a result of a direct bone marrow toxic effect and immune-mediated destruction of blood cells. After withdrawal of the drug, hematologic recovery generally occurs within 1 week. The cephalosporins may cause elevations in serum alkaline phosphatase, alanine transferase, and aspartate transferase, as well as an increase in serum urea nitrogen. False-positive Coombs' test results and false-positive urinary glucose reactions also have been documented. Third-generation cephalosporins can prolong the partial thromboplastin time and the prothrombin time by inhibiting vitamin K activation of clotting factors. Allergic skin reactions have been reported with the use of cephalexin. Cephalothin produces pain and may cause sterile abscess formation on injection. Cross-allergenicity with penicillins may occur. An additive or synergistic effect is gained against some organisms when cefoxitin is used in conjunction with the penicillins, chloramphenicol, or the aminoglycoside antibiotics. For additional information, see the specific cephalosporin.

DRUG INTERACTIONS: The cephalosporins are potentially nephrotoxic, and it is advised that these drugs be used with caution when administered concurrently with other potentially nephrotoxic drugs, e.g., aminoglycosides, amphotericin B, vancomycin, polymyxin B, or a diuretic. See specific drug.

SUPPLIED AS: See specific drug.

CEPHALOTHIN

INDICATIONS: Cephalothin (Keflin ✚ ★) is a first-generation cephalosporin.

ADVERSE AND COMMON SIDE EFFECTS: In experimental studies, cephalothin impairs platelet aggregation. However, clinical evidence of a bleeding tendency has not been demonstrated. For more information, including **DRUG INTERACTIONS**, see **CEPHALOSPORIN ANTIBIOTICS**.

SUPPLIED AS: HUMAN PRODUCT
For injection containing 1, 2, and 20 g in vials

CEPHAPIRIN

INDICATIONS: Cephapirin (Cefadyl ★) is a first-generation cephalosporin. It resists β-lactamase and has been used when a relatively short-acting, injectable, first-generation cephalosporin is indicated. For additional information, see **CEPHALOSPORIN ANTIBIOTICS**.

ADVERSE AND COMMON SIDE EFFECTS and **DRUG INTERACTIONS:** See CEPHALOSPORIN ANTIBIOTICS.

SUPPLIED AS: HUMAN PRODUCT
For injection containing 500 mg and 1, 2, 4, and 20 g powder

CEPHRADINE

INDICATIONS: Cephradine (Velosef ★) is a first-generation cephalosporin with a spectrum of activity similar to that of cephalexin. For additional information, see **CEPHALOSPORIN ANTIBIOTICS**.

ADVERSE AND COMMON SIDE EFFECTS and **DRUG INTERACTIONS:** See CEPHALOSPORIN ANTIBIOTICS.

SUPPLIED AS: HUMAN PRODUCTS
Capsules containing 250 and 500 mg

Oral suspension containing 125 mg/5 mL and 250 mg/5 mL
For injection containing 250 and 500 mg and 1 and 2 g powder

CHARCOAL, ACTIVATED

INDICATIONS: Activated charcoal (Charcodote ✦, Charcocaps ★, CharcolantiDote ★, SuperChar-Vet ★, SuperChar ★, Toxiban ★) is an excellent absorbent used in the treatment of accidental poisoning. Repetitive dosing (e.g., every 6 hours for 1 to 2 days) increases clearance of drugs already absorbed into the systemic circulation. It often is used in conjunction with emetics and gastric lavage. Activated charcoal must be of vegetable origin, not mineral or animal. A slurry is made and administered by stomach tube. A cathartic (sodium sulfate) often is given 30 minutes after the administration of charcoal. Activated charcoal is most useful when used for acetaminophen, atropine, digitalis glycosides, phenytoin, mercuric chloride, strychnine, morphine sulfate, atropine, and ethylene glycol poisoning.

ADVERSE AND COMMON SIDE EFFECTS: Vomiting (rapid ingestion of high doses), constipation, and diarrhea may occur with its use.

DRUG INTERACTIONS: Activated charcoal reportedly is not effective in the treatment of poisoning by cyanide, mineral acids, caustic alkalis, organic solvents, ethanol, lead, iron, or methanol. Syrup of ipecac should not be used with activated charcoal because ipecac negates the absorbent activity of the charcoal. If used for the relief of GI upset, other oral drugs should not be given within 2 hours. Stools will be discolored black.

SUPPLIED AS: VETERINARY PRODUCTS
Liquid formulation:
[SuperChar-Vet] 30 g in 240-mL squeeze bottles
[Toxiban Granules] containing 47.5% charcoal, 10% kaolin in 1-lb bottles and 5-kg pails
[Toxiban Suspension] containing 10.4% charcoal, 6.25% kaolin in 240-mL bottles
HUMAN PRODUCTS
[Superchar] As a powder containing 15, 30, 40, 120, and 240 g
[Charcodote] 200 mg/mL; total 50 g in 250-mL bottles and Pediatric suspension containing 200 mg/mL for a total of 25 g in 125-mL bottles
[Charcodote Aqueous] 200 mg/mL; total 50 g in 250-mL bottle and Pediatric aqueous suspension 200 mg/mL; total 25 g in 125-mL bottle

OTHER USES: Activated charcoal also has been used to absorb intestinal gases in the treatment of dyspepsia, flatulence, and gastric distention.

CHLORAMBUCIL

INDICATIONS: Chlorambucil (Leukeran ✦ ★) is an alkylating chemotherapeutic agent indicated for the treatment of lymphocytic leukemia, polycythemia vera, multiple myeloma, ovarian adenocarcinoma, and macroglobulinemia. The drug also has been used in the treatment of immune-mediated glomerulonephritis, immune-mediated nonerosive arthritis, and immune-mediated skin diseases.

ADVERSE AND COMMON SIDE EFFECTS: Alkylating agents generally cause leukopenia, thrombocytopenia, and anemia with the nadir of leukocyte counts observed 7 to 14 days after treatment and recovery noted in an additional 7 to 14 days. Bone marrow suppression occurs less often with chlorambucil than it does with cyclophosphamide. The complete blood count should be monitored on a regular basis. The drugs busulfan, cyclophosphamide, and chlorambucil also have been associated with the occurrence of bronchopulmonary dysplasia leading to pulmonary fibrosis. Hair regrowth is delayed in shaved areas, and chlorambucil may cause alopecia is some dogs (poodles, Kerry blue terriers). Gastrointestinal side effects are rare, and occasional urticarial reactions have been reported. The drug may affect spermiogenesis and cause embryotoxicity or malformations in the newborn.

DRUG INTERACTIONS: None of relevance to small-animal medicine.

SUPPLIED AS: HUMAN PRODUCT
Tablets containing 2 mg

CHLORAMPHENICOL

INDICATIONS: Chloramphenicol (Azramycine ✦, Chlor Palm ✦, Chlor Tablets ✦, Chloromycetin ✦ ★, Karomycin Palmitate ✦, Viceton ★, and many others) is a bacteriostatic antibiotic with activity against a number of pathogens including *Bacteroides*, *Staphylococcus*, *Salmonella*, *Pasteurella*, *Bordetella*, *Hemophilus*, enteric coliforms, most anaerobes, mycoplasmas, chlamydiae, rickettsiae, and some protozoa. It is well absorbed after oral administration, is distributed widely throughout the body—including the prostate, CSF, aqueous and vitreous humor, milk, and amniotic fluid, and is excreted in the bile and urine. It is used commonly in the treatment of eye, skin, urinary, and mucous membrane infections. Serum concentrations are monitored just before the next dose or 6 to 12 hours after the last dose, depending on the regimen, and after steady-state levels have been attained (21 hours in the dog and 26 hours in the cat). The therapeutic serum concentration for dogs and cats is less than or equal to 8 µg/mL (trough). Toxic levels are listed as greater than 20 µg/mL.

ADVERSE AND COMMON SIDE EFFECTS: The most common side effect after oral administration is GI upset manifested by transient depression, anorexia, nausea, vomiting, or diarrhea. Adverse reactions also may include a reversible bone marrow suppression and nonregenerative anemia, thrombocytopenia, and leukopenia. Cats are more sensitive to the adverse effects of the drug. Bone marrow changes may occur after 1 week of therapy at doses of 50 mg/kg bid. After 3 weeks of therapy, neutropenia, lymphopenia, nonregenerative anemia, and thrombocytopenia may be seen. Resolution of these changes occurs within several days after discontinuation of the drug. Toxic changes are not seen if the drug is given intermittently at a lower dose. Decreased antibody production may be a sequelae of chloramphenicol use. Other clinical signs seen have included ataxia and even death. The drug should not be used in breeding animals and should not be given to pregnant animals because the fetus is unable to metabolize it. The drug should not be used in animals with severe liver impairment or those with severe myocardial dysfunction because of myocardial depression associated with its use. Chloramphenicol should not be used in animals with extensive wounds because it interferes with protein synthesis. Chloramphenicol may cause a false-positive result for glucose in urine when glucose oxidase strips are used.

DRUG INTERACTIONS: Chloramphenicol is a hepatic microsomal enzyme inhibitor. It potentiates the activity of barbiturate drugs, codeine, cyclophosphamide, phenytoin, primidone, warfarin, inhalation anesthetics, digitalis, and aspirin, and yet phenobarbital and other barbiturates actually may reduce the efficacy of chloramphenicol if given concurrently. Its bacteriostatic action inhibits the efficacy of penicillin and cephalosporin antibiotics and the aminoglycosides.

SUPPLIED AS: VETERINARY PRODUCTS
Tablets containing 100, 250, and 500 mg, and 1 g
Oral suspension containing 25 and 50 mg/mL [Azramycine, Chlor Palm, Karomycin Palmitate]

HUMAN PRODUCTS
Capsules containing 250 mg [Chloromycetin, Kapseals]
Oral suspension containing 30 mg/mL [Chloramphenicol Palmitate]
For injection containing 100 mg/mL (chloramphenicol sodium succinate)

CHLORHEXIDINE

INDICATIONS: Chlorhexidine (Chlorasan ★, ChlorhexiDerm ★, Hibitane ♣, Nolvadent ♣ ★, Nolvasan ★, Savlon ♣) is a commonly used antiseptic and disinfectant. It is effective against *Proteus* and

Pseudomonas. Chlorhexidine can be important adjunct topical therapy in the management of pyoderma and dermatophytosis. It is an effective and nonirritating antiseptic useful for the flushing of wounds. Concentrations of 0.5% chlorhexidine in water or alcohol reduce bacterial contamination of wounds and surgical sites but tend to retard granulation tissue formation and epithelialization. Lower concentrations (0.1%) are less antiseptic, but do not inhibit wound repair. As a disinfectant, it can be used against canine infectious tracheobronchitis virus, canine distemper virus, parainfluenza virus, rabies virus, and feline respiratory viruses. Flushing dental surfaces once daily with 0.1% to 0.2% chlorhexidine may delay the accumulation of tartar.

ADVERSE AND COMMON SIDE EFFECTS: Chlorhexidine has a low order of toxicity after oral ingestion. It is poorly absorbed from the GIT or the skin. It is, however, absorbed across serous membranes, the uterus, and bladder. Sufficient quantities can be absorbed to cause intravascular hemolysis with hemoglobinemia and hemoglobinuria because of a direct effect on the erythrocyte membrane. If these signs occur, diuresis should be promoted to prevent renal damage. Deafness may occur if the product comes in contact with the middle ear.

CHLORINATED HYDROCARBONS

INDICATIONS: Included in this group are chlorpyrifos (Duratrol), cythioate (Proban), diazinon (various generic products), dichlorvos (Vapona), fenthion (Spotton, Pro-Spot), malathion (various generic products), and phosmet (Louse Kill, Vet-Kem Paramite Flea, and Tick Dip). These agents have been used in the eradication of mites, fleas, lice, mosquitoes, and some ticks in dogs.

ADVERSE AND COMMON SIDE EFFECTS: Muscarinic effects include salivation, lacrimation, miosis, pallor, cyanosis, dyspnea, vomiting, and diarrhea. Nicotinic effects include twitching of the facial and tongue muscles, progressing to all musculature and followed by paralysis. Central nervous system effects include depression and tonic–clonic seizures. Respiratory muscle paralysis, bronchoconstriction, excessive pulmonary secretions, and pulmonary edema lead to dyspnea and death.

Treatment includes removal of unabsorbed drug by cleansing the affected area of skin or inducing vomiting, followed by oral administration of activated charcoal to prevent further absorption of insecticide remaining in the GIT. This is followed by the use of atropine (0.2 mg/kg; one fourth given intravenously and the remainder given intramuscularly or subcutaneously as needed to control clinical signs) and pralidoxime chloride (20 mg/kg bid–tid; IM or slow IV;

most efficacious if given within the first 12 to 18 hours—of little benefit after 24 hours). Diazepam can be used to control seizures. In addition, diphenhydramine (4 mg/kg tid; PO) has been shown to block the effects of nicotine stimulation and prevent the receptor paralysis associated with organophosphate-induced myasthenia-like syndrome. Maintenance of fluid balance will help hasten recovery. Where indicated, ventilatory support is used. Respiratory failure is the most common cause of death.

DRUG INTERACTIONS: Other drugs that inhibit cholinesterase, e.g., physostigmine, morphine, succinylcholine, phenothiazine, pyridostigmine, and neostigmine, should be avoided.

CHLOROTHIAZIDE

INDICATIONS: Chlorothiazide (Diuril ★) is a thiazide diuretic used in the management of congestive heart failure, pulmonary edema, and systemic hypertension. Thiazide diuretics inhibit sodium and chloride absorption in the distal tubules. Potassium secretion is promoted, and loss is comparable to that seen with furosemide. The onset of action occurs within 1 hour and peaks in 4 hours. Because thiazide diuretics work in a different part of the kidney than other diuretics, the thiazides and other diuretics often are used concurrently.

ADVERSE AND COMMON SIDE EFFECTS: Hypokalemia and excessive extravascular volume depletion are the most notable concerns associated with the use of these drugs, although hypokalemia rarely is severe enough to cause clinical signs. Other possible adverse effects include vomiting, diarrhea, hematologic toxicity, hyperglycemia, hyperlipidemia, polyuria, and hypersensitivity dermal reactions.

DRUG INTERACTIONS: When used with amphotericin B or the corticosteroids, there may be enhancement of the hypokalemic effect of chlorothiazide. When chlorothiazide is used with insulin preparations, the hypoglycemic effects of the insulin may be antagonized by the hyperglycemic effect of the thiazide. Hypokalemia may predispose to digitalis toxicity when these drugs are used concurrently. The half-life of quinidine may be prolonged by thiazides. Hypercalcemia may be exacerbated if thiazides are used with vitamin D or calcium salts.

SUPPLIED AS: HUMAN PRODUCTS
Tablets containing 250 and 500 mg
Oral suspension containing 50 mg/mL
For injection in 500-mg vial

VETERINARY PRODUCT
As boluses containing 2 g

OTHER USES
Dogs
CONGENITAL NEPHROGENIC DIABETES INSIPIDUS
20 to 40 mg/kg bid (in conjunction with a salt-restricted diet)

CALCIUM OXALATE UROLITHIASIS
The thiazide diuretics have been used as adjunct therapy in the management of calcium oxalate urolithiasis to decrease urinary excretion of calcium; however, studies in dogs have not shown consistent results, high dosage (130 mg/kg) actually increased urinary calcium excretion, and long-term use may increase serum calcium levels.

CHLORPHENIRAMINE MALEATE

INDICATIONS: Chlorpheniramine (Chlor-Trimeton ★, Chlor-Tripolon ✦) may be useful in the management of pruritus in dogs and cats. It also may be of some benefit in treating feline miliary dermatitis and excessive grooming in cats. For additional information, see **ANTIHISTAMINES.**

ADVERSE AND COMMON SIDE EFFECTS: The most common adverse effects are lethargy and somnolence. Anorexia, vomiting, and diarrhea also may occur. For additional information, see **ANTIHISTAMINES.**

DRUG INTERACTIONS: Concurrent use with phenytoin may lead to increased pharmacologic effects of phenytoin. Also see **ANTIHISTAMINES.**

SUPPLIED AS: HUMAN PRODUCTS
Tablets containing 4 mg
Tablets containing 8 and 12 mg (timed-release)
Oral syrup containing 1.2 and 2.5 mg/5 mL
For injection as 10 mg/mL in 1- and 30-mL vials and 100 mg/mL in 10-mL vials

CHLORPROMAZINE

INDICATIONS: Chlorpromazine (Largactil ✦, Thorazine ★) is a phenothiazine derivative. It primarily is used as an antiemetic agent. The drug also has been used to sedate and reduce activity. It has pharmacologic properties similar to acepromazine but is less potent and has a longer duration of activity.

ADVERSE AND COMMON SIDE EFFECTS: Constipation, paradoxical aggression, hypotension, collapse, and the initiation of seizure activity in animals with epilepsy have been reported. The drug should not be used in animals with tetanus. In cats, the drug may cause extrapyramidal signs at high doses, e.g., tremors, shivering, muscle rigidity, and the patient's inability to right itself. Lethargy, diarrhea, and loss of anal sphincter tone also may be seen. For additional information, see **ACEPROMAZINE.**

DRUG INTERACTIONS: Chlorpromazine should not be used with organophosphates or strychnine toxicity. Phenothiazines should not be given within 1 month of worming with organophosphate medications because their effects may be potentiated. If used concurrently with dipyrone, serious hypothermia may result. Physostigmine toxicity may be enhanced by chlorpromazine. Other CNS depressants enhance hypotension and respiratory depression if used concurrently. The concurrent use of quinidine may cause additive cardiac depression. Antacids and antidiarrheal compounds decrease absorption of oral phenothiazines. Space administration by at least 2 hours. Atropine and other anticholinergics have additive anticholinergic potential and reduce the antipsychotic effect of phenothiazines. Barbiturate drugs increase the metabolism of phenothiazines and may reduce their effects. Barbiturate anesthetics may increase excitation (tremor, involuntary muscle movements) and hypotension. Propranolol may have additive hypotensive effects. Phenothiazines may mask the ototoxic effects of aminoglycoside antibiotics. Chlorpromazine inhibits phenytoin metabolism and increases its potential for toxicity. In humans, there is the unexplained possibility of sudden death if chlorpromazine is used concurrently with phenylpropanolamine. Tricyclic antidepressants, e.g., amitriptyline, may intensify the sedative and anticholinergic effects of chlorpromazine. Also see **ACEPROMAZINE.**

SUPPLIED AS: HUMAN PRODUCTS
Tablets containing 10, 25, 50, 100, and 200 mg [Thorazine]
Capsules (extended-release) containing 30, 75, 150, 200, and 300 mg [Thorazine Spanule]
Oral solutions available as 2, 30, 40, and 100 mg/mL
For injection containing 25 mg/mL
Rectal suppositories in 25- and 100-mg strengths

OTHER USES: Chlorpromazine raises the threshold for ventricular ectopia and may be used to protect the heart from arrhythmias. The drug also has been used as adjunct therapy in the management of pulmonary edema by its effect in decreasing venous return. In addition, chlorpromazine has been used in the treatment of feline infectious anemia (*Hemobartonella felis*), where it is believed that the drug affects erythrocyte permeability and facilitates detachment of *H. felis* from the erythrocyte membrane.

CHLORPROPAMIDE

INDICATIONS: Chlorpropamide (Diabinese ♣ ★) is an oral hypo-glycemic agent used in humans in the management of diabetes mellitus. In small animals, it has been used in the treatment of partial diabetes insipidus, where it potentiates the effect of antidiuretic hormone at the renal tubules and reduces polyuria. The efficacy in canine diabetes insipidus has been variable, with a 20% to 50% reduction in urine output reported by some and no reduction in output reported by others. The drug has been used successfully in a cat with central diabetes insipidus to control urine output. A positive response may require several consecutive days of therapy.

ADVERSE AND COMMON SIDE EFFECTS: Hypoglycemia is the most common expected side effect. Other side effects are not well documented in small animals. In humans, anorexia, drowsiness, weakness, diarrhea, and jaundice have been reported, as have anemia, leukopenia, and thrombocytopenia.

DRUG INTERACTIONS: Chloramphenicol, phenylbutazone, the salicylates, sulfonamides, and ammonium chloride may potentiate the hypoglycemic effects of chlorpropamide if given concurrently. Thiazide diuretics, sodium bicarbonate, and β-blocking agents (propranolol, atenolol) may decrease the hypoglycemic effects of chlorpropamide. The hyperglycemic actions of diazoxide may be antagonized by the concurrent use of chlorpropamide.

SUPPLIED AS: HUMAN PRODUCT
Tablets containing 100 and 250 mg

CIMETIDINE

INDICATIONS: Cimetidine (Tagamet ♣ ★), a histamine (H_2)-blocking agent, reduces gastric acid secretion and is useful in the management of gastric and duodenal ulceration associated with renal failure, liver disease, mast cell tumor, and gastrinoma. It is less effective than antacids in the treatment of acute gastrointestinal bleeding because it impairs the secretory capacity of the gastric mucosa and decreases bicarbonate concentrations. However, some researchers state that the drug also may increase luminal bicarbonate secretion, increase mucus production, and increase mucosal blood flow. Histamine (H_2) antagonists are not effective in preventing NSAID-induced gastric ulceration. The drug has been recommended to help prevent gastrointestinal side effects of corticosteroids. Cimetidine may be beneficial in cases of esophagitis and gastroesophageal reflux, where it increases caudal esophageal sphincter tone and promotes gastric emptying. In uremic dogs, cimetidine decreases the secretion of parathyroid hormone, decreases bone resorption and serum phosphate levels, and increases serum calcium levels.

ADVERSE AND COMMON SIDE EFFECTS: Adverse effects in small animals appear rare. In humans, confusion, headache, gynecomastia, and, rarely, agranulocytosis may occur. Pain at the injection site may occur. The drug should not be used in animals with significantly impaired renal or hepatic function. Histamine enhances cardiac automaticity; cimetidine blocks histamine and may cause bradycardia, hypotension, and cardiac arrest. Cimetidine has been implicated as a cause of infertility in human men (decreased sperm counts, loss of libido, decreased plasma testosterone).

DRUG INTERACTIONS: By interfering with hepatic microenzyme systems, cimetidine decreases the metabolism of many drugs, including warfarin-type anticoagulants, phenytoin, theophylline, digitoxin, and diazepam, resulting in delayed excretion. Ketoconazole concentrations are decreased if the drugs are used concurrently because ketoconazole requires adequate stomach acidity for maximal oral absorption. Propranolol, lidocaine, and morphine plasma concentrations are increased, associated with decreased metabolism caused by cimetidine-induced decreased hepatic blood flow. Tetracycline, erythromycin, penicillin G, and procainamide plasma concentrations also are increased because of better oral absorption in a stomach with lower acidity (tetracycline, erythromycin, penicillin G) and because of competitive inhibition of renal tubular secretion (procainamide). Antacids may reduce GI absorption of cimetidine and, if used, should be given no less than 1 hour before or after cimetidine. Because sucralfate can absorb drugs, it is recommended that cimetidine be given parenterally or that dosage times be staggered by approximately 2 hours. Cardiac toxicity is increased with the infusion of lidocaine.

SUPPLIED AS: HUMAN PRODUCTS
Tablets containing 200, 300, 400, 600, and 800 mg
Oral solution containing 60 mg/mL
For injection containing 150 mg/mL or premixed bag containing 300 mg cimetidine in 50 mL 0.9% saline

OTHER USES
Dogs

IMMUNOMODULATOR
10 to 25 mg bid; PO
It enhances cell-mediated immunity and suppresses T suppressor cell function and has been used in conjunction with antibiotics in dogs with chronic pyoderma and other recurrent infectious dermatoses.

PANCREATIC EXOCRINE INSUFFICIENCY
5 to 10 mg/kg tid–qid; PO 30 minutes preprandially to reduce gastric acid destruction of pancreatic enzyme preparations

RENAL FAILURE/VOMITING
5 to 10 mg/kg bid–qid; IV, PO

CIPROFLOXACIN

INDICATIONS: Ciprofloxacin (Cipro ✦ ★) is a fluoroquinolone antibiotic with activity against *E. coli, Klebsiella, Proteus, Pseudomonas, Staphylococcus, Salmonella, Shigella, Yersinia, Campylobacter,* and *Vibrio* species. It has little activity against anaerobic cocci or clostridia or *Bacteroides* organisms. The fluoroquinolone antibiotics are indicated in the treatment of genitourinary tract infections, including prostatitis, severe bacterial gastroenteritis, and infections of the respiratory tract and external auditory canal. In humans, ciprofloxacin is a preferred drug in the treatment of prostatitis. See also **FLUORO-QUINOLONE ANTIBIOTICS.**

ADVERSE AND COMMON SIDE EFFECTS: See **FLUORO-QUINOLONE ANTIBIOTICS.**

DRUG INTERACTIONS: Absorption is hindered by antacid preparations. The concomitant use of theophylline and ciprofloxacin increases the plasma concentration of theophylline. See **FLUORO-QUINOLONE ANTIBIOTICS.**

SUPPLIED AS: HUMAN PRODUCT
Tablets containing 250, 500, and 750 mg
For injection containing 200 mg/20 mL, 400 mg/40 mL, and 1,200 mg/120 mL in dextrose and vials of 20 and 40 mL containing 10 mg ciprofloxacin
Note: For IV use, dilute to concentration of 1 to 2 mg/mL.

CISAPRIDE

INDICATIONS: Cisapride (Prepulsid ✦, Propulsid ★) is chemically related to metoclopramide and may be useful in small animals in cases of gastroesophageal reflux and to stimulate GI motility in cases of primary motility disorders. It stimulates GI motility by increasing acetylcholine release. The drug increases lower esophageal pressure and lower esophageal peristalsis (in those species in which the distal esophageal muscularis is composed of smooth muscle, e.g., cat; the dog esophagus is composed entirely of striated muscle and would not be expected to respond to the drug at this level), accelerates gastric emptying, and enhances small intestinal and colonic activity. In small animals, the drug may be useful in the management of regurgitation associated with idiopathic megaesophagus, gastroparesis, idiopathic megacolon in cats (along with a stool softener and a fiber-augmented diet), gastroesophageal reflux, and postoperative ileus. It has only weak antiemetic properties. The drug generally is given 15 minutes before a meal.

ADVERSE AND COMMON SIDE EFFECTS: A single oral dose of 640 mg/kg is lethal to dogs. Signs of acute toxicosis include diarrhea, dyspnea, ptosis, tremors, loss of righting reflex, hypotonia, catalepsy, and convulsions. Use of the drug is contraindicated in those with GI hemorrhage, obstruction, or perforation.

DRUG INTERACTIONS: Because cisapride increases gastric emptying, absorption of drugs from the stomach may be decreased whereas absorption from the small bowel may be increased. Coagulation times of anticoagulant drugs may be increased if cisapride is used concurrently. The sedative effects of benzodiazepines may be enhanced. Concurrent use of cimetidine or ranitidine increases the bioavailability of cisapride. Concurrent use of anticholinergic agents, e.g., atropine, aminopentamide, and isopropamide, antagonize the beneficial effects of cisapride on the GIT.

SUPPLIED AS: HUMAN PRODUCT
Tablets containing 5, 10, and 20 mg

OTHER USES
Dogs
DELAYED GASTRIC EMPTYING
0.5 to 1.0 mg/kg

Cats
IDIOPATHIC CONSTIPATION
2.5 mg bid–tid; PO

CISPLATIN

INDICATIONS: Cisplatin (Platinol ✳ ★) is a chemotherapeutic agent that as a single agent has modest efficacy in the treatment of some adenocarcinomas, squamous cell carcinomas, and osteosarcomas. It is a reasonable choice for palliation in patients with nonresectable carcinoma or metastatic osteosarcoma and has been used in the treatment of transitional cell carcinoma of the bladder. However, in the case of transitional cell carcinoma and even at higher dosages (60 mg/m^2), none of the dogs treated achieved complete remission, suggesting that a more effective approach should be sought. Recent reports suggest that dogs treated with cisplatin alone after amputation for osteosarcoma have increased survival times. Intracavitary cisplatin chemotherapy has been used in dogs with pleural or abdominal effusion associated with neoplasia of the thoracic cavity (mesotheliomas and carcinomatosis of unknown origin). Its use resulted in rapid resolution of the effusion in five of six dogs treated.

ADVERSE AND COMMON SIDE EFFECTS: The principal side effects of cisplatin are gastrointestinal upset, nephrotoxicity, bone marrow suppression, and ototoxicity. Transient vomiting is the most common side effect reported in dogs. Dogs that receive butorphanol (0.4 mg/kg; IM) immediately after cisplatin therapy are much less likely to vomit. Anorexia and diarrhea also may occur, and seizure activity has been reported. Mild granulocytopenia and thrombocytopenia have been documented. Saline (0.9%) diuresis (18.3 mL/kg/hour over a 4-hour period) before and after (same rate for 2 hours) use of the drug is recommended to decrease the incidence of renal pathology. Several protocols involving the use of saline diuresis have been proposed, the most effective of which has not been determined. Concurrent administration of methimazole (40 mg/kg; IV over 1 minute) has been found to decrease the incidence of renal toxicity of cisplatin. Intravenous sodium thiosulfate delivered during and after intracavitary cisplatin administration has been recommended in humans to protect against renal toxicosis. The incidence of cisplatin-induced renal toxicosis is decreased if the drug is administered in the latter part of the afternoon as opposed to the morning. The concurrent use of mannitol appears to do little to further limit renal toxicity and does not appear to be required. Carboplatin, a second-generation platinum compound, is less nephrotoxic and does not require saline diuresis. Intracavitary cisplatin (50 mg/m^2 every 4 weeks), however, was not associated with toxicity in the dog. Cisplatin is quite toxic to cats. Its use has led to dose-related pulmonary edema, dyspnea, and death in this species. The drug should not be used in patients with renal disease or myelosuppression. Complete blood counts should be monitored on a weekly basis when the low-dose regimen is used and before therapy if the monthly high dose regimen is chosen. Reduction of dosage is recommended if the leukocyte count or platelet count significantly decreases or if serum creatinine or urea nitrogen increases. Use of the drug is discontinued if the leukocyte count decreases to less than 3,200/µL, if the platelet count decreases to less than 100,000/µL, or if endogenous creatinine clearance decreases to less than 1.4 mL/minute/kg.

DRUG INTERACTIONS: Concurrent use with aminoglycoside antibiotics, amphotericin B, or furosemide increases the risk of ototoxicity and nephrotoxicity. Serum phenytoin levels are decreased by cisplatin.

SUPPLIED AS: HUMAN PRODUCT
For injection containing 10 mg and 50 mg per vial
and 0.5 mg/mL [Platinol AQ 0.5 mg]
and 1 mg/mL [Platinol AQ 1 mg]

CLAVAMOX

INDICATIONS: Clavamox ✦ ★ (amoxicillin/clavulanate) is an amoxicillin and clavulanic acid combination. This combination increases efficacy against *E. coli*, *Klebsiella*, and *Proteus*. *Pseudomonas* usually is resistant. The drug is indicated in the treatment of skin and soft tissue infections caused by susceptible organisms, including β-lactamase–producing and non-β-lactamase–producing *Staphylococcus aureus* and *Staphylococcus* spp. and *E. coli*. It is useful in the treatment of cystitis, and in cats, the drug combination also is effective against *Pasteurella* spp. Amoxicillin penetrates most body tissues with the exception of the brain and spinal fluid, where entry occurs only if the meninges are inflamed. For additional information, see **PENICILLIN ANTIBIOTICS.**

ADVERSE AND COMMON SIDE EFFECTS: The drug combination is contraindicated in animals with sensitivity to the penicillins or the cephalosporin antibiotics. Also see **PENICILLIN ANTIBIOTICS.**

DRUG INTERACTIONS: See **PENICILLIN ANTIBIOTICS.**

SUPPLIED AS: VETERINARY PRODUCTS
Tablets containing 62.5, 125, 250, and 375 mg amoxicillin and 12.5, 25, 50, and 75 mg clavulanic acid, respectively
Oral suspension containing amoxicillin 50 mg/mL and clavulanic acid 12.5 mg/mL

CLEMASTINE

INDICATIONS: Clemastine (Tavist ✦ ★), an antihistamine, has been used in dogs and cats to control chronic pruritus. It is the most effective antihistamine for the control of pruritus tested to date.

ADVERSE AND COMMON SIDE EFFECTS and **DRUG INTERACTIONS:** See **ANTIHISTAMINES.**

SUPPLIED AS: HUMAN PRODUCTS
Tablets containing 1 and 2 mg
Syrup containing 5,000 µg/5 mL

CLINDAMYCIN

INDICATIONS: Clindamycin (Antirobe ✦ ★, Cleocin ★) is a lincosamide antibiotic with activity against gram-positive cocci (staphylococci and streptococci). It often is effective against gram-positive organisms that are resistant to penicillin and the cephalosporins. The drug also may be effective against *Salmonella*, *Pseudomonas*, *Klebsiella*, *Pasteurella*, *Actinomyces*, *Nocardia*, *Mycoplasma*, and *Toxoplasma* organisms, *Neospora caninum*, and anaerobic bacteria (*Bacteroides fragilis*, fusobacteria, *Propionibacterium*, eubacterium, actinomyces species, peptostreptococci, *Clostridium perfringens*) and possibly *Babesia canis* infections. It has greater activity than lincomycin but is more expensive. The drug is distributed extensively in most body tissues, and it appears that clindamycin may penetrate the CSF and ocular tissue if inflammation is present.

ADVERSE AND COMMON SIDE EFFECTS: Adverse effects may include vomiting and diarrhea (sometimes hemorrhagic) after oral use of the drug. Intramuscular injection may cause local pain. Clindamycin dosage should be reduced or the drug avoided in animals with hepatic insufficiency or cholestasis. The drug also should be used with caution in animals with renal impairment. Transient vomiting occasionally is induced by the drug in cats during the first few days of therapy. Vomiting is controlled by stopping the drug for 24 hours and then reintroducing it at a lower dosage, gradually increasing it to 25 mg/kg. Small bowel diarrhea occurs in some cats. It tends to resolve within 1 week after therapy. Caution is advised by the manufacturer if the drug is used in atopic animals. The safety of its use in pregnant and breeding animals has not been established.

DRUG INTERACTIONS: Clindamycin may potentiate the effects of neuromuscular-blocking agents (e.g., atracurium, tubocurarine, pancuronium) during anesthesia. Mutual antagonism is expected if erythromycin or chloramphenicol are used with clindamycin. Diphenoxylate [Lomotil] and the opiates, e.g., paregoric, may reduce the rate (not the extent of absorption) of clindamycin and prolong diarrhea if present.

SUPPLIED AS: VETERINARY PRODUCTS
Capsules containing 25, 75, and 150 mg
Oral solution containing 25 mg/mL

OTHER USES
Dogs
NEOSPORA CANINUM
13.5 mg/kg tid; PO

BABESIA CANIS
10 mg/kg tid; PO for 2 weeks with imidocarb dipropionate at 5 mg/kg; IM

CLONAZEPAM

INDICATIONS: Clonazepam (Klonopin ★, Rivotril ♣) is a benzodiazepine drug that is potentially useful in the management of status epilepticus. It should not, however, be considered a major anticonvulsant in the dog. Clonazepam may be used in conjunction with phenobarbital in the management of intractable epilepsy. Peak serum concentrations are reached within 3 hours.

ADVERSE AND COMMON SIDE EFFECTS: Ataxia and sedation occur at higher doses. Vomiting and pronounced ataxia were noted in dogs at doses of 0.2 mg/kg; IV. Other side effects noted in humans include bradycardia, dry mouth, anorexia, nausea, increased appetite, constipation, diarrhea, dysuria, urinary retention, dyspnea, hepatomegaly, leukopenia, anemia, and thrombocytopenia. Tolerance develops after a 3- to 9-month period.

DRUG INTERACTIONS: Cimetidine may increase the pharmacologic effects of clonazepam.

SUPPLIED AS: HUMAN PRODUCTS
Tablets containing 500 μg and 2 mg [Rivotril]
Tablets containing 0.5, 1, and 2 mg [Klonopin]

CLORAZEPATE

INDICATIONS: Clorazepate (Tranxene ♣ ★) is an anxiolytic, sedative benzodiazepine that has been used in the management of behavioral problems in dogs, e.g., anxiety and noise phobia. It also may prove useful as a secondary anticonvulsant in the management of refractory canine epilepsy in conjunction with phenobarbital.

ADVERSE AND COMMON SIDE EFFECTS: The drug is contraindicated in myasthenia gravis. In one study in dogs, mild and transient sedation and ataxia were noted only infrequently and did not recur on additional dosing. In humans, drowsiness, ataxia, paradoxical excitement, GI disturbances, hypotension, and blood dyscrasias have been reported. Safe use during pregnancy has not been established.

DRUG INTERACTIONS: Antacids delay absorption of the drug. Cimetidine may increase the pharmacologic effects of clonazepam.

SUPPLIED AS: HUMAN PRODUCT
Capsules containing 3.75, 7.5, and 15 mg

CLOTRIMAZOLE

INDICATIONS: Clotrimazole (Canesten ✦, Lotrimin ★, Mycelex ★)
is a topical imidazole useful in the treatment of localized dermatophytosis and candidal stomatitis in small animals. It also has been
used successfully in the topical treatment of nasal aspergillosis in
dogs where the drug is infused through tubes surgically implanted
by trephination into the frontal sinuses. For detailed information
concerning its use for the treatment of nasal aspergillosis, the reader
is referred to Kirk's Current Veterinary Therapy XII, page 899.

ADVERSE AND COMMON SIDE EFFECTS: Local irritation may
occur in some patients. Mild subcutaneous emphysema and inflammation associated with placement of the infusion tubes occurs in
some dogs.

DRUG INTERACTIONS: None.

SUPPLIED AS: HUMAN PRODUCTS
Topical cream containing 10 mg/g (1%) [Canesten, Lotrimin,
Mycelex]
Topical solution containing 10 mg/mL [Canesten, Lotrimin,
Mycelex]
Topical lotion containing 10 mg/g (1%) [Lotrimin]

OTHER USES
Dogs
NASAL ASPERGILLOSIS
One gram of clotrimazole is suspended in 100 mL polyethylene glycol. Trephine nasal cavity and frontal sinuses, and insert feeding
tubes. Pack back of nasopharynx with gauze to prevent spillage.
Flush with saline and then with dilute iodine solution. Instill clotrimazole over the course of 1 hour. Complete procedure by flushing
with saline, and suture skin holes.

CLOXACILLIN

INDICATIONS: Cloxacillin (Cloxapen ★, Orbenin ✦, Tegopen ✦ ★)
is a penicillin antibiotic used primarily against gram-positive, β-lactamase–producing bacteria, especially staphylococcal spp. For further information, see **PENICILLIN ANTIBIOTICS.**

ADVERSE AND COMMON SIDE EFFECTS and **DRUG INTER-
ACTIONS:** See **PENICILLIN ANTIBIOTICS.**

SUPPLIED AS: HUMAN PRODUCTS
Capsules containing 250 and 500 mg [Cloxapen, Orbenin]
Oral suspension containing 125 mg/5 mL [Orbenin, Tegopen]
For injection containing 250, 500, and 2,000 mg of base [Orbenin, Tegopen]

COAL TAR

INDICATIONS: Coal tar shampoos are keratolytic and keratoplastic. They are used in the treatment of seborrhea, to relieve pruritus, and to remove crusts and scales. Coal tar is found alone or in combination with other agents in the following products: Micro-Pearls Coal Tar ★, Mycodex Tar and Sulfur ★, Lytar ✦ ★, and Allerseb T ✦ ★.

ADVERSE AND COMMON SIDE EFFECTS: Coal tar shampoos may be irritating. Reduce frequency of use or discontinue if this occurs. These products may be toxic to cats and should not be used in this species.

DRUG INTERACTIONS: None.

SUPPLIED AS: See specific product.

CODEINE

INDICATIONS: Codeine (Methylmorphine ★, Paveral ✦, Tylenol No. 1 ✦) often is used in the management of mild to moderate pain. It is only 10% as potent an analgesic as morphine sulfate. It also is useful as an antidiarrheal agent and as an antitussive.

ADVERSE AND COMMON SIDE EFFECTS: Drowsiness, nausea, ileus, vomiting, and constipation may occur with its use. Its use is contraindicated in liver disease, intestinal obstruction, and invasive or toxigenic bowel disease. Spasm of the biliary and pancreatic ducts can occur. The respiratory depressant effects and the capacity to increase CSF pressure may be exacerbated in cases of head injury. Use of the drug is cautioned in patients with a history of seizure or cardiac arrhythmias. In cats, opiate agonists may cause CNS excitation with hyperexcitability, tremors, and seizure activity.

DRUG INTERACTIONS: The concurrent use of barbiturates, phenothiazines, and other CNS depressants potentiate CNS depression.

SUPPLIED AS: HUMAN PRODUCTS
Oral suspension containing 10 mg/mL [Paveral]

For injection containing 30 and 60 mg codeine phosphate
Caplets containing 8 mg (#1), 15 mg (#2), 30 mg (#3), and 60 mg (#4)
codeine with acetaminophen and caffeine [Tylenol with codeine]
Elixir containing 8 mg/5 mL codeine with acetaminophen [Tylenol
with codeine elixir]
Tablets containing 15, 30, and 60 mg codeine phosphate

COLCHICINE

INDICATIONS: Colchicine (generic products ✤ ★) has been recommended in the treatment of chronic hepatic fibrosis in the dog. The
drug works by decreasing collagen formation and promoting its
breakdown. Its anti-inflammatory properties are mediated by the
drug's inhibition of mononuclear cell and neutrophil migration.
Colchicine also may have hepatoprotective effects by stabilizing he-
patocyte plasma membranes and restoring hepatic enzyme activities. It also has been used in the treatment of amyloidosis. In this
condition, the drug impairs the release of serum amyloid A (SAA)
from hepatocytes, prevents the production of amyloid-enhancing
factor, and delays tissue deposition of amyloid. Because of the advanced state in which veterinary patients present, colchicine is unlikely to benefit those with amyloidosis.

ADVERSE AND COMMON SIDE EFFECTS: Reports of its use in
dogs are scant; however, no toxicity was observed in a dog treated
with the drug over a 7-month period at a dose of 0.03 mg/kg/day. In
humans, nausea, vomiting, and diarrhea are most common. Muscular weakness, hematuria, oliguria, agranulocytosis, and anemia also
have been reported with chronic use. Use of the drug is contraindicated in patients with serious GIT, renal, or cardiac disease. It is not
recommended for use in breeding or pregnant animals.

DRUG INTERACTIONS: Colchicine action is inhibited by acidifying agents and potentiated by alkalinizing agents.

SUPPLIED AS: HUMAN PRODUCT
Tablets containing 0.5, 0.6, and 1 mg colchicine

CYCLOPHOSPHAMIDE

INDICATIONS: Cyclophosphamide (Cytoxan ✤ ★, Procytox ✤) is
an alkylating agent with potent immunosuppressive properties and
has been used in small animals in the treatment of lymphosarcoma,
hemangiosarcoma, mammary gland carcinoma, mastocytoma,
transmissible venereal tumor, bladder carcinoma, macroglobulinemia, multiple myeloma, and autoimmune diseases not responsive

to other immunosuppressive agents, including autoimmune skin diseases, immune-mediated arthritis, lymphocytic–plasmacytic enteritis, autoimmune anemia, thrombocytopenia, and polymyositis. The drug impairs B- and T-cell responses and suppresses macrophage function and thus, inflammation. However, short-term use (1 week) of the drug does not affect the humoral or cell-mediated immune response. A beneficial clinical response may take 1 to 4 weeks.

ADVERSE AND COMMON SIDE EFFECTS: Bone marrow depression, hemorrhagic cystitis (especially if therapy exceeds 2 months), and an association with the induction of transitional cell carcinoma of the bladder have been documented. Measures aimed at decreasing the frequency or severity of cystitis have included administering the drug in the morning, encouraging diuresis (promoting increased water intake and the concurrent use of furosemide), administering prednisone on the same day, and intravesicular administration of 50% dimethyl sulfoxide (DMSO), 1% formalin, or acetylcysteine. Chlorambucil may be substituted should adverse effects necessitate discontinuation of the drug. Alkylating agents generally cause leukopenia, thrombocytopenia, and anemia, with the nadir of the leukocyte counts observed 7 to 14 days after treatment and recovery noted in an additional 7 to 14 days. The complete blood count should be monitored weekly for the first 2 months and monthly thereafter. Other side effects include GI inflammation causing vomiting, diarrhea, anorexia, depression, infertility, teratogenicity, alopecia (especially in poodles, old English sheepdogs), and altered wound healing. The drug should not be used for more than 4 to 5 months.

DRUG INTERACTIONS: The pharmacologic activity of digoxin may be reduced if the two drugs are used concurrently. Cyclophosphamide inhibits the metabolism of succinylcholine, potentially leading to prolonged neuromuscular-blocking activity. Barbiturate drugs including phenobarbital may increase the rate of cyclophosphamide metabolism via hepatic microsomal enzyme induction. Allopurinol and the thiazide diuretics may potentiate the myelosuppression associated with cyclophosphamide. Cyclophosphamide should be used with caution in patients receiving doxorubicin because potentiation of cardiotoxicity may occur.

SUPPLIED AS: HUMAN PRODUCTS
Tablets containing 25 or 50 mg
For injection containing either 500-, 1,000-, and 2,000-mg base lyophilized in mannitol or 100 and 200 mg nonlyophilized with sodium chloride

CYCLOSPORINE

INDICATIONS: Cyclosporine (Sandimmune ✦ ★, Optimmune ✦ ★) is an effective immunosuppressant agent. It inhibits B- and T-lymphocyte activation. It exerts its major effect on helper T cells by blocking the release of interleukin-2. Cyclosporine may be useful in the management of autoimmune disease, in perianal fistulae, and to block rejection of organ and tissue transplants. A recent study failed to demonstrate beneficial effects of the drug in dogs with glomerulonephritis. Susceptibility to infection appears to be less common than that observed with common immunosuppressive agents. A 0.2% solution (Optimmune ✦ ★) is quite effective in the treatment of dogs with keratoconjunctivitis sicca. Causes varied, but tear production improved and corneal pigmentation decreased. The drug appears to inhibit T cells within the lacrimal gland from secreting inflammatory mediators that damage lacrimal acini. Lacrimation increases, and superficial pigmentation, vascularization, and granulation decrease. Days to weeks may be required before ocular improvement is noted.

ADVERSE AND COMMON SIDE EFFECTS: In dogs, vomiting, diarrhea, anorexia, gingival hyperplasia, pyoderma, predisposition to infection, and papillomatosis have been reported. These adverse effects tend to abate when the dosage of the drug is decreased. The incidence of nephrotoxicity and hepatotoxicity in dogs appears to be less than that observed in humans and has not been demonstrated in cats. Many cats find the oral solution unpalatable, resulting in ptyalism and head shaking. Intravenous administration causes acute anaphylactoid reactions in a high percentage of dogs. Use of the ophthalmic preparation may be associated with local irritation with periocular redness, blepharospasm, and excessive rubbing. Expense and systemic toxicity may limit the use of the systemic drug in veterinary medicine.

DRUG INTERACTIONS: Gentamicin, amphotericin B, and melphalan may potentiate cyclosporine nephrotoxicity. Ketoconazole, erythromycin, and cimetidine depress hepatic metabolism of cyclosporine. Phenobarbital and phenytoin increase hepatic metabolism of cyclosporine and result in lower than anticipated blood levels.

SUPPLIED AS: HUMAN PRODUCTS
Capsules containing 25, 50, and 100 mg
Oral solution containing 100 mg/mL
Solutions for IV injection are **NOT** recommended

VETERINARY PRODUCT
Optimmune as an ointment

OTHER USES
Dogs
KERATOCONJUNCTIVITIS SICCA
Applied topically; bid
PERIANAL FISTULAE
3 to 5 mg/kg bid; PO continued for 2 weeks beyond clinical remission (not less than 8 weeks; average treatment duration 16 weeks)

CYPROHEPTADINE

INDICATIONS: Cyproheptadine (Periactin ♣ ★) is an antihistamine–antiserotonin, and acetylcholine antagonist. The drug has been used to stimulate appetite in cats (it may not be effective in dogs). Cyproheptadine may be useful in the management of bronchospasm associated with allergic airway disease in cats. It also has been used with limited success in the treatment of pituitary-dependent hyperadrenocorticism in dogs. It is ineffective in the management of allergic pruritus.

ADVERSE AND COMMON SIDE EFFECTS: Excitability and aggressive behavior have been documented in some cats. Other adverse effects sometimes noted in people include nausea, vomiting, jaundice, and drowsiness. The drug is contraindicated in patients with glaucoma, pyloric or duodenal obstruction, urinary retention, and acute asthma.

DRUG INTERACTIONS: Monoamine oxidase inhibitors, possibly amitraz and selegiline, prolong and intensify the anticholinergic effects of the drug. Central nervous system depressant drugs may have an additive effect if used concurrently with cyproheptadine.

SUPPLIED AS: HUMAN PRODUCTS
Tablets containing 4 mg
Syrup containing 2 mg/5 mL

OTHER USES
Dogs
PITUITARY-DEPENDENT HYPERADRENOCORTICISM
0.3 to 3.0 mg/kg daily for 4 to 27 weeks (8 of 10 dogs failed to improve)

CYTARABINE

INDICATIONS: Cytarabine (Cytosar ♣, Cytosar-U ★) is a chemotherapeutic agent that has been used in the treatment of lymphoreticular neoplasms, mastocytoma, and myeloproliferative disease. It also has been injected intrathecally in the treatment of lymphoma involving the CNS.

ADVERSE AND COMMON SIDE EFFECTS: Nausea, vomiting, diarrhea, and, rarely, anaphylaxis have been reported. Bone marrow suppression (nadir at 5–7 days, recovery at 7–14 days), oral ulceration, hepatotoxicity, and fever also may occur. The drug is potentially teratogenic and embryotoxic.

DRUG INTERACTIONS: Cytarabine may decrease the amount of orally administered digoxin, an effect that may persist for several days after discontinuation of cytarabine. Cytarabine may decrease the efficacy of gentamicin and flucytosine.

SUPPLIED AS: HUMAN PRODUCT
For injection containing 100- and 200-mg and 1- and 2-g vials

CYTHIOATE

INDICATIONS: Cythioate (Proban ♣ ★) is an organophosphate compound indicated in dogs and cats to control fleas. The drug also has significant activity against ticks and demodectic mites. Fleas must ingest the drug and, because it is the flea saliva that is allergenic, sensitive animals remain pruritic.

ADVERSE AND COMMON SIDE EFFECTS: There is a wide margin of safety with the use of the drug. This drug should not be used in greyhounds or animals that are sick, pregnant, or anemic. Cythioate is a cholinesterase inhibitor. With drug overdose, muscular tremor, hyperexcitability, vomiting, diarrhea, anorexia, and salivation occur. Atropine is antidotal (0.22 mg/kg; IM at 15- to 30-minute intervals).

DRUG INTERACTIONS: See ORGANOPHOSPHATES.

SUPPLIED AS: VETERINARY PRODUCT
Tablets containing 30 mg
Oral liquid containing 1.6%

DACARBAZINE

INDICATIONS: Dacarbazine (DTIC ♣ ★) is a chemotherapeutic agent with alkylating and antimetabolite properties. It has been used primarily in the treatment of lymphoreticular neoplasms.

ADVERSE AND COMMON SIDE EFFECTS: Nausea, anorexia, vomiting, diarrhea, and cytopenia have been reported. A burning sensation may occur when injected intravenously, and extravascular injection may cause tissue damage and severe pain. Anaphylaxis has been reported in some patients. Delayed toxicity may cause alopecia, photosensitivity, and renal and hepatic impairment.

DRUG INTERACTIONS: None reported.

SUPPLIED AS: HUMAN PRODUCT
For injection in vials containing 100 and 200 mg

DACTINOMYCIN

INDICATIONS: Dactinomycin, or actinomycin-D (Cosmegen ♣ ★), is a potent antibiotic used in the treatment of bone and soft tissue sarcomas, anal sac adenocarcinoma, perianal adenocarcinoma, squamous cell carcinoma, thyroid carcinoma, transitional cell carcinoma, lymphoma, and malignant melanomas. It has been recommended as a rescue drug for dogs with lymphoma after traditional combination chemotherapy studies have failed to demonstrate a beneficial effect.

ADVERSE AND COMMON SIDE EFFECTS: In dogs, GI (anorexia, vomiting, diarrhea) and hematologic (thrombocytopenia, neutropenia) toxicity are reported. At this point, no toxicity has been documented in the limited number of cats on which the drug has been used. Dactinomycin is contraindicated in patients with viral infections, and use is cautioned in patients that have had radiation therapy within the past 3 to 6 weeks, bone marrow suppression, infections, obesity, and renal or hepatic impairment.

DRUG INTERACTIONS: Dactinomycin may cause elevations in uric acid levels if used concurrently with allopurinol. Potentiation of myelosuppression may occur if the drug is used concurrently with other myelosuppressive agents. Radiation may potentiate the effects of dactinomycin and vice versa. Dactinomycin decreases vitamin K effects, leading to prolonged clotting time and potential hemorrhage.

SUPPLIED AS: HUMAN PRODUCT
For injection containing 500 µg/vial

DANAZOL

INDICATIONS: Danazol (Danocrine ★, Cyclomen ♣) is a modified androgen. It has been shown to be effective in the treatment of canine immune-mediated thrombocytopenia and anemia in conjunction with prednisolone or prednisone. When combined with corticosteroids, the immunomodulating effects are synergistic. Response to danazol reduces the need for other therapies and may replace them when remission is achieved. A clinically significant response may not be apparent for 2 to 3 months. A recent study in dogs with autoimmune hemolytic anemia given prednisone and azathioprine failed to show additional benefit when danazol was added to the regimen. Danazol decreases immunoglobulin G production, cell-bound immunoglobulin, and complement. It also modulates the balance between T suppressor and helper cells. The therapeutic effects reportedly are slow. In cases of autoimmune hemolytic anemia (AIHA), elevations in packed cell volume may not be apparent for 1 to 3 weeks. Also see **ANABOLIC STEROIDS.**

ADVERSE AND COMMON SIDE EFFECTS: In humans, side effects are rare but may include virilization and hepatic dysfunction. Hepatopathy also has been documented in dogs.

DRUG INTERACTIONS: None reported.

SUPPLIED AS: HUMAN PRODUCT
Capsules containing 50, 100, and 200 mg

DANTROLENE

INDICATIONS: Dantrolene (Dantrium ✚ ✶) is a skeletal muscle relaxant that may be useful in reducing external urethral sphincter tone in cases of urinary incontinence associated with urethral hypertonia. Dantrolene also is used in the prevention and treatment of malignant hyperthermia.

ADVERSE AND COMMON SIDE EFFECTS: Sedation, nausea, vomiting, constipation, and, possibly, hypotension occur. Drug overdose may cause generalized muscle weakness. Hepatotoxicity has been documented in humans after long-term drug therapy.

DRUG INTERACTIONS: Concurrent use of other CNS depressants may cause additive CNS depression. Use of calcium channel-blocking agents, e.g., verapamil, diltiazem, may predispose to ventricular fibrillation.

SUPPLIED AS: HUMAN PRODUCTS
Capsules containing 25, 50, and 100 mg
For injection containing 20 mg

OTHER USES
Dogs
FUNCTIONAL URETHRAL OBSTRUCTION
i)   1 to 5 mg/kg tid; PO

ii) 3 to 15 mg/kg div. bid–tid; PO

ADJUNCTIVE THERAPY FOR BLACK WIDOW SPIDER BITES
1 mg/kg; IV; followed by 1 mg/kg every 4 hours; PO

Cats
FUNCTIONAL URETHRAL OBSTRUCTION
i)   0.5 to 2 mg/kg tid; PO
ii) 1 mg/kg; PO in conjunction with prazosin (0.03 mg/kg; IV)

DAPSONE

INDICATIONS: Dapsone (Avlosulfon ♣ and generic products ★) is an anti-inflammatory, antibacterial agent that has been used in the dog for treatment of pemphigus foliaceus, dermatitis herpetiformis, sub-corneal pustular dermatosis, leprosy, and leukocytoclastic vasculitis.

ADVERSE AND COMMON SIDE EFFECTS: In dogs, hepatotoxicity, mild anemia and neutropenia, severe thrombocytopenia, GI signs, and skin reactions may occur. Gastrointestinal signs usually can be reduced or eliminated by giving the drug with food. A complete blood count and serum biochemistry should be performed every other week during the first 6 weeks of therapy and reduced in frequency after the dose is reduced.

DRUG INTERACTIONS: Pyrimethamine increases the risk of adverse dapsone-induced hematologic effects. Rifampin lowers dapsone blood levels by increasing plasma clearance. Higher doses of dapsone may be required.

SUPPLIED AS: HUMAN PRODUCT
Tablets containing 25 and 100 mg

DEHYDROCHOLIC ACID

INDICATIONS: Dehydrocholic acid (Atrocholin ★, Dycholium ♣, Decholin ★) is a bile acid that may stimulate flow of watery bile and help alleviate cholestasis. The drug only should be used once a positive diagnosis of biliary sludge or precipitation has been established. Dehydrocholic acid is used until urine is negative for bilirubin. Dehydrocholic acid in conjunction with fluid therapy may improve biliary flow, although it does not hasten the clearance of jaundice. Because biliary sludging and precipitation may be associated with infection, the drug always should be used in conjunction with fluid therapy and antibiotics. There is little evidence that this drug is of benefit in cats with cholestatic disorders. Ursodeoxycholic acid may be more effective.

ADVERSE AND COMMON SIDE EFFECTS: The drug is not to be used in the presence of jaundice, hepatic insufficiency, or cholelithiasis, or in complete mechanical obstruction of the common bile duct. Nausea, vomiting, diarrhea, abdominal discomfort, and dizziness are observed in people.

DRUG INTERACTIONS: None reported.

SUPPLIED AS: HUMAN PRODUCTS
Tablets containing 300 mg [Dycholium]
Tablets containing 130 mg [Atrocholin]
Tablets containing 250 mg [Decholin]

DEMECLOCYCLINE

INDICATIONS: Demeclocycline (Declomycin ♣ ★) is an intermediate-acting tetracycline antibiotic. For more information, see **TETRACYCLINE ANTIBIOTICS.**

ADVERSE AND COMMON SIDE EFFECTS: Demeclocycline has been shown to induce a reversible nephrogenic diabetes insipidus in humans. Experience with the drug in small animals is limited.

DRUG INTERACTIONS: See **TETRACYCLINE ANTIBIOTICS.**

SUPPLIED AS: HUMAN PRODUCTS
Tablets containing 150 and 300 mg
Capsules containing 150 mg

DERM CAPS

INDICATIONS: Derm caps ♣ ★ are a fatty acid nutritional supplement containing eicosapentaenoic, linoleic, and gamma-linolenic acid. It may be of benefit in lessening or eliminating pruritus associated with atopic disease in some dogs. The anti-inflammatory action is likely the result of the decreased production of inflammatory eicosanoids. The drug also has been used to treat idiopathic seborrhea in dogs and may be effective in controlling seborrhea and pruritus in cats. Pruritus was eliminated in 40% of cats with nonlesional pruritus or miliary dermatitis, and approximately 67% of cats with eosinophilic granuloma complex responded favorably to the drug.

ADVERSE AND COMMON SIDE EFFECTS: Side effects are rare. Vomiting, lethargy, diarrhea, urticaria, and increased pruritus have been reported in a few dogs. Although not well documented, these agents may induce pancreatitis in animals predisposed to the disease.

DRUG INTERACTIONS: None reported.

SUPPLIED AS: VETERINARY PRODUCTS
DERM CAPS capsules for small and medium breeds
DERM CAPS ES capsules for medium and large breeds
DERM CAPS ES liquid for medium and large breeds
DERM CAPS liquid for small and medium breeds

OTHER USES
Cats

NONLESIONAL PRURITUS or MILIARY DERMATITIS and
EOSINOPHILIC GRANULOMA COMPLEX
1 mL per 9.1 kg daily; PO for 14 days

DESMOPRESSIN

INDICATIONS: Desmopressin acetate (DDAVP ✦ ★) is a vasopressin
analog used in the management of central diabetes insipidus and type
I von Willebrand's disease [quantitative deficiency of von Willebrand
factor (vWF)]. DDAVP exerts its maximal effect in diabetes insipidus
in 2 to 8 hours, and the duration of activity lasts from 8 to 24 hours. It
causes an increase in factor VIII:C and vWF by stimulating the release
of preformed factor VIII from storage sites. Maximal levels are attained within 30 minutes, but the duration of effect of DDAVP in von
Willebrand's disease is only 2 to 4 hours. Multiple doses of DDAVP
are not effective because release of preformed vWF depletes its storage pool, decreasing subsequent responses. Because not all dogs with
von Willebrand's disease respond to DDAVP, a response test should
be performed in dogs. Buccal mucosal bleeding time and plasma vWF
are measured before and after administration of DDAVP and before
surgical procedures or possible future hemorrhagic events. DDAVP is
not effective in the management of hemophilia A.

ADVERSE AND COMMON SIDE EFFECTS: Side effects in small
animals are rare; however, hypersensitivity reactions and fluid retention leading to hyponatremia are a possibility. At the doses required for hemostasis, adverse effects may include a decrease in
blood pressure, peripheral vasodilation, and tachycardia. German
short-haired pointers (GSHPs) typically have type II von Willebrand's disease, a qualitative vWF disorder, and if this breed reacts
as humans with type II disease do, GSHPs may respond to DDAVP
with platelet aggregation and thrombocytopenia.

DRUG INTERACTIONS: The use of demeclocycline, lithium, or epinephrine may decrease the antidiuretic response. Carbamazepine,
chlorpropamide, and clofibrate may prolong the antidiuretic effect
of desmopressin.

SUPPLIED AS: HUMAN PRODUCTS
For injection in ampules containing 4 µg/mL
For intranasal use containing 10 µg/0.1 mL metered spray and 100 µg/mL as drops*
Tablets containing 0.1 and 0.2 mg

OTHER USES:
Dogs
MODIFIED WATER DEPRIVATION TEST
After the failure to concentrate urine after water deprivation, 2 µg of DDAVP is given subcutaneously or intravenously, or 20 µg (approximately 4 drops of the 100 µg/mL intranasal solution) is given intranasally or conjunctivally. Urine-specific gravity or osmolality are monitored every 2 hours for a total of 6 to 10 hours. Further increases in urine osmolality greater than 10% are supportive of central diabetes insipidus (DI) or partial nephrogenic DI. Increases less than 10% are suggestive of complete nephrogenic DI or psychogenic polydipsia.

DESOXYCORTICOSTERONE

INDICATIONS: Desoxycorticosterone acetate [DOCA (Percorten acetate)] and desoxycorticosterone pivalate [DOCP (Percorten pivalate)] are mineralocorticoid preparations that have been used in the management of hypoadrenocorticism. DOCA (where available) is used in the management of the acute crisis of the disease, and DOCP is used for maintenance therapy.

ADVERSE AND COMMON SIDE EFFECTS: DOCP is well tolerated even at higher than recommended dosages. Hypokalemia, hypernatremia, muscle weakness, and hypertension are reported in some patients.

DRUG INTERACTIONS: None reported.

SUPPLIED AS: VETERINARY PRODUCT
DOCP (25 mg/mL) in 4-mL vials

DEXAMETHASONE

INDICATIONS: Dexamethasone (Azium ♣ ★, Azium SP ♣ ★, Dex-5 ♣) is a glucocorticoid used in the treatment of nonspecific dermatosis and inflammatory conditions involving the joints (in the absence of structural damage). It also is used in the management of hy-

---

* NB: In small animals, conjunctival application is preferred; the injectable form is costly and has a short duration of activity.

drocephalus in toy breeds, as adjunctive therapy in cranial and spinal trauma—including intervertebral disc disease associated with paraparesis, in the reduction of intracerebral pressure and edema, as adjunctive therapy of fibrocartilaginous embolic myopathy, for the treatment of shock, for the management of acute hypoadrenocortical insufficiency, for treatment of acquired thrombocytopenia, and as adjunctive therapy in endotoxemia secondary to gastric dilation-volvulus and cholecalciferol toxicity. Dexamethasone sodium phosphate is used in the diagnosis of hyperadrenocorticism. For further information, see **GLUCOCORTICOID AGENTS.**

ADVERSE AND COMMON SIDE EFFECTS and **DRUG INTERACTIONS:** See GLUCOCORTICOID AGENTS.

SUPPLIED AS: VETERINARY PRODUCTS
For injection containing 2 mg/mL dexamethasone [Azium solution]
For injection containing dexamethasone 21-isonicotinate
1 mg/mL [Voren ★]
For injection containing 4 mg/mL [Azium-SP], 2 mg/mL [Dex-2], and 5 mg/mL [Dex-5] as dexamethasone sodium phosphate
Tablets containing 0.25 mg [Azium, Dextab ♣]

DEXTRANS

INDICATIONS: Dextran 70 (Macrodex ♣ ★) and dextran 40 (Rheomacrodex ♣ ★) are polysaccharide solutions of high molecular weight that are used for plasma volume expansion and the treatment of hypovolemic shock (dextran 70). Dextran 40, with its smaller molecular size, has a greater osmotic effect per gram. Dextran 70 has a particle size similar to that of albumin. The half-lives of both dextrans are approximately 25 hours. Infusion of 1 L of dextran 70 expands plasma volume by 800 mL. Less than 30% of the product is retained within the vascular compartment, leading to a rapid (4–6 hour) dissipation of its initial volume-expanding effect. Infusion of 1 L of 10% dextran 40 in normal saline increases plasma volume by 1,000 mL for approximately 2 to 6 hours. The smaller molecular weight of dextran 40 compared with that of dextran 70 accounts for its shorter duration of vascular volume expansion and its rapid removal from the intravascular compartment.

ADVERSE AND COMMON SIDE EFFECTS: Hypervolemia, hyperviscosity, hemorrhagic diathesis (abnormal platelet function, precipitation of coagulation factors, increased fibrinolytic activity, decrease in vWF), and anaphylaxis are reported. Dextran 70 may exacerbate intravascular erythrocyte sludging. These effects are rare in dogs and usually are the result of too rapid or excessive administration. Dextrans should be used with caution in cases with cardiac decompensation, and with oliguric or anuric renal failure. Dextran 40 has been associated more often with renal failure. Large volumes of dextran may cause a dilutional lowering of plasma protein levels. Dextrans may interfere with cross-matching of blood and cause artifactual increases in serum glucose.

DRUG INTERACTIONS: Rheomacrodex 10% in dextrose should not be given through the same apparatus as blood because globulin precipitation and erythrocyte aggregation may occur. Rheomacrodex in saline is not associated with this problem.

SUPPLIED AS: HUMAN PRODUCTS
Dextran 70:
For injection containing 6 g dextran 70 and 900 mg sodium chloride per 100 mL [Macrodex-Saline]
For injection containing 6 g dextran 70 and 5 g dextrose per 100 mL [Macrodex-Dextrose]

Dextran 40:
For injection containing 10 g dextran 40 and 900 mg saline per 100 mL [Rheomacrodex-Saline]
For injection containing 10 g dextran 40 and 5 g dextrose per 100 mL [Rheomacrodex-Dextrose]

OTHER USES
Dogs
SHOCK
7% saline in 6% dextran 70 at a dosage of 5 mL/kg, given slowly over a 5-minute period; IV, followed by lactated Ringer's solution at a dosage of 20 mL/kg/hour

DEXTROAMPHETAMINE

INDICATIONS: Dextroamphetamine (Dexedrine ♣ ★) is an isomer of amphetamine. In dogs, the drug has been used in the treatment of hyperkinesis and narcolepsy.

ADVERSE AND COMMON SIDE EFFECTS: Amphetamines are potent stimulators of the CNS and the cardiovascular system. The drug is contraindicated in glaucoma, hyperthyroid disease, significant heart disease, or hypertension, or within 14 days of having used an MAO inhibitor, possibly amitraz and selegiline. Side effects may include hyperexcitability, hyperesthesia, tachycardia, hypertension, hyperthermia, panting, mydriasis, vomiting, diarrhea, trembling, and seizures. Amphetamines also have been implicated as a potential cause of thrombocytopenia. Treatment of drug overdose may include diazepam (2.5–20 mg; IV, as needed).

DRUG INTERACTIONS: Ammonium chloride and other urinary acidifiers may reduce the pharmacologic effect of the drug by enhancing urinary excretion. Phenothiazines are mutually antagonistic with amphetamines. Furazolidone increases the risk of dextroamphetamine toxicity from an additive pressor response.

SUPPLIED AS: HUMAN PRODUCTS
Capsules containing 5, 10, and 15 mg
Tablets containing 5 and 10 mg

DEXTROMETHORPHAN

INDICATIONS: Dextromethorphan (Broncho-Grippol-DM ✦, Balminil DM ✦, Benylin DM ✦ ★) is a non-narcotic opiate with antitussive activity equal to that of codeine but is 15 to 20 times less potent than butorphanol.

ADVERSE AND COMMON SIDE EFFECTS: In humans, nausea and drowsiness are infrequent complaints. With large doses, confusion, nervousness, irritability, and excitability may occur.

DRUG INTERACTIONS: Other CNS depressants may potentiate CNS depression.

SUPPLIED AS: HUMAN PRODUCT
Syrup containing 15 mg/5 mL

DIAZEPAM

INDICATIONS: Diazepam (Valium ✦ ★, Valrelease ★) is an effective anticonvulsant for the control of seizure in status epilepticus. For cats with more long-term use of the drug, the recommended therapeutic range for benzodiazepine concentration, measured 2 weeks after the initiation of treatment, is 500 to 700 ng/mL. Because of the development of tolerance, the oral form is less useful as an anticonvulsant. It also is useful in the management of toxicity associated with metaldehyde and methylxanthine (chocolate and caffeine), nicotine, amphetamine, strychnine, chlorinated hydrocarbon, and salicylate poisoning. Diazepam has been used in functional urethral obstruction and in canine and feline behavioral problems, including noise phobias, fear-induced and defensive aggression, destructive behavior, excessive grooming, anxiety, and urine spraying. The drug is useful as adjunctive therapy to promote relaxation in cases with tetanus. The drug also is used as a preanesthetic. Diazepam is used to stimulate appetite. It is more effective in cats than dogs for this purpose, but oxazepam (Serax) actually is even more effective than diazepam in stimulating appetite. Flurazepam (Dalmane) also is an effective appetite stimulant, and it has a longer duration of action. The use of benzodiazepines to stimulate appetite in cats with hepatic disease should be viewed with caution. These drugs require hepatic biotransformation for elimination and produce sedation in addition to appetite stimulation and, finally, a benzodiazepine receptor has been characterized as one of the causal factors in the development of hepatic encephalopathy.

ADVERSE AND COMMON SIDE EFFECTS: The benzodiazepines generally are safe drugs. They have minimal cardiopulmonary effects and are short-acting. Dose-related sedation, ataxia, excitement, and sometimes paradoxical aggression may occur. The benzodiazepines should not be used for more than 2 days to stimulate appetite. Acute fulminant hepatic necrosis has been associated with the ingestion of 1.25 to 2 mg once or twice daily in cats. Many cats became lethargic, ataxic, anorectic, and jaundiced within 96 hours of administration. Death may ensue. An idiosyncratic drug reaction is suspected. The authors recommend baseline serum ALT and AST be completed before and within 5 days of initiation of diazepam treatment.

DRUG INTERACTIONS: Metabolism may be decreased and excessive sedation may occur if diazepam is given with cimetidine, erythromycin, ketoconazole, or propranolol. Additive CNS effects may be anticipated if diazepam is given with barbiturates, narcotics, or anesthetics. Antacids may slow the rate of drug absorption. The pharmacologic effects of digoxin may be potentiated. Rifampin may induce hepatic microsomal enzyme activity and decrease the efficacy of diazepam. An increase in the duration and intensity of respiratory depression may occur if diazepam is used with pancuronium or succinylcholine.

SUPPLIED AS: HUMAN PRODUCTS
Tablets containing 2, 5, and 10 mg
Timed-release tablets containing 15 mg [Valrelease]
Oral solution containing 1 mg/mL in 500-mL containers [PMS-Diazepam ✦] and unit dose (5 and 10 mg) 5 mg/mL in 30-mL dropper bottles [Diazepam Intensol ★]
For injection containing 5 mg/mL

OTHER USES
Dogs
SCOTTY CRAMP
0.5 to 2 mg/kg to effect; IV, or tid; PO
It decreases the clinical signs associated with the disease and its recurrence.

WHITE DOG SHAKER SYNDROME
0.25 mg/kg tid–qid; PO
It is used to reduce tremors associated with this syndrome.

Cats

URINE SPRAYING

1 to 2 mg bid; PO for an initial 2-week period. If therapy is successful, then this dose is continued for 6 to 8 weeks. After the treatment period, diazepam is reduced gradually, and if spraying does not recur, further treatment is not given. Recurrences are treated at the previous effective dose. If spraying does not subside, the dose is increased to 2 to 3 mg bid; PO for an additional 2-week trial period. For cats that respond to the increased dose, treatment is continued for 6 to 8 weeks. If cats still spray urine at this dose, diazepam is decreased gradually over the next 2 weeks and then discontinued. It is reported that a better response can be expected from female cats with diazepam (approximately 50% of cats respond) than with progestins (approximately 20% of cats respond), whereas the response of male cats is approximately the same for both drugs (approximately 50% of cats respond).

DIAZOXIDE

INDICATIONS: Diazoxide (Proglycem ✦ ★) is an antihypertensive agent. In dogs, it has been used for the management of hypoglycemia associated with islet cell tumors (insulinomas). It inhibits pancreatic insulin secretion, enhances epinephrine-induced glycogenolysis, and inhibits peripheral glucose use.

ADVERSE AND COMMON SIDE EFFECTS: Side effects primarily are anorexia, vomiting, and diarrhea. Other possible side effects include diabetes mellitus, anemia, agranulocytosis, thrombocytopenia, sodium and fluid retention, and cardiac arrhythmias.

DRUG INTERACTIONS: Diazoxide in conjunction with frequent small meals and prednisone (1 mg/kg/day div.) transiently controls hypoglycemia in most dogs with islet cell neoplasia. Hydrochlorothiazide (2–4 mg/kg/day) may potentiate the hyperglycemic effects of diazoxide if diazoxide alone is not effective. Phenothiazines may enhance the hyperglycemic effects. Diazoxide may increase the metabolism or decrease the protein binding of phenytoin, and the risk of hyperglycemia may be increased when these two drugs are used concurrently. Diazoxide may potentiate the hypotensive effects of other hypotensive agents, e.g., hydralazine and prazosin.

SUPPLIED AS: HUMAN PRODUCTS
Capsules containing 50 mg
Oral suspension containing 50 mg/mL

DICHLORPHENAMIDE

INDICATIONS: Dichlorphenamide (Daranide ★) is a carbonic anhydrase inhibitor used in the management of glaucoma.

ADVERSE AND COMMON SIDE EFFECTS: The drug is contraindicated in significant liver disease, obstructive pulmonary disease, renal or adrenocortical insufficiency, hyponatremia, hypokalemia, and hyperchloremic acidosis. Long-term use of the drug is contraindicated in chronic, noncongestive angle-closure glaucoma because the drug may mask the severity of the disease by lowering intraocular pressure.

Adverse effects may include GI upset, sedation, depression, excitement, bone marrow depression, dysuria, polyuria, crystalluria, hypokalemia, hyponatremia, hyperglycemia, hepatic insufficiency, skin rash, and hypersensitivity.

DRUG INTERACTIONS: The drug may inhibit primidone absorption from the GIT. Primidone or phenytoin used concurrently with dichlorphenamide may cause osteomalacia. Concurrent use of corticosteroids, amphotericin B, or diuretics may enhance potassium depletion. This may be especially important to patients receiving digitalis compounds. Carbonic anhydrase preparations may interfere with the efficacy of insulin.

SUPPLIED AS: HUMAN PRODUCT
Tablets containing 50 mg

DICHLORVOS

INDICATIONS: Dichlorvos (Task ★) is a cholinesterase inhibitor anthelmintic used for the elimination of *Toxocara canis, Toxascaris leonina, Ancylostoma caninum, Uncinaria stenocephalia,* and *Trichuris vulpis.*

ADVERSE AND COMMON SIDE EFFECTS and **DRUG INTER-ACTIONS:** See ORGANOPHOSPHATES.

SUPPLIED AS: VETERINARY PRODUCTS
Capsules containing 68, 136, and 204 mg
Packet containing 136, 204, and 544 mg
Tablets containing 10 and 25 mg

DICLOXACILLIN

INDICATIONS: Dicloxacillin (Dynapen ★) is a β-lactamase–resistant penicillin antibiotic with activity against gram-positive bacteria. Also see **CLOXACILLIN.**

ADVERSE AND COMMON SIDE EFFECTS: See PENICILLIN ANTIBIOTICS.

DRUG INTERACTIONS: Tetracyclines and other bacteriostatic antibiotics may interfere with the antibacterial activity of penicillin antibiotics.

SUPPLIED AS: HUMAN PRODUCT
Capsules containing 125, 250, and 500 mg

DIETHYLCARBAMAZINE

INDICATIONS: Diethylcarbamazine; DEC (Carbam ★, Filaribits ✦ ★) is recommended for the prevention of heartworm disease and as an aid in the treatment of ascarid infection in dogs and cats. Filaribits Plus combines DEC and oxibendazole and is used for the elimination of heartworms (*Dirofilaria immitis*), roundworms (*Toxocara canis*), hookworms (*Ancylostoma caninum*), and whipworms (*Trichuris vulpis*) in dogs.

ADVERSE AND COMMON SIDE EFFECTS: Vomiting and diarrhea occasionally are noted. Administration with food reduces this problem. Low sperm counts have been reported in dogs receiving the drug. If given to dogs with microfilaremia, hypersensitivity or anaphylaxis and death may occur. The use of Filaribits Plus has been associated with a hepatopathy that is potentially fatal. The drug should not be given to dogs with a history of liver disease.

DRUG INTERACTIONS: Levamisole and pyrantel may enhance the toxic effects of DEC, and vice versa.

SUPPLIED AS: VETERINARY PRODUCTS
Oral liquid containing 60 mg/mL [Carbam]
Tablets containing 50, 100, 200, 300, and 400 mg [Carbam]
Tablets containing 60, 120, and 180 mg DEC [Filaribits]

DIETHYLSTILBESTROL

INDICATIONS: Diethylstilbestrol; DES (Stilboestrol ✦) is used in the management of estrogen-responsive urinary incontinence, vaginitis, perianal gland adenoma, and benign prostatic gland hyperplasia. It is not effective when used alone to prevent pregnancy.

ADVERSE AND COMMON SIDE EFFECTS: Thrombocytopenia may be observed approximately 2 weeks after the initiation of treatment with estrogens. Leukocytosis with a left shift may develop at approximately 16 to 20 days, and anemia may become gradually apparent. Leukopenia may follow at approximately 22 to 25 days. Bone marrow suppression is unlikely at doses recommended to control urinary incontinence. There is considerable variation in sensitivity to the adverse effects of DES. Feminization or the induction of estrus also is possible. Estrogens induce squamous metaplasia and fibromuscular proliferation of the prostate gland, which predisposes to fluid stasis and infection.

DRUG INTERACTIONS: Estrogen activity may be decreased if the drug is used concurrently with rifampin, phenytoin, or barbiturate drugs. Estrogens may enhance glucocorticoid activity, necessitating adjustment of the glucocorticoid dose.

SUPPLIED AS: VETERINARY PRODUCT
Tablets containing 1 mg

HUMAN PRODUCTS
Tablets containing 1 and 5 mg ★
Tablets (enteric-coated) containing 0.1, 0.5, 1, and 5 mg

OTHER USES
Dogs
PERIANAL GLAND ADENOMA AND PROSTATIC HYPERPLASIA
0.1 to 1 mg every 24 to 48 hours; PO

DIGITOXIN

INDICATIONS: Digitoxin (Crystodigin ★, Digitaline ✤) is a cardiac glycoside used in the treatment of supraventricular tachyarrhythmias (atrial flutter or fibrillation), premature atrial contractions, and tachycardia. Because the drug has less parasympathetic activity than digoxin, it is less effective in the management of supraventricular arrhythmias. However, it is preferred to digoxin in patients with renal dysfunction. Measurements of serum concentrations are taken after steady-state levels are attained (after approximately 5 days of therapy). Normal serum values are 15 to 35 ng/mL, 6 to 8 hours after treatment. Toxicity generally is noted when serum levels exceed 40 ng/mL.

ADVERSE AND COMMON SIDE EFFECTS: Anorexia, vomiting, diarrhea, depression, atrioventricular block, ectopia, and junctional tachycardia have been documented. Patients with hypokalemia, hypernatremia, and hypercalcemia are predisposed to toxicity. Because of the exceedingly long half-life in the cat (greater than 100 hours), it is not recommended in this species.

DRUG INTERACTIONS: See DIGOXIN.

SUPPLIED AS: HUMAN PRODUCTS
Tablets containing 0.05 and 0.1 mg digitoxin [Crystodigin]
Tablets containing 0.1 and 0.2 mg [Digitaline]

DIGOXIN

INDICATIONS: Digoxin (Lanoxin ★, Cardoxin ♣ ★) decreases sympathetic nerve activity and is a positive inotropic and negative chronotropic agent. Its chronotropic properties make it a popular choice in the management of supraventricular tachyarrhythmias, e.g., atrial flutter and fibrillation and sinus tachycardia associated with congestive heart failure. Its inotropic value is questionable. However, digoxin is used in an effort to improve cardiac output in conditions of congestive heart failure and cardiomyopathy. Samples for the determination of serum blood concentration should be taken after steady-state levels have been attained (greater than 7 days in dogs and cats). Blood samples are taken just before the next dose or at least 8 hours after the previous dose. Normal serum concentrations are between 0.9 and 3 ng/mL in dogs and between 0.9 and 2 ng/mL in cats. Concurrent measurement of serum electrolytes helps interpret the digoxin concentration and its effect on the patient.

ADVERSE AND COMMON SIDE EFFECTS: Toxic serum levels are in excess of 3 ng/mL in dogs and in excess of 2.4 ng/mL in cats. Vomiting, diarrhea, anorexia, lethargy, ataxia, arrhythmias, and conduction abnormalities may occur. Toxicity is enhanced by hypokalemia, hypercalcemia, decreased glomerular filtration, and hyperthyroid states. It does not appear necessary to adjust drug doses in hypothyroid dogs. Doberman pinschers with dilated cardiomyopathy appear to be more sensitive to digitalis intoxication. Acute increases in serum digoxin levels are better tolerated than prolonged high concentrations.

Intoxication can be managed by preventing further digoxin absorption from the GIT with activated charcoal that binds digoxin, correction of electrolyte imbalances and acid–base status, and management of arrhythmias. In addition, a specific digoxin/digitoxin antidote (Digoxin Immune Fab) can be given. The only drawback to the use of this antidote is its high cost.

DRUG INTERACTIONS: Furosemide, quinidine, and verapamil may potentiate digoxin toxicity. Serum digoxin levels also may increase with the concurrent use of spironolactone, diltiazem, triamterene, erythromycin, and prazosin. Antacid preparations, cimetidine, metoclopramide, oral neomycin, cyclophosphamide, doxorubicin, Vinca alkaloids, and cytarabine decrease GIT digoxin absorption. Drugs that inhibit hepatic microsomal activity, e.g., chloramphenicol, quinidine, and tetracycline, decrease digoxin excretion and should be used with caution if given concurrently. Drugs that predispose to hypokalemia, e.g., amphotericin B, glucocorticoids, laxatives, sodium polystyrene sulfonate, and high-dose dextrose solutions, may potentiate digoxin toxicity.

SUPPLIED AS: VETERINARY PRODUCT
Elixir containing 0.05 and 0.15 mg/mL [Cardoxin]

HUMAN PRODUCTS
Capsules containing 0.05, 0.1, and 0.2 mg [Lanoxicaps ★]
Tablets containing 0.0625, 0.125, 0.25, and 0.5 mg [Lanoxin]
Elixir containing 0.05 mg/mL [Lanoxin]
For injection containing 0.05, 0.1, and 0.25 mg/mL [Lanoxin]

DIGOXIN IMMUNE FAB (OVINE)

INDICATIONS: Digoxin Immune Fab (Digibind ✦ ★) uses purified
fragments of antibodies specific for digoxin (but also effective for
digitoxin) to bind the drug and prevent further intoxication. The
complex then is eliminated in the urine. Each 40-mg vial binds approximately 0.6 mg of digoxin or digitoxin. It is used for the treatment of potentially life-threatening cases of digitalis intoxication.
The dose of drug necessary to counteract digoxin intoxication is calculated as in the following equation. These calculations are based on
adult human pharmacokinetic parameters and may not be appropriate in animals.

Acute ingestion of a known amount:

Number of vials required =
Total digitalis body load in mg ÷ 0.6 mg of digitalis bound/vial

For toxicity from acute ingestion, total body load in milligrams
will be approximately equal to the amount ingested in milligrams
for digoxin capsules and digitoxin, or the amount ingested in milligrams times 0.80 for digoxin tablets (reduced absorption).

With chronic toxicity, i.e., after steady-state levels have been attained, the dose of Digibind required can be calculated as follows:

Number of vials required =
[serum digoxin (ng/mL) × body weight (kg)] ÷ 100

ADVERSE AND COMMON SIDE EFFECTS: The drug is contraindicated in patients in renal or cardiac failure. Cardiac status
may deteriorate with therapy as inotropic activity of digitalis is withdrawn. Patients should be monitored closely for congestive heart
failure, arrhythmias, and an increase in heart rate. After treatment
with digoxin immune Fab, potassium shifts back into cells,
resulting in possible hypokalemia. Interpretation of serum digoxin
levels after therapy is inaccurate and is not advised. Reversal of
signs of digitalis intoxication become clinically apparent 15 to 60
minutes after administration in people. If the patient fails to respond
within this time, other causes for the clinical signs should be considered.

DRUG INTERACTIONS: None established.

SUPPLIED AS: HUMAN PRODUCT
For injection containing 40 mg/vial

DIHYDROSTREPTOMYCIN

INDICATIONS: Dihydrostreptomycin (Ethamycin ✤) is an amino-glycoside antibiotic used for the treatment of leptospirosis. For information on INDICATIONS, ADVERSE AND COMMON SIDE EFFECTS, and DRUG INTERACTIONS, see **AMINOGLYCOSIDE ANTIBIOTICS.**

SUPPLIED AS: VETERINARY PRODUCT
For injection containing 500 mg/mL

DIHYDROTACHYSTEROL

INDICATIONS: Dihydrotachysterol (DHT ★, Hytakerol ✤ ★) is used in the treatment of hypocalcemia. The time required for the drug to exert its maximal effect may not be attained for 2 to 4 weeks, and the duration of effect after cessation of therapy may be as long as 1 week.

ADVERSE AND COMMON SIDE EFFECTS: Hypercalcemia leading to polyuria, polydipsia, listlessness, depression, anorexia, vomiting, nephrocalcinosis, muscle weakness, and trembling or muscle twitching may occur. Serum calcium levels should be monitored every 2 weeks.

DRUG INTERACTIONS: None established.

SUPPLIED AS: HUMAN PRODUCTS
Tablets containing 0.125, 0.2, and 0.4 mg [DHT]
Capsules containing 0.125 mg [Hytakerol]
Oral concentrate containing 0.2 mg/mL [DHT Intensol] and 0.25 mg/mL [Hytakerol ★]

DILTIAZEM

INDICATIONS: Diltiazem (Cardizem ✤ ★), like nifedipine and verapamil, is a calcium channel-blocking agent. Calcium channel-blocking agents decrease heart rate, myocardial contractility, and oxygen demand, decrease systolic pressure gradients, improve myocardial relaxation, and dilate coronary blood vessels. Diltiazem decreases afterload, prolongs atrioventricular conduction (although not as much as verapamil), and is a less potent negative inotrope than verapamil or nifedipine. The drug appears to be useful in the treatment of supraventricular tachycardia, e.g., atrial fibrillation and hypertrophic cardiomyopathy. Diltiazem causes less peripheral arterial vasodilation and reflex tachycardia than verapamil or nifedipine. The drug also may be useful in the management of congestive cardiomyopathy because it decreases ventricular response to atrial fibrillation, decreases peripheral resistance and afterload, and has minimal cardiodepressant effects. Because they inhibit angiotensin II and α-adrenergic–mediated vasoconstriction, calcium channel-blocking agents have renoprotective effects, the extent and clinical utility of which in veterinary medicine have yet to be determined.

ADVERSE AND COMMON SIDE EFFECTS: Bradycardia appears to be the most common side effect in dogs. Diltiazem also can cause depression and hypotension and can contribute to heart failure. Acute toxicity can be managed with 10% calcium gluconate infusion (1 mL/10 kg; IV) or the administration of a positive inotrope, e.g., dopamine. The drug has been used at standard doses without side effects in most cats.

DRUG INTERACTIONS: Diltiazem is reported to increase serum digoxin levels in humans. Diltiazem and verapamil inhibit hepatic microsomal enzyme, affecting the clearance of propranolol, theophylline, and quinidine. Cimetidine increases serum levels. Prolongation of atrioventricular conduction is potentiated by the concurrent use of β-blockers, e.g., propranolol and atenolol, or digoxin.

SUPPLIED AS: HUMAN PRODUCTS
Tablets containing 30, 60, 90, and 120 mg
Capsules (sustained-release) containing 60, 90, and 120 mg
Capsules (controlled-delivery) containing 180, 240, and 300 mg

DIMETHYL SULFOXIDE

INDICATIONS: Dimethyl sulfoxide; DMSO (Domoso ♣ ★) is reported to have a number of beneficial properties, yet little scientific evidence is available to support these claims. The drug often is used to help transport drugs across the skin into the general circulation. It has anti-inflammatory activity and is a potent diuretic, local analgesic, muscle relaxant, vasodilator, and inotropic agent. Dimethyl sulfoxide inhibits platelet aggregation, decreases fibroplasia, and is bacteriostatic and antifungal. The drug is recommended for topical treatment in dogs with acute and chronic musculoskeletal disease, otitis externa, and ophthalmic disease. It also has been recommended in the treatment of trauma to the head and spine and in renal amyloidosis, where the beneficial effects are attributed to its anti-inflammatory activity.

ADVERSE AND COMMON SIDE EFFECTS: Topical application can lead to erythema, edema, pruritus, vesiculation, and pain. Dryness of the skin and oyster-like breath odor also may be noted. Toxicity after IV injection may include sedation, hematuria, seizure, coma, dyspnea, and pulmonary edema. Intravascular injection of concentrations greater than 20% leads to severe hemolysis. Side effects of repeated administration of DMSO in dogs may include perivascular inflammation and local thrombosis (if used in undiluted form), reversible hemolytic anemia (when given repeatedly intravenously), and reduced lucency of the lens cortex (which resolves with discontinuation of the drug). The drug is potentially teratogenic during the first trimester of pregnancy. Dimethyl sulfoxide should not be given to animals with ocular, renal, or liver disease, or those with a history of allergy, and it should not be used in animals weighing less than 4.5 kg.

DRUG INTERACTIONS: None established.

SUPPLIED AS: VETERINARY PRODUCTS
Gel 90% in 60- and 120-g tubes and 425-g jars
Topical solution 90% in 4-oz (=/- spray bottle), 16-oz, and 1-gal bottle
Otic preparation containing DMSO 60% [Synotic ♣ ★]

OTHER USES
Dogs
CYCLOPHOSPHAMIDE-INDUCED HEMORRHAGIC CYSTITIS
10 mL of 50% DMSO solution diluted in equal volume of sterile saline instilled in urinary bladder for 20 minutes; repeat in 1 week
RENAL AMYLOIDOSIS
80 mg/kg 3 times weekly; SC

DIPHENHYDRAMINE

INDICATIONS: Diphenhydramine (Benadryl ♣ ★) is an antihistamine used as an antiemetic and to help alleviate urticaria and angioedema, canine atopy, canine pruritus, and to guard against the effects of histamine release from mast cell tumors. Diphenhydramine also is used to prevent allergic reactions in animals receiving doxorubicin. This drug also has been used to manage a number of behavioral problems, e.g., compulsive scratching, self-trauma, and waking at night. It has mild sedative properties. Diphenhydramine also may be useful in the treatment of organophosphate and carbamate poisoning, where nicotinic signs predominate, e.g., muscular twitching. For further information, refer to **ANTIHISTAMINES.**

SUPPLIED AS: HUMAN PRODUCTS
Capsules containing 25 and 50 mg
Tablets containing 25 and 50 mg
Elixir and syrup containing 12.5 mg/mL
For injection containing 10 and 50 mg/mL
Solution and cream containing 1% and 2% w/v diphenhydramine

OTHER USES
Dogs
PREMEDICATION FOR DOGS RECEIVING DOXORUBICIN
10 mg before doxorubicin; IV (dogs ≤ 9 kg)
20 mg before doxorubicin; IV (dogs 9–27 kg)
30 mg before doxorubicin; IV (dogs > 27 kg)

PREOPERATIVE THERAPY FOR SPLENIC MAST CELL TUMOR
2.2 mg/kg bid; IM (with cimetidine 5 mg/kg tid–qid; PO, IV)

ANTIPRURITIC
25 to 50 mg bid–tid; PO

ANTIEMETIC
2 to 4 mg/kg tid; PO

BEHAVIORAL DISORDERS
2 to 4 mg/kg bid–tid; PO

Cats
ANTIEMETIC
2 to 4 mg/kg tid; PO

BEHAVIORAL DISORDERS
2 to 4 mg/kg bid–tid; PO

DIPHENOXYLATE

INDICATIONS: Diphenoxylate (Lomotil ✤ ★) is indicated for the management of diarrhea. The drug increases intestinal segmentation, decreases the frequency of bowel movements, decreases abdominal pain and tenesmus, and possibly inhibits fluid secretion.

ADVERSE AND COMMON SIDE EFFECTS: Constipation, bloating, and sedation may occur. It should only be used for a 36- to 48-hour period and should not be used in cases with infectious enteritis. In cats, the use of opiate antidiarrheal preparations may cause excitement.

DRUG INTERACTIONS: Diphenoxylate may potentiate the action of barbiturates, phenothiazines, antihistamines, and anesthetic agents.

SUPPLIED AS: HUMAN PRODUCTS
Tablets containing 2.5 mg diphenoxylate with atropine (0.025 mg)

Oral liquid containing 2.5 mg/5 mL diphenoxylate with atropine (0.025 mg)

DIPYRONE

INDICATIONS: Dipyrone (Novolate ♣ and generic products ★) is an anti-inflammatory, antipyretic, antispasmodic, and analgesic agent. It is prescribed for the relief of pain, reducing fever, and relaxing smooth muscle.

ADVERSE AND COMMON SIDE EFFECTS: Sedation is common. Subcutaneous injection may cause irritation and is not recommended. At high doses or with prolonged therapy, agranulocytosis and leukopenia may develop. Nausea, vomiting, skin rashes, pain at the injection site, hemolytic anemia, tremors, GI hemorrhage, and prolongation of bleeding times also may occur. Novolate may discolor urine red. The drug should not be used in animals with a history of blood dyscrasias.

DRUG INTERACTIONS: Phenothiazines may predispose to hypothermia in patients given dipyrone. The drug should not be used in animals receiving phenylbutazone or barbiturates because of drug interaction involving hepatic microsomal systems.

SUPPLIED AS: VETERINARY PRODUCT
For injection containing 500 mg/mL

DISOPYRAMIDE PHOSPHATE

INDICATIONS: Disopyramide (Norpace ♣ ★) is an antiarrhythmic drug used for the management of ventricular tachyarrhythmias. It has anticholinergic effects and is a potent negative inotrope. Although disopyramide has been of benefit in humans with supraventricular tachycardia, e.g., atrial fibrillation, it does not appear to be as effective for this use in the dog.

ADVERSE AND COMMON SIDE EFFECTS: Disopyramide should be avoided in patients in congestive heart failure or shock because of its negative inotropic effects. Dry mouth, vomiting, urinary retention, glaucoma, depression, atrioventricular block, sinus node depression, and multiform ventricular tachycardia also may occur. Hyperkalemia potentiates its myocardial depressant effects, and hypokalemia reduces its therapeutic effects.

DRUG INTERACTIONS: Dilantin and other drugs that induce hepatic microsomal enzymes may increase the metabolism of disopyramide.

SUPPLIED AS: HUMAN PRODUCTS
Capsules containing 100 and 150 mg
Tablets (controlled-release) containing 150 mg

DOBUTAMINE

INDICATIONS: Dobutamine (Dobutrex ✣ ★) is a rapid-acting synthetic catecholamine that predominantly stimulates β_1-receptors and is useful for short-term increases in cardiac output in conditions of shock, congestive heart failure, and cardiomyopathy.

ADVERSE AND COMMON SIDE EFFECTS: Generally the drug has little effect on heart rate and blood pressure, except at higher doses. Sinus tachycardia and ventricular arrhythmias may occur. An increase in atrioventricular conduction may occur. Animals with atrial fibrillation should be pretreated with a cardiac glycoside or calcium channel-blocking agent, e.g., diltiazem. The drug is contraindicated in animals with aortic stenosis. Vomiting and seizure activity have been reported in some cats.

DRUG INTERACTIONS: Propranolol, atenolol, and metoprolol may negate the effects of dobutamine. Halothane may increase the likelihood of arrhythmias. Insulin requirements may increase in diabetic patients.

SUPPLIED AS: HUMAN PRODUCT
For injection containing 12.5 mg/mL in 20-mL vials and 12.5 mg/mL in 40-mL vials

DOCUSATE CALCIUM

INDICATIONS: Docusate calcium (Surfak ✣ ★) is an anionic surface-active agent with emulsifying and wetting properties. Detergent action lowers surface tension, permitting water and fats to penetrate and soften stools. It is used for the prevention and treatment of constipation. The drug acts at the small and large bowel and generally takes 12 to 72 hours to work effectively.

ADVERSE AND COMMON SIDE EFFECTS: Mild, transient cramping may occur. A bitter taste, nausea, vomiting, and diarrhea also are reported. The drug should not be administered with mineral oil because increased absorption of the oil may occur, resulting in tumor-like deposits. Liquid preparations may cause throat irritation.

DRUG INTERACTIONS: None established.

SUPPLIED AS: HUMAN PRODUCT
Capsules containing 50 and 240 mg

DOCUSATE SODIUM

INDICATIONS: Docusate sodium (Colace ♣ ★). For INDICATIONS, ADVERSE AND COMMON SIDE EFFECTS, and DRUG INTERACTIONS, see **DOCUSATE CALCIUM.**

SUPPLIED AS: VETERINARY PRODUCTS
Liquids available in gallon formulations containing 50 mg/mL (Refer to Part II, Section 6, Large Animal Preparations, for further discussion.)
Enema containing 250 mg in 12 mL glycerin [Docu-Soft Enema ★]

HUMAN PRODUCTS
Capsules containing 50, 100, 240, and 250 mg
Syrup containing 50 and 60 mg/15 mL
Solution containing 10 and 50 mg/mL
Tablets containing 50 and 100 mg

DOPAMINE

INDICATIONS: Dopamine (Intropin ♣ ★) is an endogenous precursor of norepinephrine that stimulates β_1-receptors and dopaminergic receptors. Dopaminergic receptors are located predominantly in renal, mesenteric, coronary, and cerebral arterioles. Intermediate dosages (3–10 µg/kg/minute) increase cardiac output with little change in heart rate or blood pressure. High infusion rates (10–20 µg/kg/minute) stimulate α- and β-adrenergic receptors and lead to an increase in cardiac contractility, heart rate, and blood pressure. It is indicated in cases of acute or chronic congestive heart failure and shock unresponsive to other methods. The drug also is used as adjunctive therapy in oliguric and anuric renal failure to promote renal vasodilation and an improvement in glomerular filtration. The drug also has been used experimentally to protect against hemorrhagic pancreatitis in cats when it was given up to 12 hours after initiation of the insult.

ADVERSE AND COMMON SIDE EFFECTS: Nausea, vomiting, hypotension or hypertension, and dyspnea may occur. Overdose may cause tachycardia, increases in blood pressure, and ventricular ectopia. Extravascular injection may cause tissue necrosis and sloughing. Should perivascular injection occur, the site should be infiltrated with phentolamine (5–10 mg) in 10 to 15 mL of saline. The drug is contraindicated in patients with ventricular arrhythmias.

DRUG INTERACTIONS: Phenytoin may decrease the effects of dopamine, leading to hypotension and bradycardia.

SUPPLIED AS: HUMAN PRODUCTS
For injection containing 40, 80, and 160 mg/mL in 5-mL vials or additive syringes

For infusion containing 0.8, 1.6, 3.2, and 6.4 mg/mL in D_5W in 250- and 500-mL bags

OTHER USES
OLIGURIC RENAL FAILURE
1 to 3 µg/kg/minute

Cats

HEMORRHAGIC PANCREATITIS
5 µg/kg/minute; IV, continued for 6 hours

DOXAPRAM

INDICATIONS: Doxapram (Dopram-V ♣ ★) is used to stimulate respiration in patients with postanesthetic respiratory depression or apnea and to encourage the return of laryngopharyngeal reflexes in patients with mild to moderate respiratory and CNS depression due to anesthetic overdose. In the neonate, doxapram may be used to stimulate respiration after dystocia or Cesarean-section birth.

ADVERSE AND COMMON SIDE EFFECTS: Cough, dyspnea, and laryngospasm may occur. Overdose may cause tremor, lacrimation, excessive salivation, occasional vomiting, diarrhea, and stiffness of the extremities. Excessive doses may initiate hyperventilation and respiratory alkalosis. Arrhythmias and urinary retention may occur, and seizure activity may be provoked in epileptic patients.

DRUG INTERACTIONS: Do not mix with alkaline solutions. The concomitant use with sympathomimetic agents or MAO inhibitors (possibly amitraz and selegiline) may lead to serious increases in blood pressure and arrhythmias. Halothane and enflurane may precipitate arrhythmias. It is recommended that doxapram use be delayed approximately 10 minutes after discontinuation of these anesthetic agents.

SUPPLIED AS: VETERINARY PRODUCT
For injection containing 20 mg/mL

DOXORUBICIN

INDICATIONS: Doxorubicin (Adriamycin ♣ ★) is a chemotherapeutic agent used in the treatment of lymphoma, osteosarcoma (30 mg/m^2 every 2 weeks; IV), thyroid carcinomas, mammary gland adenocarcinoma (in one case at a dose of 30 mg/m^2 every 3 weeks; IV), and other solid tumors. It has been suggested that six treatments of doxorubicin (30 mg/m^2) may be more advantageous in maintaining longer remission length than three treatments for cases of canine lymphoma. Preliminary results in cats have shown response with lymphoma, mammary adenocarcinoma, and fibrosarcoma.

ADVERSE AND COMMON SIDE EFFECTS: A study in 1994 suggested that dose based on body weight, as opposed to body surface area, results in more uniform therapeutic and predictable toxic responses in the dog. In the dog, doxorubicin toxicity can be classified as acute, short-term, and chronic. Acute toxicity occurs during or immediately after treatment and includes head-shaking, pruritus, erythema, and occasionally acute collapse. Diphenhydramine (Benadryl) given at a dose of 2.2 mg/kg intramuscularly 20 minutes before doxorubicin use has been recommended to prevent anaphylactic reactions. The efficacy of this precaution is unknown. Severe local tissue damage occurs if the drug is injected extravascularly. The drug may discolor urine orange or red for 1 to 2 days after treatment.

Short-term toxicity occurs 5 to 10 days after treatment and includes myelosuppression, anorexia, vomiting, diarrhea, and weight loss. Bone marrow suppression peaks 10 to 14 days after the initiation of treatment, followed by recovery in 21 days. Complete blood counts should be monitored 10 days after initiation of therapy and before each dose. If neutrophil counts decrease to less than 2,000/µL or platelet numbers decrease to less than 50,000/µL, the drug should be discontinued until counts return to normal. Alopecia also may occur within a few weeks of therapy and most commonly occurs in curly-coated breeds. Dose-dependent congestive cardiomyopathy is reported, and dose-independent cardiac arrhythmias occur with chronic toxicity. Do not exceed a cumulative dose of 250 mg/m^2. Prolongation of infusion time to greater than 6 hours or using a low-dose weekly schedule may be helpful in reducing cardiotoxicity by decreasing peak plasma concentrations. In addition, it has been suggested that carnitine supplementation also may reduce the cardiac toxicity of chronic doxorubicin therapy, although the efficacy of this recommendation has yet to be established.

In cats, short-term toxicities include neutropenia (nadir 8–11 days) and poikilocytosis. Neutrophil counts return to normal within 14 days in the cat. Thrombocytopenia is uncommon and mild when it does occur. A complete blood count and platelet numbers should be completed on days 1 and 8 of each treatment cycle. Anorexia, vomiting, diarrhea, and weight loss also have been reported in some cats. No clinical evidence of cardiotoxicity has been seen. Mild azotemia also has been reported. Other uncommon adverse effects have included whisker loss and testicular atrophy.

DRUG INTERACTIONS: Barbiturates may decrease pharmacologic effects by increasing hepatic metabolism. Streptozocin may prolong doxorubicin half-life, necessitating a decrease in dose.

SUPPLIED AS: HUMAN PRODUCTS
For injection containing 10, 20, 50, 100, and 150 mg
For injection containing 2 mg/mL in 5-, 10-, and 25-mL vials

DOXYCYCLINE

INDICATIONS: Doxycycline (Vibramycin ♣ ★, Vibravet ♣) is a sec-ond-generation, long-acting, lipid-soluble tetracycline antibiotic used in the treatment of actinomycosis, ehrlichiosis, *chlamydia*, lep-tospirosis, borreliosis, Rocky Mountain spotted fever, toxoplasmo-sis, and hemobartonella infections. Doxyciline and minocycline have greater activity against anaerobes and facultative intracellular bacteria such as *Brucella canis* than other tetracyclines. It is a useful tetracycline in patients with renal failure. For more information, see **TETRACYCLINE ANTIBIOTICS.**

ADVERSE AND COMMON SIDE EFFECTS: The most common side effects of oral tetracycline use in small animals are vomiting and diarrhea. Mixing the drug with food decreases the incidence of these reactions. See also **TETRACYCLINE ANTIBIOTICS.**

DRUG INTERACTIONS: Barbiturate drugs and carbamazepine de-crease the serum half-life of doxycycline. Antacid preparations con-taining aluminum, calcium, iron, or magnesium, antidiarrheal com-pounds containing kaolin and pectin or bismuth, and laxatives reduce GIT absorption of doxycycline. Sodium bicarbonate inter-feres with gastric absorption of oral tetracyclines. Schedule doxy-cycline 1 to 2 hours before use of these preparations.

SUPPLIED AS: VETERINARY PRODUCT
Oral suspension containing 5 mg/mL after reconstitution [Vibravet]
HUMAN PRODUCTS
Tablets and capsules containing 50 and 100 mg
Oral suspension containing 5 mg/mL after reconstitution
Oral syrup containing 10 mg/mL
For injection in 100- and 200-mg vials

ECONAZOLE

INDICATIONS: Econazole (Ecostatin ♣ ★, Spectazole ★) is a topical imidazole used in the eradication of localized demodicosis. In hu-mans, it also is used in the treatment of dermatophytosis and candi-dal infections.

ADVERSE AND COMMON SIDE EFFECTS: Occasionally, local skin irritation with burning, pruritus, and erythema may occur.

DRUG INTERACTIONS: None.

SUPPLIED AS: HUMAN PRODUCT
Cream containing 1% econazole

EDROPHONIUM CHLORIDE

INDICATIONS: Edrophonium chloride (Tensilon ♣ ★) is a cholinesterase inhibitor. It is used in the diagnosis of myasthenia gravis and in the treatment of curare poisoning and unresponsive atrial tachycardia.

ADVERSE AND COMMON SIDE EFFECTS: Cholinergic reactions, including bradycardia, pupillary constriction, laryngospasm, bronchiolar constriction, nausea, vomiting, diarrhea, and muscle weakness, may occur. In the case of accidental overdose, atropine should be administered. The drug should be used with caution in patients with asthma or cardiac arrhythmias.

DRUG INTERACTIONS: The anticholinergic properties of procainamide and quinidine may antagonize the cholinergic effects of edrophonium.

SUPPLIED AS: HUMAN PRODUCT
For injection containing 10 mg/mL in 10-mL vials

EFA-CAPS ♣, EFA CAPS HP ♣, EFA-VET PLUS ♣, EFA LIQUID ★ AND EFA-Z PLUS ♣ ★

INDICATIONS: These products are dietary multivitamin and mineral supplements containing fatty acids derived from primrose and fish oil. They have useful anti-inflammatory properties and may be used in the management of seborrhea and pruritus in dogs and cats. Potential beneficial effects of omega-3 fatty acid supplementation include the alleviation of pain, control of pruritus, suppression of inflammation and autoimmune disease, decrease in serum triglyceride levels, decreased formation of thrombi, antiarrhythmogenesis, and inhibition of tumorigenesis. Supplementation of diets with linoleic acid increases glomerular filtration rate and decreases proteinuria. Diets containing fish oil can decrease blood pressure. However, clinical relevance of these claims remains to be established.

ADVERSE AND COMMON SIDE EFFECTS: Although rare, use of these products may be associated with GIT disorders (softening of the stools and diarrhea), increased pruritus, and urticaria. Although the cutaneous bleeding time may be slightly prolonged, the risk of bleeding is low. Although not well documented, these agents may induce pancreatitis in animals predisposed to the disease.

DRUG INTERACTIONS: None.

SUPPLIED AS: VETERINARY PRODUCTS
These products are available in liquid formulations and as capsules.

ENALAPRIL

INDICATIONS: Enalapril (Enacard ♣ ★, Vasotec ♣ ★) is an angiotensin converting enzyme (ACE) inhibitor. Peak concentrations occur 4 to 6 hours after oral administration. It has a longer duration of action than captopril. Angiotensin-converting enzyme inhibitors are used for their vasodilatory properties in the treatment of congestive heart failure, systemic hypertension, renal disease, and shock. Angiotensin-converting enzyme inhibitors may significantly improve even mild cases of congestive heart failure. Experimentally, ACE inhibitors actually may slow the progression of renal disease via decreasing glomerular pressures (which contribute to the progression of renal disease) and possibly by limiting the growth/proliferation of glomerular cells.

ADVERSE AND COMMON SIDE EFFECTS: Hypotension causing lethargy, anorexia, weakness, and difficulty rising, possibly in association with dehydration or azotemia, has been reported. Vomiting, diarrhea, sinus tachycardia, and hyperkalemia also have been documented. In addition, in people, pruritus, proteinuria, bone marrow-induced neutropenia, and deterioration of renal function have been noted with the use of ACE inhibitors. Doses should be reduced in patients with renal disease. Drug overdose may be treated with a β-agonist, e.g., dobutamine. Bradyarrhythmias may respond to atropine or glycopyrrolate. Unlike captopril, enalapril requires hepatic hydrolysis to become activated. Therefore, captopril is a better choice in patients with liver disease. Use of the drug in pregnant bitches is not recommended.

DRUG INTERACTIONS: Indomethacin may decrease the antihypertensive activity of the drug. Potassium-sparing diuretics, e.g., spironolactone, may potentiate the hyperkalemia associated with enalapril use. Vomiting may occur in patients given digoxin in combination with enalapril. Low-salt diets and accelerated salt loss induced by loop diuretics may predispose to renal insufficiency associated with ACE inhibitor use. Drugs that cause volume depletion e.g., diuretics, may predispose to azotemia. If clinical signs of hypotension or azotemia develop, the dose of the diuretic should be reduced first. If signs persist, it may be necessary to further decrease the dose of the diuretic, or discontinue it altogether. Persistence of clinical signs necessitate reduction of the dosing frequency or discontinuation of enalapril.

SUPPLIED AS:
Tablets containing 1, 2.5, 5, 10, and 20 mg

ENILCONAZOLE

INDICATIONS: Enilconazole (Imaverol ♣) is a topical imidazole antifungal agent successfully used intranasally in the dog for the treatment of nasal aspergillosis. It also has activity against *Penicillium* and is recommended for the treatment of dermatophyte infections.

ADVERSE AND COMMON SIDE EFFECTS: Side effects are rare. Sneezing and salivation occur with intranasal use. Because of extensive destruction caused by the fungus, some animals may continue to have a mucopurulent nasal discharge, even with successful elimination of the fungus. Secondary bacterial infection may respond to appropriate antibiotic therapy. Slight weight loss may occur. Anorexia may occur at higher doses.

DRUG INTERACTIONS: Unknown.

SUPPLIED AS: VETERINARY PRODUCT
Solution containing 100 mg/mL

ENROFLOXACIN

INDICATIONS: Enrofloxacin (Baytril ♣ ★) is a fluoroquinolone antibiotic with activity against *E. coli, Klebsiella pneumoniae, Staphylococcus aureus* and *epidermidis, Pasteurella multocida,* and *Proteus mirabilis,* as well as *Mycoplasma* spp, *Rickettsia rickettsii,* and atypical mycobacteria. The fluoroquinolone antibiotics are indicated in the treatment of genitourinary tract infections, including prostatitis, dermal infections, and infections of the respiratory tract in the dog. Enrofloxacin has limited activity against anaerobes, although it is reported to have activity against some obligate anaerobic bacteria.

ADVERSE AND COMMON SIDE EFFECTS: Isolated incidents of vomiting and anorexia occur at higher than recommended (e.g., 10 times) doses. Oral treatment of 15- to 28-week-old puppies at doses of 25 mg/kg (recommended dose is 2.5 mg/kg bid) induced abnormal carriage of the carpal joints and weakness in the hindquarters. Significant improvement followed drug withdrawal. Cartilage damage occurred after treatment for 30 days at 5, 15, and 25 mg/kg in this age group. Cartilaginous lesions did not occur in puppies 29- to 34-weeks-old after treatment at 25 mg/kg for a 30-day period. The drug is contraindicated in small and medium breeds of dogs during the rapid growth phase (between 2 and 8 months). Large breed dogs may be in the rapid growth phase for as long as 1 year and giant breeds for up to 18 months. Because of the risk of induction of cartilage defects, the drug is not recommended for use in pregnant animals. Other side effects may include GI upset, polydipsia, and CNS dysfunction, i.e., seizures. No drug-related side effects were documented in cats, although doses of 50 mg/kg have been reported to cause CNS dysfunction. See also **FLUOROQUINOLONE ANTIBIOTICS.**

DRUG INTERACTIONS: Absorption is hindered by antacid preparations and sucralfate. Nitrofurantoin may antagonize the effects of enrofloxacin. Fluoroquinolone antibiotics may potentiate the nephrotoxicity of cyclosporine. In humans, concurrent use of NSAID drugs may promote CNS-related side effects. See **FLUORO-QUINOLONE ANTIBIOTICS.**

SUPPLIED AS: VETERINARY PRODUCTS
Tablets containing 5.7, 22.7, and 68 mg
For injection containing 22.7 and 50 mg/mL

OTHER USES
Dogs and Cats
ATYPICAL MYCOBACTERIA
5 to 15 mg/kg bid; PO for 3 to 4 weeks

Dogs
PSEUDOMONAS AERUGINOSA
5.5 mg/kg bid; PO is effective, although 11 mg/kg bid; PO may be more efficacious

EPHEDRINE

INDICATIONS: Ephedrine sulfate is an α-receptor stimulant. It is useful in the management of urinary incontinence, as a bronchodilator, as a nasal decongestant, and in the management of hypotension.

ADVERSE AND COMMON SIDE EFFECTS: Tachycardia, hypertension, tremors, restlessness, anxiety, hyperexcitability, and urine retention may occur. The drug is minimally arrhythmogenic.

DRUG INTERACTIONS: Sodium bicarbonate may increase the pharmacologic effects of ephedrine with excessive CNS stimulation and cardiovascular effects. Use with amitriptyline may potentiate α-adrenergic effects, leading to hypertension and fever.

SUPPLIED AS: HUMAN PRODUCTS
Capsules containing 25 and 50 mg [generic products ★]
For injection containing 25 and 50 mg/mL [generic products ✦ ★]

OTHER USES
Dogs and Cats
NASAL DECONGESTANT
1 drop per nostril tid–qid (0.5% solution)

Dogs
NASAL DECONGESTANT
5 to 15 mg tid–qid; PO

Cats
NASAL DECONGESTANT
2 to 5 mg tid–qid; PO

EPINEPHRINE

INDICATIONS: Epinephrine is indicated for the treatment of cardiac arrest associated with ventricular standstill. It accelerates atrial and ventricular rates. A topical solution (2%) is used to treat glaucoma.

ADVERSE AND COMMON SIDE EFFECTS: Fear, anxiety, excitability, vomiting, hypertension, and arrhythmias are reported. The topical preparations are locally irritating, resulting in conjunctival hyperemia, chemosis, and blepharospasm.

DRUG INTERACTIONS: The use of other sympathomimetic agents, e.g., isoproterenol, may have additive and potentially toxic effects. The antihistamines diphenhydramine and chlorpheniramine and l-thyroxine also may potentiate the effects of epinephrine. Epinephrine potentiates halothane-induced arrhythmias, especially with the concurrent use of barbiturate or xylazine anesthesia. Acepromazine given 20 minutes before anesthesia may decrease the incidence of epinephrine-induced arrhythmias. Propranolol, metoprolol, and atenolol may potentiate hypertension and antagonize the effect of epinephrine on the heart and bronchi. Nitrates, α-blocking agents, and diuretics may mitigate the pressor effects of the drug.

SUPPLIED AS: VETERINARY AND HUMAN PRODUCT ♣ ★
For injection containing 0.1 mg/mL (1:10,000) and 1.0 mg/mL (1:1,000) epinephrine

OTHER USES
Dogs
BRONCHODILATION AND ANAPHYLAXIS
0.02 mg/kg; IV, SC, IM

Cats
ASTHMA AND ANAPHYLAXIS
0.1 mg every 4 to 6 hours; SC or 0.2 mg in 100 mL D_5W bid–tid PRN; IV

EPSIPRANTEL

INDICATIONS: Epsiprantel (Cestex ♣ ★) is an anthelmintic used for the eradication of *Dipylidium caninum* and *Taenia pisiformis* in dogs and *Dipylidium caninum* and *Taenia taeniaeformis* in cats.

ADVERSE AND COMMON SIDE EFFECTS: The drug should not be given to puppies and kittens less than 7 weeks of age. Significant side effects at recommended doses are unreported.

DRUG INTERACTIONS: None reported.

SUPPLIED AS: VETERINARY PRODUCT
Tablets containing 12.5, 25, 50, and 100 mg

ERYTHROMYCIN

INDICATIONS: Erythromycin (Erythro-100 ★) is a macrolide antibiotic with primary activity against gram-positive bacteria. It is effective against streptococci, staphylococci, Erysipelothrix, Clostridium, Bacteroides, Borrelia, Fusobacterium, Pasteurella, and Bordetella. The drug also has activity against *Campylobacter fetus*, mycoplasmas, chlamydiae, rickettsiae, spirochetes, some atypical mycobacteria, *Leptospira*, and amoebae. At lower dosages, the drug may be used to treat gastroesophageal reflux and reflux esophagitis in cats and perhaps dogs, to promote gastric emptying, and to stimulate intestinal motility.

ADVERSE AND COMMON SIDE EFFECTS: Adverse effects are rare, but nausea, vomiting, abdominal pain, anorexia, and diarrhea may occur with oral use of the drug. Liver dysfunction and/or abnormal liver function tests may be noted. Erythromycin estolate and ethylsuccinate have been associated with an increased risk of cholestasis and hepatotoxicity. Allergic reactions, including urticaria, mild skin eruptions, and anaphylaxis, have been reported. All parenteral preparations are irritating at the site of injection.

DRUG INTERACTIONS: Kaolin, pectin, and bismuth decrease GI absorption of the drug. Because of competitive protein binding, erythromycin should not be used in patients given chloramphenicol, lincomycin, or clindamycin. At low doses, erythromycin may antagonize the antimicrobial action of the penicillins. Increased serum levels leading to toxicity may occur in those concurrently receiving theophylline. There is the possibility of increased digitalis effect in humans using both drugs. The occurrence in small animals is unknown. Erythromycin may cause prolongation of bleeding times in those receiving warfarin therapy. Methylprednisolone metabolism may be inhibited by erythromycin. Concurrent use of erythromycin with terfenadine (Seldane) may predispose to severe and life-threatening cardiac arrhythmias in humans.

SUPPLIED AS: VETERINARY PRODUCT
For injection containing 100 mg/mL [Erythro-100 ★] and 200 mg/mL [Erythro-200 ✦ ★] for use in large animals

HUMAN PRODUCTS
Tablets (enteric-coated) containing 250, 333, and 500 mg as erythromycin base [E-Mycin ♣ ★]
Tablets (film-coated) containing 250 and 500 mg as erythromycin stearate
Capsules containing 250 and 333 mg as erythromycin base [Eryc ♣ ★]
Oral drops containing 100 mg/mL and oral suspension containing 25 and 50 mg/mL as erythromycin estolate [Ilosone ♣ ★]
Note: There are several other human preparations available.

OTHER USES
Dogs and Cats
GASTROINTESTINAL STIMULANT
0.5 to 1 mg/kg tid; PO

ERYTHROPOIETIN

INDICATIONS: Human recombinant erythropoietin (Epogen ★, Eprex ♣) is used to stimulate the production of erythrocytes in patients with anemia due to renal failure. The product also has been used successfully in dogs and cats. Improved appetite (may precede increases in hematocrit), increased activity levels, weight gain, reduced sleep requirements, and improved grooming behavior also have been reported in cats.

ADVERSE AND COMMON SIDE EFFECTS: Although rare, skin rash at the injection site, fever, arthralgia, and mucocutaneous ulcers have been reported. Autoantibodies may develop in 20% of dogs and 30% of cats, leading to a progressive decline in the hematocrit. In humans, additional adverse effects may include systemic hypertension, hyperkalemia, iron deficiency, and seizures. In cats, polycythemia, systemic hypertension, iron depletion, mucocutaneous reactions, and seizures have been reported. Seizures have been reported in cats with severe azotemia or hypertension.

DRUG INTERACTIONS: None reported.

SUPPLIED AS: HUMAN PRODUCT
For injection in vials containing 2,000, 4,000, and 10,000 units

ESTRADIOL CYPIONATE

INDICATIONS: Estradiol cypionate (ECP ♣ ★) has been used in the prevention of pregnancy. It likely causes expulsion of the ova into the uterus or delays transport of the ova through the oviduct, predisposing to its degeneration. This agent also has been used in the treatment of urinary incontinence in spayed female dogs and for palliation of benign anal tumors in aged male dogs.

ADVERSE AND COMMON SIDE EFFECTS: Feminization or the induction or prolongation of estrus may occur. Estrogens predispose to the development of cystic endometrial hyperplasia and pyometra. Thrombocytopenia may be observed approximately 2 weeks after the initiation of treatment with estrogens. Leukocytosis with a left shift may develop at approximately 16 to 20 days, and anemia may become gradually apparent. Leukopenia may follow at approximately 22 to 25 days. There is considerable variation in sensitivity to the adverse effects of estrogens. In some dogs, severe and fatal myelotoxicosis develops, whereas others may have only mild to moderate reversible marrow damage. Bone marrow hypoplasia appears more likely to occur after repeated use or high doses of long-acting preparations such as ECP. Estrogens induce squamous metaplasia and fibromuscular proliferation of the prostate gland, which predisposes to fluid stasis and infection.

DRUG INTERACTIONS: Estrogen activity may be decreased if the drug is used concurrently with rifampin, phenytoin, or barbiturate drugs. Estrogens may enhance glucocorticoid activity, necessitating adjustment of the glucocorticoid dose.

SUPPLIED AS: For injection containing 1 ♣, 2 ★, and 4 mg/mL ♣

OTHER USES
Dogs
MISMATING
i)   0.02 mg/kg; IM within 72 hours of mating
ii) 0.044 mg/kg; IM once during 3 to 5 days of standing heat or within 72 hours of mating

Cats
MISMATING
0.125 to 0.25 mg; IM within 40 hours of mating

ETHACRYNIC ACID

INDICATIONS: Ethacrynic acid (Edecrin ♣ ★) is a loop diuretic similar in action to furosemide.

ADVERSE AND COMMON SIDE EFFECTS: Urinary potassium loss and hypokalemia may occur. In humans, nausea, vomiting, diarrhea, and abdominal pain occur in a small number of individuals with chronic use of the drug. There is little information concerning side effects in small animals.

DRUG INTERACTIONS: In humans, aminoglycosides increase the risk of ototoxicity. Amphotericin B increases the potential for ototoxicity, nephrotoxicity, and hypokalemia. Indomethacin may reduce the diuretic and antihypertensive effect.

SUPPLIED AS: HUMAN PRODUCTS
For injection containing 50 mg ethacrynate sodium
Tablets containing 25 and 50 mg ethacrynic acid

ETIDRONATE

INDICATIONS: Etidronate (Didronel ✤ ★) is potentially useful in the management of refractory hypercalcemia.

ADVERSE AND COMMON SIDE EFFECTS: In humans, nausea, diarrhea, and loose stools may occur. With drug overdose, hypocalcemia may occur. Absorption is decreased by food and dairy products.

DRUG INTERACTIONS: None.

SUPPLIED AS: HUMAN PRODUCTS
Tablets containing 200 and 400 mg
For injection containing 50 mg/mL ✤ ★

ETRETINATE

INDICATIONS: Etretinate (Tegison ✤ ★) is a synthetic retinoid with anti-inflammatory properties. It is useful for disorders of keratinization, abnormalities in follicular keratinization, and quantitative or qualitative disorders of sebaceous gland secretion. It is stored in the liver and has a prolonged elimination time. The drug has been used successfully to treat idiopathic seborrhea, especially in the cocker spaniel, canine lamellar ichthyosis, solar-induced precancerous lesions in bull terriers and Dalmatians, and multiple keratoacanthomas (intracutaneous cornifying epitheliomas). The drug also may be beneficial in the treatment of actinic keratosis and squamous cell carcinoma in the dog.

ADVERSE AND COMMON SIDE EFFECTS: Little information is available concerning its use in veterinary medicine. Side effects have included vomiting, conjunctivitis, joint stiffness, ventral abdominal erythema, and cracking of the foot pads. Additional side effects reported with the use of retinoids include pruritus, polydipsia, and swollen tongue. Biochemical abnormalities may include elevations in serum alanine transferase, alkaline phosphatase, and hypertriglyceridemia. The drug is teratogenic.

DRUG INTERACTIONS: It should not be used with other vitamin A preparations, e.g., isotretinoin, because additive toxic effects may result. In humans, methotrexate may increase the risk of hepatotoxicity and the use of tetracyclines may increase the risk of increased CSF pressure and cerebral edema.

SUPPLIED AS: HUMAN PRODUCT
Capsules containing 10 and 25 mg

OTHER USES
Dogs
IDIOPATHIC SEBORRHEA
0.75 to 1 mg/kg/day (benefit should be noted by 2 to 3 months, maximal improvement may take 4 to 6 months)
Once maximal improvement has been achieved, the dose can be decreased to lowest daily dose required to control the problem, e.g., 10 mg every other day. The ceruminous otitis that often accompanies this problem is not benefited by etretinate therapy, and etretinate has not been effective in treating idiopathic seborrhea seen in West Highland white terriers and basset hounds.

SOLAR-INDUCED PRECANCEROUS LESIONS
0.5 mg/kg/day
New tumors (squamous cell carcinomas) were noted to form even in the face of this therapy.

MULTIPLE KERATOACANTHOMAS
1 to 2 mg/kg/day

Cats
SOLAR-INDUCED PRECANCEROUS LESIONS
2 mg/kg/day

FAMOTIDINE

INDICATIONS: Famotidine (Pepcid ✚ ✦) is a histamine (H_2) receptor antagonist. Although it is more potent than cimetidine, studies have not indicated that it actually is more efficacious than cimetidine or ranitidine in the management of gastric hyperacidity and gastrointestinal ulcer.

ADVERSE AND COMMON SIDE EFFECTS: In humans, depression, anxiety, insomnia, conjunctival injection, nausea, vomiting, anorexia, dry mouth, diarrhea, arthralgia, bronchospasm, pruritus, fever, and thrombocytopenia have been reported. There is little experience with use of the drug in small animals.

DRUG INTERACTIONS: None.

SUPPLIED AS: HUMAN PRODUCTS
Tablets containing 20 and 40 mg
For injection containing 10 mg/mL

FENBENDAZOLE

INDICATIONS: Fenbendazole (Panacur ♣ ★) is an anthelmintic recommended for the elimination of roundworms (*Toxocara canis, Toxascaris leonina*), hookworms (*Ancylostoma caninum, Uncinaria stenocephala*), whipworms (*Trichuris vulpis*), and tapeworms (*Taenia pisiformis*). The drug also has been shown to reduce the burden of *Ancylostoma caninum* and *Toxocara canis* in newborn pups when the bitch is treated during the last trimester of pregnancy. Fenbendazole is effective and safe for treating *giardia* in dogs. The drug also may have some efficacy against crenosomiasis. It also has been used to treat the fluke *Eurytrema procyonis* in cats.

ADVERSE AND COMMON SIDE EFFECTS: Although the drug generally does not have side effects, vomiting and diarrhea may occur.

DRUG INTERACTIONS: None in small animals.

SUPPLIED AS: VETERINARY PRODUCT
Granules (222 mg fenbendazole/g) to be mixed with food

OTHER USES
Dogs
CAPILLARIA AEROPHILA
25 to 50 mg/kg bid for 10 to 14 days; PO

CAPILLARIA PLICA
i) 50 mg/kg once daily for 3 days; PO, repeat in 3 weeks
ii) 50 mg/kg once daily for 3 to 10 days; PO

CRENOSOMA VULPIS
50 mg/kg once daily; PO for 3 days

FILAROIDES HIRTHI
50 mg/kg once daily for 14 days; PO
Note: Clinical signs may worsen during therapy, ostensibly because of reaction to dying worms.

PARAGONIMUS KELLICOTTI
50 to 100 mg/kg div. bid for 10 to 14 days; PO

TRICHURIS VULPIS COLITIS
50 mg/kg once daily for 3 days; repeat in 2 to 3 weeks and again in 2 months

GIARDIA CANIS
50 mg/kg once daily; PO for 3 doses

Cats

ASCARIDS, HOOKWORMS, STRONGYLOIDES, and TAPE-
WORMS (*Taenia* spp.)
50 mg/kg for 5 days; PO

AELUROSTRONGYLUS ABSTRUSUS
i)   20 mg/kg once daily for 5 days; repeat 5 days later
ii) 25 to 50 mg/kg bid for 10 to 14 days; PO

CAPILLARIA AEROPHILA
50 mg/kg for 10 days; PO

CAPILLARIA FELISCATI
25 mg/kg bid for 10 days; PO

PARAGONIMUS KELLICOTTI
50 mg/kg daily for 10 days; PO

EURYTREMA PROCYONIS
30 mg/kg daily for 6 days

FENTANYL

INDICATIONS: Fentanyl (Duragesic ❖ ★, Sublimaze ❖ ★) is a synthetic narcotic with an analgesic potency approximately 100 times
that of morphine and 500 times that of meperidine. Its onset of action
is rapid. The drug induces profound analgesia, sedation, and respiratory depression within 6 to 8 minutes after injection. It has a short
duration of action; peak effects last approximately 30 to 45 minutes.
Fentanyl can be reversed by narcotic antagonists.

   Its use in the form of a transdermal slow-release formulation also
has been described in the dog and cat. Plasma concentrations of 1 to
2 ng/mL are considered analgesic in dogs. Some authors recommend that the 75- and 100-µg/hour patches be used in dogs weighing 20 kg. There may be a wide range of variation in analgesic effect
because of differences in absorption of the product. For management
of postoperative pain, the patch should be placed 12 to 24 hours before surgery to attain effective concentrations at the time of surgery.

ADVERSE AND COMMON SIDE EFFECTS: Fentanyl is eliminated by hepatic biotransformation, and most of its metabolites are
excreted in the urine. Its use in patients with compromised hepatic
or renal function may be contraindicated. It should not be used in
patients with compromised respiratory function, increased intracranial pressure, brain tumors, or altered consciousness. It should be
used with caution in those with bradyarrhythmias. In humans, side
effects may include sedation, respiratory depression, bronchoconstriction, constipation, muscle rigidity, miosis, suppression of the
cough reflex, bradycardia, and mood changes. Tolerance to the drug
may occur. Concurrent administration of atropine prevents brady-

cardia. In cats given the transdermal patches, no adverse effects were noted.

DRUG INTERACTIONS: Barbiturates, other narcotics, and general anesthetics potentiate cerebral and respiratory depression associated with its use.

SUPPLIED AS: HUMAN PRODUCTS
Patches delivering 25, 50, 75, and 100 μg/hour as fentanyl (Duragesic ♣ ★)
For injection containing 50 μg as fentanyl citrate (Sublimaze ♣ ★)

OTHER USES
Cats
CHRONIC PAIN CONTROL
Shave dorsal cervical region (avoid abrading skin), and press patch firmly on skin for 10 to 20 seconds; exposed amount of patch to skin should deliver 0.004 mg/kg or 4 μg/kg.

Dogs
PAIN CONTROL
Clip hair, cleanse area, and apply patch.
75 or 100 μg/hr patches (dog around 20 kg.)

FENTANYL–DROPERIDOL

See **INNOVAR-VET.**

FERROUS SULFATE

INDICATIONS: Ferrous sulfate (Fer-In-Sol, Slow-Fe, and others, as listed below) is used for the treatment and prevention of iron-deficiency anemia.

ADVERSE AND COMMON SIDE EFFECTS: Mild GIT upset may occur. The drug is contraindicated in patients with GIT ulcers, enteritis, colitis, and hemolytic anemia.

DRUG INTERACTIONS: Oral iron supplements may interfere with the absorption of tetracycline antibiotics. Antacids decrease iron absorption from the GIT. Chloramphenicol and cimetidine may delay the hematologic response to iron. Iron may decrease the efficacy of penicillamine by decreasing its absorption.

SUPPLIED AS: HUMAN PRODUCTS
Tablets (20% elemental iron) containing 195 mg (39 mg iron), 300 mg (60 mg iron), and 325 mg (65 mg iron) as ferrous sulfate

Tablets containing 195 mg [Mol-Iron ★]
Tablets containing 300 mg ferrous sulfate [Apo-Ferrous ♣], 525 mg
(105 mg elemental iron) in timed-release form
[Fero-Grad ♣, Film tabs], 160 mg (50 mg elemental iron)
[Slow-Fe ♣]
Capsules (timed-release) containing 150 mg (30 mg iron) and 250 mg
(50 mg iron) [Ferospace ★, Ferralyn Lana caps ★, Ferra-TD ★]
Syrup containing 18 mg/mL (3.6 mg iron/mL) [Fer-In-Sol ★]
Elixir containing 44 mg/mL (8.8 mg iron/mL) [Feosol ★]
Drops containing 125 mg/mL (25 mg iron/mL) [Fer-Iron Drops ★]

FLUCONAZOLE

INDICATIONS: Fluconazole (Diflucan ♣ ★) is an azole derivative
that has been used to treat canine nasal aspergillosis and penicilliosis infections. It has demonstrated efficacy against *Blastomyces, Candida, Coccidioides, Cryptococcus,* and *Histoplasma* infections. Fluconazole has greater water solubility, better oral bioavailability, higher
plasma extravascular levels, and a longer plasma half-life than ketoconazole and penetrates the CSF and brain tissue. Overall, fluconazole is successful in approximately half the dogs treated, which is
similar to what can be expected with thiabendazole or ketoconazole
treatment of the same condition. Therefore, fluconazole is recommended only if topical treatment (i.e., enilconazole or clotrimazole)
is not feasible. The drug also has been used to treat systemic cryptococcosis in the cat.

ADVERSE AND COMMON SIDE EFFECTS: Although experience
with the drug in small animals is limited, no adverse effects were
noted in dogs during therapy. In subacute toxicity studies in dogs, a
dose of 30 mg/kg caused slight increases in plasma transaminase activity. In humans, adverse effects may include nausea, vomiting, diarrhea, abdominal pain, skin rash, and elevations in serum ALT, alkaline phosphatase, and AST.

DRUG INTERACTIONS: High doses of fluconazole may increase
serum cyclosporine levels. Fluconazole also increases serum phenytoin levels. Prothrombin time may increase if used concurrently with
warfarin. Hydrochlorothiazide increases fluconazole plasma levels.
Rifampin decreases serum levels of fluconazole, necessitating an increase in fluconazole drug dosages. Fluconazole decreases the elimination of oral sulfonylurea drugs, e.g., glipizide, predisposing to
hypoglycemia.

SUPPLIED AS: HUMAN PRODUCTS
For injection containing 2 mg/mL

Tablets containing 50, 100, and 200 mg
Oral suspension containing 10 and 40 mg/mL

FLUCYTOSINE

INDICATIONS: Flucytosine (Ancobon ★, Ancotil ♣) has been recommended for the treatment of cryptococcosis and candidiasis. It also has been used in combination with amphotericin B and ketoconazole in the treatment of cryptococcosis. *Aspergillus* spp. has an intermediate sensitivity to the drug. It is deaminated to 5-fluorouracil in fungal cells.

ADVERSE AND COMMON SIDE EFFECTS: Leukopenia and thrombocytopenia (which may occur within days of onset of treatment), hepatotoxicity, cutaneous eruption, rash, nausea, diarrhea, and abdominal pain have been reported. The drug is teratogenic and should not be given to pregnant animals. Resistance to the drug develops rapidly, especially when low doses are used.

DRUG INTERACTIONS: An additive or synergistic response may be expected when used with amphotericin B; however, toxicity of flucytosine may be increased with this combination because of decreased renal clearance. Combination therapy with flucytosine and ketoconazole in cats is especially toxic.

SUPPLIED AS: HUMAN PRODUCT
Capsules containing 250 and 500 mg [Ancobon] and 500 mg [Ancotil]

OTHER USES
Dogs
URINARY TRACT CANDIDIASIS
200 mg/kg/day div. tid–qid; PO. The drug is continued at least 2 to 3 weeks beyond clinical resolution of the disease.

FLUDROCORTISONE

INDICATIONS: Fludrocortisone (Florinef ♣ ★) is a long-acting steroid with potent mineralocorticoid and moderate glucocorticoid activity. It is indicated in the treatment of hypoadrenocorticism, where it promotes sodium retention and urinary potassium excretion. In larger doses, it inhibits endogenous cortisol secretion.

ADVERSE AND COMMON SIDE EFFECTS: Adverse effects are rare but with overdose may include sodium retention causing edema and hypertension, hypokalemia, and muscle weakness. At higher drug dosages clinical signs of glucocorticoid excess may become apparent, e.g., polyuria, polydipsia, or urinary incontinence. To help resolve these problems, switch the patient to DOCP and then gradually taper the dog off fludrocortisone over a 4 to 5 day period.

DRUG INTERACTIONS: The likelihood of hypokalemia is increased with the concurrent use of amphotericin B, thiazide diuretics, and furosemide. The drug may increase insulin requirements of diabetic patients.

SUPPLIED AS: HUMAN PRODUCT
Tablets containing 0.1 mg

OTHER USES
Dogs
HYPERKALEMIA
0.1 to 1 mg/dog per day (as adjunctive therapy)

FLUMETHASONE

INDICATIONS: Flumethasone (Flucort ✤ ★) is a long-acting glucocorticoid recommended for use in dogs and cats for inflammatory musculoskeletal conditions, acute and chronic dermatoses to help control pruritus, irritation and inflammation associated with these disorders, in allergic states, in shock, and in cats for appetite stimulation along with B-complex vitamins. For further information on INDICATIONS, ADVERSE AND COMMON SIDE EFFECTS, and DRUG INTERACTIONS, see **GLUCOCORTICOID AGENTS.**

SUPPLIED AS: VETERINARY PRODUCT
For injection containing 0.5 mg/mL in 100-mL vials

FLUNIXIN MEGLUMINE

INDICATIONS: Flunixin meglumine (Banamine ✤ ★) is a potent antiprostaglandin with anti-inflammatory and antipyretic properties that make it useful in the treatment of inflammation and pain associated with musculoskeletal disease. Its analgesic properties are considered superior to those of aspirin, meperidine, pentazocine, codeine phosphate, and phenylbutazone. The drug also has been recommended as adjunctive therapy in the treatment of shock in the dog. In addition, flunixin has been used for the short-term relief of ocular inflammation, e.g., conjunctivitis, corneal trauma, uveitis, chorioretinitis, and panophthalmitis.

ADVERSE AND COMMON SIDE EFFECTS: Increased serum concentrations of ALT, nephrotoxicity, and gastric ulceration may be noted. Gastric ulceration may be exacerbated by the concurrent use of prednisone. At higher doses, salivation, panting, vomiting, and tremors have been reported. Kidney necrosis may occur in patients with preexisting kidney disease. Intramuscular injection can be irritating.

DRUG INTERACTIONS: None established. Concurrent use of methoxyflurane may predispose to acute renal tubular necrosis.

SUPPLIED AS: VETERINARY PRODUCTS
Granules containing 25 mg/g
Paste containing 50 mg/g
For injection containing 50 mg/mL

FLUOROQUINOLONE ANTIBIOTICS

INDICATIONS: Norfloxacin (Noroxin ♣ ★), enrofloxacin (Baytril ♣ ★), ciprofloxacin (Cipro ♣ ★), and orbifloxacin (Orbax ♣ ★) constitute the fluoroquinolone group. These antibiotics have activity against *Escherichia coli, Enterobacter, Klebsiella, Proteus, Pseudomonas,* some *Staphylococcus, Salmonella, Shigella, Vibrio, Yersinia,* and *Campylobacter* organisms. They have little activity against anaerobic cocci, *Bacteroides,* or clostridial organisms. Resistance does occur, especially with *Pseudomonas, Klebsiella, Acinetobacter,* and Enterococcus organisms. Ciprofloxacin has more activity than other quinolones against *Pseudomonas* and *Acinetobacter.* Streptococci (particularly enterococci) generally are resistant, which may limit the use of fluoroquinolone antibiotics in the treatment of respiratory infections, where streptococci often are present. Orbifloxacin appears more effective than enrofloxacin in the treatment of urinary tract infection and equally as effective as enrofloxacin in the treatment of skin wounds and abscesses in dogs. Fluoroquinolone antibiotics may be effective against atypical mycobacteria (*M. fortuitum* and *M. chelonei*), although higher dosages may be needed. The fluoroquinolone antibiotics are effective in the treatment of respiratory tract infections, bronchopneumonia, enteric infections, bacterial prostatitis, bacterial meningoencephalitis, osteomyelitis, and skin and soft tissue infections.

ADVERSE AND COMMON SIDE EFFECTS: Side effects are rare but may include vomiting and diarrhea. Rapid IV injection in anesthetized dogs or cats may cause hypotension related to histamine release. At high doses, renal toxicity may develop from crystalluria and crystal deposition in renal tubules. Drug dose should be decreased in patients with renal disease. Fluoroquinolone antibiotics also may cause erosion of cartilage and a permanent lameness in young animals, and they are not recommended between 2 and 8 months of age in small and medium-sized breeds of dogs, before 1 year in large breeds, and before 18 months in giant breed dogs. These drugs should not be given to lactating bitches. The drugs are potentially teratogenic and should not be given to pregnant animals. Seizure activity may be precipitated with the concurrent use of NSAIDs. Dogs given high doses have had subcapsular cataract formation of the lens and associated inflammatory response after treatment for 8 to 12 months. Cats given high doses of ciprofloxacin developed erythema of the pinnae, vomiting, and clonic muscle spasm.

DRUG INTERACTIONS: Food impairs absorption of these drugs. Absorption also is hindered by antacid preparations, multivitamin compounds and sucralfate, and agents containing divalent and trivalent cations, e.g., iron, aluminum, calcium, magnesium, and zinc. Nitrofurantoin may impair pharmacologic efficacy. Enrofloxacin and ciprofloxacin may increase plasma theophylline levels. Fluoroquinolones may exacerbate the nephrotoxic potential of cyclosporine. Antibiotic synergism may occur if these agents are used with aminoglycosides, third-generation cephalosporins, and extended-spectrum penicillins.

SUPPLIED AS: See specific product.

FLUOROURACIL

INDICATIONS: Fluorouracil (Adrucil ✤ ★) is an antimetabolite chemotherapeutic agent that has been used in the treatment of various canine carcinomas and sarcomas.

ADVERSE AND COMMON SIDE EFFECTS: Nausea, vomiting, and diarrhea may occur. Oral and GI ulceration, leukopenia, thrombocytopenia, anemia, cerebellar ataxia, and alopecia also have been reported. The drug is extremely neurotoxic to cats and should not be used in this species.

DRUG INTERACTIONS: The concurrent use of other myelosuppressive agents or radiation therapy may require adjustment of drug dose.

SUPPLIED AS: HUMAN PRODUCT
For injection containing 50 mg/mL

FOLIC ACID

INDICATIONS: Folic acid (Folvite ✤ ★ and generic products ✤ ★) is a member of the vitamin B complex group and is essential for the maintenance of normal erythropoiesis. Folic acid deficiency may occur with blood loss, prolonged malabsorption, or sulfonamide administration. It may be indicated in cases in which pyrimethamine is used on a long-term basis.

ADVERSE AND COMMON SIDE EFFECTS: The drug is reportedly nontoxic.

DRUG INTERACTIONS: Chloramphenicol may antagonize the hematologic response.

SUPPLIED AS: HUMAN PRODUCTS
Tablets containing 100, 400, 800 µg and 1 and 5 mg
For injection containing 5 and 10 mg/mL

FOMEPIZOLE

INDICATIONS: Fomepizole (Antizol-Vet ★) is a synthetic alcohol dehydrogenase inhibitor used in the treatment of ethylene glycol (antifreeze) toxicity in dogs. Its chemical name is 4-methylpyrazole, and it is a more potent inhibitor of alcohol dehydrogenase than ethanol. Once inhibition of alcohol dehydrogenase has been effected, the remaining unmetabolized ethylene glycol and its metabolites are excreted in the urine. This agent is only effective if it is used before complete metabolism of ethylene glycol. Likely efficacy of the product can be determined before the initiation of therapy by measuring serum creatinine and BUN after clinical dehydration has been corrected. Blood urea nitrogen levels in excess of 40 mg/dL (14.28 mmol/L) and serum creatinine levels greater than 1.8 mg/dL (159.12 µmol/L) imply that ethylene glycol has been metabolized completely and that significant renal impairment probably has occurred. However, if urine output can be maintained, treatment with fomepizole still may be beneficial. Experimental studies with 4-methylpyrazole have indicated that most dogs survive if treatment is begun within 8 hours of ingestion of ethylene glycol. In another study, all dogs treated within 5 hours of antifreeze ingestion survived. 4-methylpyrazole does not appear to be as effective as ethanol in the treatment of ethylene glycol toxicity in cats.

ADVERSE AND COMMON SIDE EFFECTS: At higher-than-recommended dosages, fomepizole can cause CNS depression. Dosages of 25 mg/kg resulted in decreased food consumption, weight loss, and a sweet breath. At 30 mg/kg, the drug caused hypoactivity. At 50 mg/kg, ataxia, hypoactivity, hypothermia, tremors and/or prostration, injected sclera, ptosis, protruding tongues, and decreased defecation were noted. Anaphylaxis, as documented by tachypnea, gagging, excessive salivation, and trembling, is rare. Safe use of the drug in pregnant or breeding dogs has not been established.

DRUG INTERACTIONS: There are no specific drug interactions documented to date. Supportive care, in the form of maintaining adequate hydration status, and normal acid–base and electrolyte balance are vital to successful outcome.

SUPPLIED AS: VETERINARY PRODUCT
For injection containing 1.5 mL (1.5 g) giving 50 mg/mL once reconstituted with sodium chloride

FUROSEMIDE

INDICATIONS: Furosemide (Lasix ✦ ★) is a potent loop diuretic effective in reducing preload and pulmonary edema in patients with congestive heart failure. The drug also may be used after adequate rehydration to promote diuresis in patients with oliguria. It promotes significant sodium and water excretion by inhibiting chloride resorption in the ascending loop of Henle. It also redistributes blood flow from the juxtamedullary region of the kidney to the cortex and may act as a venous vasodilator by increasing systemic and venous capacitance. The drug is beneficial in the management of systemic hypertension. Activity is noted 5 minutes after IV injection and 1 hour after oral use. Peak activity occurs 30 minutes after IV injection and 1 to 2 hours after oral dosing. Duration of activity is 2 hours after IV injection and 6 hours after oral administration.

ADVERSE AND COMMON SIDE EFFECTS: Dehydration, hypokalemia, hyponatremia, and hypochloremic alkalosis may occur. The drug should not be used in patients with anuria or with progressive renal disease in the face of increasing azotemia. Ototoxicity may occur in cats, especially with high IV doses. Other side effects may include GI upset, anemia, leukopenia, weakness, and restlessness.

DRUG INTERACTIONS: Furosemide-induced hypokalemia may enhance the toxic potential of digitalis. The likelihood of hypokalemia may be increased if used with amphotericin B or the glucocorticoids. Pharmacologic effects of theophylline may be increased with furosemide. Ototoxicity and nephrotoxicity of the aminoglycosides may be potentiated. Competition for renal excretory sites may require adjustment of aspirin doses. Furosemide may inhibit muscle relaxation produced by tubocurarine, but it may enhance the effects of succinylcholine. Adjustments in insulin requirements also may need to be addressed. With continuous use, the loss of water-soluble vitamins may occur, and it may be advisable to supplement these patients with B-complex vitamins.

SUPPLIED AS: VETERINARY PRODUCTS
Tablets containing 20 and 40 mg ✦
Tablets containing 12.5 and 50 mg ★
Oral solution containing 10 mg/mL ★
For injection containing 50 mg/mL ✦★

GENTAMICIN

INDICATIONS: Gentamicin (Gentocin ✦ ★) is an aminoglycoside antibiotic. For information on ADVERSE AND COMMON SIDE EFFECTS and DRUG INTERACTIONS, see **AMINOGLYCOSIDE ANTIBIOTICS.**

Steady-state levels are achieved in 6.5 hours in the dog and 6.8 hours in the cat. Serum concentrations are measured 1 hour after dosing and just before the next dose (trough). Therapeutic drug levels should be based on 4 to 5 times the MIC of the offending organism. Therapeutic peak drug levels are 8 to 10 µg/mL, and trough levels are 1 µg/mL. Toxic drug levels are greater than 15 µg/mL (peak concentration) and greater than 2 µg/mL (trough concentration).

SUPPLIED AS: VETERINARY PRODUCTS
Ophthalmic preparation containing 5 mg/mL or 3 mg/mL that includes betamethasone
Otic preparation containing 3 mg/mL gentamicin as well as betamethasone
For injection containing 50 mg/mL and 100 mg/mL gentamicin

GLIPIZIDE

INDICATIONS: Glipizide (Glucotrol ★) is an oral sulfonylurea hypoglycemic agent. It stimulates functioning pancreatic β-cells to secrete insulin within 10 minutes of oral administration. Indirectly, glipizide leads to increased insulin binding at receptor sites, and it causes inhibition of hepatic glucose production and a reduction in serum glucagon levels. The drug has been used successfully in some cats with type II (noninsulin-dependent) diabetes mellitus. More than 50% and as many as 65% of cats may be responsive to oral hypoglycemic agents when used in conjunction with dietary therapy and correction of obesity. In a more recent study, 44% of diabetic cats improved. Response often is not apparent during the first 2 to 6 weeks of therapy. If response does occur, it usually is apparent by week 8 of treatment, although some cats require up to 12 weeks of therapy before clinical response occurs. It has been reported that cats that respond well to the drug tend to have preprandial serum glucose levels of less than 200 mg/dL (11.1 mmol/L). Identifying a high preprandial serum insulin concentration or an increase in serum insulin during a glucose tolerance test is supportive of a diagnosis of noninsulin-dependent diabetes mellitus and the cases that are likely to benefit from the use of an oral sulfonylurea agent. A more recent study determined that body weight, serum glucose, and insulin were not reliable predictors of response to glipizide. Response to glipizide does not rule out the possible need for exogenous insulin in the future. The drug also has been used in some cases of type II and type III canine diabetes, but most dogs tend to be type I (insulin-dependent) diabetics, undermining the effect of the drug. In addition, some type II and type III diabetic animals have insulin antagonism as a result of hyperadrenocorticism or excessive growth hormone secretion. The cause of the diabetes should be determined before therapy is instituted.

ADVERSE AND COMMON SIDE EFFECTS: The drug is contraindicated in diabetic ketoacidosis. Caution is advised in patients with impaired renal or hepatic function and those with adrenal or pituitary insufficiency. Experience with the drug in small animals is limited; however, adverse reactions in cats have included anorexia, vomiting, hypoglycemia, icterus, and increased serum alanine aminotransferase levels. Chronic treatment may result in decreased insulin content in β cells and decreased nutrient-stimulated insulin secretion. The drug should be discontinued and insulin treatment initiated if clinical signs of the disease worsen; if the cat becomes ill or develops ketoacidosis or neuropathy; if blood glucose levels remain greater than 350 mg/dL (19.4 mmol/L); or if owners become dissatisfied with the treatment. If cats suffer from side effects of the drug but the owners wish to try the drug again, these cats may be started at a lower dose, e.g., 2.5 mg every other day or once daily, slowly increasing the dose on a weekly basis.

In humans, other side effects may include nausea, diarrhea, constipation, cholestatic jaundice, leukopenia, thrombocytopenia, hemolytic anemia, agranulocytosis, and pruritus.

DRUG INTERACTIONS: Oral anticoagulants, cimetidine, chloramphenicol, phenylbutazone, salicylates, and sulfonamides may potentiate the hypoglycemic action of the drug. β-adrenergic–blocking agents may increase the frequency and severity of hypoglycemia, and if these drugs must be used, a selective β-1–blocking agent, e.g., atenolol or metoprolol, is recommended. Diazoxide and the thiazide diuretics may antagonize the action of glipizide, decreasing its hypoglycemic effect.

SUPPLIED AS: HUMAN PRODUCT
Tablets containing 5 and 10 mg

GLUCOCORTICOID AGENTS

INDICATIONS: Glucocorticoid agents are recommended for the treatment of allergic and immune-mediated diseases, pruritus, cardiogenic and septic shock, and trauma and edema of the CNS and spinal cord. The benefit of steroid use in traumatic shock has not been proven to decrease morbidity or mortality. Corticosteroids are absorbed by cells wherein they affect the formation of new mRNA and initiate new protein synthesis. The newly formed proteins mediate the effects of these drugs. Beneficial effects include stabilization of lysosomal and capillary membranes; decrease in activation of the complement and clotting cascades; binding of endotoxin; positive inotropic effect; dilation of precapillary sphincters; prevention of GI mucosal ischemia associated with shock; increase in glucogenesis; inhibition of the formation of vasoactive substances (kinins, prostaglandins); decreased chemotaxis, phagocytosis, and bactericidal activity; depressed T-cell responses and interleukin-2 production; decrease in collagen and scar formation; and decrease in the accumulation of phagocytes at areas of inflammation. In autoimmune disease, glucocorticoids have a rapid onset of action. They interfere with the F_c receptors of immunoglobulin G and C_{3b} receptors on macrophages and decrease immunoglobulin affinity for erythrocytes in cases of autoimmune hemolytic anemia. In large doses, they decrease antibody production. They do not decrease the concentration of antibody already present. Analgesic activity is only related to prostaglandin inhibition. These agents do not possess direct analgesic activity.

The glucocorticoids are classified according to their duration of action. As biologic half-life increases, anti-inflammatory potency increases and mineralocorticoid potency decreases. Short-acting drugs (less than 12 hours) include hydrocortisone and cortisone acetate. Intermediate-acting drugs (12–36 hours) include prednisone, prednisolone, methylprednisolone, and triamcinolone. The long-acting steroids (more than 48 hours) include paramethasone, flumethasone, betamethasone, and dexamethasone. Topical corticosteroids are used for their local anti-inflammatory, antipruritic, and vasoconstrictive effects.

ADVERSE AND COMMON SIDE EFFECTS: Polyuria, polydipsia, polyphagia, panting, lethargy, weakness, and bilateral symmetrical alopecia are the most common clinical signs of glucocorticoid excess. Changing to a corticosteroid with little or no mineralocorticoid activity (methylprednisolone, dexamethasone, triamcinolone) can reduce or eliminate excessive polyuria–polydipsia. Weight loss, anorexia, and diarrhea may follow use of these drugs. Hemorrhagic gastroenteritis, pancreatitis, glomerulonephritis, and hepatopathy have been reported with the use of corticosteroids. In one study, although daily doses of prednisone (4 mg/kg; PO or IM) caused an increase in serum lipase values (and a decrease in serum amylase), the drug did not induce pancreatitis. Urine protein to creatinine ratios may increase (generally values less than 3) in dogs treated with large doses of prednisone over long-term use. Laboratory changes noted with these drugs may include elevations in serum alanine transferase, alkaline phosphatase, gamma-glutamyl transpeptidase, hyperglycemia, hypokalemia, hypocalcemia, a stress leukogram, and increases in red blood cell numbers. Glucocorticoid drugs suppress inflammation, reduce fever, and increase protein catabolism and their conversion to carbohydrates, leading to a negative nitrogen balance, promote sodium retention and potassium diuresis, retard wound healing, lower resistance to infection, and cause a reduction in the number of circulating lymphocytes. Only prolonged or high-dose therapy started before surgery actually delays wound healing, an effect potentiated by starvation or protein depletion. Once the inflammatory phase is established, usually within 1 to 3 days of injury, glucocorticoid therapy has little effect on subsequent healing. If preoperative corticosteroid use is necessary, vitamin A or zinc supplementation may help counter the effects of the steroids on collagen production and metabolism. An increase in the incidence of osteoporosis may be noted, especially in older dogs, with prolonged use of these drugs. Their use during the healing phase of bone fractures is not recommended. Iatrogenic hyperadrenocorticism may follow prolonged use of parenteral as well as topical glucocorticoid agents. Glucocorticoids are contraindicated in animals with acute or chronic bacterial infections unless therapeutic doses of an effective bactericidal agent is used concurrently. Corticosteroids may mask signs of infection, such as elevation in body temperature. These drugs should be used with caution in animals with congestive heart failure, diabetes mellitus, and renal disease. These drugs may retard growth if given to young growing animals. Corticosteroids have been associated with an increased incidence of cleft palate and other congenital malformations. In addition, their use may be associated with the induction of the first stage of parturition, when administered during the last trimester of pregnancy, and may precipitate premature parturition followed by dystocia, fetal death, retained placenta, and metritis.

DRUG INTERACTIONS: Glucocorticoids may decrease the efficacy of bacteriostatic antibiotics by decreasing the inflammatory response and diminishing the phagocytic activity of leukocytes. Amphotericin B, furosemide, and the thiazide diuretics may potentiate hypokalemia. Hypokalemia may predispose to digitalis toxicity. Glucocorticoids may reduce serum salicylate levels. Phenytoin, phenobarbital, and rifampin may increase the metabolism of glucocorticoids, and insulin requirements of diabetic patients may increase. Hepatic metabolism of methylprednisolone may be inhibited by erythromycin. The concomitant use of glucocorticoids and cyclosporine may lead to increases in serum levels of both drugs. The dose of steroids used in animals receiving mitotane may have to be increased. Live attenuated-virus vaccines generally should not be given to animals receiving glucocorticoid drugs. Concurrent use of NSAIDs may increase the potential for GIT ulceration. Estrogens may potentiate the effects of hydrocortisone and other glucocorticoids.

SUPPLIED AS: See specific product.

GLYBURIDE

INDICATIONS: Glyburide (Diaβeta ✦ ★, Micronase ★) is an oral sulfonylurea hypoglycemic drug with indications similar to those of glipizide. The drug has a longer duration of effect (24 hours) in people than glipizide (10–16 hours). The practitioner is advised that experience with use of this specific agent is limited in small animals. Also see **GLIPIZIDE**.

ADVERSE AND COMMON SIDE EFFECTS: Experience with use of this oral sulfonylurea hypoglycemic agent is limited. See **GLIPIZIDE.**

DRUG INTERACTIONS: Glyburide is less likely to be displaced or cause the displacement of highly protein-bound drugs than glipizide. Phenylbutazone may potentiate the hypoglycemic effects of the drug. Thiazide diuretics may exacerbate diabetes mellitus, increasing the dosage requirement of the sulfonylurea drugs. Nonselective-blocking agents may potentiate the hypoglycemic effects of these drugs. These effects may be mitigated by the use of selective β_1-blocking agents. Monamine oxidase inhibitors (possibly amitraz and selegiline) may enhance the hypoglycemic effect of sulfonylurea agents. Drugs that may decrease the hypoglycemic effect include furosemide, corticosteroids, phenothiazines, estrogens, thyroid agents, phenytoin, calcium channel-blocking drugs, rifampin, and sympathomimetic agents.

SUPPLIED AS: Tablets containing 1.25, 2.5, and 5 mg

GLYCOPYRROLATE

INDICATIONS: Glycopyrrolate (Robinul-V ★, Robinul ✦ ★) is an anticholinergic agent used in preanesthetic regimens to reduce salivary, tracheobronchial, and pharyngeal secretions, to reduce the volume and acidity of gastric secretion, and to inhibit cardiac vagal inhibitory reflexes during anesthetic induction and intubation.

ADVERSE AND COMMON SIDE EFFECTS: Mydriasis and xerostomia may be noted with its use. Excretion of the drug may be prolonged in animals with impaired renal or gastrointestinal function. It should not be given to pregnant animals. Refer also to ADVERSE AND COMMON SIDE EFFECTS of **ATROPINE,** which are similar.

DRUG INTERACTIONS: As for atropine, interactions include enhancement of activity if used with antihistamines, procainamide, quinidine, meperidine, benzodiazepines, and phenothiazines. Adverse effects may be potentiated by primidone, disopyramide, nitrates, and long-term corticosteroid use (via increasing intraocular pressure). Glycopyrrolate may enhance the actions of nitrofurantoin, thiazide diuretics, and sympathomimetic agents. The drug may antagonize the activity of metoclopramide.

SUPPLIED AS: VETERINARY PRODUCT
For injection containing 0.2 mg/mL ★

HUMAN PRODUCTS
Tablets containing 1 and 2 mg
For injection containing 0.2 mg/mL

OTHER USES
Dogs
REDUCE SECRETIONS
0.01 mg/kg PRN; SC

PREANESTHETIC
0.01 to 0.02 mg/kg; SC, IM

Cats
PREANESTHETIC
0.011 mg/kg; IM (15 minutes before anesthetic)

GONADORELIN

INDICATIONS: Gonadorelin (Cystorelin ✤ ★) has been used experimentally in dogs to diagnose reproductive failure and to identify intact animals from neutered ones by maximally stimulating follicle-stimulating hormone (FSH) and luteinizing hormone (LH) production. It also has been used experimentally via pulse-dosing to induce estrus in dogs. The drug has been used to induce estrus in cats with prolonged anestrus.

ADVERSE AND COMMON SIDE EFFECTS: None reported.

DRUG INTERACTIONS: VETERINARY PRODUCT
For injection in 50 µg/mL [Cystorelin]

HUMAN PRODUCT
For injection in 100 and 500 µg/vial [Factrel ✤ ★]

GRANULOCYTE COLONY-STIMULATING FACTOR

INDICATIONS: Filgrastim (Neupogen ✤ ★) is a human granulocyte colony-stimulating factor that has been used to manage dogs and cats with chemotherapy-induced neutropenia. More specifically, it is indicated in animals with febrile neutropenia (counts less than 1,000/µL), prolonged (more than 72 hours) severe neutropenia (counts less than 500/µL), or a history of febrile neutropenia associated with previous dosages of chemotherapy. Canine recombinant granulocyte colony-stimulating factor, although not commercially available at this time, is effective in dogs and cats.

ADVERSE AND COMMON SIDE EFFECTS: Neutrophilia accompanied by a left shift, Dohle bodies, vacuolation, and toxic granulation of leukocytes are to be expected with use of the product and do not necessarily indicate sepsis. Increases in alkaline phosphatase activity also has been reported in people receiving this therapy. Initially, a significant and rapid (within 12 hours and steadily rising over a 2-week period) increase in neutrophil numbers is to be expected. In healthy dogs and cats, the increase in neutrophil numbers is followed by a decrease in neutrophil numbers (after 23 days in dogs and as early as day 14) and (after 17 to 21 days in cats) which in the case of healthy dogs is due to the formation of antibodies directed against the product. Antibody formation apparently does not occur in dogs with cancer that are receiving the drug. It is suggested that the drug only be used as aforementioned, for short courses only, and that it be discontinued 2 days after segmented neutrophil numbers exceed 3,000/µL. The most common adverse effect reported in people is medullary bone pain, which in most cases is readily controlled with nonopioid analgesics. Other less common adverse effects in people include exacerbation of skin disease (psoriasis, cutaneous vasculitis), hematuria, proteinuria, and thrombocytopenia. Long-term (up to 4.5 years) adverse effects in people include osteoporosis.

DRUG INTERACTIONS: Because of the potential sensitivity of rapidly dividing myeloid cells to cytotoxic chemotherapy, filgrastim should not be given 24 hours before or after cytotoxic chemotherapy is administered. The efficacy of this agent in patients receiving nitrosourea compounds or with myelosuppressive dosages of 5-fluorouracil or cytosine arabinoside has not been established. Nor has filgrastim's safety and efficacy been established in those undergoing concurrent radiation therapy. There is the possibility that filgrastim may potentiate the growth of certain tumor types, particularly myeloid malignancies.

SUPPLIED AS: HUMAN PRODUCT
For injection containing 300 µg/mL

GRISEOFULVIN

INDICATIONS: Griseofulvin (Fulvicin U/F ✤ ★) is used for the treatment of dermatophyte infections. The drug is detectable in the skin within 4 to 8 hours of oral administration. High dietary fat facilitates absorption.

ADVERSE AND COMMON SIDE EFFECTS: Nausea, vomiting, and diarrhea are the most common side effects. Hepatotoxicity and photosensitization also have been reported but are rare. Cats, especially kittens, are more sensitive to the adverse effects of the drug. Anemia and panleukopenia also have been documented. Seropositive cats with FIV are at increased risk for griseofulvin-associated neutropenia. Anorexia, dehydration, edema of the skin and mucosae, pruritus, and ataxia also have been reported in cats. The drug may inhibit spermatogenesis and is potentially teratogenic and mutagenic in a number of species and may cause cleft palate, skeletal, and brain malformations in kittens if administered during the first trimester of pregnancy.

DRUG INTERACTIONS: Phenobarbital decreases absorption of the drug. Coumarin anticoagulant activity may be reduced by griseofulvin. Vaccination or viral infection induce interferon synthesis, which in turn inhibits hepatic enzyme systems and may prolong the elimination of griseofulvin.

SUPPLIED AS: VETERINARY PRODUCT
Tablets (microsize) containing 250 and 500 mg ★
HUMAN PRODUCT
Tablets (microsize) containing 125, 250, and 500 mg ♣ ★

GUAIFENESIN

INDICATIONS: Guaifenesin (Guailaxin ★), formerly glyceryl guaiacolate, is used as an adjunct to anesthesia to induce muscle relaxation and restraint for short procedures. In humans, the drug is used as an expectorant in the management of dry, unproductive cough. It stimulates gastric receptors that initiate a reflex secretion of bronchial glands, thereby increasing the volume and decreasing the viscosity of bronchial secretions. Its efficacy in improving mucociliary clearance, however, is questionable.

ADVERSE AND COMMON SIDE EFFECTS: A mild decrease in blood pressure and an increase in heart rate may occur. Thrombophlebitis has been reported, and perivascular injection may cause tissue reaction. Hemolysis may occur if solutions greater than 5% concentration are used. If overdose occurs, apneustic breathing, nystagmus, hypotension, and paradoxical muscle rigidity have been noted. With oral preparations, nausea, gastric upset, and drowsiness are reported in people. The drug may prolong activated clotting time and impair platelet function. It should be avoided in animals with bleeding tendencies.

DRUG INTERACTIONS: Physostigmine and other cholinesterase agents, e.g., neostigmine, pyridostigmine, and edrophonium, are contraindicated with its use.

SUPPLIED AS: VETERINARY PRODUCTS
For IM injection containing 75 mg guaiacol
[Guaitex ♣]—small and large animals
For injection containing 50 g, for reconstitution [Guailaxin]—horses only

HALOTHANE

INDICATIONS: Halothane (Fluothane ✦ ★, Halothane ✦ ★) is an inhalant anesthetic agent. It is a fast, potent anesthetic that allows for smooth induction without excitement and a quick uneventful recovery.

ADVERSE AND COMMON SIDE EFFECTS: Dose-dependent hypotension has been documented. Hepatic necrosis, although rare, may occur with the use of halothane, the incidence of which increases with each use of this agent. Should unexplained fever, jaundice, or other signs of liver dysfunction occur after use of the drug, its subsequent use in that animal is contraindicated. High doses of halothane may cause uterine atony and postpartum bleeding, and generally, it is not recommended for obstetric procedures unless uterine relaxation is required.

DRUG INTERACTIONS: The drug is potentially arrhythmogenic, especially in the presence of epinephrine and the thiobarbiturates. D-tubocurare causes a marked decrease in blood pressure.

SUPPLIED AS: VETERINARY AND HUMAN PRODUCT
Halothane is supplied in 250-mL bottles

HEPARIN

INDICATIONS: Heparin may be indicated in cases of aortic and venous thrombosis, pulmonary thromboembolic disease, and disseminated intravascular coagulation (DIC). It inactivates thrombin, blocks the conversion of fibrinogen to fibrin, and—in combination with antithrombin III—inactivates factors IX, X, XI, and XII and prevents the formation of a stable fibrin clot via the inactivation of factor XIII. Heparin does not lyse clots. The drug promotes resolution of thromboemboli by preventing deposition of fibrin and platelets on the thrombin surface, inhibiting thrombus formation and allowing natural thrombolytic mechanisms to decrease the size of the thrombus. In the case of burn victims, heparin has been used to increase the effectiveness of repair mechanisms, decrease thrombosis and the development of gangrene, and protect against the development of DIC.

ADVERSE AND COMMON SIDE EFFECTS: Bleeding and thrombocytopenia are the most common adverse effects of the drug, leading to prolonged activated partial thromboplastin time. Protamine zinc may be used to reverse the adverse effects of bleeding. Intramuscular injection can result in hematoma formation. Other side effects reported have included osteoporosis with long-term use, diminished renal function after long-term use, high dose therapy, rebound hyperlipidemia, hyperkalemia, alopecia, suppressed aldosterone synthesis, and priapism.

DRUG INTERACTIONS: Heparin may antagonize the action of corticosteroids, insulin, and ACTH and increase serum levels of diazepam. Antihistamines, IV nitroglycerin, digoxin, and tetracyclines may antagonize the effects of heparin. Heparin should be used with caution with other drugs that may adversely affect coagulation, e.g., aspirin, phenylbutazone, dipyridamole, or warfarin.

SUPPLIED AS: HUMAN PRODUCTS
For injection containing 1,000, 5,000, 10,000, 20,000, and 40,000 U/mL [Liquaemin Sodium ★]
For injection containing 100, 1,000, 10,000, and 25,000 U/mL [Heparin Leo ♣]
For injection containing 5,000 U/0.2-mL syringe, 12,500 U/0.5 mL, and 20,000 U/0.8 mL [Calciparine ♣ ★]

OTHER USES
Dogs
HEARTWORM DISEASE
300 U/kg tid; SC (prevention of pulmonary thromboembolism associated with adulticide therapy)

HEPARIN STIMULATION TEST
100 U/kg; IV to stimulate lipoprotein lipase
A lack of increase in lipolytic activity is suggestive of lipoprotein lipase inactivity.

DISSEMINATED INTRAVASCULAR COAGULATION
i)   5 to 10 U/kg/hour by continuous intravenous infusion
ii) 75 U/kg tid; SC

Monitoring of activated partial thromboplastin time (APTT) at these dosages is not necessary because the risk of bleeding is minimal.

PULMONARY THROMBOEMBOLISM
200 U/kg; IV followed by 100 to 200 U/kg qid; SC or 15 to 20 U/kg/hour IV infusion adjusted to prolong APTT by 1.5 to 2.0 times baseline values. Warfarin is recommended if anticoagulant therapy is required for longer periods. Warfarin requires 2 to 7 days to become effective. A dose of 0.2 mg/kg; PO is used initially, followed by 0.05 to 0.10 mg/kg/day to maintain prothrombin time (PT) 1.5 to 2 times baseline values. Heparin therapy is tapered gradually and discontinued when desired PT is achieved.

Cats
ACUTE ARTERIAL EMBOLIZATION
100 U/kg tid; SC

AORTIC THROMBOEMBOLISM
Heparin 100 U/kg; tid; SC in conjunction with warfarin 0.5 mg/day;
PO. Discontinue heparin after 3 to 4 days. Adjust warfarin dose to
maintain international normalized ratio (INR) PT, which is the patient's PT divided by control PT, to 2 to 3.

HETACILLIN

INDICATIONS: Hetacillin (Hetacin-K ✤ ★) is a broad-spectrum
penicillin antibiotic with activity against a number of gram-positive
organisms, including α- and β-hemolytic streptococci, staphylococci, enterococci, and clostridia and gram-negative organisms, including *Proteus mirabilis*, *Salmonella*, *Shigella*, *E. coli*, *Brucella* spp.,
and *Pasteurella multocida*. After oral ingestion, the drug is broken
down in the body into ampicillin. Hetacillin is susceptible to β-
lactamase.

For more information, including ADVERSE AND COMMON
SIDE EFFECTS and DRUG INTERACTIONS, see **PENICILLIN
ANTIBIOTICS.**

SUPPLIED AS: VETERINARY PRODUCT
Tablets containing 55, 110, and 220 mg

HETASTARCH

INDICATIONS: Hetastarch or hydroxyethyl starch (Hespan ✤ ★) is
a colloidal plasma volume expander used in cases requiring intravascular volume expansion, e.g., shock. It also has been used successfully to manage patients with hypoalbuminemia with or without
accompanying peripheral edema or body cavity transudates. The
product is eliminated primarily by the kidneys. Hetastarch has a
longer half-life in plasma than dextran because of its larger molecular size. Intravenous infusion of 1 L of hetastarch expands plasma
volume by approximately 700 mL, with 40% of the resultant increase
in plasma volume persisting approximately 24 to 36 hours. A recent
study in dogs with hypoalbuminemia, however, demonstrated that
a single dose of hetastarch raised colloid oncotic pressure for less
than 12 hours, indicating that multiple doses may be required to prolong the beneficial effects.

ADVERSE AND COMMON SIDE EFFECTS: Large volumes may
adversely affect coagulation and cause a decrease in platelet numbers and a prolongation of prothrombin time, partial thromboplastin time, and clotting times. Large volumes may decrease the hematocrit and cause dilution of plasma proteins. Hypervolemia may
occur, and patients with congestive heart failure or anuric renal failure are at increased risk. Because the product is eliminated via the

kidneys, caution is advised if it is used in patients with renal insufficiency. Other adverse effects reported in people include vomiting, pruritus, chills, elevated body temperature, muscle pain, edema of the extremities, and anaphylaxis.

DRUG INTERACTIONS: None established.

SUPPLIED AS: HUMAN PRODUCT
For injection containing 6 g hetastarch in 0.9% sodium chloride

OTHER USES
Dogs
HYPOALBUMINEMIA
25 to 30 mL/kg over 6 to 8 hours; IV. A second dose may be given immediately after the first without concurrent crystalloid fluid administration in cases of severe hypoalbuminemia combined with intravascular volume depletion and moderate to marked peripheral edema or body cavity effusions. In less severe cases, give concurrent crystalloids at approximately two thirds of the daily dosing requirements. Most dogs require at least 2 doses of hetastarch given 12 to 24 hours apart.

HYDRALAZINE

INDICATIONS: Hydralazine (Apresoline ♣ ★) is an arterial vasodilator. It facilitates increased cardiac output and decreases mitral regurgitation and left atrial size. It helps alleviate the cough associated with compression of the left principal bronchus from enlargement of the left atrium secondary to mitral valvular regurgitation. The drug also is used to manage systemic hypertension, often in conjunction with a diuretic and a β-blocker.

ADVERSE AND COMMON SIDE EFFECTS: Hypotension, increases in heart rate, sodium and water retention, vomiting, diarrhea, and tolerance to the drug have been described. Initial weakness and lethargy, which generally resolve in 3 to 4 days, may be noted.

DRUG INTERACTIONS: Phenylpropanolamine may exacerbate the tachycardia associated with use of hydralazine. Hydralazine may increase the absorption of propranolol and other β-blockers; in addition, the concurrent use of β-blockers or diazoxide may predispose to hypotension. The pressor response to epinephrine may be mitigated by hydralazine.

SUPPLIED AS: HUMAN PRODUCTS
Tablets containing 10, 25, 50, and 100 mg
For injection containing 20 mg/mL

HYDROCHLOROTHIAZIDE

INDICATIONS: Hydrochlorothiazide (HydroDiuril ✤ ★) is a diuretic used to decrease pulmonary edema in patients with congestive heart failure and cardiomyopathy. It is a less potent diuretic than furosemide. The drug also may be beneficial in reducing the recurrence of calcium oxalate urolithiasis, especially when used concurrently with Prescription Diet u/d.

ADVERSE AND COMMON SIDE EFFECTS: Hypokalemia, hypochloremic alkalosis, dilutional hyponatremia, and loss of water-soluble vitamins may occur with chronic use. Other side effects may include vomiting, diarrhea, polyuria, hyperglycemia, hyperlipidemia, hypotension, and hypersensitivity/dermatologic reactions.

DRUG INTERACTIONS: Concurrent use with corticosteroids or amphotericin B may predispose to hypokalemia. Thiazide hypokalemia predisposes to digitalis toxicity, and hydrochlorothiazide may prolong the half-life of quinidine. Sulfonamides may potentiate the action of hydrochlorothiazide. Hydrochlorothiazide may increase the activity of tubocurarine. The concurrent use of diazoxide may predispose to hyperglycemia, hypotension, and hyperuricemia. This drug also may alter the requirements of insulin.

SUPPLIED AS: HUMAN PRODUCT
Tablets containing 25, 50, and 100 mg

OTHER USES
Dogs
NEPHROGENIC DIABETES INSIPIDUS
i)   0.5 to 1 mg/kg bid; PO

ii) 2.5 to 5 mg/kg bid; PO

SYSTEMIC HYPERTENSION
2 to 4 mg/kg once to twice daily; PO (along with dietary salt restriction)

HYPOGLYCEMIA
2 to 4 mg/kg bid; PO (along with diazoxide)

HYDROCODONE

INDICATIONS: Hydrocodone (Hycodan ✤ ★) is a narcotic antitussive that is especially useful in the control of cough not responsive to other agents. The drug also has been used to treat compulsive, behaviorally related skin disorders.

ADVERSE AND COMMON SIDE EFFECTS: Sedation, vomiting, and constipation with chronic use may occur. In cats, opiate agonists may cause CNS excitation with hyperexcitability, tremors, and seizure activity.

DRUG INTERACTIONS: Antihistamines, phenothiazines, barbiturates, and other CNS depressants may potentiate CNS depression.

SUPPLIED AS: HUMAN PRODUCTS
Tablets containing 5 mg
Syrup containing 1 mg/mL

OTHER USES
Dogs
BEHAVIORAL DISORDERS
0.22 mg/kg bid–tid; PO

Cats
BEHAVIORAL DISORDERS
0.25 to 1 mg/kg bid–tid; PO

HYDROCORTISONE SODIUM SUCCINATE

INDICATIONS: Hydrocortisone sodium succinate (Solu-Cortef ✿ ★) is a glucocorticoid used primarily in cases of shock, feline asthma, and animals in acute hypoadrenocortical crisis. For information concerning ADVERSE AND COMMON SIDE EFFECTS and DRUG INTERACTIONS, see **GLUCOCORTICOID AGENTS.**

SUPPLIED AS: HUMAN PRODUCT
For injection containing 100, 250, 500, and 1,000 mg/vial

HYDROXYUREA

INDICATIONS: Hydroxyurea (Hydrea ✿ ★) is a chemotherapeutic agent used in the treatment of leukemia, mastocytoma, and primary polycythemia (polycythemia vera).

ADVERSE AND COMMON SIDE EFFECTS: In the dog, anorexia, vomiting, arrest of spermatogenesis, bone marrow hypoplasia, and sloughing of the nails have been reported. A complete blood count and platelet count should be done every 7 to 14 days until the hematocrit has normalized and repeated every 3 to 4 months thereafter. If leukopenia, thrombocytopenia, or anemia develop, the drug should be discontinued until blood counts return to normal. The drug should then be resumed at a lower dose. Other side effects may include alopecia, stomatitis, and dysuria.

DRUG INTERACTIONS: None established.

SUPPLIED AS: HUMAN PRODUCT
Capsules containing 500 mg

OTHER USES
Dogs
PRIMARY POLYCYTHEMIA
30 mg/kg daily for 5 to 7 days, then 15 mg/kg daily; PO

HYDROXYZINE

INDICATIONS: Hydroxyzine (Atarax ✿ ★) is an anxiolytic, antihistaminic agent. It has been used to manage some behavioral disorders, e.g., compulsive scratching and self-trauma, and to provide
mild sedation. The drug also has anticholinergic, antiemetic, and
bronchodilator effects. It has been used in small animals primarily
for its antihistaminic properties. For more information concerning
ADVERSE AND COMMON SIDE EFFECTS and DRUG INTERAC-
TIONS, see **ANTIHISTAMINES.**

ADVERSE AND COMMON SIDE EFFECTS: Transitory drowsiness is the most common side effect. Other adverse effects may include fine rapid tremors, seizures, xerostomia, hypotension, diarrhea, and decreased appetite.

DRUG INTERACTIONS: Barbiturates and other sedatives may potentiate CNS depression.

SUPPLIED AS: HUMAN PRODUCTS
Capsules containing 10, 25, 50, and 100 mg
Syrup containing 10 mg/5 mL
For injection containing 25 and 50 mg/mL

IBUPROFEN

INDICATIONS: Ibuprofen (Advil ✿ ★, Motrin ✿ ★) is a nonsteroidal
anti-inflammatory agent with antipyretic and analgesic properties
that make it useful in the management of joint pain secondary to degenerative joint disease. However, the drug is not routinely recommended because of its GI side effects and the availability of other
safer NSAIDs, e.g., aspirin.

ADVERSE AND COMMON SIDE EFFECTS: The drug appears to
cause gastric irritation and ulceration more frequently in dogs than
it does in people. Toxicity develops in dogs at a dosage of 50 to 125
mg/kg and may include vomiting, depression, diarrhea, anorexia,
ataxia and incoordination, and melena. Polyuria–polydipsia may
occur. Hemorrhagic gastroenteritis can be severe and lead to per-

foration. Less often, ataxia and stupor have been reported. Cats appear less prone to gastroenteritis, but are more apt to show tachypnea.

DRUG INTERACTIONS: Use of heparin and other anticoagulants may augment ibuprofen's inhibition of platelet aggregation, predisposing to bleeding. The pharmacologic activity of lithium may be increased if both drugs are used concurrently.

SUPPLIED AS: HUMAN PRODUCT
Tablets containing 200, 300, 400, and 600 mg

IMIPENEM–CILASTATIN

INDICATIONS: Imipenem–cilastatin (Primaxin ✤ ★) is a fixed combination of a β-lactam antibiotic and cilastatin, an inhibitor of dipeptidase inactivation of imipenem. This drug combination has the widest antibacterial spectrum of any β-lactam antibiotic, surpassing even that of the third-generation cephalosporins. The spectrum of activity includes gram-positive, gram-negative, anaerobic bacteria, and *Pseudomonas aeruginosa*. Infections resistant to cephalosporins, penicillins, and aminoglycosides often respond favorably to this combination.

ADVERSE AND COMMON SIDE EFFECTS: The drug combination is contraindicated in patients with hypersensitivity to penicillins or cephalosporins. Cautious use is recommended in patients with a history of seizures, brain lesions, recent head injury, or renal impairment. Drug dosage should be reduced in cases of renal failure. Nausea, vomiting, diarrhea, phlebitis at the infusion site, fever, pruritus, tachycardia, hypotension, and seizure activity have been reported. Safe use in pregnancy has not been established.

DRUG INTERACTIONS: The antibacterial effect of imipenem and aminoglycosides is additive or synergistic against some gram-positive bacteria. Imipenem antagonizes the antibacterial activity of other β-lactam antibiotics, including most cephalosporins and extended spectrum penicillins against *Pseudomonas aeruginosa* and some strains of *Enterobacter* and *Klebsiella*. Chloramphenicol may antagonize the bactericidal activity of imipenem.

SUPPLIED AS: HUMAN PRODUCT
For injection containing 250 and 500 mg

IMIPRAMINE

INDICATIONS: Imipramine (Tofranil ✤ ★) is a tricyclic antidepressant, structurally related to phenothiazines and used in dogs for the treatment of canine narcolepsy/cataplexy, separation anxiety, and lick granuloma. The drug also has been used to manage cases of urinary sphincter incontinence.

ADVERSE AND COMMON SIDE EFFECTS: In humans, hypotension, tachycardia, arrhythmias, anxiety, ataxia, seizure, constipation, mydriasis, urinary retention, pruritus, anorexia, vomiting, diarrhea, jaundice, and bone marrow suppression leading to granulocytopenia and thrombocytopenia have been documented. Experience with the drug in small animals is limited.

DRUG INTERACTIONS: Barbiturates potentiate the adverse effects but decrease serum levels of imipramine. Cimetidine increases serum levels. Phenothiazines may enhance the drug's effects. Thyroid medication may potentiate tachycardia and arrhythmias.

SUPPLIED AS: HUMAN PRODUCT
Tablets containing 10, 25, 50, and 75 mg

OTHER USES
Dogs
URINARY SPHINCTER INCONTINENCE
5 to 15 mg bid; PO

BEHAVIORAL PROBLEMS
2.2 to 4.4 mg/kg once to twice daily; PO

Cats
URINARY SPHINCTER INCONTINENCE
2.5 to 5 mg bid; PO

BEHAVIORAL PROBLEMS
1 to 2 mg/kg bid–tid; PO

IMMUNOGLOBULIN

INDICATIONS: Pooled human immunoglobulin, primarily IgG (Iveegam ✦ ★, Gamimune ✦ ★), has been used in the treatment of autoimmune hemolytic anemia and immune-mediated thrombocytopenia. It blocks the F_c receptor on macrophages, enhances C_8 function, causes suppression of polyclonal B biosynthesis, inhibits inflammation, and blocks the uptake of antibody-coated cells in the spleen. In one study, the drug improved short-term survival of dogs with autoimmune hemolytic anemia, but it did not improve long-term survival, i.e., survival longer than 1 year. In another study, an 85% response rate was observed in dogs unresponsive to conventional immunosuppressive therapy alone.

ADVERSE AND COMMON SIDE EFFECTS: Experience with use of the drug in small animals is limited. However, no adverse effects have been documented with its use in dogs thus far. In humans, IV use has been associated with nausea, chills, wheezing, skeletal pain, abdominal cramps, and anaphylaxis.

DRUG INTERACTIONS: Antibodies in immunoglobulin may interfere with response to live virus vaccines. In humans, it is recommended that live virus vaccines be given 14 days before or 3 months after use of this agent.

SUPPLIED AS: HUMAN PRODUCT
For injection containing 4.5% to 5.5% protein containing approximately 50 mg/mL protein

INDOMETHACIN

INDICATIONS: Indomethacin (Indocid ♣ ★, Indocin ★) is a nonsteroidal anti-inflammatory agent recommended by some clinicians for the management of joint pain secondary to degenerative joint disease. Use of the drug, however, has been associated with hepatotoxicity in dogs and cats and fatal GI hemorrhage in dogs, and because of the availability of other suitable NSAID agents, it is not recommended by this author for use in small animals.

INNOVAR-VET

INDICATIONS: Innovar-Vet ♣ ★ is a combination of droperidol and fentanyl citrate. The drug has tranquilizing and analgesic properties and is used as a preanesthetic sedative or as an anesthetic induction agent. Given intramuscularly, it provides 30 to 40 minutes of analgesia.

ADVERSE AND COMMON SIDE EFFECTS: Respiratory depression and centrally mediated vagal bradycardia occur. A standard dose of atropine may be used to reverse or prevent the bradycardia. Naloxone (0.4 mg; IM, IV, SC) counters the respiratory depression of 0.4 mg fentanyl. Intramuscular injection may be associated with local pain, nystagmus, flatulence, and defecation. Salivation and bradycardia may occur, especially in those not pretreated with atropine. Innovar-Vet may cause panting. Some patients still may respond to loud noises and mechanical stimulation. Analgesia and tranquillity may not be obtained in some dogs with this drug combination, especially Australian terriers. Behavioral changes, including aggression, have been reported in some dogs after its use. The drug should not be used in animals with significant renal or hepatic disease or in those in which respiration is depressed. Perivascular injection is irritating to surrounding tissues. Overdose may cause tonic–clonic convulsions and long-lasting extension and rigidity of the neck, which may be antagonized by small IV doses (6.6 mg/kg) of sodium pentobarbital. The drug causes CNS excitation in cats and is not recommended in this species.

DRUG INTERACTIONS: Tranquilizers, antitussives, or analgesics must not be given in conjunction with or for at least 8 hours after use of Innovar-Vet. Sodium pentobarbital has an additive effect and should not be used for 4 hours after use of Innovar-Vet.

SUPPLIED AS: VETERINARY PRODUCT
For injection containing 0.628 mg/mL fentanyl citrate and 20 mg/mL droperidol

INSULIN

INDICATIONS: Insulin preparations ♣ ★ are used in the management of diabetes mellitus. The various types of beef/pork insulin and their properties are indicated in the table below. Although the clinical significance of insulin resistance due to insulin antibodies in small animals is unknown, dog insulin and pork insulin are identical in structure, and pork insulin may be expected to be less antigenic than beef insulin. In the cat, beef insulin is more similar to cat insulin. Regardless, where available, combination beef/pork insulin is recommended initially.

Regular insulin has the fastest onset of action and the shortest duration. Semilente also is classified as a short-acting insulin but is only available as a component of Lente insulin.

Intermediate-acting insulins include isophane insulin suspension (NPH) and insulin zinc suspension (Lente insulin). Lente is a mixture of Semilente (3 parts) and Ultralente insulin (7 parts). Lente insulin is the insulin of choice for the dog with uncomplicated diabetes. If the duration of effect of NPH or Lente or Ultralente insulin is 10 to 14 hours, administer it twice daily. If the duration of NPH or Lente insulin is less than 10 hours, switch to Ultralente insulin given once or twice daily. If NPH or Lente insulin has a duration of effect of 16 to 20 hours and clinical signs of hyperglycemia are present, consider changing to Ultralente insulin.

Long-acting formulations include Ultralente insulin. Human insulin preparations appear better absorbed than beef/pork insulin in cats. The dosage of Ultralente Humulin insulin is approximately 1 to 4 units per cat. Ultralente is the insulin of choice for the uncomplicated diabetic cat. If Ultralente insulin has a duration of effect of 16 to 20 hours in the dog and clinical signs of hyperglycemia are present, consider a supplemental dose of regular insulin administered in the late evening. Otherwise, discontinue the Ultralente insulin and replace it with Lente or NPH administered twice daily.

Peak effect and duration of activity, as listed below, serve as guidelines only and will vary according to individual response and the effects of diet, exercise, and concurrent illness. Caninsulin is a product specifically designed for use in dogs and cats. It is a purified porcine insulin consisting of 30% amorphous and 70% crystalline zinc insulin. The amorphous fraction reaches its maximum effect approximately 3 hours after SC injection, and the total duration of effect lasts about 8 hours. The crystalline zinc portion has an onset of action of 7 to 12 hours and a total duration of activity of approximately 24 hours.

Insulin mixtures of rapid-acting and intermediate-acting insulins also are available. Some authors have used insulin mixtures in diabetic dogs that required twice daily NPH insulin. In these patients, a mixture of 1 part regular insulin and 3 parts Ultralente was effective. Early peak activity was noted within 2 to 4 hours, a second peak occurred 10 to 12 hours later, and total duration of activity was 20 to 24 hours. When mixing insulins in the same syringe, the short-acting insulin should be drawn up first. Feeding several small meals is preferable to feeding one large meal. For diabetics receiving one injection per day, a suitable feeding schedule would consist of three equally sized meals fed at 6-hour intervals. Dogs receiving two injections of insulin per day would benefit best from four equally sized meals: immediately after each insulin injection, at midafternoon, and at late evening.

Insulin Type	Route	Onset of Activity	Peak Effect		Duration	
			Dog	Cat	Dog	Cat
Regular	IV	Instant	½ to 2 hrs	Same	1 to 4 hrs	Same
	IM	10 to 30 min	1 to 4 hrs	Same	3 to 8 hrs	Same
	SC	10 to 30 min	1 to 5 hrs	Same	4 to 10 hrs	Same
NPH	SC	½ to 3 hrs	2 to 10 hrs	2 to 8 hrs	6 to 24 hrs	4 to 12 hrs
Lente	SC	Instant	2 to 10 hrs	2 to 10 hrs	8 to 24 hrs	6 to 18 hrs
Ultralente	SC	4 to 12 hr (cat) or 2 to 8 hrs	4 to 16 hrs	4 to 16 hrs	8 to 28 hrs	8 to 24 hrs

ADVERSE AND COMMON SIDE EFFECTS: Overdose may cause hypoglycemia, leading to disorientation, weakness, hunger, seizure, coma, and death. If overdose occurs, the animal should be fed sugar with water or food. If seizures occur, dextrose solutions should be given intravenously until seizure activity stops. If poor SC absorption is present, changing the type of insulin to a more potent form may be useful. Insulins in increasing order of potency include Ultralente, Lente, NPH, Semilente, and regular crystalline insulin.

DRUG INTERACTIONS: Anabolic steroids, including stanozolol, β-blocking agents, including propranolol and metoprolol, phenylbutazone, tetracycline, aspirin, and other salicylates may potentiate hypoglycemia induced by insulin. Glucocorticoids, dobutamine, epinephrine, estrogens, progesterones, furosemide, and thiazide diuretics may antagonize the hypoglycemic effects of insulin. Similarly, thyroid preparations may increase blood glucose levels in diabetic patients when thyroid preparations are first initiated. Insulin preparations may alter serum potassium levels, which is of importance in those receiving digitalis, especially if the patient also is receiving a diuretic.

SUPPLIED AS: HUMAN PRODUCTS
Regular insulin containing 100 U/mL (beef/pork combinations) [regular Iletin I] and 100 U/mL (pork source only)
Regular insulin (purified) containing 100 U/mL (pork source only) [Velosulin, Iletin II] and 500 U/mL Novolin R and Humulin R containing 100 U/mL (human)
Isophane insulin (NPH) containing 100 U/mL (beef and pork sources) [Iletin I NPH]
Isophane insulin (purified) containing 100 U/mL (pork source only) [Iletin II]
Intermediate-acting isophane, human semisynthetic insulin containing 100 U/mL [Insulatard (NPH), Novolin-NPH, Humalin-N]
Ultralente containing 100 U/mL (beef and pork sources)
Long-acting human insulin preparations containing 100 U/mL [Novolin-Ultralente, Humalin-U]
Caninsulin ✦ containing 40 U/mL (pork source). See manufacturers instructions for dosage and use of the product.
Note: The trend in human medicine is to move to the use of human insulin preparations that are chemically, physically, biologically, and immunologically similar to human insulin. Protamine zinc is no longer available, and the long-term supply of Semilente and Ultralente beef/pork insulins cannot be guaranteed.

OTHER USES
Dogs

ADJUNCTIVE TREATMENT OF HYPERKALEMIA
5 U/kg/hour regular insulin; IV with 2 g glucose/unit of insulin given

Cats
ADJUNCTIVE TREATMENT OF HYPERKALEMIA
0.5 U/kg regular insulin; IV with 2 g of glucose/unit of insulin

INTERFERON

INDICATIONS: Interferon (Roferon A ♣ ★) has immunomodulating and antiproliferative capabilities and antiviral activity. It has been used in the treatment of FeLV infection. Treated cats improved clinically, and hematocrit values returned to normal. In another study, cats also improved clinically (increased appetite, weight gain, increased physical activity, loss of fever), peripheral blood values improved, and recovery from secondary bacterial infections improved as well when antibiotics were also used. Despite treatment, 95% of cats remained persistently viremic. However, because adequate controls were not included in these studies, definitive conclusions concerning the efficacy of this agent in this disease cannot be made. Experimentally, the drug also has been used alone or in combination with *Propionibacterium acnes* in cats with feline infectious peritonitis, where the combination apparently suppressed clinical signs of the disease and prolonged survival. The drug combination did not prevent death.

ADVERSE AND COMMON SIDE EFFECTS: None were observed in the cats in these studies. In humans, however, hypersensitivity may develop, and nausea, anorexia, vomiting, diarrhea, fever, somnolence, depression, seizure, and coma are reported.

DRUG INTERACTIONS: Interferon α-2a may affect CNS function, and interaction with other centrally acting drugs is possible.

SUPPLIED AS: HUMAN PRODUCT
Solution containing 3 million IU/mL
Note: Dilute the 3 million IU into 1 L of sterile saline, which then can be divided into aliquots of 1 to 10 mL and frozen. The original stock solution (3 million IU) can be frozen for years without losing activity. Once reconstituted, it can be stored in a refrigerator (4°C) for several months without losing activity. The activity of dilute solution after frozen storage is unknown.

IPECAC

INDICATIONS: Syrup of ipecac ♣ ★ is a useful emetic agent. It acts via gastric irritation and stimulation of the medullary chemoreceptor trigger zone. Only half of the patients that the formulation is given to will vomit.

ADVERSE AND COMMON SIDE EFFECTS: At regular doses, side effects are rare but may include lacrimation, salivation, and an increase in bronchial secretions. In humans, diarrhea and lethargy also may occur. With drug overdose, syrup of ipecac is potentially cardiotoxic, leading to arrhythmias, hypotension, and fatal myocarditis. The total dose should not exceed 15 mL (1 tablespoon).

DRUG INTERACTIONS: Syrup of ipecac should not be used with activated charcoal because the charcoal will decrease the activity of ipecac. Vomiting may be induced initially with syrup of ipecac and then followed by activated charcoal.

SUPPLIED AS: HUMAN PRODUCT
Oral syrup available in 15- and 30-mL and pint and gallon bottles

IRON DEXTRAN

INDICATIONS: Iron dextran is indicated for the treatment of iron deficiency anemia.

ADVERSE AND COMMON SIDE EFFECTS: Intramuscular injection can be irritating. Allergic reactions and anaphylaxis occasionally have been reported in humans.

DRUG INTERACTIONS: Clinical response may be delayed in patients concurrently receiving chloramphenicol.

SUPPLIED AS: VETERINARY PRODUCT
For injection containing 100 and 200 mg elemental iron/mL [Ferrodex ★, Ironol-100 ♣, and generic products]

ISOFLURANE

INDICATIONS: Isoflurane (Forane ♣ ★, Isoflo ♣ ★) is an inhalant anesthetic agent that is especially useful for short surgical procedures. It is well tolerated in debilitated patients and those with hepatic or renal impairment. Induction and recovery times are more rapid with isoflurane than with halothane. Cardiovascular status is better maintained with isoflurane, and isoflurane does not sensitize the heart to epinephrine-induced cardiac arrhythmias, as does halothane.

ADVERSE AND COMMON SIDE EFFECTS: Dose-dependent cardiac and respiratory depression occurs. Hypotension, respiratory depression, arrhythmias, nausea, vomiting, and postoperative ileus have been reported.

DRUG INTERACTIONS: Isoflurane potentiates the effects of muscle relaxants.

SUPPLIED AS: VETERINARY AND HUMAN PRODUCT
Supplied in 100-mL bottles

ISOPROTERENOL

INDICATIONS: Isoproterenol (Isuprel ♣ ★) is a β-adrenergic agent used for the short-term management of incomplete heart block, sinus bradycardia, and sick sinus syndrome. The drug increases atrioventricular conduction and ventricular excitability. It also causes peripheral vascular dilation and bronchial smooth muscle relaxation and is used to promote bronchodilation.

ADVERSE AND COMMON SIDE EFFECTS: Vomiting, nervous excitation, weakness, tachycardia, and ectopic beat formation are reported. The drug is considered more arrhythmogenic than dopamine or dobutamine, so it rarely is used in the treatment of heart failure or shock.

DRUG INTERACTIONS: Digitalis and amitriptyline may have additive effects and lead to arrhythmias if used with isoproterenol. The use of β-blockers, e.g., propranolol or metoprolol, may antagonize the β-adrenergic effects of isoproterenol. If used with theophylline, there is a possibility of increased cardiotoxic effects.

SUPPLIED AS: HUMAN PRODUCTS
For injection containing 0.2 mg/mL (1:5,000)
For inhalation delivering 125 µg/dose
1:200 (5 mg/mL) concentration

OTHER USES
Dogs and Cats
BRONCHODILATION
0.1 to 0.2 mg qid; IM, SC

ISOTRETINOIN

INDICATIONS: Isotretinoin (Accutane ♣ ★) appears to be useful in the treatment of disorders of keratinization, abnormalities in follicular keratinization, and quantitative or qualitative disorders of sebaceous gland secretion, e.g., seborrhea. It appears to cause a reduction in sebum production, has an anti-inflammatory effect, an effect on the microflora population, and an antikeratinizing effect. It has been used successfully to treat sebaceous adenitis in standard poodles, canine lamellar ichthyosis, Schnauzer comedo syndrome, intracutaneous cornifying epitheliomas, multiple epidermal inclusion cysts, idiopathic seborrheic disorders, and cutaneous T-cell lymphoma (mycosis fungoides).

ADVERSE AND COMMON SIDE EFFECTS: The incidence of adverse effects appears to be low. Lethargy, anorexia, vomiting, conjunctivitis, pruritus, polydipsia, erythema of mucocutaneous junctions and feet, hyperactivity, abdominal distension, collapse, and a swollen tongue have been reported. All side effects were reversible on discontinuation of the drug. Occasional laboratory changes include increases in serum triglyceride and cholesterol levels, accompanied by corneal lipid deposits, increases in alanine aminotransferase levels, and thrombocytosis. A higher incidence of side effects has been noted in cats. Erythema, periocular crusting, epiphora, blepharospasm, and diarrhea have been reported. The drug is potentially teratogenic and may inhibit spermatogenesis and should not be used in breeding animals.

DRUG INTERACTIONS: In humans, minocycline and tetracycline may increase the risk of papilledema and cerebral edema.

SUPPLIED AS: HUMAN PRODUCT
Capsules containing 10, 20, and 40 mg

OTHER USES
Dogs
SEBACEOUS ADENITIS
1 mg/kg once daily; PO (Vizslas)
CUTANEOUS LYMPHOMA
3 to 4 mg/kg once daily
INTRACUTANEOUS CORNIFYING EPITHELIOMA
1 to 2 mg/kg daily

ITRACONAZOLE

INDICATIONS: Itraconazole (Sporanox ♣ ★) is active against histoplasmosis, blastomycosis, coccidioidomycosis, and cryptococcosis. It is more effective than amphotericin B or ketoconazole in the treatment of canine nasal aspergillosis. The drug also is active against *Microsporum, Trichophyton, Sporothrix, Pythium, Candida* spp., *Leishmania* sp., and *Trypanosoma cruzi*. Unlike ketoconazole, itraconazole may reach adequate levels in the CNS at therapeutic doses. Itraconazole is best absorbed when given with a fatty meal.

ADVERSE AND COMMON SIDE EFFECTS: Minimal toxicity has been seen in dogs. Anorexia secondary to hepatotoxicity and vasculitis characterized by ulcerative dermatitis has been reported. If adverse effects occur, the drug should be discontinued until the appetite returns. Treatment then can be reinstituted at half the dose. It appears that adequate serum concentrations can be maintained at this decreased dose level. Anorexia and hepatotoxicity, with a concurrent mild to moderate increase in serum alanine aminotransferase activity, are the most frequently observed adverse effects reported in cats. Teratogenic effects have been documented in rat studies. The potential risk versus the benefit must be ascertained in pregnant animals before the drug is used.

DRUG INTERACTIONS: Concurrent use with terfenadine is contraindicated. Rare cases of ventricular tachycardia and death have been reported in people.

SUPPLIED AS: HUMAN PRODUCTS
Capsules containing 100 mg
Liquid containing 10 mg/mL

OTHER USES
Cats
MICROSPORUM CANIS
i) 10 mg/kg daily; PO

ii) 20 mg/kg every other day; PO

HISTOPLASMOSIS
5 mg/kg bid; PO for 60 or more days

IVERMECTIN

INDICATIONS: Ivermectin (Heartgard ✣ ★, Ivomec ✣ ★, Eqvalan ✣ ★) is used for the eradication of demodectic, sarcoptic, otodectic, and *Cheyletiella* mites in dogs. It also has been used in the treatment of *Capillaria aerophila* and is marketed for the prevention of canine heartworm [Heartgard]. The drug has been used as a microfilaricide in heartworm disease. In fact, ivermectin has been shown to be effective against heartworm infection when 1 year of monthly prophylactic dosing is started as late as 4 months after infection. In cats, the drug has been used in the treatment of ear mites, *Cheyletiella blakei*, *Physaloptera preputialis*, *Demodex*, and fleas.

ADVERSE AND COMMON SIDE EFFECTS: Ivermectin has a wide margin of safety. In dogs, mydriasis and tremors were noted at doses of 5,000 µg/kg, and more pronounced tremors and ataxia were reported at doses of 10,000 µg/kg. Some collies and related breeds have a variable sensitivity to the drug. In approximately 5% of dogs with microfilaremia, vomiting, trembling, tachypnea, and collapse develop within 1 to 4 hours of use of the drug. Fatalities are rare. The drug is not recommended for use in puppies younger than 6 weeks of age.

DRUG INTERACTIONS: None.

SUPPLIED AS: VETERINARY PRODUCTS
For injection Ivomec 1% (10 mg/mL) (for use in cattle, sheep, and swine)
Oral paste 1.87% (for equine use)
Ivermectin liquid 1% (10 mg/mL) [Eqvalan] (for equine use)
Tablets containing 68, 136, and 272 µg [Heartgard]

OTHER USES
Dogs
OTODECTES CYNOTIS and *SARCOPTES SCABEI*
Single dose 200 µg/kg; SC, PO, repeat in 14 days

SARCOPTES SCABEI
0.2 to 0.3 mg/kg; PO, SC given twice 2 weeks apart

DIROFILARIA IMMITIS
i) 50 µg/kg 3 to 4 weeks after adulticide therapy (microfilaricide)

ii) 50 to 200 µg/kg as a single oral dose

iii) 6 µg/kg once monthly; PO (preventative dose)

CHEYLETIELLA YASGURI
300 µg/kg once; SC, repeat in 3 weeks if required

GENERALIZED DEMODICOSIS
i)   400 µg/kg weekly; SC (total of 8 treatments)—efficacy questionable

ii) 0.6 mg/kg daily; PO (median duration of treatment was 10 weeks)

CAPILLARIA SPP.
0.2 mg/kg once; PO

ROUNDWORMS, HOOKWORMS, and WHIPWORMS
Single dose 200 µg/kg; PO

PNEUMONYSSUS CANINUM
i)   200 µg/kg; SC, repeat in 3 weeks

ii) 200 to 400 µg/kg; SC, PO

STRONGYLOIDES STERCORALIS
200 µg/kg; PO. A second treatment at the same dose may be required.

Cats

ANCYLOSTOMA BRAZILIENSE and *TUBAEFORME*
24 µg/kg; PO

OTODECTES CYNOTIS
Single dose 200 µg/kg; SC

NOTOEDRES CATI and *CHEYLETIELLA* MITES
Single dose 400 µg/kg; SC

CHEYLETIELLA BLAKEI
300 µg/kg twice at 5 week intervals; SC

DEMODEX
300 µg/kg; SC, 2 weeks apart with concurrent use of 2.5% lime sulfur

PHYSALOPTERA PREPUTIALIS
Single dose 200 µg/kg; SC

KANAMYCIN

INDICATIONS: Kanamycin (Kantrim ★) is an aminoglycoside antibiotic with activity against *Staphylococcus aureus* and *albus*, *Klebsiella pneumonia*, *Salmonella*, *Pasteurella*, *Corynebacterium*, *Bacillus anthracis*, *Proteus*, *E. coli*, and *A. aerobacter*. It penetrates most body fluids other than spinal fluid. Also see **AMINOGLYCOSIDES.**

ADVERSE AND COMMON SIDE EFFECTS: Impairment of vestibular function or irreversible hearing loss may occur if dosage is excessive or use prolonged. Nephrotoxicity may occur, especially in toxic, poorly hydrated patients. At higher doses, local irritation at the injection site may occur. The drug also has been shown to decrease cardiac output and produce hypotension and bradycardia. Cardiac arrest has been reported in humans receiving overdoses of the drug. Also see **AMINOGLYCOSIDES.**

DRUG INTERACTIONS: The potential for ototoxicity increases if kanamycin is used with other aminoglycosides. Furosemide potentiates ototoxicity. Amphotericin B, cisplatin, methoxyflurane, vancomycin, and succinylcholine may have an additive neuromuscular blocking effect. Calcium gluconate can be given intravenously to reverse aminoglycoside-induced neuromuscular blockade or myocardial depression and to restore blood pressure. Penicillins and aminoglycosides should not be mixed in the same syringe because inactivation of the aminoglycoside may result. Also see **AMINOGLYCOSIDES.**

SUPPLIED AS: VETERINARY PRODUCT
For injection containing 50 and 200 mg/mL

KAOLIN–PECTIN

INDICATIONS: Kaolin–pectin (Kaopectate ♣ ★, others) is a GI protectant used in the management of diarrhea. It coats the surface of the gut and exerts a mild demulcent and absorbent effect. It actually is relatively ineffective in absorbing toxins produced by enteropathogenic bacteria. It appears to act by adding particulate matter to the feces, which serves to improve consistency until the disease spontaneously resolves. Kaolin is a potent coagulation activator and may be of some benefit in treating diarrhea associated with mucosal disruption and hemorrhage.

ADVERSE AND COMMON SIDE EFFECTS: Kaolin–pectin may cause constipation, especially in poorly hydrated patients.

DRUG INTERACTIONS: The absorption of lincomycin is decreased if given concurrently with kaolin–pectin. Administer kaolin–pectin 2 hours before or 3 to 4 hours after lincomycin. Absorption of digoxin also may be hindered by kaolin–pectin.

SUPPLIED AS: VETERINARY PRODUCTS
Oral suspensions containing:

Kaolin 197 mg and pectin 4.33 mg per mL (large animal preparation) [Kaopectate ✤, Kaopectolin ★]
Kaolin 7 g/oz and pectin 259 mg/oz = 233 mg kaolin/mL and 8.6 mg pectin/mL [K-P-Sol ★]

KETAMINE

INDICATIONS: Ketamine (Ketaset ✤ ★, Vetalar ✤ ★) is a nonbarbiturate anesthetic used in cats. It generally is used for chemical restraint or anesthesia of short duration. Additional doses can be given, providing anesthesia for 6 hours or more. The drug is characterized by a rapid onset of action, profound analgesia, maintenance of normal muscle tone and laryngeal reflex, mild cardiac stimulation, and respiratory depression. Recovery generally is smooth and uneventful, especially if animals are not stimulated by sound or handling during recovery. At lower doses, recovery is complete within 4 to 5 hours. At high doses, complete recovery may take as long as 24 hours or more, especially if the patient is in poor condition or suffering from renal impairment. In cats, ketamine often is combined with acepromazine or midazolam. The combination provides dependable chemical restraint with minimal cardiovascular effects. In addition, ketamine may be combined with atropine to decrease respiratory and salivary secretions. Somatic analgesia is moderate and only of short duration; it provides little to no visceral analgesia.

ADVERSE AND COMMON SIDE EFFECTS: Pain on IM injection may occur. The use of ketamine is associated with increased muscle tone and should not be used as the sole anesthetic for procedures requiring muscle relaxation. Used alone, ketamine may induce seizure activity in dogs and in up to 20% of cats. In fact, the drug should not be used in dogs or cats with a history of seizure disorders. The incidence of seizure can be reduced if ketamine is combined with diazepam or midazolam. Dose-dependent respiratory depression and hypotension may occur with larger doses. The drug is eliminated via the kidney and should be used with caution in patients with renal impairment. The drug may cause elevations in CSF pressure and should not be used in cases with suspect increases in CSF or trauma to the head. Ketamine should not be used in animals with increased intraocular pressure or trauma to the globe, or for procedures involving the pharynx, larynx, and trachea. Eyes remain open after ketamine induction and should be protected from drying with an ophthalmic lubricant.

At high doses, respiratory depression, vomiting, vocalization, erratic and prolonged recovery, dyspnea, spastic jerking movements, convulsions, muscular tremors, hypertonicity, opisthotonos, and cardiac arrest may occur. In the cat, the myoclonic jerking and clonic–tonic convulsions can be controlled by ultrashort-acting barbiturates or acepromazine given slowly intravenously and to effect.

DRUG INTERACTIONS: Concurrent barbiturate, narcotic, or diazepine use may prolong recovery time after ketamine use. Ketamine may potentiate the neuromuscular blocking action of tubocurarine. Concomitant use of halothane can cause cardiac depression. Chloramphenicol may prolong the anesthetic actions of ketamine. With the use of thyroid medications, marked hypertension and tachycardia after induction with ketamine has been documented in people.

SUPPLIED AS: VETERINARY PRODUCT
For injection containing 100 mg/mL

OTHER USES
SHORT, PAINFUL SURGICAL PROCEDURES
1 to 2 mg/kg; IV

KETOCONAZOLE

INDICATIONS: Ketoconazole (Nizoral ✤ ★) has been used in the treatment of *Trichophyton mentagrophytes* and *Microsporum canis* infections, candidiasis, coccidioidomycosis, cryptococcosis, blastomycosis, histoplasmosis, and canine nasal aspergillosis. The drug also has been used effectively in the treatment of Malassezia infection in dogs and cats. Therapeutic concentrations are achieved in all body fluids except the skin, bone, bile, brain, testes, and eye. However, some authors report that doses of 30 to 40 mg/kg/day are likely to achieve therapeutic concentrations in the brain and CSF. The drug also has been used in the treatment of canine hyperadrenocorticism.

Ketoconazole effectively blocks cortisol synthesis in dogs with pituitary-dependent hyperadrenocorticism and those with adrenocortical tumor. Long-term administration of the drug does not suppress plasma cortisol concentrations in clinically normal cats.

ADVERSE AND COMMON SIDE EFFECTS: Nausea, anorexia, vomiting, diarrhea, lightening of the hair coat, transient elevations in liver enzymes, and jaundice have been reported. Gastrointestinal side effects may be prevented by administering the drug with food (which also may serve to increase its absorption) and by dividing the daily dose and administering the drug 2 to 4 times daily. In the management of hyperadrenocorticism, overdose of the drug could result in hypocortisolism and resultant vomiting, diarrhea, anorexia, weakness, and depression. The drug should not be given to pregnant animals because its use has been associated with stillbirths and mummified fetuses. In addition, decreased libido and impotence occur in humans and may occur in dogs.

DRUG INTERACTIONS: Antacids, cimetidine, and ranitidine decrease the absorption of ketoconazole. Phenytoin may antagonize the actions of ketoconazole. Rifampin and isoniazid reduce the antifungal effects of ketoconazole. Mitotane and ketoconazole should not be used concurrently in the treatment of hyperadrenocorticism because the adrenolytic effects of mitotane may be inhibited by ketoconazole's inhibition of cytochrome P-450 enzymes. Ketoconazole may increase the anticoagulant effects of warfarin. The duration of activity of methylprednisolone is prolonged with ketoconazole. Ketoconazole may decrease serum concentrations of theophylline in some patients. Cyclosporine levels may be increased by ketoconazole. Concurrent use of ketoconazole and terfenadine (Seldane) or astemizole (Hismanal) may predispose to severe and life-threatening cardiac arrhythmias in humans.

SUPPLIED AS: HUMAN PRODUCTS
Tablets containing 200 mg
Suspension containing 20 mg/mL

OTHER USES
Dogs
ASPERGILLOSIS
Ketoconazole 20 mg/kg for at least 6 weeks; long-term maintenance may be required

BLASTOMYCOSIS
i) Ketoconazole 10 mg/kg bid; PO (15–20 mg/kg bid; PO if CNS involvement) for at least 3 months with amphotericin B, initially at 0.25 to 0.5 mg/kg every other day; IV. If tolerated, increase dose to 1 mg/kg until 4 to 5 mg/kg total dose is attained.

ii) Ketoconazole 20 mg/day; once daily or div. bid PO; 40 mg/kg div. bid for ocular or CNS involvement (for at least 2 to 3 months or until remission, then start maintenance) with amphotericin B 0.15 to 0.5 mg/kg; IV 3 times a week. When the total dose of amphotericin reaches 4 to 6 mg/kg, start maintenance dose of amphotericin at 0.15 to 0.25 mg/kg; IV, once a month, or use ketoconazole at 10 mg/kg once daily or div. bid; PO or ketoconazole at 2.5 to 5 mg/kg once daily; PO. If ocular or CNS involvement, use ketoconazole at 20 to 40 mg/kg div. bid; PO.

CANDIDAL STOMATITIS
10 mg/kg tid; PO until lesions resolve

COCCIDIOIDOMYCOSIS
i) 5 to 10 mg/kg bid; PO (systemic disease)

ii) 15 to 20 mg/kg bid; PO (CNS disease)
Continue treatment for 3 to 6 months. Those with bony lesions or relapses may require lifelong treatment at 5 mg/kg every other day; PO.

CRYPTOCOCCOSIS
Amphotericin B 0.15 to 0.4 mg/kg 3 times a week; IV with flucytosine at 150 to 175 mg/kg div. tid–qid; PO. When total dose of amphotericin B reaches 4 to 6 mg/kg, start maintenance dose of amphotericin B at 0.15 to 0.25 mg/kg once monthly; IV or with ketoconazole at 10 mg/kg once daily or div. bid; PO.

HISTOPLASMOSIS
i) 10 mg/kg once daily or bid; PO for at least 3 months. Continue treatment for at least 30 days beyond complete remission. If relapse occurs, retreat as indicated and put on maintenance of 5 mg/kg every other day indefinitely.

ii) Ketoconazole 10 to 20 mg/kg once daily; PO or div. bid (for at least 2 to 3 months or until remission, then start maintenance) with amphotericin B at 0.15 to 0.5 mg/kg; IV 3 times weekly. When a total dose of amphotericin B reaches 2 to 4 mg/kg, start maintenance dose of amphotericin B at 0.15 to 0.25 mg/kg once a month; IV, or use ketoconazole at 10 mg/kg once daily or div. bid; PO or at 2.5 to 5 mg/kg once daily; PO.

MALASSEZIA
5 to 10 mg/kg bid; PO for 30 to 45 days

HYPERADRENOCORTICISM
i) 30 mg/kg once daily or div. bid; PO

ii) Initially at 10 mg/kg bid; PO for 7 to 10 days. Discontinue drug for 24 to 48 hours if adverse reactions occur. Reevaluate ACTH stimulation at end of 7- to 10-day period. If response is inadequate, increase dose to 15 mg/kg bid; PO, and reevaluate again in 7 to 10 days. Once controlled, continue on that dose long term.

iii) Initially at 5 mg/kg bid; PO for 7 days to evaluate for side effects. If none, increase dose to 10 mg/kg bid; PO for 14 days. Perform ACTH stimulation 1 to 3 hours after last dose. If no improvement noted, increase dose again to 15 mg/kg bid; PO and reevaluate in 14 days.

Cats

ASPERGILLOSIS

20 mg/kg; PO for at least 6 weeks; long-term maintenance therapy may be required

BLASTOMYCOSIS

i) Ketoconazole at 10 mg/kg bid; PO (15–20 mg/kg bid if CNS involvement) for at least 3 months with amphotericin B, initially at 0.25 to 0.5 mg/kg every other day; IV. If tolerated, increase dose to 1 mg/kg until a total dose of 4 to 5 mg/kg is attained.

ii) Ketoconazole at 10 mg/kg bid; PO (for at least 2 months) with amphotericin B at 0.25 mg/kg in 30 mL D_5W IV over 15 minutes every 48 hours. Continue amphotericin until total dose of 4 mg/kg is attained or until BUN is greater than 50 mg/dL (18 mmol/L). If renal toxicity does not occur, increase amphotericin dose to 0.5 mg/kg.

iii) Ketoconazole at 10 mg/kg once daily; PO or div. bid (for at least 2 to 3 months or until clinical remission, then start maintenance) with amphotericin B at 0.15 to 0.5 mg/kg 3 times a week; IV. When total amphotericin B dose reaches 4 to 6 mg/kg, start maintenance dose of 0.15 to 0.25 mg/kg once monthly; IV, or use ketoconazole at 10 mg/kg once daily; PO or div. bid or ketoconazole at 2.5 to 5 mg/kg once daily; PO. For ocular or CNS disease, use ketoconazole at 20 to 40 mg/kg div. bid; PO.

COCCIDIOIDOMYCOSIS

i) 5 to 10 mg/kg bid; PO (systemic disease)
   15 to 20 mg/kg bid; PO (CNS disease)

Continue treatment for 3 to 6 months. Those with relapses or with bony lesions may require lifelong therapy at 5 mg/kg every other day; PO.

ii) 10 mg/kg once or twice daily; PO for at least 6 months

iii) 50 mg/day; PO (in several cases treatment periods continued 28 to 43 months)

CRYPTOCOCCOSIS

i) 10 mg/kg once or twice daily; PO for 3 months or for at least 30 days beyond clinical remission

ii) 10 to 20 mg/kg div. bid; PO (20–30 mg/kg/day if CNS involvement). Continue for at least 3 to 4 weeks beyond clinical remission.

iii) Amphotericin B at 0.15 to 0.4 mg/kg 3 times a week; IV with flucytosine at 125 to 250 mg/kg div. tid–qid; PO. Start maintenance dose of amphotericin of 0.15 to 0.25 mg/kg once a month; IV after a total dose of 4 to 6 mg/kg has been reached along with flucytosine at the dose indicated or with ketoconazole at 10 mg/kg once daily or div. bid; PO.

HISTOPLASMOSIS

i)   10 mg/kg once or twice daily; PO for at least 3 months. Continue for at least 30 days after clinical remission. If relapse occurs, retreat as indicated and maintain on 5 mg/kg every other day; PO indefinitely.

ii) Ketoconazole at 10 mg/kg bid; PO with amphotericin at 0.25 mg in 30 mL of D₅W; IV given over 15 minutes every 48 hours. Continue amphotericin for 4 to 8 weeks or until BUN is greater than 50 mg/dL (18 mmol/L). If BUN increases to greater than 50 mg/dL (18 mmol/L), continue ketoconazole alone for at least 6 months.

iii) Ketoconazole at 10 mg/kg once daily or div. bid; PO (for at least 2 to 3 months or until clinical remission is apparent, then start maintenance dose) with amphotericin B at 0.15 to 0.5 mg/kg 3 times a week; IV. When total amphotericin B dose reaches 2 to 4 mg/kg, start maintenance dose of 0.15 to 0.25 mg/kg once a month; IV, or use ketoconazole at 10 mg/kg once daily or div. bid or at 2.5 to 5 mg/kg once daily; PO.

MALASSEZIA

5 mg/kg every 24 to 48 hours; PO for a minimum of 30 days

Dogs and Cats

DERMATOPHYTOSIS

10 mg/kg once to twice daily; PO with food

Continue treatment until lesions have resolved and fungal cultures yield no growth (median duration of treatment 6 weeks).

Note: Griseofulvin may be more effective than ketoconazole in the treatment of dermatophytosis.

KETOPROFEN

INDICATIONS: Ketoprofen (Anafen ✤, Ketofen ★) is an NSAID with potent analgesic and antipyretic properties. The drug inhibits the cyclooxygenase and lipoxygenase inflammatory pathways. Most NSAIDs only inhibit the cyclooxygenase pathway. Ketoprofen is used in the management of fever and acute, subacute, and chronic pain associated with musculoskeletal disease. Onset of activity of the drug occurs within 30 minutes of parenteral administration and 1 hour after oral use. The terminal half-life in cats and dogs is 2 to 3 hours. It reportedly can be used for several months for the management of chronic pain in dogs and cats. The drug is 50 to 100 times more potent than phenylbutazone as an analgesic. Ketoprofen is more effective and longer lasting than oxymorphone or butorphanol in the management of postoperative orthopedic pain.

ADVERSE AND COMMON SIDE EFFECTS: Ketoprofen has a wide margin of safety. In dogs, mild and self-limiting cases of vomiting, diarrhea, anorexia, melena, increased thirst, and weight loss have been documented with drug overdose. Although for the most part cats did not demonstrate adverse drug effects, occasional vomiting may result. The drug should not be given to animals with GI ulceration, or impaired renal or hepatic function, or those with coagulation disorders. It may be inadvisable to use the drug before surgical procedures in which noncompressible hemorrhage may be a problem (e.g., laparotomy, laminectomy, rhinotomy). The effect(s) of ketoprofen on breeding animals in not known.

DRUG INTERACTIONS: Concomitant use of ketoprofen and high-dose methotrexate may cause prolonged excretion and increased serum levels predisposing to methotrexate toxicity. Ketoprofen may impair platelet aggregation and prolong bleeding times. Concurrent use of aspirin decreased ketoprofen protein binding and increased plasma clearance. Patients taking diuretic agents are at greater risk of developing renal failure because of prostaglandin production. Ketoprofen is highly protein bound and may compete with sulfonamides, warfarin, phenylbutazone, oral hypoglycemic agents, and phenytoin for binding sites.

SUPPLIED AS:
For injection containing 10 mg/mL
Tablets containing 5, 10, and 20 mg

KETOROLAC

INDICATIONS: Ketorolac tromethamine (Toradol ✦ ★) is a non-steroidal anti-inflammatory analgesic with antipyretic properties. It is used in the management of moderate to severe pain. Its principle mode of action is via prostaglandin inhibition. The analgesic properties of the drug are estimated to be approximately 180 to 350 times greater than those of aspirin. In humans and apparently in dogs, the onset of analgesia after IM injection is apparent within 10 minutes and peaks within 75 to 150 minutes, and analgesia may be maintained for 8 to 12 hours. The duration of analgesia is greater than that observed with morphine or meperidine. For the management of anticipated postsurgical pain, the drug is best given at least 30 minutes before extubation.

ADVERSE AND COMMON SIDE EFFECTS: Like other NSAIDs, ketorolac has the potential to adversely affect renal function, inhibit platelet aggregation, and cause gastric mucosal damage, which may result in ulceration and bleeding. However, the incidence of these side effects is less common than that observed with other NSAIDs.

Drug dose should be cut in half in patients with renal impairment, and the drug should only be used when the apparent benefits outweigh the risks of the drug. Patients have been reported to recover from renal injury after discontinuation of the drug. The drug should be used with caution in dehydrated/hypovolemic or hypotensive patients. Fluid retention and edema have been reported in humans with congestive heart failure.

DRUG INTERACTIONS: Ketorolac may be used concurrently with morphine or meperidine in the management of moderate to severe pain. The combined use results in reduced opiate analgesic requirements. Diuretic use increases the risk of renal injury. Ketorolac may decrease the diuretic response to furosemide. Ketorolac may increase serum lithium concentrations. It also may increase serum methotrexate concentrations, predisposing to toxicity by decreasing its clearance.

SUPPLIED AS: HUMAN PRODUCTS
For injection containing 10, 15, and 30 mg/mL
Tablets containing 10 mg

LACTULOSE

INDICATIONS: Lactulose (Cephulac ✦ ★, Chronulac ✦ ★) is a synthetic nonabsorbable disaccharide. It acts as a mild osmotic laxative, increases the rate of passage of ingesta, and leads to the reduction of bacterial production of ammonia, making it useful in the management of hepatic encephalopathy. Enteric bacteria ferment lactulose to acidic by-products, decrease intraluminal pH, and favor the formation of ammonium ions, which are poorly absorbed.

ADVERSE AND COMMON SIDE EFFECTS: Transient gastric distention, flatulence, and abdominal cramping may occur. With excessive doses, diarrhea may occur. The preparation is distasteful to cats and may be difficult to administer.

DRUG INTERACTIONS: Antacids decrease the efficacy of the drug. Neomycin and other oral antibiotics may inhibit lactulose activity by reduction or removal of resident colonic bacteria. However, clinical experience suggests that combined therapy in hepatic encephalopathy actually may be synergistic.

SUPPLIED AS: HUMAN PRODUCT
Syrup containing 10 g/15 mL

LEVAMISOLE

INDICATIONS: Levamisole (Levasole ✦ ★, Ripercol ✦, Tramisol ✦ ★) is an anthelmintic licensed for use in large animals. It also has been used for the elimination of *Dirofilaria immitis* microfilaria and for the treatment of *Filaroides osleri*, *Crenosoma vulpis*, and *Capillaria* infection in dogs and *Aelurostrongylus abstrusus*, *Capillaria aerophila*, and *Ollulanus tricuspis* infection in cats. Levamisole may help restore immune function by increasing the number and function of T lymphocytes and macrophages. It also has been reported to stimulate antibody production, increase macrophage phagocytosis, inhibit tumor growth, and stimulate suppressor cell activity.

ADVERSE AND COMMON SIDE EFFECTS: Vomiting, diarrhea, anorexia, salivation, agranulocytosis, depression, panting, head shaking, muscular tremors, and agitation are reported in dogs. In cats, hypersalivation, excitement, mydriasis, and vomiting are reported. Atropine is only partially effective as an antidote. If toxicity progresses to flaccid paralysis, respiratory assistance should be given until recovery has occurred.

DRUG INTERACTIONS: The concurrent use of chloramphenicol has led to death in some cases. Pyrantel, diethylcarbamazine, and organophosphate drugs may enhance the toxic effects of levamisole.

SUPPLIED AS: VETERINARY PRODUCTS (large animal products)
For injection containing 136.5 mg/mL
Soluble drench powder containing 11.7 g/packet [Levasole]
Soluble drench containing 46.8 and 93.6 g/packet [Tramisol]
Oral tablets/boluses containing 184 mg and 2.19 g bolus

OTHER USES
Dogs

AS AN IMMUNOSTIMULANT
i)   For recurrent skin infections, use 2.2 mg/kg every other day; PO along with appropriate antibiotic therapy.
ii) As adjunctive therapy for chronic pyoderma, give 0.5 to 1.5 mg/kg 2 to 3 times weekly; PO.

MICROFILARICIDE
11 mg/kg for 6 to 12 days; PO
Examine blood on day 6, discontinue therapy when microfilaria are negative. Retching and vomiting is common. Discontinue if ataxia or abnormal behavior occurs.

CRENOSOMA VULPIS
8 mg/kg once; PO

CAPILLARIA
7 to 12 mg/kg once daily for 3 to 7 days; PO

FILAROIDES OSLERI
7 to 12 mg/kg once daily for 20 to 45 days; PO

Cats

LUNGWORMS
Aelurostrongylus abstrusus: 100 mg daily every other day for 5 treatments; PO; give atropine (0.5 mg; SC, 15 minutes before levamisole) or 15 mg/kg every other day for 3 treatments, then 3 days later, 30 mg/kg; PO, then 2 days later, 60 mg/kg; PO

CAPILLARIA AEROHPILA
4.4 mg/kg; SC for 2 days, then 8.8 mg/kg once 2 weeks later; or 5 mg/kg once daily for 5 days, followed by 9 days without therapy; repeat twice.

OLLULANUS TRICUSPIS
5 mg/kg; SC

MICROFILARICIDE
10 mg/kg for 7 days; PO

EOSINOPHILIC GRANULOMA
5 mg/kg 3 times weekly; PO

LEVOTHYROXINE

INDICATIONS: Levothyroxine (Eltroxin ✦ ★, Synthroid ✦ ★) is a synthetic form of T_4 used in the treatment of hypothyroid disease. Peak serum concentrations are reached in 4 to 12 hours. Some animals require the drug twice daily. Serum levels can be measured after steady-state levels have been attained (as early as 5 to 10 days, but preferably 1 month because the increased metabolism may change the rate of T_4 catabolism). For those on once-daily treatment, serum samples are taken 24 hours after the last dose. Timing is not as important for those on twice-daily dosing. Individual response to recommended starting dosages is quite variable and should be evaluated. Levothyroxine also has been used (at standard doses) in the management of dogs with hypothyroidism, von Willebrand's disease, and problems of platelet dysfunction. The drug causes an increase in vWF antigen (vWF:Ag) and platelet adhesiveness and platelet production and release, corresponding to a correction in bleeding times. However, other reports have not demonstrated decreased vWF:Ag in hypothyroid patients or an increase in plasma vWF:Ag with levothyroxine therapy. Therapy may actually exacerbate the deficiency.

ADVERSE AND COMMON SIDE EFFECTS: Thyroid replacement should be undertaken with caution in animals with hypoadrenocorticism, diabetes mellitus, or congestive heart failure. The increase in metabolism may place undue stress on the heart. Increased metabolism of adrenal hormones may precipitate a hypoadrenocortical crisis, and increased metabolism may enhance ketone production and potentiate ketoacidosis in animals with diabetes mellitus. Clinical signs consistent with drug overdose include polyuria, polydipsia, polyphagia, weight loss, panting, vomiting, diarrhea, abnormal pupillary light reflexes, nervousness, and tachycardia. Clinical signs resolve 1 to 3 days after discontinuation of the drug. After this time, levothyroxine can be reinstituted at a lower dose and serum levels reevaluated in 2 to 4 weeks. Levothyroxine overdose in recently exposed dogs, without clinical signs of toxicity, can be managed by the induction of vomiting followed by the administration of activated charcoal (1–2 g/kg; PO) and a saline cathartic (e.g., 250 mg/kg; PO of magnesium sulfate or sodium sulfate). Repeated administration of activated charcoal (every 4 to 8 hours at a reduced dose of 0.5 to 1 g/kg) may further reduce the reabsorption of thyroxine by interfering with enterohepatic recirculation. A saline cathartic may be used with the second dose of activated charcoal at one half the initial dose. Further cathartic use is not recommended. Propranolol may be useful in the management of significant tachycardia.

DRUG INTERACTIONS: The activity of epinephrine and norepinephrine increases with the use of levothyroxine. Insulin requirements may increase, and the therapeutic effects of digitalis products may decrease. With the use of thyroid medications, marked hypertension and tachycardia after induction with ketamine have been documented in humans.

SUPPLIED AS: VETERINARY PRODUCTS (United States only)
Tablets containing 0.1, 0.2, 0.3, 0.4, 0.5, 0.6, 0.7, and 0.8 mg [Soloxine, Thyro-Tabs]
Tablets (chewable) containing 0.2, 0.5, and 0.8 mg [Thyro-Form]
HUMAN PRODUCTS
Tablets containing 25, 50, 75, 88, 100, 112, 125, 150, 175, 200, and 300 µg [Eltroxin, Synthroid]
For injection containing 200- and 500-µg vials [Synthroid ★]

OTHER USES
Dogs
HEMOSTATIC DEFECTS, including von WILLEBRAND'S DISEASE
22 µg/kg bid; PO

LIDOCAINE

INDICATIONS: Lidocaine ✿ ★ is licensed as a local anesthetic in small animals. It also is the drug of choice for the management of ventricular premature contractions or tachycardia. Serum concentrations are measured after steady-state levels have been attained (5 hours in the dog). Therapeutic serum concentrations in dogs range from 2 to 6 µg/mL. Toxic levels are in excess of 8 µg/mL.

ADVERSE AND COMMON SIDE EFFECTS: With drug overdose, drowsiness, vomiting, tremors, nystagmus, seizure (especially in cats), excitation, hypotension, and increased atrioventricular conduction with atrial flutter and fibrillation have been reported. The neurologic signs can be controlled with diazepam. Hypokalemia reduces antiarrhythmic effects.

DRUG INTERACTIONS: Cimetidine, propranolol, metoprolol, and quinidine increase the activity of lidocaine. Barbiturates decrease lidocaine action via enzyme induction. Phenytoin increases the cardiac depressant effect of lidocaine. Procainamide may have additive neurologic and cardiac effects.

SUPPLIED AS: VETERINARY PRODUCT
For injection containing 10 mg/mL (1%) and 20 mg/mL (2%)
To prepare IV infusion (without epinephrine) using 2% veterinary solution, add 1 g (50 mL) of 2% solution to 1 L of D_5W, thus providing 1 mg/mL (1,000 µg/mL).
With a minidrop (60 drops/mL) IV set, each drop will contain approximately 17 µg.

HUMAN PRODUCTS
For injection containing 0.2%, 0.4%, or 0.8% in 5% dextrose and 2% in disposable syringes
Topical 5% cream containing 25 mg lidocaine and 25 mg prilocaine [Emla ✚ ★]
Patch containing 1 g of emulsion [Emla patch ✚ ★]

OTHER USES
Dogs
SYSTEMIC ANALGESIA
40 to 70 µg/kg/minute; constant rate IV infusion (without epinephrine)

LINCOMYCIN

INDICATIONS: Lincomycin (Lincocin ✚ ★) is a lincosamide antibiotic with activity against gram-positive cocci, particularly *Streptococcus* spp. and *Staphylococcus* spp. It also is active against *Clostridium tetani* and *perfringens, Mycoplasma* spp., *Leptospira pomona,* and *Erysipelothrix insidiosa.* In dogs, the drug is indicated in the treatment of upper respiratory infections and skin infections, nephritis, and metritis. In cats, lincomycin is indicated in the treatment of localized infections, such as abscesses. Lincomycin is effective against penicillinase-producing staphylococci. Significant concentrations of the drug are achieved in most tissues of the body other than CSF. The drug is excreted in the bile and urine.

ADVERSE AND COMMON SIDE EFFECTS: Vomiting and loose stools may occur. Hemorrhagic diarrhea is infrequent in dogs. Pain at the injection site is reported.

DRUG INTERACTIONS: Kaolin, pectin, and bismuth subsalicylate decrease GI absorption. Chloramphenicol and erythromycin may be mutually antagonistic with lincomycin. Lincomycin has intrinsic neuromuscular blocking properties and should be used with caution with other neuromuscular blocking agents.

SUPPLIED AS: VETERINARY PRODUCTS
Tablets containing 100, 200, and 500 mg
Drops containing 50 mg/mL [Lincocin Aquadrops]
For injection containing 100 mg/mL [Lincocin ★]
For injection containing 50 and 100 mg [Lincomix ♣] (licensed for use in swine only)

LIOTHYROXINE

INDICATIONS: Liothyroxine or liothyronine (Cytobin ♣, Cytomel ♣ ★) is a synthetic form of T_3 that has been used in the treatment of some forms of hypothyroid disease. Specifically it is indicated in animals with an inability to convert thyroxine (T_4) to triiodothyronine (T_3), e.g., animals on corticosteroid therapy, and in those with impaired absorption of thyroxine from the GIT. Conversion abnormalities in small animals are rare, if they occur at all. Peak serum concentrations occur 2 to 5 hours after oral administration. Serum T_3 levels are measured just before and 2 to 4 hours after administration (T_4 levels will be low to undetectable because of negative feedback suppression on the remaining functional thyroid tissue).

ADVERSE AND COMMON SIDE EFFECTS: As for **LEVOTHYROXINE.** Clinical signs of drug overdose resolve within 1 to 2 days after discontinuation of the drug. After this time, liothyroxine can be reinstituted at a lower dose.

DRUG INTERACTIONS: As for **LEVOTHYROXINE.**

SUPPLIED AS: VETERINARY PRODUCT
Tablets containing 60 and 120 μg [Cytobin]
HUMAN PRODUCT
Tablets containing 5, 25, and 50 μg [Cytomel]

LOPERAMIDE

INDICATIONS: Loperamide (Imodium ✚ ★) is a narcotic analgesic useful for the management of diarrhea in dogs. It also has been used in the treatment of acute colitis and malabsorption/maldigestion.

ADVERSE AND COMMON SIDE EFFECTS: The drug is relatively safe. Sedation, constipation, and ileus may occur. Dose-dependent vomiting (doses greater than 0.63 mg/kg) is reported. With chronic use, soft stools, bloody diarrhea, vomiting, and weight loss also have been reported. The drug should not be used to treat cases of suspect invasive bacterial enteritis such as *Salmonella,* because decreased intestinal transit can delay clearance of the pathogen. Loperamide also is contraindicated in patients with liver disease, obstructive GI disease, glaucoma, and obstructive uropathy. The drug should be discontinued if diarrhea has not been controlled within 48 hours. Use of opiate antidiarrheal products in cats may be associated with CNS excitation.

DRUG INTERACTIONS: None established.

SUPPLIED AS: HUMAN PRODUCTS
Capsules containing 2 mg
Oral liquid containing 0.2 mg/mL

MAGNESIUM HYDROXIDE

INDICATIONS: Magnesium hydroxide (Phillips' Milk of Magnesia ✚ ★) acts as an antacid at low doses and as a mild laxative at higher doses. For more information on ADVERSE AND COMMON SIDE EFFECTS and DRUG INTERACTIONS, see **ANTACIDS.**

SUPPLIED AS: VETERINARY PRODUCTS (large animal preparations)
Oral powder containing 310 g of magnesium hydroxide/lb of powder [Magnalax ★]
Oral boluses containing 27 g [Carmilax ✚, Magnalax ★]

HUMAN PRODUCTS
Oral suspension containing 408 mg/5 mL
Tablets containing 310 mg

MAGNESIUM SULFATE

INDICATIONS: Magnesium maintains the electrolyte balance across all membranes. Magnesium deficiency may occur with GI, renal, and endocrine disease and other miscellaneous causes. Magnesium-deficient states predispose to ventricular arrhythmias. Magnesium slows the rate of sinoatrial node impulse formation and prolongs conduction time. Clinical signs of hypomagnesemia may include muscle weakness. Hypokalemia and hyponatremia may be seen in association with hypomagnesemia. Animals at greater risk for the development of hypomagnesemia include critically ill animals on peritoneal dialysis and dogs with congestive heart failure being treated with furosemide.

ADVERSE AND COMMON SIDE EFFECTS: Clinical signs of drug overdose include depression, weakness, hypotension, loss of deep tendon reflexes, and prolongation of PR and QRS intervals on electrocardiograms. At toxic levels, respiratory depression and coma may be observed. Treatment of hypermagnesemia includes IV calcium (antagonizes magnesium) and fluid therapy with concurrent use of furosemide to enhance excretion.

DRUG INTERACTIONS: Magnesium sulfate can be diluted in normal saline, 2.5% dextrose in 0.45% saline, or 5% dextrose in water. Concurrent administration of CNS depressants (barbiturates, opiates, general anesthetics) may augment CNS depression. Magnesium sulfate may enhance the neuromuscular blockade of agents used to induce neuromuscular blockade. Cautious use of the drug is recommended in patients on digitalis therapy.

SUPPLIED AS: HUMAN PRODUCT
For injection at various concentrations, e.g., 20%, 50%

MANNITOL

INDICATIONS: Mannitol (Osmitrol ♣ ★) is a potent osmotic diuretic agent. It is used in the prevention and treatment of oliguria and acute glaucoma and in the management of acute cerebral edema. The use of the drug in animals with intracranial injury is controversial. These patients may have a damaged blood–brain barrier that allow the drug to leak across into the damaged brain and cause the area to swell further. The drug also has been used to enhance the renal elimination of toxins, such as aspirin, ethylene glycol, some barbiturates, and bromides.

ADVERSE AND COMMON SIDE EFFECTS: Volume overload and pulmonary edema may occur, especially in patients with compromised renal or cardiac function. With drug overdose, hyponatremia and seizures have been reported. Other side effects may include nausea, vomiting, and dizziness.

DRUG INTERACTIONS: Mannitol may increase the renal elimination of lithium.

SUPPLIED AS: HUMAN PRODUCT
For injection containing 5%, 10%, and 15% [Osmitrol]

OTHER USES
Dogs and Cats
ACUTE GLAUCOMA
1 to 2 g/kg over a 15- to 20-minute period; IV (withhold water for 30 to 60 minutes after administration)

ACUTE CEREBRAL EDEMA
Mannitol (20%) 2 g/kg once; slowly IV

OLIGURIC RENAL FAILURE
Mannitol (20–25%) 0.5 g/kg; slowly IV after adequate rehydration; repeat dose at 15-minute intervals up to 1.5 g/kg total dose.

MEBENDAZOLE

INDICATIONS: Mebendazole (Telmin ✤) is an anthelmintic used for the elimination of *Toxocara canis, Ancylostoma caninum, Uncinaria stenocephala, Trichuris vulpis,* and *Taenia pisiformis* in dogs.

ADVERSE AND COMMON SIDE EFFECTS: Although rare, vomiting and diarrhea are the most common side effects. Hepatotoxicity is rare. The drug is contraindicated in dogs with a history of hepatic disease.

DRUG INTERACTIONS: None established.

SUPPLIED AS: VETERINARY PRODUCT
Paste containing 200 mg mebendazole (for horses)
HUMAN PRODUCT
Tablets (chewable) containing 100 mg [Vermox ✤ ★]

MECLOFENAMIC ACID

INDICATIONS: Meclofenamic acid (Arquel ✤ ★) is a nonsteroidal anti-inflammatory agent with analgesic and antipyretic properties. The drug may act by inhibiting the migration of monocytes from inflamed blood vessels, their phagocytic activity, and the release of prostaglandins. Centrally, meclofenamic acid may raise the pain threshold. It has been used to treat inflammatory conditions of the musculoskeletal system in dogs.

ADVERSE AND COMMON SIDE EFFECTS: Anorexia, vomiting, diarrhea with or without blood, small intestinal ulcers, anemia, and leukocytosis may occur. Drug dosage should not exceed 1.1 mg/kg. The drug should not be used in animals with GI, hepatic, asthma, or renal disease. The drug may delay parturition and should be avoided in the last stages of pregnancy.

DRUG INTERACTIONS: The drug is highly protein bound and may displace other agents, e.g., phenytoin, salicylates, sulfonamides, and oral anticoagulants, resulting in increased serum levels of these drugs. Aspirin may decrease plasma levels of meclofenamic acid and increase the likelihood of adverse GIT effects.

SUPPLIED AS: VETERINARY PRODUCTS
Granules containing 50 mg/g [Arquel] (for use in the horse)
Tablets containing 10 and 20 mg (approved by the FDA for use in the dog, but not available at time of this writing)

MEDETOMIDINE

INDICATIONS: Medetomidine (Domitor ✦ ★) is an α-2 agonist pre-anesthetic agent with sedative and analgesic properties. When used with barbiturates, ketamine, or inhalation anesthetics, it produces safe and reliable sedation (1–2 hours), muscle relaxation, and analgesia. The drug should not be used alone. Medetomidine should only be used in young healthy animals undergoing routine or diagnostic procedures not requiring muscle relaxation or tracheal intubation.

ADVERSE AND COMMON SIDE EFFECTS: Paradoxical excitation, prolonged sedation, bradycardia, cyanosis, vomiting, apnea, death from circulatory failure, and recurrence of sedation have been reported. Urination during recovery is common, and adrenergic-induced hyperglycemia is seen. The drug should not be used in animals with cardiac, respiratory, renal, or liver disease, dogs in shock, debilitated patients, or dogs stressed due to extremes in heat, cold, or fatigue. Acutely stressed dogs may not respond to medetomidine and if they should not, repeat dosing is discouraged. Bradycardia, second-degree heart block, marked sinus arrhythmia, decreased respiratory rate, pain on injection, muscle jerking, and vomiting have been reported. Atipamezole, an α-2 adrenergic antagonist, shortens the recovery times of medetomidine in dogs.

DRUG INTERACTIONS: Medetomidine should be used with caution with other analgesic or sedative agents. Clinical effects may be enhanced. Atropine and glycopyrrolate given at the same time as or after medetomidine may induce bradycardia, heart block, premature ventricular contractions, and sinus tachycardia.

SUPPLIED AS: VETERINARY PRODUCT
For injection containing 1 mg/mL

MEDIUM CHAIN TRIGLYCERIDE (MCT) OIL

INDICATIONS: MCT oil ♣ ★ is used in the management of patients that cannot efficiently digest and absorb long chain food fats, e.g., animals with lymphangiectasia. Medium chain triglycerides are absorbed directly into mucosal cells and transported to the liver by the portal system.

ADVERSE AND COMMON SIDE EFFECTS: The oil is distasteful. It should be mixed with small amounts of food. It may lead to signs of hepatic encephalopathy in patients with advanced cirrhosis or portacaval shunts and should not be used in these patients. The hyperosmolality may worsen diarrhea, so it is best introduced gradually.

DRUG INTERACTIONS: None established.

SUPPLIED AS: HUMAN PRODUCT
Oil in 500-mL bottles

MEDROXYPROGESTERONE ACETATE

INDICATIONS: Medroxyprogesterone (Depo-Provera ♣ ★, Provera ♣ ★) is a synthetic prolonged-action progestational compound that suppresses secretion of FSH and LH, thus arresting the development of Graafian follicles and corpora lutea within the ovary. The drug has been used to treat benign prostatic hyperplasia in the dog. It also has been used to treat feline endocrine alopecia, eosinophilic granuloma complex, psychogenic alopecia and dermatitis, miliary dermatitis, stud tail, intermale aggression, and urine spraying by male cats.

ADVERSE AND COMMON SIDE EFFECTS: Overdose or prolonged treatment may cause cystic endometritis. Transient or permanent diabetes mellitus, acromegaly, mammary hyperplasia or adenocarcinoma, adrenocortical suppression, polydipsia, polyphagia, depression, immunosuppression, suppression of fibroblast function (which may delay healing), inhibition of spermatogenesis, and pyometra in intact females also are reported. Injection may cause temporary local alopecia, cutaneous atrophy, and pigmentary changes. Use the inguinal area for injection. Medroxyprogesterone acetate also has been associated with causing calcinosis circumscripta in two poodle bitches at the site of injection. The lesions were successfully removed surgically.

DRUG INTERACTIONS: None established.

SUPPLIED AS: HUMAN PRODUCTS
Tablets containing 2.5, 5, 10, and 100 mg [Provera]
For injection containing 50, 100, and 400 mg/mL [Depo-Provera]

OTHER USES
Dogs
ADJUNCTIVE THERAPY TO AGGRESSIVE BEHAVIOR
10 mg/kg; IM, SC as indicated (not to exceed 3 injections per year)

BENIGN PROSTATIC HYPERPLASIA
3 mg/kg; SC, repeat in 4 to 6 weeks if needed or if relapse occurs

Cats
RECURRENT ABORTION
1 to 2 mg once weekly; IM. Stop treatment 7 to 10 days before parturition.

TO ALLEVIATE SIGNS OF ESTRUS AND MATING ACTIVITY
i)   5 mg once daily; PO for up to 5 days; alleviates signs in 24 hours

ii) 25 mg injected every 6 months to postpone estrus

LONG-TERM REPRODUCTIVE CONTROL
2.5 to 5 mg once weekly; PO

BEHAVIORAL DISORDERS
Male cats: 100 mg; IM initially, then reduce dose by 1/3 to 1/2 and repeat every 30 days
Female cats: 50 mg; IM initially, then reduce dose by 1/3 to 1/2 and repeat every 30 days

PSYCHOGENIC ALOPECIA
75 to 150 mg; IM, SC, repeat PRN, but not more often than every 2 to 3 months

URINE SPRAYING
100 mg; SC for male cats
50 mg; SC for female cats

MEGESTROL ACETATE

INDICATIONS: Megestrol acetate (Ovaban ✦ ✦, Ovarid ✦) is a progestational compound marketed for the postponement of estrus and the alleviation of false pregnancy in bitches. The drug also is used to treat acral lick dermatitis and dominance aggression in dogs. In cats, the drug has been used to treat neurodermatitis (psychogenic alopecia), eosinophilic granuloma complex, eosinophilic keratitis, miliary dermatitis, pemphigus foliaceus, endocrine alopecia, hyperesthesia, urine spraying, intermale aggression, and aggression toward people. It also has been used in cats to prevent or postpone estrus.

ADVERSE AND COMMON SIDE EFFECTS: The drug should not be given to bitches with reproductive problems, pregnant bitches, or bitches with mammary tumors. Polyphagia, polydipsia, weight gain, and a change in behavior are common side effects. Overdose or prolonged use may result in cystic endometritis. Transient or permanent diabetes mellitus, mammary hyperplasia or adenocarcinoma, adrenocortical suppression (especially in cats), immunosuppression, suppression of fibroblast function (which may delay healing), and pyometra are other possible side effects. Rare reports of jaundice and hepatotoxicity in cats have been documented.

DRUG INTERACTIONS: None established.

SUPPLIED AS: VETERINARY PRODUCT
Tablets containing 5 and 20 mg

OTHER USES
Dogs
UNACCEPTABLE MASCULINE BEHAVIOR
1.1 to 2.2 mg/kg once daily; PO for 2 weeks, then 0.5 to 1.1 mg/kg once daily for 2 weeks (used in conjunction with behavior modification)

Cats
EOSINOPHILIC KERATITIS
0.5 mg/kg/day; PO until a response is seen, then maintain on 1.25 mg 2 to 3 times weekly to prevent recurrence

EOSINOPHILIC ULCERS
5 to 10 mg every other day for 10 to 14 treatments, then every 2 weeks; PO (alone or with methylprednisolone acetate)

URETHRITIS: FELINE LOWER URINARY TRACT INFLAMMATION
2.5 to 5 mg once daily to every other day; PO

IMMUNE SKIN DISEASE
2.5 to 5 mg once daily for 10 days, then every other day; PO

URINE SPRAYING, ANXIETY, INTRASPECIES AGGRESSION
5 mg once daily for 5 to 7 days, then once weekly; PO

MELARSOMINE

INDICATIONS: Melarsomine (Immiticide ★) is indicated in the treatment of heartworm disease caused by immature (4-month-old, stage L_5) to mature adult infections of *Dirofilaria immitis* in dogs. The drug causes greater worm mortality than thiacetarsamide and is associated with fewer complications.

ADVERSE AND COMMON SIDE EFFECTS: Melarsomine has a low margin of safety. Three times the recommended dosage may cause pulmonary inflammation, edema, and death. Pain and irritation at the injection site accompanied by swelling, tenderness, and reluctance to move occurs in up to 30% of dogs. Recovery from signs occurs over 1 week to 1 month. Firm nodules may persist indefinitely. Other adverse effects may include coughing, gagging, depression, lethargy, anorexia, fever, lung congestion, and vomiting. Hypersalivation and panting are infrequent. Safety for use in pregnant bitches or lactating or breeding animals has not been established.

DRUG INTERACTIONS: None reported.

SUPPLIED AS: VETERINARY PRODUCT
For injection containing 25 mg/mL

MELPHALAN

INDICATIONS: Melphalan (Alkeran ♣ ★) is an alkylating chemotherapeutic agent indicated in the treatment of lymphoreticular neoplasms, osteosarcoma, mammary and lung tumors, ovarian adenocarcinoma, and multiple myeloma.

ADVERSE AND COMMON SIDE EFFECTS: Nausea, anorexia, and vomiting have been reported. Leukopenia, thrombocytopenia, and anemia also may occur. The complete blood count should be monitored on a regular basis. Pulmonary infiltrates and fibrosis are reported.

DRUG INTERACTIONS: In humans, the concomitant use of melphalan and cyclosporine has resulted in nephrotoxicity.

SUPPLIED AS: HUMAN PRODUCTS
Tablets containing 2 mg
For injection containing 50 mg/vial

MEPERIDINE

INDICATIONS: Meperidine (Demerol ♣ ★) is a short-acting narcotic analgesic used for the relief of moderate to severe pain or as a preanesthetic. It has minimal sedative effects and is only approximately one eighth as potent as morphine in providing pain relief. It has a more rapid onset of action and shorter duration than morphine, causes less depression of the cough reflex, and is spasmolytic for some smooth muscle-containing tissues. Given orally, its onset of action is 15 minutes, with a peak effect in 1 hour. The analgesic effect is only approximately one half as effective when given orally as opposed to that given parenterally. Given parenterally, the onset of analgesia is 10 minutes, and the duration of effect is 2 to 4 hours. In cats, its duration of action is short (60 minutes). Meperidine is the only narcotic with depressant effects on the heart, and it also may cause histamine release.

ADVERSE AND COMMON SIDE EFFECTS: Nausea, vomiting, and decreased peristalsis are reported. With drug overdose, respiratory depression, cardiovascular collapse, hypothermia, skeletal muscle hypotonia, and seizure are possible side effects. Naloxone should be used to reverse the respiratory depression. Bronchoconstriction after IV use in dogs has been reported. The drug is quite irritating given subcutaneously. Meperidine should not be given to animals with head trauma because it may increase intracranial pressure. It should be used with caution in animals with adrenocortical insufficiency, hypothyroid disease, and renal disease, in geriatrics, in those with respiratory disease, and in debilitated patients. Meperidine may potentiate the toxicity of venom of the scorpion *Centruroides sculpturatus*. In cats, the drug may cause CNS excitation with hyperexcitability, tremors, and seizure activity at doses greater than 20 mg/kg.

DRUG INTERACTIONS: Central nervous system depression or stimulation induced by meperidine may be potentiated by amphetamines, barbiturates, or cimetidine. Phenytoin may increase meperidine toxicity and decrease its analgesic effects.

SUPPLIED AS: HUMAN PRODUCTS
Tablets containing 50 and 100 mg
Syrup containing 10 and 25 mg/mL
For injection containing 50-, 75-, and 100-mg/mL single- or multiple-dose units and 25-, 75-, and 100-mg single-dose ampules

MERCAPTOPURINE

INDICATIONS: Mercaptopurine (Purinethol ♣ ★) is an antimetabolite chemotherapeutic agent used in the treatment of lymphosarcoma, acute lymphocytic and granulocytic leukemia, and rheumatoid arthritis. In humans, the drug also has been used to treat granulomatous and ulcerative colitis unresponsive to corticosteroids or sulfasalazine.

ADVERSE AND COMMON SIDE EFFECTS: Nausea, vomiting, and diarrhea have been reported. Leukopenia is rare. In addition, cholestasis (rarely necrosis), oral and intestinal ulcers, and pancreatitis have been documented in humans.

DRUG INTERACTIONS: Allopurinol delays the metabolism of mercaptopurine and enhances its antineoplastic effect and toxicity. Mercaptopurine may reverse the neuromuscular blocking effect of tubocurarine.

SUPPLIED AS: HUMAN PRODUCT
Tablets containing 50 mg

METAMUCIL

INDICATIONS: Metamucil ♣ ★ is a psyllium hydrophilic mucilloid used for the management of constipation and colitis. It may require 12 to 24 hours to be effective.

ADVERSE AND COMMON SIDE EFFECTS: Side effects are minimal. Temporary cramping, flatulence, and bloating may occur. It should not be used in patients with abdominal pain, vomiting, nausea, or fecal impaction.

DRUG INTERACTIONS: None established.

SUPPLIED AS: HUMAN PRODUCT
Powder containing 3.4 to 3.6 g psyllium hydrophilic mucilloid/packet and 3.4 g psyllium hydrophilic mucilloid per rounded teaspoonful

METHENAMINE MANDELATE

INDICATIONS: Methenamine mandelate (Mandelamine ♣ ★, Rena-Tone ♣) is a urinary antibacterial agent. It is used in the management of urinary tract infection. In the presence of an acid urine (pH less than 6), the drug is hydrolyzed to formaldehyde. Concurrent use of a urinary acidifier is common. It also is effective against fungal urinary tract infections.

ADVERSE AND COMMON SIDE EFFECTS: The drug may cause GI upset and dysuria (due to urinary tract irritation). It should not be given to patients with renal insufficiency.

DRUG INTERACTIONS: Methenamine should not be given to patients receiving sulfamethizole because formaldehyde and sulfamethizole form insoluble precipitates in acid urine. Drugs that increase urine pH, e.g., acetazolamide and sodium bicarbonate, prevent hydrolysis of methenamine and decrease its antimicrobial efficacy.

SUPPLIED AS: VETERINARY PRODUCT
Liquid containing 60 gr [Rena-Tone]

HUMAN PRODUCT
Tablet containing 500 mg and 1 g [Mandelamine]

METHIMAZOLE

INDICATIONS: Methimazole (Tapazole ♣ ★) is the drug of choice for the medical management of feline hyperthyroid disease. It is safer and more potent than propylthiouracil in blocking thyroid hormone synthesis. Use of the drug generally will bring serum T_4 into normal ranges within 2 to 3 weeks. The drug also is used to decrease renal toxicity of cisplatin in dogs. Its efficacy in this regard is probably related to its antioxidant properties.

ADVERSE AND COMMON SIDE EFFECTS: Adverse effects have been observed in approximately 15% of cats and generally are transient. Anorexia, vomiting, and transient lethargy have been reported. Serum antinuclear antibodies develop in many cats with long-term use of the drug. A glucocorticoid-responsive pruritus involving the face, ears, and neck may occur. In less than 2% of cases, thrombocytopenia and agranulocytosis have been reported in cats treated with the drug. Withdrawal of the drug and provision of care for thrombocytopenia or agranulocytosis generally results in resolution of the drug reaction. Cats on chronic methimazole therapy should be rechecked every 3 to 6 months to assay serum T_4 levels and to check for signs of drug toxicity.

DRUG INTERACTIONS: The activity of anticoagulants may be potentiated by methimazole.

SUPPLIED AS: HUMAN PRODUCT
Tablets containing 5 and 10 mg

METHIONINE

INDICATIONS: Methionine (Methio-Tabs ❤ ★, Methigel ❤) is a urinary acidifying agent used in the treatment and prevention of struvite urolithiasis and to control urine odor. Urine acidification also may be effective adjunctive therapy to optimize the efficacy of certain antibiotics, e.g., penicillin, ampicillin, carbenicillin, tetracycline, and nitrofurantoin, in the treatment of urinary tract infections.

ADVERSE AND COMMON SIDE EFFECTS: The drug is contraindicated in patients with renal failure or pancreatic disease. The drug has no place in the treatment of hepatic lipidosis unless it is caused by choline deficiency, as with pancreatic exocrine insufficiency. It may potentiate clinical signs of hepatic encephalopathy by leading to the increased production of mercaptan-like compounds. The drug is not recommended for use in kittens.

DRUG INTERACTIONS: Methionine may increase the renal excretion of quinidine. The antibacterial efficacy of the aminoglycosides and erythromycin may be decreased in the presence of an acid urine produced by methionine.

SUPPLIED AS: VETERINARY PRODUCTS
Tablets containing 200 and 500 mg
Gel containing 400 mg/5 g [Methigel]

METHOCARBAMOL

INDICATIONS: Methocarbamol (Robaxin-V ★, Robaxin ♣ ★) is a central-acting muscle relaxant that may be used as adjunct therapy to rest and physical therapy in the treatment of musculoskeletal injury. It also has been used to reduce muscular spasm associated with tetanus and metaldehyde or strychnine poisoning.

ADVERSE AND COMMON SIDE EFFECTS: Excessive salivation, sedation, vomiting, muscular weakness, and ataxia have been reported. Extravascular injection may cause tissue necrosis. The drug should not be given to animals with renal dysfunction, nor should it be used in pregnant animals.

DRUG INTERACTIONS: Other CNS depressants may potentiate CNS depressive effects of methocarbamol.

SUPPLIED AS: VETERINARY PRODUCTS (United States only)
Tablets containing 500 mg
For injection containing 100 mg/mL

HUMAN PRODUCTS ♣ ★
Tablets containing 500 and 750 mg
For injection containing 100 mg/mL

METHOTREXATE

INDICATIONS: Methotrexate ♣ ★ is an antimetabolite chemotherapeutic agent that has been recommended in the treatment of lymphoreticular neoplasms, myeloproliferative disease, osteosarcoma, transmissible venereal tumor, and Sertoli cell tumor.

ADVERSE AND COMMON SIDE EFFECTS: Vomiting, nausea, diarrhea, leukopenia, thrombocytopenia, and anemia are reported. Delayed toxicity may be associated with oral and GI ulceration, renal tubular necrosis, hepatic necrosis, alopecia, pulmonary infiltrates and fibrosis, encephalopathy, and anaphylactoid reactions with high doses. Leucovorin calcium, a reduced folate, given at 3 mg/m² within 3 hours of methotrexate administration, helps ameliorate these effects. Methotrexate may adversely affect spermiogenesis and may cause embryotoxicity or congenital malformations.

DRUG INTERACTIONS: Chloramphenicol, salicylates, sulfonamides, phenylbutazone, phenytoin, tetracyclines, and para-aminobenzoic acid

(PABA) displace methotrexate from plasma proteins, causing increased toxicity. Oral aminoglycoside antibiotics may reduce GIT absorption. Penicillin and probenecid increase methotrexate plasma levels predisposing to toxicity.

SUPPLIED AS: HUMAN PRODUCTS
Tablets containing 2.5 mg [Rheumatrex ✦]
For injection (parenteral solution) containing equivalent of 2.5, 10, and 25 mg/mL methotrexate
Lyophilized powder equivalent to 20, 25, 50, 100, 250, and 1000 mg/vial

METHOXYFLURANE

INDICATIONS: Methoxyflurane (Metafane ✦ ★) is used for induction and maintenance of general anesthesia. Because induction time for methoxyflurane alone is slow (5–10 minutes), an ultrashort-acting IV anesthetic generally is used for induction.

ADVERSE AND COMMON SIDE EFFECTS: The drug should be used cautiously in animals with liver disease. Minimal hepatic damage may occur with drug overdose. Hypoxia at deep levels of anesthesia predisposes to hepatic damage. The drug is potentially nephrotoxic. Nephrotoxicity is enhanced by dehydration and the concurrent use of other potentially nephrotoxic drugs, e.g., flunixin meglumine.

DRUG INTERACTIONS: Large doses of epinephrine may produce atrioventricular block and arrhythmias. Vomiting is infrequent and mild when it does occur. The drug will cross the placental barrier and depress the fetus. If depression of a newborn does occur, administration of oxygen usually brings about prompt recovery.

SUPPLIED AS: VETERINARY PRODUCT
Available in 118-mL bottles

METHYLENE BLUE

INDICATIONS: Methylene blue ✦ ★ is used in the treatment of methemoglobinemia. It also has been used for the intraoperative identification of parathyroid and pancreatic islet cell tumors in dogs.

ADVERSE AND COMMON SIDE EFFECTS: The drug is contraindicated in patients with renal insufficiency. Methylene blue may cause Heinz body hemolytic anemia and possibly acute renal failure. Cats are especially sensitive to Heinz body formation.

In people, additional side effects may include bladder irritation, nausea, vomiting, diarrhea, and abdominal pain. With large IV doses, fever, cardiovascular abnormalities, methemoglobinemia, and profuse sweating has been recorded in humans.

DRUG INTERACTIONS: None reported.

SUPPLIED AS: HUMAN PRODUCT
For injection containing 10 mg/mL

OTHER USES
Dogs
TO STAIN ISLET CELL TUMORS
3 mg/kg in 250 mL saline over 30 to 40 minutes intraoperatively; IV. Tumors appear reddish-violet against a dusky blue background.

TO STAIN PARATHYROID TUMORS
Dose as aforementioned; tumor staining becomes evident starting 15 minutes after infusion. Tumors appear dark blue.

METHYLPHENIDATE

INDICATIONS: Methylphenidate (Ritalin ♣ ★) is used in dogs in the management of narcolepsy (as a supplement to imipramine) and hyperkinesis.

ADVERSE AND COMMON SIDE EFFECTS: In humans, nervousness, anorexia, and tachycardia are reported. Overdose may cause vomiting, tremors, muscle twitching, convulsions, arrhythmias, mydriasis, and dryness of the mucous membranes. The drug tends to lose its effect over time. Experience with the drug in small animals is limited. Signs of toxicosis reported in a cat included muscle tremors, mydriasis, agitation, and tachycardia. In severe toxicosis, supportive treatment, anxiolytic drugs, e.g., diazepam, and the use of an adrenergic blocking agent, e.g., propranolol, may be required.

DRUG INTERACTIONS: Combination with MAO inhibitors, e.g., possibly amitraz and selegiline, may cause hypertension.

SUPPLIED AS: HUMAN PRODUCTS
Tablets (sustained-release) containing 20 mg
Tablets containing 5, 10, and 20 mg

METHYLPREDNISOLONE

INDICATIONS: Methylprednisolone (Medrol ♣ ★, Depo-Medrol ♣ ★) is an intermediate-acting glucocorticoid used for its anti-inflammatory properties, to control autoimmune skin diseases in dogs, as adjunctive therapy in spinal cord trauma, and in the treatment of shock. In cats, it also is used to treat eosinophilic ulcers, plasma cell gingivitis-pharyngitis, and for the adjunctive treatment of asthma.

ADVERSE AND COMMON SIDE EFFECTS and **DRUG INTERACTIONS:** See **GLUCOCORTICOID AGENTS.**

SUPPLIED AS: VETERINARY PRODUCTS
Tablets containing 1 and 4 mg [Medrol]
For injection containing 20 and 40 mg/mL methylprednisolone acetate [Depo-Medrol]
HUMAN PRODUCTS
Tablets containing 2, 4, 8, 16, 24, and 32 mg [Medrol ✤ ★]
For injection containing 40 mg/mL, 125 mg/2 mL, 500 mg/8 mL, 1,000 mg/16 mL, and 2,000 mg/32 mL methylprednisolone sodium succinate [Solu-Medrol ✤ ★]

OTHER USES
Dogs
ANTI-INFLAMMATORY DOSE
i) 1 mg/kg tid; PO methylprednisolone
ii) 1.1 mg/kg; SC, IM methylprednisolone acetate (lasts 1 to 3 weeks in skin conditions)

AUTOIMMUNE SKIN DISEASE "PULSE THERAPY"
Methylprednisolone sodium succinate 11 mg/kg in 250 mL D_5W infused over 1 hour for 3 consecutive days. Maintenance therapy includes oral prednisone at 1.1 mg/kg every 1 to 2 days and azathioprine (2.2 mg/kg daily for 2 weeks, then every 48 hours). Cimetidine may be given concurrently to reduce the incidence of GIT ulcerations.

Cats
ANTI-INFLAMMATORY AGENT
Methylprednisolone acetate 5.5 mg/kg; IM or SC (effects for skin conditions may last from 1 week to 6 months)

EOSINOPHILIC ULCER
Methylprednisolone acetate 20 mg; SC every 2 weeks for 2 to 3 doses

PLASMA CELL GINGIVITIS/PHARYNGITIS
Methylprednisolone acetate 10 to 20 mg PRN; SC

INFLAMMATORY BOWEL DISEASE
i) Methylprednisolone acetate 20 mg; SC, IM, repeated at 1- to 2-week intervals for 2 to 3 doses, then given every 2 to 4 weeks PRN
ii) 20 mg; IM every 2 to 4 weeks

FELINE ASTHMA
Methylprednisolone acetate 1 to 2 mg/kg; IM

METOCLOPRAMIDE

INDICATIONS: Metoclopramide (Maxeran ♣, Reglan ♣ ★) is an antiemetic agent with central (chemoreceptor trigger zone) and peripheral activity. It contributes to lower esophageal sphincter competence and promotes gastric emptying. It is useful in the management of vomiting, gastroesophageal reflux, and gastric motility disorders.

ADVERSE AND COMMON SIDE EFFECTS: Metoclopramide should not be used in patients with gastric outlet obstruction or those with a history of epilepsy. Renal disease may increase blood levels of the drug. Central nervous system reactions include increased frequency of seizure activity, vertigo, hyperactivity, depression, and disorientation.

DRUG INTERACTIONS: Phenothiazine drugs may potentiate CNS effects. Digoxin, cimetidine, tetracycline, narcotic agents, and sedatives enhance CNS effects. Digoxin absorption also may be decreased, whereas acetaminophen, aspirin, diazepam, and tetracycline absorption may be accelerated. Atropine will block the effects of the drug on GIT motility.

SUPPLIED AS: HUMAN PRODUCTS
Tablets containing 5 and 10 mg
Syrup containing 1 mg/mL
For injection containing 5 mg/mL

OTHER USES
Dogs
DISORDERS OF GASTRIC MOTILITY
0.2 to 0.4 mg/kg tid; PO, SC given 30 minutes before meals
ESOPHAGEAL REFLUX
i) 0.5 mg/kg tid; PO
ii) 0.2 to 0.5 mg/kg tid; PO, SC given 30 minutes before meals and at bedtime

Cats
GASTRIC MOTILITY DISORDERS AND ESOPHAGEAL REFLUX
0.2 to 0.4 mg/kg tid–qid; PO

METOPROLOL

INDICATIONS: Metoprolol (Lopressor ♣ ★) is a selective β_1-blocking agent equal in potency to propranolol. It is the preferred β-blocker in patients with pulmonary disease such as asthma. The drug also is useful in the management of supraventricular tachyarrhythmias, ventricular premature contractions, and hypertrophic cardiomyopathy.

ADVERSE AND COMMON SIDE EFFECTS: Depression, lethargy, bradycardia, impaired atrioventricular conduction, and congestive heart failure have been reported with the use of β-blocking drugs. Glycopyrrolate and dopamine may be used to counter bradycardia. The drug should be used with caution in patients with renal insufficiency.

DRUG INTERACTIONS: Barbiturates and rifampin may decrease the pharmacologic effects of metoprolol. Cimetidine, methimazole, and propylthiouracil may increase the pharmacologic effects of metoprolol. Digitalis may potentiate bradycardia associated with metoprolol. The pharmacologic effects of hydralazine and metoprolol may be increased if both drugs are used concurrently. Indomethacin may cause a decrease in the antihypertensive effects of the drug.

SUPPLIED AS: HUMAN PRODUCTS
Tablets containing 50 and 100 mg
Tablets (slow-release) containing 100 and 200 mg
For injection containing 1 mg/mL

METRONIDAZOLE

INDICATIONS: Metronidazole (Flagyl ♣ ★) is a synthetic antibacterial, antiprotozoal agent that has been used in the treatment of giardiasis, trichomoniasis, amoebiasis, balantidiasis, and trypanosomiasis. It is as effective and is better tolerated than quinacrine for the treatment of giardiasis, but it is not as safe or as efficacious as albendazole. It is bactericidal to many anaerobic bacteria, including *Bacteroides* spp., *Fusobacterium, Clostridium* spp., *Veillonella, Peptococcus,* and *Peptostreptococcus.* It has been used in the treatment of septicemia, meningitis, peritonitis, biliary infections, colitis, and gingivostomatitis, in which anaerobic bacteria are involved. The drug also may have immunosuppressive or immunostimulatory properties.

ADVERSE AND COMMON SIDE EFFECTS: Clinical signs generally begin 7 to 12 days after initiation of therapy. Nausea, anorexia, vomiting, lethargy, weakness, and dose-dependent neurologic signs (ataxia, nystagmus, seizure, head tilt, bradycardia, rigidity, and stiffness) have been reported. Neutropenia and hematuria also have been seen in some dogs. It is potentially hepatotoxic. The tablets have a bitter taste and should **NOT** be crushed before use. The drug also may be mutagenic and should not be given to pregnant animals.

DRUG INTERACTIONS: Blood levels may be decreased by concurrent use of phenobarbital or phenytoin, and blood levels may be increased by cimetidine use.

SUPPLIED AS: HUMAN PRODUCTS
Tablets containing 250 and 500 mg
Capsules containing 500 mg
For injection containing 500 mg/vial and 500 mg in 100 mL of isotonic saline

OTHER USES
Dogs
LYMPHOCYTIC/PLASMOCYTIC ENTERITIS–COLITIS
i)   30 to 60 mg/kg once daily; PO
ii) 10 to 30 mg/kg 1 to 3 times daily for 2 to 4 weeks; PO (refractory cases)

ANAEROBIC INFECTIONS
i)   30 mg/kg/day div. tid–qid; PO
ii) 25 to 50 mg/kg bid; PO (bacterial meningitis)

GIT BACTERIAL OVERGROWTH
20 to 40 mg/kg once daily; PO (in food)

AMOEBIASIS, BALANTIDIASIS
60 mg/kg once daily; PO for 5 days

ADJUNCTIVE THERAPY IN HEPATIC ENCEPHALOPATHY
i)   20 mg/kg tid; PO
ii) 7.5 mg/kg tid for 2 to 4 weeks; PO

CHOLANGITIS
i)   7.5 mg/kg tid; PO
ii) 25 to 30 mg/kg bid; PO (may be used with chloramphenicol); 4 to 6 weeks of therapy may be required

STOMATITIS
15 mg/kg tid; PO

Cats
ANAEROBIC INFECTION
i)   10 mg/kg once daily; PO (adjunctive therapy of plasmocytic/lymphocytic enteritis)
ii) 25 to 30 mg/kg bid; PO for 2 to 3 weeks (adjunctive therapy of hepatic lipidosis—efficacy unknown)

PLASMA CELL GINGIVITIS/PHARYNGITIS
50 mg/kg once daily; PO for 5 days (antibacterial effects)

INFLAMMATORY BOWEL DISEASE
10 to 20 mg/kg bid–tid; PO with prednisone 2 mg/kg/day; PO (refractory cases)

BALANTIDIUM
10 to 25 mg/kg once to twice daily; PO for 5 days

MEXILETINE

INDICATIONS: Mexiletine (Mexitil ♣ ★) is an analog of lidocaine with electrophysiologic properties similar to those of tocainide. The drug has been used in dogs to treat ventricular arrhythmias, including premature contractions and runs of tachycardia.

ADVERSE AND COMMON SIDE EFFECTS: Side effects are uncommon but may include vomiting. In humans, gastric irritation, anorexia, and tremor are reported infrequently and discontinue with cessation of therapy.

DRUG INTERACTIONS: Mexiletine may be used in combination with quinidine (6.6–22 mg/kg) in those cases refractory to either drug alone. Enhanced activity and a reduction in toxicity are noted when these drugs are used concurrently. Antacids, cimetidine, and narcotic analgesics may slow GI absorption. Hepatic enzyme inducers, e.g., phenobarbital, phenytoin, and rifampin, may increase drug clearance. Mexiletine may increase theophylline levels because of decreased hepatic metabolism of theophylline.

SUPPLIED AS: HUMAN PRODUCT
Capsules containing 100, 150, and 200 mg

MIBOLERONE

INDICATIONS: Mibolerone (Cheque Drops ★) is an androgenic, anabolic, antigonadotropic agent used for the prevention of estrus in adult female dogs.

ADVERSE AND COMMON SIDE EFFECTS: Mibolerone is contraindicated in female dogs with perianal adenoma, perianal adenocarcinoma, and liver and renal disease. The drug also is not recommended for use in Bedlington terriers. The drug should not be given to pregnant bitches because it will cause masculinization of the female fetus. In prepuberal females, the drug may cause premature closure of epiphyses, clitoral enlargement, and vaginitis. In the adult bitch, adverse effects may include mild clitoral enlargement, vulvovaginitis, and abnormal behavior, including riding behavior, urinary incontinence, exacerbation of seborrhea oleosa, and epiphora. Significant hepatic disease is rare, and renal changes generally are not pathologic. With the exception of mild residual clitoral enlargement, all changes resolve after discontinuation of the drug.

In the cat, dosages of 60 µg/day induced hepatic dysfunction, and dosages of 120 µg/day caused death. Other adverse effects noted in cats include clitoral enlargement, thyroid dysfunction, cervical dermis thickening, and pancreatic dysfunction. Although not approved for use in cats, the drug has been used to prevent estrus at doses of 50 µg/day. The potential for adverse side effects, however, is great. The drug may incite seizure activity in dogs predisposed to seizures.

DRUG INTERACTIONS: Mibolerone should not be used in conjunction with estrogen or progestin products.

SUPPLIED AS: VETERINARY PRODUCT
Oral drops containing 100 µg/mL

OTHER USES
Dogs
PSEUDOCYESIS
16 µg/kg once daily for 5 days; PO
GALACTORRHEA
8 to 18 µg/kg once daily for 5 days; PO (once discontinued galactorrhea may resume because of effects of prolactin)

MIDAZOLAM

INDICATIONS: Midazolam (Versed ♣ ★) is a short-acting parenteral benzodiazepine, CNS depressant with sedative-hypnotic, anxiolytic, muscle-relaxing, and anticonvulsant properties useful in small animals as a preanesthetic agent. The drug is two to three times more potent than diazepam and has a shorter half-life.

ADVERSE AND COMMON SIDE EFFECTS: No significant cardiovascular effects are noted. Respiratory depression and dose-dependent sedation occur.

DRUG INTERACTIONS: Barbiturates prolong respiratory depression predisposing to apnea and underventilation. Fentanyl and droperidol (Innovar-Vet) increase the hypnotic effect. Hypotension has been reported with the concurrent use of meperidine.

SUPPLIED AS: HUMAN PRODUCT
For injection containing 1 and 5 mg/mL

MILBEMYCIN

INDICATIONS: Milbemycin oxime (Interceptor ♣ ★) is an anthelmintic used in dogs for the prevention of heartworm caused by *Dirofilaria immitis,* as a microfilaricide, and for the control of hookworm (*Ancylostoma caninum*) and roundworm (*Toxocara canis*) infections. It also may be effective against *Trichuris vulpis* infections. The drug also prevents the development of infection in cats by larvae of *Dirofilaria immitis* and has been used in the treatment of generalized demodicosis in adult dogs.

ADVERSE AND COMMON SIDE EFFECTS: At therapeutic doses, no adverse effects are seen. With drug overdose (5 times recommended dose), the only adverse effects seen were transient ataxia and trembling in 8-week-old puppies. If milbemycin is administered to heartworm-infected dogs, a mild shock-like reaction may occur.

DRUG INTERACTIONS: None reported.

SUPPLIED AS: VETERINARY PRODUCT
Tablets containing 2.3, 5.75, 11.5, and 23 mg

OTHER USES
Dogs
JUVENILE GENERALIZED DEMODICOSIS
11.5 mg/22.7 kg once daily. Treat until no mites are detected and then 30 days after. If mite counts are still high after 90 days, double the dose. Resolution has been reported in 83% of previously untreated cases, and cure is reported in 60% of cases.

ADULT CHRONIC GENERALIZED DEMODICOSIS
i)   0.52 to 3.8 mg/kg once daily; PO for 30 days after mites are no longer detected on skin scraping
NB: relapse may occur

ii) 1 mg/kg per day; PO until 30 days after skin scraping fails to detect mites. If the mite count has not decreased by 25%, increase the drug dose to 2 mg/kg/day.

DIROFILARIA IMMITIS
500 µg/kg 3 to 4 weeks after adulticide therapy (microfilaricide)

Cats
DIROFILARIA IMMITIS
0.5 to 0.9 mg/kg 60 and 90 days after inoculation with infective larvae prevents development of infection

MINERAL OIL

INDICATIONS: Mineral oil ♣ ★ is used for the relief of constipation. It softens stools by coating the feces and preventing the colonic absorption of water. The agent works at the level of the colon and may take 6 to 12 hours to work effectively. It also has been used to retard the absorption of lipid-soluble toxins (kerosene, metaldehyde).

ADVERSE AND COMMON SIDE EFFECTS: Mineral oil is contraindicated in patients with nausea, vomiting, abdominal pain, intestinal obstruction, or dysphagia. A small amount of oil is absorbed, but it generally is of no clinical significance. Because of the lack of taste, accidental aspiration and subsequent pneumonia may occur. Occasionally, pruritus ani may occur. Interference with postoperative anorectal wound healing may occur. Prolonged use may cause anorexia and vomiting.

DRUG INTERACTIONS: Increased absorption may occur if mineral oil is given concurrently with docusate sodium or docusate calcium. Mineral oil may interfere with the absorption of fat-soluble vitamins and should only be given between meals. Mineral oil may interfere with action of nonabsorbable sulfonamides.

SUPPLIED AS: VETERINARY PRODUCTS
Several products are available, including generic mineral oil as well as petrolatum preparations, Kit-Lax ♣ ★, Dislax ♣, and many others.

MINOCYCLINE

INDICATIONS: Minocycline (Minocin ♣ ★) is a second-generation, long-acting, lipid-soluble tetracycline. It is more active against anaerobes and several facultative intracellular bacteria, such as *Brucella canis,* than other tetracyclines except for doxycycline. It is more active against *Nocardia* and staphylococcus than other tetracyclines. The drug has been used in the treatment of actinomycosis, canine ehrlichiosis, nocardiosis, and Rocky Mountain spotted fever. Minocycline does not reach high enough concentrations in the urine to be effective in treating urinary tract infection. Also see **TETRA-CYCLINE ANTIBIOTICS.**

ADVERSE AND COMMON SIDE EFFECTS: Hypotension, shock, and urticaria developed in dogs given rapid doses of minocycline. Doses of 10 to 20 mg/kg per day caused the erythrocyte count to decrease and alanine transferase (ALT) activity to increase in dogs. Daily IV doses of 40 mg/kg caused decreased appetite and weight loss. None of these side effects were noted at similar oral doses.

DRUG INTERACTIONS: Minocycline and doxycycline are less affected by the presence of food. In fact, these two agents often are given with food to decrease GIT irritation.

SUPPLIED AS: HUMAN PRODUCT
Capsule containing 50 and 100 mg

MISOPROSTOL

INDICATIONS: Misoprostol (Cytotec ✦ ★) is a synthetic prostaglandin E_1 analog used to prevent gastric ulceration. It mitigates nonsteroidal anti-inflammatory drug-induced gastroduodenal injury. Although partial protection is provided, gastritis still may occur and contribute to vomiting. The drug decreases gastric acid secretion, increases bicarbonate and mucus secretion, increases epithelial cell turnover, and increases mucosal blood flow. The drug did not prevent gastric hemorrhage in dogs treated with methylprednisolone.

ADVERSE AND COMMON SIDE EFFECTS: Vomiting, diarrhea, flatulence, and abdominal pain are reported. The incidence of diarrhea can be minimized by adjusting the dose, by administering the drug after food, and by avoiding the administration of misoprostol with magnesium-containing antacids. The drug may induce abortion in pregnant animals. Experience with the drug in small animals is limited.

DRUG INTERACTIONS: No clinically significant drug interactions have been reported.

SUPPLIED AS: HUMAN PRODUCT
Tablets containing 100 and 200 µg

MITOTANE

INDICATIONS: Mitotane or o,p'-DDD (Lysodren ✦ ★) is indicated in the treatment of pituitary-dependent hyperadrenocorticism in dogs. It causes selective necrosis of the zona fasciculata and reticularis in the adrenal gland. Damage to the zona glomerulosa is slight. The drug also is used to manage primary adrenal hyperadrenocorticism, but patients with adrenal tumors causing hyperadrenocorticism appear more resistant and require higher drug doses.

ADVERSE AND COMMON SIDE EFFECTS: Mitotane is effective and relatively safe for treatment of canine pituitary-dependent hyperadrenocorticism. More than 80% of dogs are reported to have a good to excellent response. Lethargy, vomiting, weakness, anorexia, and diarrhea are reported. In approximately 5% of dogs, adrenal insufficiency develops. Although cats appear more sensitive to the chlorinated hydrocarbons, the drug has been used in this species. It is well tolerated by 75% of cats and results in adrenocortical suppression in half.

DRUG INTERACTIONS: Spironolactone may decrease pharmacologic effects of the drug. Mitotane may induce hepatic microsomal enzymes and increase the metabolism of barbiturates and warfarin. Insulin requirements in diabetic patients may be decreased as the hyperadrenocortical situation is brought under control. Additive depression may occur if the drug is used concurrently with CNS depressants.

SUPPLIED AS: HUMAN PRODUCT
Tablets containing 500 mg

OTHER USES
Dogs
ADRENAL TUMORS CAUSING HYPERADRENOCORTICISM
50 to 75 mg/kg for 10 to 14 days (induction) with prednisone at 0.2 mg/kg/day; PO; maintenance regimen is 75 to 100 mg/kg/week

MITOXANTRONE

INDICATIONS: Mitoxantrone (Novantrone ✚ ★) is a chemotherapeutic agent related to doxorubicin. It has been used in dogs to treat various malignancies, including lymphoma, fibrosarcoma, thyroid carcinomas, transitional cell carcinoma, hemangiopericytoma, and renal adenocarcinoma. The drug also has been used in cats with malignant tumors.

ADVERSE AND COMMON SIDE EFFECTS: The drug is considered safe and effective. The most common signs of toxicosis noted in dogs include depression, vomiting, diarrhea, anorexia, and sepsis secondary to myelosuppression. Use of the drug has not been associated with cardiotoxicity, as noted with doxorubicin. Toxicity is not dose dependent in dogs. Neutropenia may occur (nadir on day 10). The use of recombinant canine granulocyte colony-stimulating factor (Amgen, Thousand Oaks, CA) at a dosage of 5 µg/kg/day SC for 20 days after infusion of mitoxantrone reduces the severity and duration of myelosuppression and neutropenia. Also see **GRANULOCYTE COLONY-STIMULATING FACTOR** (Neupogen).
  The most common adverse effects in cats include vomiting, anorexia, diarrhea, lethargy, sepsis secondary to myelosuppression, and seizures. The drug even may cause death in some cats. In cats with signs of toxicosis during the first 21-day interval, signs of toxicosis are more likely to develop between the second and third doses during the 21-day interval.

DRUG INTERACTIONS: Mitoxantrone should not be mixed with heparin because precipitates may form.

SUPPLIED AS: HUMAN PRODUCT
For injection containing 2 mg/mL

MORPHINE

INDICATIONS: Morphine (Astramorph ★, Duramorph ★, Roxanol ★, M.S. Contin ✦ ★, M.O.S. ✦ ★, Morphitec ✦, Statex ✦) is a very effective analgesic narcotic agent. It is used for the management of acute pain and as a preanesthetic agent. Analgesia lasts 4 to 6 hours after IM injection. In addition to analgesia, morphine produces CNS depression with sedation or sleep. It increases cardiac output and decreases pulmonary edema associated with congestive heart failure and cardiomyopathy. The drug also has been administered via epidural injection to relieve somatic or visceral pain, especially of the hind limbs, but as far forward as the neck. It particularly is useful after hind limb, fore limb, and pelvic orthopedic surgery. The onset of action is 30 to 60 minutes, and the duration of analgesia is 6 to 24 hours.

ADVERSE AND COMMON SIDE EFFECTS: In dogs, it may produce initial excitement, restlessness, panting, salivation, nausea, vomiting, urination, defecation, and hypotension. Subsequently, CNS depression, constipation, urinary retention, bradycardia, respiratory depression, hypothermia, and miosis occur. Morphine should be used with caution in animals with biliary tract disease because it will increase bile duct luminal pressure. In cats, analgesia and CNS depression occur at lower doses (0.1 mg/kg qid). At doses of 1 mg/kg, hyperexcitability, tonic spasms, seizure activity, ataxia, aggression, vomiting, and even death may occur. The depressive effects of the drug are antagonized by naloxone (0.1 mg/kg; IV). The drug should not be used in animals with renal failure or a history of seizures or in those in hypovolemic shock. Pruritus may occur after epidural injection.

DRUG INTERACTIONS: Phenothiazines, amitriptyline, antihistamines, fentanyl, and parenteral magnesium sulfate may potentiate the depressant effects of morphine.

SUPPLIED AS: HUMAN PRODUCTS
For injection containing 0.5, 1, 2, 4, 5, 8, 10, 15, 25, and 50 mg/mL
Tablets containing 5, 10, 15, 20, 25, 30, and 50 mg
Tablets (slow-release) containing 15, 30, 60, 100, and 200 mg
Syrup containing 1, 5, and 10 mg/mL
Oral solution containing 2, 4, 20, and 50 mg/mL

OTHER USES
Dogs
POSTOPERATIVE ANALGESIC
0.25 to 1 mg/kg PRN; IM, IV

EPIDURAL ANALGESIA
0.1 mg/kg diluted in 0.2 mL/kg of sterile saline injected into the lumbosacral space

PREANESTHETIC
0.1 to 0.2 mg/kg; SC

SUPRAVENTRICULAR PREMATURE BEATS
0.2 mg/kg; IM, SC

NAFCILLIN

INDICATIONS: Nafcillin (Unipen ♣ ★) is a β-lactamase–resistant parenterally administered penicillin effective against gram-positive bacteria, especially staphylococcal bacteria. For information see **PENICILLIN ANTIBIOTICS.**

ADVERSE AND COMMON SIDE EFFECTS: Nausea, vomiting, and diarrhea are reported in humans. Rash, pruritus, urticaria, and thrombophlebitis with IV injection also are reported. Intraoperative use of the drug may be associated with the development of acute azotemia in dogs. Experience with the drug in small animals is limited. Also see **PENICILLIN ANTIBIOTICS.**

DRUG INTERACTIONS: Also see **PENICILLIN ANTIBIOTICS.**

SUPPLIED AS: HUMAN PRODUCT
For injection containing 0.5, 1, 2, and 10 g powder
Capsules containing 250 mg [Unipen ★]
Tablets containing 500 mg [Unipen ★]

NALOXONE

INDICATIONS: Naloxone (P/M Naloxone ♣ ★) is a narcotic antagonist. It is the preferred agent for reversal of narcotic-induced depression, including respiratory depression induced by morphine, oxymorphone, meperidine, or fentanyl. Survival times have been shown to increase and mortality rates decrease in animals in endotoxic shock given naloxone. Naloxone increases cardiac output and arterial blood pressure, decreases hemoconcentration and metabolic acidosis, and helps prevent hypoglycemia.

ADVERSE AND COMMON SIDE EFFECTS: At recommended doses, the drug is relatively free of adverse effects. At high doses, seizure activity has been reported. The duration of its action may be less than that of the opioid it is antagonizing; consequently, animals should be monitored for signs of returning narcosis. The safety of the drug in pregnant animals has not been established, although reproductive studies in rats did not reveal any adverse effects.

DRUG INTERACTIONS: Naloxone also reverses the effects of butorphanol and pentazocine. One milliliter (0.4 mg) of P/M Naloxone counteracts the following narcotic dosages: 1.5 mg oxymorphone, 15 mg morphine sulfate, 100 mg meperidine, and 0.4 mg fentanyl.

SUPPLIED AS: VETERINARY PRODUCT
For injection containing 0.4 mg/mL

NANDROLONE

INDICATIONS: Nandrolone decanoate (Deca-Durabolin ✤ ★) is an anabolic steroid that has been recommended for the treatment of nonresponsive anemia. The efficacy of anabolic steroids in promoting a positive nitrogen balance, in stimulating appetite, and in stimulating an increase in erythrocyte mass is questionable. The positive nitrogen balance that has been linked with their use is a reflection of an increase in appetite rather than an alteration in the patient's metabolism. Also see **ANABOLIC STEROIDS.**

ADVERSE AND COMMON SIDE EFFECTS: Prolonged use of anabolic steroids may result in hepatotoxicity. Also see **ANABOLIC STEROIDS.**

DRUG INTERACTIONS: None of clinical importance.

SUPPLIED AS: HUMAN PRODUCT
For injection containing 50, 100, and 200 mg/mL

OTHER USES
Dogs
APPETITE STIMULANT
5 mg/kg weekly; IM (maximum 200 mg/week)

NEOMYCIN

INDICATIONS: Neomycin (Biosol-M ✤, Mycifradin ✤ ★), an aminoglycoside antibiotic, generally is less effective against many bacteria than amikacin or gentamicin. It is used most often as a topical antibiotic and orally for its local antibiotic effects. Systemic use of the drug is very toxigenic.

ADVERSE AND COMMON SIDE EFFECTS: Neomycin is the most nephrotoxic aminoglycoside. The drug also is potentially toxic to the vestibular and auditory nerves. Ototoxicity is especially a concern if the drug is instilled into external ear canals with ruptured tympanic membranes. It also may cause a contact hypersensitivity and otitis externa. Neomycin may decrease cardiac output and produce hypotension.

DRUG INTERACTIONS: Orally administered, neomycin may decrease the absorption of digitalis, methotrexate, penicillin VK, and vitamin K.

SUPPLIED AS: VETERINARY PRODUCTS
Oral liquid containing 35 mg/mL [Biosol-M Aquadrops]
Tablets containing 70 mg [Biosol-M]

HUMAN PRODUCTS
Oral solution containing 25 mg/mL [Mycifradin]
Tablets containing 500 mg [Mycifradin]

OTHER USES
Dogs
HEPATIC ENCEPHALOPATHY
i)   22 mg/kg tid–qid; PO
ii) After evacuation enema, instill 10 to 20 mg/kg neomycin sulfate diluted in water as an enema for emergency treatment of hepatic encephalopathy.

Cats
HEPATIC ENCEPHALOPATHY
10 to 20 mg/kg bid; PO

NEOSTIGMINE

INDICATIONS: Neostigmine methylsulfate (Prostigmin ✦ ⋆) is a cholinesterase inhibitor used in the diagnosis and treatment of myasthenia gravis. There is marked clinical variability in response to dose.

ADVERSE AND COMMON SIDE EFFECTS: Salivation, urination, and diarrhea may occur if the drug dose is too high. With severe overdose, generalized weakness similar in appearance to that which occurs with myasthenia gravis occurs. A test dose of edrophonium will differentiate between the two. A cholinergic crisis should be treated with atropine.

DRUG INTERACTIONS: Corticosteroids and magnesium administration may decrease the anticholinesterase activity of neostigmine.

Aminoglycosides, which have some neuromuscular blocking activity, may decrease the efficacy of neostigmine in the diagnosis and treatment of myasthenia gravis. Neostigmine antagonizes the action of pancuronium and tubocurarine. Atropine antagonizes the muscarinic effects of neostigmine and often is used to treat adverse effects of the drug.

SUPPLIED AS: HUMAN PRODUCTS
Tablets containing 15 mg neostigmine bromide
For injection containing 0.25, 0.5, 1, and 2.5 mg/mL neostigmine methylsulfate

NITROFURANTOIN

INDICATIONS: Nitrofurantoin (Apo-Nitrofurantoin ✤, Equifur ✤, Furadantin ★, Macrodantin ✤ ★, Novofuran ✤) is bacteriostatic or bactericidal, depending on susceptibility of the organisms and the concentration of the drug at the site of infection. It is active against *E. coli, Klebsiella, Enterobacter,* Enterococci, *Staphylococcus aureus* and *epidermidis, Citrobacter, Salmonella, Shigella,* and *Corynebacterium.* The drug is used in the treatment of canine tracheobronchitis (kennel cough) and urinary tract infections. Treatment should continue for 4 to 7 days in cases of canine tracheobronchitis, 7 to 10 days for acute infections, and 10 to 14 days for chronic infections.

ADVERSE AND COMMON SIDE EFFECTS: The drug is contraindicated in patients with significant renal impairment, including anuria and oliguria. Cautious use is advised if the drug is to be given to patients with a history of asthma, anemia, diabetes, or electrolyte imbalance. Nausea, vomiting, hypersensitivity reactions, peripheral nervous system toxicity (weakness, numbness), polymyositis, and hepatopathy have been reported. The drug can cause yellow discoloration of permanent teeth if given before tooth eruption.

DRUG INTERACTIONS: Drugs that tend to alkalinize urine (acetazolamide, thiazides) may decrease the effect of nitrofurantoin. Antacids may delay absorption of nitrofurantoin. Magnesium-containing drugs may decrease the antimicrobial efficacy of the drug. Concomitant administration of probenecid or sulfinpyrazone may increase serum nitrofurantoin concentrations predisposing to toxicity. Nitrofurantoin may interfere with the action of fluoroquinolone antibiotics, and it may antagonize the effects of nalidixic acid. Food and anticholinergic drugs may increase bioavailability of the drug.

SUPPLIED AS: VETERINARY PRODUCT ✤
Oral suspension containing 15 mg/mL [Equifur]

HUMAN PRODUCTS
Tablets and capsules containing 50 and 100 mg [Furadantin, Novofuran]
Capsules (macrocrystals) containing 25, 50, and 100 mg [Macrodantin]
Oral suspension containing 5 mg/mL [Furadanin, Novofuran]

NITROGLYCERIN

INDICATIONS: Nitroglycerin (Nitro-Bid ✤ ★, Nitrol ✤ ★) is a venous vasodilator used to treat cases of congestive heart failure, especially those with pulmonary edema.

ADVERSE AND COMMON SIDE EFFECTS: Rash and hypotension are reported.

DRUG INTERACTIONS: Use of calcium channel-blocking agents, e.g., verapamil and diltiazem; β-blocking agents, e.g., propranolol, atenolol, or metoprolol; and phenothiazine drugs may potentiate hypotension.

SUPPLIED AS: HUMAN PRODUCT
Topical ointment containing 2% nitroglycerin

NITROPRUSSIDE

INDICATIONS: Nitroprusside sodium (Nitropress ★, Nipride ✤ ★) is a potent arterial and venous vasodilator used in refractory cases of heart failure and life-threatening mitral regurgitation caused by rupture of the chordae tendineae.

ADVERSE AND COMMON SIDE EFFECTS: The drug should be used with caution in patients with hepatic insufficiency, renal impairment, hypothyroid disease, and hyponatremia. Hypotension is the most serious side effect, but it is reversed readily within 10 minutes of discontinuation of the drug. The drug may be irritating if injected extravascularly.
   In humans, prolonged use may result in cyanide toxicity. Monitoring of serum thiocyanate levels is recommended. Levels greater than 100 μg/mL are considered toxic. The administration of hydroxocobalamin (vitamin B_{12}) prevents cyanide toxicity.

DRUG INTERACTIONS: Hypotensive effects are potentiated by the use of β-blockers, e.g., propranolol; ACE inhibitors, e.g., captopril and enalapril; and general anesthetics, e.g., halothane or enflurane.

SUPPLIED AS: HUMAN PRODUCT
For injection containing 50 mg/vial

NITROSCANATE

INDICATIONS: Nitroscanate (Lopatol ♣) is an anthelmintic agent used for the eradication of *Toxocara canis, Toxascaris leonina, Ancylostoma caninum, Uncinaria stenocephala, Taenia* spp., and *Dipylidium caninum* in dogs. It also has been used to eliminate *Echinococcus* and *Trichuris* in dogs and *Ancylostoma* and *T. cati* in cats.

ADVERSE AND COMMON SIDE EFFECTS: The drug is considered to be safe. Vomiting may occur. To help limit the occurrence of vomiting, food should be given 15 minutes before administration of the drug. With drug overdose, depression and anorexia may occur. The drug should not be given to severely debilitated animals. The drug is safe in breeding and pregnant dogs. Some cats given in excess of 400 mg/kg developed a reversible hind-limb paralysis.

DRUG INTERACTIONS: Nitroscanate should not be administered concurrently with other anthelmintics.

SUPPLIED AS: VETERINARY PRODUCT
Tablets containing 100 and 500 mg

NORFLOXACIN

INDICATIONS: Norfloxacin (Noroxin ♣ ★) is a fluoroquinolone antibiotic. It has been recommended for the treatment of urinary tract infections and bacteremia. Also see **FLUOROQUINOLONE ANTIBIOTICS.**

ADVERSE AND COMMON SIDE EFFECTS: See **FLUOROQUINOLONE ANTIBIOTICS.**

DRUG INTERACTIONS: Absorption is impaired by magnesium- and aluminum-containing antacids and sucralfate. Nitrofurantoin may decrease the antibacterial effects of norfloxacin in the urinary tract. Also see **FLUOROQUINOLONE ANTIBIOTICS.**

SUPPLIED AS: HUMAN PRODUCT
Tablet containing 400 mg

NOVOBIOCIN

INDICATIONS: Novobiocin is active against gram-positive cocci, including staphylococci and some streptococci. Variable effectiveness has been found against *Proteus, Pseudomonas,* and *Pasteurella multocida.* It is marketed for small animals in combination with tetracycline (Albaplex ★) and with tetracycline and prednisolone (Delta-Albaplex ♣ ★).

ADVERSE AND COMMON SIDE EFFECTS: Nausea, vomiting, diarrhea, rashes, and blood dyscrasias are reported.

DRUG INTERACTIONS: Novobiocin may decrease the elimination of penicillin drugs and the cephalosporins.

SUPPLIED AS: VETERINARY PRODUCTS
Tablets containing 60 mg novobiocin with 60 mg tetracycline [Albaplex]
Tablets containing 180 mg novobiocin with 180 mg tetracycline [Albaplex 3X]
Tablets containing 60 mg novobiocin, 60 mg tetracycline, and 1.5 mg prednisolone [Delta-Albaplex]
Tablets containing 180 novobiocin, 180 mg tetracycline, and 4.5 mg prednisolone [Delta-Albaplex 3X ★]

NUTRI-SOL EFA

INDICATIONS: Nutri-Sol EFA ♣ is a dietary supplement containing omega-3 and omega-6 essential fatty acids, vitamin A, vitamin E, and zinc. A lack of these nutrients may result in excessive shedding, pruritus, flaky skin, and a dull hair coat. The product is recommended for the maintenance of healthy skin and hair coat.

ADVERSE AND COMMON SIDE EFFECTS and **DRUG INTERACTIONS:** None reported.

SUPPLIED AS: VETERINARY PRODUCT
Liquid containing the aforementioned nutrients in 112-mL bottles

NYSTATIN

INDICATIONS: Nystatin (Mycostatin ♣ ★, Nilstat ♣ ★) is used for the treatment of candidal infections of the skin, mucous membranes, and intestinal tract. The drug also has been recommended for the treatment of otitis externa caused by *Microsporum canis*. It is only partially effective against *Aspergillus* infections.

ADVERSE AND COMMON SIDE EFFECTS: Rarely, topical application causes contact dermatitis. In humans, large oral doses have been associated with diarrhea, nausea, and vomiting. The drug is too toxic for parenteral use in small animals.

DRUG INTERACTIONS: None of clinical significance in small animals.

SUPPLIED AS: HUMAN PRODUCTS
Oral suspension containing 100,000 U/mL
Tablets containing 500,000 U
Cream containing 100,000 U/g
Ointment containing 100,000 U/g

OMEPRAZOLE

INDICATIONS: Omeprazole (Prilosec ★, Losec ✦) is a proton pump-inhibitor used for the treatment of esophagitis, erosive gastritis, and gastric ulcers. The drug is 5 to 10 times more potent than cimetidine in inhibiting gastric acid secretion and has a long duration of action (24 hours or more). The drug is more effective than cimetidine in controlling aspirin-induced gastric erosions in dogs. It has cytoprotective (by enhancing mucosal cell prostaglandin production) and acid-reducing properties and may be useful in decreasing gastric hyperacidity.

ADVERSE AND COMMON SIDE EFFECTS: In humans, nausea, vomiting, flatulence, and diarrhea are reported. Long-term, high-dose administration does not cause clinical, hematologic, or biochemical abnormalities in dogs. However, it can result in reversible gastric mucosal hypertrophy as a result of sustained hypergastrinemia, which occurs with prolonged gastric acid suppression. No adverse reactions were noted in cats at doses of 0.7 mg/kg/day.

DRUG INTERACTIONS: The elimination time of diazepam, phenytoin, and warfarin is increased with chronic administration of omeprazole.

SUPPLIED AS: HUMAN PRODUCT
Capsules containing 20 mg

ONDANSETRON

INDICATIONS: Ondansetron (Zofran ✦ ★) is a potent antiemetic agent. It has been used in human medicine for the control of vomiting in patients undergoing chemotherapy with cisplatin, a drug that frequently causes nausea and vomiting. Ondansetron blocks selective serotonin S_3 receptors (mediators of the vomiting reflex) on neurons located in either the peripheral or central nervous systems. This drug is not effective in preventing motion-induced nausea and vomiting in people.

ADVERSE AND COMMON SIDE EFFECTS: Adverse effects in dogs are uncommon but may include sedation, lip licking, and head shaking. The drug dose should be reduced in patients with reduced liver function.

DRUG INTERACTIONS: Unknown.

SUPPLIED AS: HUMAN PRODUCTS
For injection containing 2 mg/mL
Tablets containing 4 and 8 mg

OTHER USES
Dogs

CISPLATIN CHEMOTHERAPY
0.5 to 1 mg/kg; PO 30 minutes before and 90 minutes after commencing cisplatin

ORBIFLOXACIN

INDICATIONS: Orbifloxacin (Orbax ♣ ★) is a synthetic broad-spectrum bactericidal antibiotic with activity against many gram-positive and gram-negative organisms, including *Staphylococcus intermedius*, coagulase-positive staphylococci, *Pasteurella multocida*, *E. coli*, *Pseudomonas aeruginosa*, *Proteus mirabilis*, and *Streptococcus-hemolytic* (grp G).

ADVERSE AND COMMON SIDE EFFECTS: Adverse effects in dogs at standard recommended dosages are not seen. Dosages greater than five times the recommended maximum daily dose did not produce any treatment-related adverse effects. As with other fluoroquinolone antibiotics, orbifloxacin should be given to young growing dogs, i.e., between 2 and 8 months of age in small and medium-sized breeds and up to 18 months of age in large and giant breed dogs. These drugs are known to cause arthropathy in immature dogs. Fluoroquinolone antibiotics may predispose to seizure activity and should be used with caution in dogs with CNS pathology. Safe use of the drug in pregnant or breeding animals has not been established.

DRUG INTERACTIONS: Absorption of the drug is hindered by sucralfate, antacids, multivitamin compounds, and agents containing divalent and trivalent cations, e.g., calcium, iron, aluminum, magnesium, and zinc.

SUPPLIED AS: VETERINARY PRODUCT
Tablets containing 5.7, 22.7, and 68 mg

ORGANOPHOSPHATES

INDICATIONS: Organophosphate agents include chlorpyrifos, cythioate, diazinon, dichlorvos, fenthion, malathion, parathion, phosmet, ronnel, safrotin, and tetrachlorvinphos. Some have been used in the treatment of Cheyletiella and sarcoptic mange, fleas, ticks, and lice. Not all drugs listed are recommended for use in small animals. All, however, have been associated with toxicity in dogs and cats.

ADVERSE AND COMMON SIDE EFFECTS: These agents, other than malathion, are not approved for use in cats. Cats are especially sensitive to toxicity from organophosphate compounds. In dogs, the greyhound appears more sensitive to the adverse effects of these drugs. Signs of intoxication are due to cholinesterase inhibition resulting in overstimulation of the parasympathetic nervous system and include bradycardia, salivation, vomiting, diarrhea, muscle tremors, convulsions, pupillary constriction, bronchoconstriction, respiratory depression, and paralysis. Death may occur. Some organophosphates are associated with a delayed neurotoxicity characterized by muscular weakness and ataxia that progresses to flaccid paralysis of the hind limbs and occasionally all four limbs 8 to 21 days after administration.

If topical application has resulted in toxicity, the skin should be cleansed. If the drug was ingested within the last 2 hours and the patient is not exhibiting clinical signs of toxicosis, vomiting should be induced as with 3% hydrogen peroxide (2 mL/kg; maximum 45 mL). Otherwise, gastric lavage followed by the oral administration of activated charcoal (2 g/kg) is indicated. In all cases, atropine should be given (0.2 mg/kg). One fourth of the total dose is given intravenously, and the balance is given intramuscularly or subcutaneously. In addition, pralidoxime chloride may be useful (20 mg/kg; IM or IV, repeat every 12 hours as indicated). In addition, the antihistamine diphenhydramine (Benadryl) (4 mg/kg tid; PO) may effectively block the effects of nicotine-receptor stimulation. Although diazepam has been used to augment the effects of atropine and reportedly has aided recovery, some authors suggest that diazepam actually may potentiate toxic signs and should *not* be used.

DRUG INTERACTIONS: Drugs that inhibit cholinesterase, including morphine, neostigmine, physostigmine, pyridostigmine, phenothiazines, and succinylcholine, should be avoided.

SUPPLIED AS: See specific product.

OXACILLIN

INDICATIONS: Oxacillin (Bactocill ★, Prostaphlin ★) is a penicillin antibiotic used in the treatment of gram-positive infections, including staphylococcal infections and infections caused by β-lactamase–producing bacteria. The drug has been used in the treatment of pyoderma, bacterial endocarditis, and blepharitis. Also see **PENICILLIN ANTIBIOTICS.**

For information concerning ADVERSE AND COMMON SIDE EFFECTS and DRUG INTERACTIONS, see **PENICILLIN ANTIBIOTICS.**

SUPPLIED AS: HUMAN PRODUCTS
Capsules containing 250 and 500 mg
Oral solution containing 250 mg/5 mL
For injection in 250- and 500-mg and 1-, 2-, 4-, and 10-g vials

OXAZEPAM

INDICATIONS: Oxazepam (Serax ♣ ★) is an anxiolytic-sedative benzodiazepine drug that is used to stimulate appetite. Feeding usually commences within 20 minutes. Also see **DIAZEPAM.**

ADVERSE AND COMMON SIDE EFFECTS: Mild sedation and ataxia may be seen. These drugs are metabolized in the liver and should be used cautiously in animals with liver or renal dysfunction. Oxazepam occasionally may exacerbate grand mal seizures. Abrupt withdrawal in these patients should be avoided. Also see **DIAZEPAM.**

DRUG INTERACTIONS: Phenothiazines and barbiturates may potentiate the action of oxazepam. Also see **DIAZEPAM.**

SUPPLIED AS: HUMAN PRODUCT
Tablets containing 10, 15, and 30 mg

OXTRIPHYLLINE

INDICATIONS: Oxtriphylline (Choledyl ♣ ★) contains 64% theophylline, which accounts for its pharmacologic effects. The drug is a bronchodilator used in the management of chronic cough.

ADVERSE AND COMMON SIDE EFFECTS: Anorexia, vomiting, restlessness, tachypnea, arrhythmias, and, rarely, seizures are reported.

DRUG INTERACTIONS: Serum levels are increased by cimetidine and erythromycin. Oxtriphylline potentiates the action of thiazide diuretics and the cardiac effects of digitalis. Synergism with ephedrine has been documented. Theophylline antagonizes the effect of propranolol. The concomitant use of morphine or curare may antagonize the effect of theophylline, and because this drug stimulates the release of histamine, bronchoconstriction may result. Acidifying agents increase the urinary excretion and inhibit the action of theophylline. Alkalinizing agents potentiate its effects.

SUPPLIED AS: HUMAN PRODUCTS
Tablets containing 100, 200, and 300 mg [Choledyl]
Tablets containing 400 and 600 mg [Choledyl SA]
Elixir containing 100 mg/5 mL [Choledyl]
Syrup containing 50 mg/5 mL

OXYBUTININ

INDICATIONS: Oxybutinin (Ditropan ♣ ★) is an anticholinergic agent with direct antispasmodic activity and antimuscarinic activity on smooth muscle. In addition, the drug exerts an analgesic and local anesthetic effect. It is useful in the management of detrusor hyperreflexia.

ADVERSE AND COMMON SIDE EFFECTS: Dry mouth, urinary hesitancy, retention of urine, pupillary dilation, tachycardia, syncope, weakness, nausea, vomiting, anorexia, and constipation may occur. In small animals, diarrhea and sedation are the most common side effects reported. In the case of drug overdose, the stomach should be emptied of any remaining drug, and physostigmine should be given.

Oxybutinin is contraindicated in patients with hyperthyroidism, prostatic disease, glaucoma, myasthenia gravis, partial or complete GIT obstruction, ileus, megacolon, severe colitis, or unstable cardiovascular status.

DRUG INTERACTIONS: None of clinical significance to small animals.

SUPPLIED AS: HUMAN PRODUCTS
Tablets containing 5 mg
Syrup containing 5 mg/5 mL

OXYMETHOLONE

INDICATIONS: Oxymetholone (Anadrol 50 ★, Anapolon 50 ♣) is an anabolic steroid used to stimulate erythrocyte production in cases of nonresponsive anemia. For more discussion on the use of these agents, including ADVERSE AND COMMON SIDE EFFECTS and DRUG INTERACTIONS, see **ANABOLIC STEROIDS.**

SUPPLIED AS: HUMAN PRODUCT
Tablets containing 50 mg

OXYMORPHONE

INDICATIONS: Oxymorphone (Numorphan ♣ ★, P/M Oxymorphone ★) is a narcotic agent used for sedation, preanesthesia, and the management of pain in the dog. Pain relief lasts 2 to 4 hours after IM or IV injection. It is approximately 10 times more potent an analgesic than morphine, causes less sedation, and does not suppress the cough reflex.

ADVERSE AND COMMON SIDE EFFECTS: Respiratory depression and bradycardia are reported. Cats are more sensitive to the drug and may exhibit dose-dependent excitement. The drug should not be used in animals with head trauma because it may increase CSF pressure; it should be used with caution in patients with hypothyroid disease, hepatic impairment, significant respiratory disease, adrenocortical insufficiency, and renal disease, and in the severely debilitated or geriatric animal. Oxymorphone should not be given to animals with diarrhea caused by a toxic agent.

With overdose, profound respiratory and/or CNS depression may occur, as may cardiovascular collapse, hypothermia, and skeletal muscle hypotonia. Adverse effects of the drug can be reversed with naloxone. In cats, use of the drug may be associated with ataxia, hyperesthesia, and behavioral changes. If used at higher doses in this species, it is recommended that it be given with a tranquilizing agent.

DRUG INTERACTIONS: Antihistamines, phenothiazines, barbiturates, and anesthetic agents may potentiate CNS or respiratory depression of the drug. In cats, the drug may be used concurrently with diazepam (0.1–0.2 mg/kg; IV, IM) to offset adverse effects of excitement and hyperalgesia.

SUPPLIED AS: VETERINARY PRODUCT
For injection containing 1.5 mg/mL (P/M Oxymorphone)
HUMAN PRODUCT
For injection containing 1.0 and 1.5 mg/mL (Numorphan)

OTHER USES
Dogs
ANALGESIA
Postoperative dose: 0.05 to 0.1 mg/kg; IM, IV

PREANESTHESIA
0.1 to 0.2 mg/kg; IM, IV (with acepromazine and atropine or glycopyrrolate)

Cats
RESTRAINT/SEDATION
0.02 to 0.03 mg/kg; IM, IV

ANALGESIA/PREANESTHESIA
0.1 to 0.4 mg/kg; IV

POSTOPERATIVE ANALGESIA
0.05 to 0.15 mg/kg; IM, IV (with acepromazine)

OXYTETRACYCLINE

INDICATIONS: Oxytetracycline (Liquamycin ✚ ★, Terramycin ✚ ★) is a short-acting, water-soluble tetracycline. The drug reaches high concentrations in the lung, liver, kidney, and mononuclear phago-cyte system and is better tolerated orally by cats. For more information, see **TETRACYCLINE ANTIBIOTICS.**

ADVERSE AND COMMON SIDE EFFECTS: Oxytetracycline may cause discoloration of the teeth in young animals. High doses or prolonged use may cause delayed bone growth and healing. Tetracyclines cause nausea, anorexia, vomiting, and diarrhea in small animals. In addition, in cats, toxicity may present as fever, colic, hair loss, and depression.

DRUG INTERACTIONS: Antidiarrheal preparations, including kaolin and pectin or bismuth, reduce absorption of tetracyclines. Medications containing aluminum, calcium, iron, magnesium, or zinc, such as antacids, laxatives, mineral supplements, and iron preparations, reduce absorption of oral tetracycline drugs. Methoxyflurane may potentiate the nephrotoxicity of tetracyclines. Sodium bicarbonate may interfere with gastric absorption by increasing gastric pH. Tetracyclines may interfere with the bactericidal activity of the penicillins, cephalosporins, and aminoglycosides. Tetracyclines may increase the bioavailability of digoxin and predispose to digitalis toxicity. Gastrointestinal tract side effects may be increased if the drug is administered concurrently with theophylline. Tetracyclines reportedly have reduced insulin requirements in diabetic patients.

SUPPLIED AS: VETERINARY PRODUCTS (large animal products)
For injection containing 50 and 100 mg/mL
[generic products ♣ ★]
Tablets containing 250 mg ★
For injection containing long-acting formula 200 mg/mL
[Liquamycin-LA]

HUMAN PRODUCTS [Terramycin ★]
Capsules containing 250 mg
For injection containing 500 mg (IV only)
For injection containing 50 and 125 mg/mL (IM only)

OXYTOCIN

INDICATIONS: Oxytocin (Pitocin ★, Syntocinon ♣ ★) is a hormone of the posterior pituitary gland and is used for the induction of parturition, for uterine prolapse in dogs and cats, and to stimulate milk letdown in bitches.

ADVERSE AND COMMON SIDE EFFECTS: The drug is contraindicated in animals with dystocia due to abnormal presentation of the fetus or in those with a closed cervix. Full relaxation of the cervix should be accomplished naturally or with the use of estrogen before oxytocin use. Overdose may precipitate intense labor, uterine rupture, fetal injury, or death. Water intoxication may occur if large doses are infused, especially in the presence of electrolyte-free fluid therapy. Intoxication may be manifested by listlessness, depression, seizures, coma, and death. Severe intoxication may be treated with mannitol or dextrose, with or without furosemide.

DRUG INTERACTIONS: Concurrent use of ephedrine or other vasopressors may result in postpartum hypertension.

SUPPLIED AS: VETERINARY PRODUCT
For injection containing 20 IU/mL (products are listed generically)
HUMAN PRODUCTS
For injection containing 5 and 10 IU/mL [Pitocin, Syntocin]
Nasal spray containing 40 IU/mL [Syntocin]

PANCREATIC ENZYME REPLACEMENT

INDICATIONS: Pancreatic enzyme replacement therapies (Pancrease-V ♣, Pancrezyme ★) are mixtures containing porcine pancreatic enzymes, especially lipase and amylase. Other products also may include protease, esterase, peptidase, nuclease, and elastase enzyme supplements. These products are used for the management of pancreatic exocrine insufficiency.

ADVERSE AND COMMON SIDE EFFECTS: Overdose can cause nausea, cramping, and diarrhea.

DRUG INTERACTIONS: Antacids (magnesium hydroxide, calcium carbonate) may diminish efficacy. Concurrent use of cimetidine may improve efficacy.

SUPPLIED AS: VETERINARY PRODUCTS
Available in tablets and as a powder

PANCURONIUM BROMIDE

INDICATIONS: Pancuronium (Pavulon ♣ ★) is a synthetic nondepolarizing neuromuscular blocking agent. It is used as an adjunct to general anesthesia to promote muscle relaxation during surgery and to facilitate mechanical ventilation and endotracheal intubation.

ADVERSE AND COMMON SIDE EFFECTS: The drug should be used with caution in patients with compromised renal function and in those in whom tachycardia may be hazardous. Lower doses are recommended in patients with hepatobiliary disease. It should be used with caution in those with myasthenia gravis. Adverse effects may include tachycardia, increases in blood pressure, hypersalivation in those not pretreated with an anticholinergic, and profound muscle weakness and respiratory depression. Drug toxicity may be treated with mechanical support of ventilation and the use of atropine (0.02 mg/kg; IV) followed by neostigmine (0.06 mg/kg; IV).

DRUG INTERACTIONS: Neuromuscular blockade may be potentiated by aminoglycoside antibiotics (amikacin, gentamicin, kanamycin, neomycin, streptomycin, tobramycin), bacitracin, clindamycin, enflurane, halothane, isoflurane, lincomycin, magnesium sulfate, polymyxin B, and quinidine. Succinylcholine may hasten the onset of action of pancuronium and potentiate neuromuscular blockade. The action of pancuronium is antagonized by acetylcholine, anticholinesterases, and potassium ions. Theophylline may inhibit or reverse the neuromuscular blocking effect of pancuronium and precipitate arrhythmias. Azathioprine may reverse the neuromuscular blocking effect of the drug.

SUPPLIED AS: HUMAN PRODUCT
For injection containing 1 and 2 mg/mL

PENICILLAMINE

INDICATIONS: Penicillamine (Cuprimine ♣ ★, Depen ♣ ★) is a thiol compound that chelates cystine, lead, and copper and promotes their excretion in the urine. It is used in the management of cystine urolithiasis, lead poisoning, and hepatitis associated with progressive copper accumulation. The very slow rate of copper dispersion makes use of this drug ineffective in advanced cases of hepatic copper storage disease and in cirrhosis. Trientine is recommended if vomiting remains a problem for animals given penicillamine. Although no more effective than penicillamine, it does have fewer side effects. A dose of 15 to 30 mg/kg bid, PO, given 1 hour before meals has been recommended in dogs. Penicillamine also has been recommended for the treatment of hepatic cirrhosis, where it may work by lessening the formation of collagen and promoting its breakdown.

ADVERSE AND COMMON SIDE EFFECTS: Lethargy, vomiting, oral lesions, anorexia, proteinuria, and thrombocytopenia have been reported. The drug decreases the strength of skin wound closure by its effect on collagen and should only be used after wound healing is complete. Finally, the drug has been used experimentally in the treatment of renal amyloidosis.

DRUG INTERACTIONS: Gold therapy and phenylbutazone may potentiate hematologic and renal toxicity of the drug. Oral iron may inhibit absorption of the drug.

SUPPLIED AS: HUMAN PRODUCTS
Tablets containing 250 mg [Depen]
Capsules containing 125 and 250 mg [Cuprimine]

OTHER USES
Dogs

BEDLINGTON COPPER STORAGE DISEASE
125 mg bid; PO given 30 minutes before eating

PENICILLIN ANTIBIOTICS

INDICATIONS: Penicillin antibiotics, including penicillin G and V, ampicillin, amoxicillin, cloxacillin, carbenicillin, ticarcillin, hetacillin, and nafcillin, are effective bactericidal antibiotics used for the treatment of gram-positive and gram-negative infections. Penicillin drugs are distributed extensively throughout the body to most body fluids and bone except the brain and CSF unless inflamed. Penicillin G is effective against most gram-positive organisms. Penicillin V has the same spectrum but is more reliably absorbed from the GIT. Ampicillin has an extended activity against *E. coli, Shigella,* and *Proteus.* Hetacillin is hydrolyzed to ampicillin in most body fluids. Amoxicillin is similar to ampicillin but is absorbed more readily and persists for a longer period of time within the body. It also is available in combination with clavulanate potassium (Clavamox), which effectively protects the drug from β-lactamase–producing staphylococci. Cloxacillin is penicillinase-resistant and is useful in the treatment of staphylococcal infections. Carbenicillin also is active against *Pseudomonas* and *Proteus.* Ticarcillin is more effective than carbenicillin against *Pseudomonas* and can be given at a lower dose.

ADVERSE AND COMMON SIDE EFFECTS: Toxicity is rare in dogs and cats. Rapid IV injection may cause neurologic signs and seizures. Hypersensitivity reactions, including hives, fever, joint pain, and anaphylaxis, have been reported in dogs and cats. Sensitivity to one penicillin confers sensitivity to all penicillins. Penicillin and its derivatives may exacerbate clinical signs associated with Scotty cramp.

DRUG INTERACTIONS: Food and antacids decrease the absorption of orally administered penicillins. The drug should be given 1 hour before or 2 hours after feeding. Neomycin blocks the absorption of oral penicillins. The bacteriostatic action of chloramphenicol, erythromycin, and the tetracyclines may antagonize the bactericidal activity of the penicillins. Aspirin, indomethacin, and phenylbutazone may increase serum levels of the penicillins by displacing them from plasma protein-binding sites. Penicillins should not be mixed with aminoglycosides because both will become inactivated.

PENTASTARCH

INDICATIONS: Pentastarch (Pentaspan ✦ ★) is a colloid used for plasma volume expansion. It has an average molecular weight of 200,000 to 300,000. Volume expansion persists for approximately 18 to 24 hours in people and is expected to improve hemodynamic status for 12 to 18 hours. Infusion of 500 mL results in a 700-mL (140%) increase in plasma volume within 30 minutes. Comparatively, the amount of volume expansion appears greatest with 10% pentastarch followed by 6% dextran 70, 6% hetastarch, and 5% albumin. Pentastarch is especially useful in the management of shock. It was developed to provide a colloidal solution with fewer adverse effects and greater osmotic properties.

ADVERSE AND COMMON SIDE EFFECTS: This agent is contraindicated in patients with bleeding disorders or with congestive heart failure in which volume overload is a potential problem. Large volumes of the drug also may predispose to coagulopathy, although this should not be expected at recommended dosages. The drug should not be used in oliguric or anuric renal failure not related to hypovolemia. Administration of large volumes of pentastarch will decrease hemoglobin concentrations and dilute plasma proteins. Hypersensitivity (wheezing and urticaria) also has been reported in humans. This agent should not be used in pregnant small animals unless the benefit outweighs the risk because it has been demonstrated to be embryocidal at large doses in experimental studies using rabbits and mice. Elevation in serum amylase levels in humans has been noted, but it has not been associated with pancreatitis.

DRUG INTERACTIONS: None established.

SUPPLIED AS: HUMAN PRODUCT
For injection containing 10 g pentastarch in 0.9 g saline

PENTAZOCINE

INDICATIONS: Pentazocine (Talwin-V ★, Talwin ✦ ★) is a narcotic agonist used in the management of moderate to severe pain in dogs. Its analgesic properties are approximately one fourth as potent as those of morphine and are equivalent to those of meperidine. Onset of action is rapid, and duration of analgesia is at least 3 hours in most patients. In cats, an IV dose of 0.75 mg/kg provides visceral analgesia of approximately 22 minutes. The duration of analgesia is increased at doses of 1.5 mg/kg, but mydriasis and apprehension are noted. The drug does not depress respiration and produces little or no sedation at therapeutic doses.

ADVERSE AND COMMON SIDE EFFECTS: In dogs, the most common side effect is profuse salivation. Other side effects may include tremors, vomiting, and swelling at the injection site. At high doses (6 mg/kg), ataxia, tremors, and seizures have been reported in dogs. In cats, the drug appears to cause dysphoria and is not recommended by some clinicians for use in this species. Others believe that the drug can be used safely in cats. Side effects can be reversed with naloxone. Use of the drug is contraindicated in patients with head injury or increased intracranial pressure. Cautious use is recommended in animals with impaired renal or hepatic function, adrenocortical insufficiency, hypothyroid disease, and respiratory depression, and in severely debilitated animals, geriatrics, and those with nausea or vomiting.

DRUG INTERACTIONS: Do not mix pentazocine with soluble barbiturates because precipitation will occur.

SUPPLIED AS: VETERINARY PRODUCT
For injection containing 30 mg/mL

HUMAN PRODUCTS
Tablets containing 50 mg [Talwin ✤]
For injection containing 30 mg/mL [Talwin ✤]

PENTOBARBITAL

INDICATIONS: Pentobarbital (Somnotol ✤, generic products ★) is a short-acting barbiturate used for promoting sedation and general anesthesia. Anesthesia is induced in 3 to 5 minutes and lasts 45 to 90 minutes, with the animal remaining quiet for several hours afterward. It is used to control intractable seizures in dogs and cats, other than those seizures induced by lidocaine intoxication. For more information on this class of drug, see **BARBITURATES.**

ADVERSE AND COMMON SIDE EFFECTS: Respiratory depression is the most common concern with the use of the drug. It also may cause excitement in the dog during recovery from anesthetic doses. The use of sodium bicarbonate to increase renal excretion of the drug is not effective with pentobarbital.

DRUG INTERACTIONS: Antihistamines, phenothiazines, narcotic agents, and chloramphenicol may potentiate the effects of the drug. Pentobarbital may decrease the effects of corticosteroids, β-blockers (e.g., propranolol, metoprolol), quinidine, metronidazole, and theophylline. Barbiturates may interfere with the metabolism of phenytoin, thus altering its serum levels. Unexplained death has occurred when dogs intoxicated with lidocaine were treated with pentobarbital.

SUPPLIED AS: VETERINARY PRODUCT
For injection containing 65 mg/mL

OTHER USES
Dogs
STATUS EPILEPTICUS
5 to 15 mg/kg to effect; IV

Cats
ANESTHETIC
25 mg/kg; IV; an additional 10 mg/kg may be given if initial dose is inadequate
STATUS EPILEPTICUS
5 to 15 mg/kg to effect; IV

PENTOSAN POLYSULFATE SODIUM

INDICATIONS: Pentosan polysulfate sodium (Cartrophen Vet ✤) possesses anti-inflammatory and antiarthritic chondroprotective properties. It is recommended in the treatment of osteoarthritis. The drug stimulates chondrocytes to synthesize cartilage matrix and synoviocytes to synthesize hyaluronic acid. It inhibits cartilage-damaging enzymes, mobilizes thrombi and fibrin deposits in synovial tissues and subchondral blood vessels to facilitate perfusion of the joint, and mobilizes lipids and cholesterol in synovial and subchondral blood vessels.

ADVERSE AND COMMON SIDE EFFECTS: Side effects are rare but may include abdominal bleeding (1 animal had splenic hemangiosarcoma, and another had liver disease), vomiting, and diarrhea. It should not be used in animals with coagulation defects, abdominal cancer, or infection. Drug overdose may exacerbate stiffness and discomfort.

DRUG INTERACTIONS: None reported.

SUPPLIED AS: VETERINARY PRODUCT
For injection containing 100 mg/mL in 10-mL vials

PHENOBARBITAL

INDICATIONS: Phenobarbital is the drug of choice for the control of seizure activity in small animals. It is effective in controlling seizures in most dogs when adequate serum concentrations are maintained. Serum levels should be monitored after steady-state levels have been reached (14 days in the dog, 9 days in the cat). Serum samples are collected just before the next dose. Effective serum levels are in the range of 65 to 170 µmol/L (15–40 µg/mL or, according to another source, 14 to 45 µg/mL). The drug also is used for its sedative properties. Also see **BARBITURATES.**

ADVERSE AND COMMON SIDE EFFECTS: Initially, sedation and ataxia may be noted, especially at higher doses. These effects tend to resolve with continued treatment. Polyuria, polydipsia, and polyphagia are reported. Phenobarbital is a hepatic enzyme inducer. It may increase the biotransformation of drugs metabolized by the liver. Phenobarbital has been implicated as causing hepatotoxicity, especially with chronic use. Anemia is a rare adverse effect documented in dogs. Activated charcoal is given in cases of drug overdose, even when it has been administered parenterally. In addition, sodium bicarbonate increases the renal excretion of the drug and is potentially useful in cases of drug overdose.

DRUG INTERACTIONS: Antihistamines, phenothiazines, narcotic agents, and chloramphenicol may potentiate the effects of the drug. Phenobarbital may decrease the effects of doxycycline, chloramphenicol, corticosteroids, β-blockers (e.g., propranolol, metoprolol), quinidine, metronidazole, and theophylline. Phenobarbital may decrease the absorption of griseofulvin. Barbiturates may interfere with the metabolism of phenytoin, thus altering its serum levels.

SUPPLIED AS: HUMAN PRODUCTS

In the United States
Tablets containing 8, 15, 16, 30, 32, 60, 65, and 100 mg
Capsules containing 16 mg
Elixir containing 15 and 20 mg/5 mL
For injection containing 30, 60, 65, and 130 mg/mL
Powder for injection containing 120 mg/amp

In Canada
Tablets containing 15, 30, 60, and 100 mg
For injection containing 30 and 120 mg/mL

OTHER USES
Dogs
SEDATION
2.2 to 6.6 mg/kg bid; PO

Cats
IDIOPATHIC EPILEPSY
i)   8 to 15 mg once to twice daily; PO
ii) 2.2 to 4.4 mg/kg/day div. bid or tid; PO

PHENOXYBENZAMINE

INDICATIONS: Phenoxybenzamine (Dibenzyline ★) is a long-acting α-adrenergic blocking agent. The drug may be of use in reducing urethral sphincter tone, thus facilitating urine flow. Several days of treatment may be required for a desirable effect.

ADVERSE AND COMMON SIDE EFFECTS: Hypotension, reflex tachycardia, weakness, miosis, increased intraocular pressure, nausea, and vomiting are reported.

DRUG INTERACTIONS: Phenoxybenzamine will antagonize the effects of α-adrenergic agonists, e.g., phenylephrine.

SUPPLIED AS: HUMAN PRODUCT
Capsules containing 10 mg

OTHER USES
Dogs
PHEOCHROMOCYTOMA
Presurgical stabilization of blood pressure
0.2 to 1.5 mg/kg bid; PO for 10 to 14 days before surgery

PHENYLBUTAZONE

INDICATIONS: Phenylbutazone (Butazone ❧, Butazolidin ❧, Bute ❧, Phenylbutazone ❧ ★) has analgesic, antipyretic, and anti-inflammatory properties that make it useful in the treatment of osteoarthritis, rheumatism, and inflammation of the skin and soft tissue. The drug also has been used for the short-term management of corneal injury, acute uveitis, chorioretinitis, endophthalmitis, and trauma to the globe.

ADVERSE AND COMMON SIDE EFFECTS: Gastric irritation with vomiting and GI ulceration may occur. Misoprostol may be effective in the prevention and treatment of the adverse GI side effects of the drug. Thrombocytopenia, leukopenia, and nonregenerative anemia also are reported. Adverse effects are unpredictable and unrelated to dose. Intramuscular or SC injection is irritating and should be avoided. Use of phenylbutazone may exacerbate clinical signs of Scotty cramp. The drug is toxic to cats and is not recommended in this species.

DRUG INTERACTIONS: Phenylbutazone is a hepatic enzyme inducer and may increase the metabolism of digitoxin and phenytoin. Conversely, barbiturates, corticosteroids, chlorpheniramine, and diphenhydramine may decrease the plasma half-life of phenylbutazone. Metabolism of phenylbutazone may be accelerated by hepatic enzyme inducers such as phenobarbital, griseofulvin, and phenytoin. Phenylbutazone may increase the plasma half-life of penicillin G and lithium. The drug also may antagonize the effects of furosemide. Concurrent use with other NSAIDs increases the potential for drug toxicity.

SUPPLIED AS: VETERINARY PRODUCTS
For injection containing 200 mg/mL ♣ ★
Tablets containing 100 mg ★
Tablets containing 1 g (horses only) ♣ ★
HUMAN PRODUCT
Tablets containing 100 mg [Butazolidin ♣]

OTHER USES
Dogs
OPHTHALMIC DISEASE
40 mg/kg tid; PO

Cats
OPHTHALMIC DISEASE
10 to 14 mg/kg bid; PO

PHENYLPROPANOLAMINE

INDICATIONS: Phenylpropanolamine (Ornade ♣ ★, Contac.C ♣ ★, Dexatrim ★, Diadax ★, Entex ♣ ★, Westrim ★) is an α-adrenergic stimulant. The drug is useful in the treatment of urinary incontinence in the dog. Excellent results are reported in 73% to 90% of dogs. Dogs older at the onset of clinical signs (median 5 years) and those with a longer period from the time of ovariohysterectomy to the onset of urinary incontinence (median 2.5 years) respond best. It is preferred to ephedrine because side effects are less severe; ephedrine has greater cardiovascular side effects and it tends to lose effectiveness over time. Phenylpropanolamine also may be useful in the management of nasal congestion.

ADVERSE AND COMMON SIDE EFFECTS: Anorexia, restlessness, irritability, tremors, tachycardia, cardiac arrhythmias, hypertension, and urine retention are reported. With drug overdose, nausea, anorexia, vomiting, tachycardia, disorientation, and mydriasis may occur.

DRUG INTERACTIONS: Phenylpropanolamine enhances the pressor effects of tricyclic antidepressants, e.g., amitriptyline; NSAIDs, including aspirin and indomethacin, also increase the potential for hypertension. Arrhythmias are more likely in those administered halogenated anesthetic agents. Ephedrine may potentiate sympathetic nervous system stimulation, causing toxicity. An unexplained mechanism leading to the possibility of death is reported in humans taking chlorpromazine with phenylpropanolamine.

SUPPLIED AS: HUMAN PRODUCTS
Tablets containing 25 and 50 mg [Propagest and generics ★]
Tablets (film-coated) containing 37.5 mg [Westrim]
Capsules containing 75 mg phenylpropanolamine and 8 mg chlorpheniramine [Contac.C, Ornade]
Tablets containing 75 mg phenylpropanolamine and 600 mg guaifenesin [Entex]
Capsules containing 12.5 mg phenylpropanolamine, 500 mg acetaminophen, 15 mg dextromethorphan, and 2 mg chlorpheniramine [Contac.C Cold Care]
Liquid containing 15 mg phenylpropanolamine and 1.5 mg chlorpheniramine per 5 mL [Ornade]

PHENYTOIN

INDICATIONS: Phenytoin, or diphenylhydantoin (Dilantin ✦ ★), is an anticonvulsant. Phenytoin stops the propagation and spread of neural excitation. Because of undesirable pharmacologic activity of the drug in small animals, it has lost favor as a single agent for long-term control of seizure activity. It is used as an alternative or adjunctive drug in dogs that have not responded to or that have developed adverse reactions to phenobarbital or primidone. Serum concentrations are measured just before the next dose and after steady-state levels have been attained (22 hours in the dog). Effective serum concentration levels are in the range of 39.6 to 79.2 µmol/L (10–20 µg/mL or, according to another source, 10–30 µg/mL). The drug also is useful in the management of digitalis-induced tachyarrhythmias and atrioventricular block. The drug may be used with other antiarrhythmic agents to control difficult ventricular arrhythmias or in the place of lidocaine or procainamide for refractory ventricular arrhythmias.

ADVERSE AND COMMON SIDE EFFECTS: Vomiting, ataxia, tremors, depression, hypotension, and atrioventricular block are reported. Gingival hyperplasia is an uncommon side effect. The drug is toxic to cats and is not recommended in this species.

DRUG INTERACTIONS: Antacids (aluminum, calcium, and magnesium compounds), antihistamines, cisplatin, vinblastine, bleomycin, barbiturates, calcium gluconate, carbamazepine, folic acid, oxacillin, and rifampin decrease serum levels of phenytoin. Serum levels are increased (and the potential for toxicity and loss of seizure control) by chloramphenicol, cimetidine, allopurinol, theophylline, anticoagulants, benzodiazepines, dexamethasone, estrogens, methyl-phenidate, nitrofurantoin, pyridoxine, phenothiazines, sulfon-amides, salicylates, and phenylbutazone. Phenytoin may decrease the activity of corticosteroids, disopyramide, doxycycline, estrogens, quinidine, dopamine, and furosemide. The analgesic properties of meperidine may be decreased and its toxicity enhanced by pheny-toin. Additive hepatotoxicity may occur if phenytoin is used in con-junction with primidone or phenobarbital. Pyridoxine (vitamin B_6) may decrease serum phenytoin levels. Lidocaine and propranolol may have additive cardiac depressant effects. Valproic acid may in-crease or decrease serum concentrations.

SUPPLIED AS: VETERINARY ★ and HUMAN PRODUCTS ✦ ★
Capsules (extended) containing 30 and 100 mg ✦ ★
Oral suspension containing 6 and 25 mg/mL ✦ ★
Tablets containing 50 mg ✦ ★
For injection containing 50 mg/mL ✦ ★
Capsules containing 100 mg phenytoin with 15 mg phenobarbital ✦
and 100 mg phenytoin with 30 mg phenobarbital ✦
Capsules containing 100 mg phenytoin with 16 mg phenobarbital ★
and 100 mg phenytoin with 32 mg phenobarbital ★

PHOSPHATE ENEMAS

INDICATIONS: Phosphate-containing enemas (Fleet ✦ ★) are used for the relief of constipation in the dog. Osmotic action draws water into the intestinal lumen.

ADVERSE AND COMMON SIDE EFFECTS: These agents should not be used in the presence of dehydration, abdominal pain, nausea, vomiting, cardiac disease, or severe debility. Their use is contraindi-cated in cats, small dogs, and those with significant renal disease. Clinical signs of toxicity occur within 1 hour of use and include de-pression, ataxia, tetany, seizure, vomiting, hemorrhagic diarrhea, tachycardia, pallor, and stupor. Associated biochemical abnormali-ties may include hyperphosphatemia, hypernatremia, hypocal-cemia, hyperglycemia, hyperosmolality, and metabolic acidosis with a high anion gap (increased lactic acid). Death has been reported with the use of these agents in cats.

DRUG INTERACTIONS: None reported.

SUPPLIED AS: HUMAN PRODUCT
Rectal use containing 16 g sodium phosphate and 6 g dibasic sodium phosphate per 100 mL sodium: 8.09 mmol (186 mg) per 5 mL

PIPERAZINE

INDICATIONS: Piperazine (Hartz Once a Month ★, Once a Month Roundworm Treatment ♣, Pipa-Tabs ★, Purina Liquid Wormer ★) is an anthelmintic used for the eradication of roundworms.

ADVERSE AND COMMON SIDE EFFECTS: The most common clinical signs of toxicity, in decreasing order of frequency, are tremors, ataxia, seizures, vomiting, and weakness. For recent ingestion, activated charcoal and a saline or osmotic cathartic are recommended. The drug should not be given to animals with chronic liver or renal disease.

DRUG INTERACTIONS: Piperazine and chlorpromazine may precipitate seizure activity if used at the same time. Piperazine may exaggerate the extrapyramidal effects of phenothiazines. Pyrantel/morantel antagonize the efficacy of piperazine. The concurrent use of laxatives is not recommended because these agents may cause elimination of the drug before it has had an opportunity to work effectively.

SUPPLIED AS: VETERINARY PRODUCTS
Tablets equivalent to 50 mg or 250 mg base [Pipa-Tabs] or
80 and 125 mg base [Once a Month Treatment] or
80 and 303 mg base [Hartz Once a Month]

PIROXICAM

INDICATIONS: Piroxicam (Feldene ♣ ★) is a nonsteroidal anti-inflammatory agent with analgesic, antipyretic, and anti-inflammatory properties. Piroxicam has been used in dogs for the management of pain associated with degenerative joint disease. In humans, it appears equivalent in efficacy to aspirin in the treatment of osteoarthritis and rheumatoid arthritis. The drug also has been used successfully in dogs for the management of transitional cell carcinoma of the bladder (median survival in dogs 181 days in 1 report) and for inducing partial remission of squamous cell carcinoma in dogs.

ADVERSE AND COMMON SIDE EFFECTS: Piroxicam is contraindicated in hemophilia and GI ulceration or bleeding. Caution is advised in patients with renal or cardiac dysfunction, predisposition to fluid retention, hypertension, or coagulation disorders. Standard dosages may cause anorexia, melena, vomiting, anemia, mild to moderate leukocytosis, and a mild increase in serum urea nitrogen in dogs. Use of the drug in dogs at doses of 1 mg/kg has been associated with GI ulceration, peritonitis, and renal papillary necrosis.

DRUG INTERACTIONS: Concurrent use of aspirin may cause a slight reduction in piroxicam plasma levels. Anticoagulants may cause a slight increase in hypoprothrombinemic response. Diazepam, propranolol, and phenylbutazone may be displaced by piroxicam, leading to increased therapeutic and possibly toxic serum levels.

SUPPLIED AS: HUMAN PRODUCT
Capsules containing 10 and 20 mg

OTHER USES
Dogs
TRANSITIONAL CELL CARCINOMA OF THE BLADDER
0.3 mg/kg/day; PO

PLICAMYCIN

INDICATIONS: Plicamycin, formerly known as mithramycin, (Mithracin ★), has been used in dogs to treat hypercalcemia of malignancy and hypercalcemia secondary to vitamin D toxicosis. Clinical effectiveness peaks 1 to 2 days after a single IV dose of 25 µg/kg. The drug has antitumor activity independent of its calcium-lowering effect. Although the drug has minimal immunosuppressive activity, its high toxicity and low therapeutic index have limited its clinical use in human medicine.

ADVERSE AND COMMON SIDE EFFECTS: No significant side effects were documented at a dose of 25 µg/kg. A dose of 100 µg/kg induced severe hepatic necrosis and death. Prolonged daily administration of the drug has been associated with hypocalcemia, hypokalemia, azotemia, and increased liver enzyme activities. These side effects are reversible on discontinuation of the drug. At an IV dose of 0.1 mg/kg (in 250 mL saline), dogs may exhibit shivering and mild pain in the injected leg. In humans, other adverse effects worth noting include thrombocytopenia and bleeding diathesis, anorexia, nausea, vomiting, diarrhea, and stomatitis.

DRUG INTERACTIONS: Concurrent administration of vitamin D may enhance hypercalcemia.

SUPPLIED AS: HUMAN PRODUCT
For injection containing 2.5 mg

POLYMYXIN B

INDICATIONS: Polymyxin B (Aerosporin ♣ ★) is used in the treatment of gram-negative infections, especially those caused by Pseudomonas, Pasteurella, Klebsiella, Salmonella, Bordetella, and

Shigella organisms. Proteus and Brucella organisms frequently are resistant. The drug is used frequently as a topical preparation for treating localized infections of the ear, eye, bowel, and urinary tract. Systemically, it is used to treat infections resistant to aminoglycosides. The drug often is combined with neomycin and bacitracin or tetracycline to broaden its spectrum of activity.

ADVERSE AND COMMON SIDE EFFECTS: Pain at the site of injection, nephrotoxicity, CNS signs, and neuromuscular blockade have been reported.

DRUG INTERACTIONS: Aminoglycoside antibiotics, bacitracin, quinidine, quinine, and sodium citrate intensify the nephrotoxic and neurotoxic potential of polymyxin B. Succinylcholine and tubocurarine may prolong neuromuscular blockade and precipitate respiratory paralysis associated with the use of polymyxin B.

SUPPLIED AS: HUMAN PRODUCT
For injection containing 500,000 units per vial equivalent to 50 mg polymyxin standard

POLYSULFATED GLYCOSAMINOGLYCANS

INDICATIONS: Polysulfated glycosaminoglycans (Adequan IM ♣ ★, Cosequin ★) may be beneficial in the treatment of osteoarthritis. Administration of the compound to growing pups susceptible to hip dysplasia resulted in better coxofemoral congruity and fewer pathologic changes. The drug stimulates the synthesis of glycosaminoglycans, inhibits collagen and proteoglycan catabolism, and inhibits neutrophil migration into synovial fluid. These agents also inhibit potentially destructive enzymes including cathepsin, collagenase, hyaluronidase, and stromelysin. They have fibrinolytic activity and stimulate hyaluronic acid synthesis. Circulation to subchondral bone and perivascular tissue may improve. To maximize therapeutic benefit treatment should begin soon after the inciting traumatic event.

ADVERSE AND COMMON SIDE EFFECTS: Some studies have reported a potentiation of antithrombin III activity leading to a dose-dependent prolongation of activated partial thromboplastin time, prothrombin time, and activated coagulation time. Recent studies of Cosequin in dogs, however, failed to demonstrate clinically significant adverse changes in hematologic, hemostatic or biochemical parameters under investigation. Adequan should be used with caution in animals with renal and/or hepatic dysfunction. It should not be used in breeding animals because the effects on fertility and reproductive function have not been determined.

DRUG INTERACTIONS: The concurrent use of glucocorticoids or NSAIDs may mask clinical signs of joint sepsis. Use with caution in dogs on long-term NSAIDs.

SUPPLIED AS: For injection containing 100 mg/mL [Adequan] Capsules containing 250 mg glucosamine and 200 mg sodium chondroitin sulfate [Cosequin] and 500 mg glucosamine and 400 mg sodium chondroitin sulfate [Cosequin DS]

POTASSIUM CHLORIDE

INDICATIONS: Potassium chloride ♣ ★ is indicated in the treatment of hypokalemia in the dog and cat.

ADVERSE AND COMMON SIDE EFFECTS: Infusion of potassium-containing fluids, especially those containing glucose, may initially decrease serum potassium levels further as a result of dilution, increased distal renal tubular flow, and cellular uptake of potassium. To minimize the likelihood of this complication, begin oral potassium supplementation 12 to 24 hours before fluid therapy, use a fluid that does not contain glucose, and administer fluids at an appropriate rate. Infusion of potassium fluid concentrations in excess of 40 mEq/L may be associated with pain and sclerosis of peripheral veins.

Hyperkalemia and cardiac arrest may occur, and patients with impaired ability to excrete potassium, e.g., renal impairment, are at increased risk. Potassium may exacerbate heart block. The drug is contraindicated in patients with renal failure and oliguria, adrenal insufficiency, acute dehydration, and hyperkalemia of any cause. In patients on a low-salt diet, hypokalemic hypochloremic alkalosis may occur that may require calcium supplementation in addition to potassium. Potassium chloride is acidifying and may exacerbate pre-existing metabolic acidosis. Clinical signs of hyperkalemia may include muscular weakness, bradycardia, vomiting, and diarrhea.

DRUG INTERACTIONS: The concurrent use of potassium-sparing diuretics, e.g., spironolactone and triamterene, may predispose to severe hyperkalemia, as may the concurrent use of penicillin G potassium.

SUPPLIED AS: HUMAN PRODUCTS
Tablets containing 750 mg potassium chloride equivalent to 10 mEq potassium and tablets containing 1,500 mg equivalent to 20 mEq
Capsules containing 600 mg potassium chloride equivalent to 8 mEq and 750 mg equivalent to 10 mEq potassium
For injection containing 2 mEq/mL in 10-mL (20 mEq) and 20-mL (40 mEq) vials
For injection containing 10, 20, 30, 40, 60, and 90 mEq

Each 7.8 g dose contains 1.85 g [25 mmol (mEq)] potassium and 25 mmol (mEq) chloride [K-Lyte/Cl ✦]

Guidelines for Routine Intravenous Supplementation of Potassium in Dogs and Cats

Serum Potassium (mEq/L)	mEq KCl to Add to 250 mL Fluid	mEq KCl to Add to 1 L Fluid	Maximal Fluid Rate (mL/kg/hr)
< 2.0	20	80	6
2.1 to 2.5	15	60	8
2.6 to 3.0	10	40	12
3.1 to 3.5	7	28	18
3.6 to 5.0	5	20	25

From: DiBartola SP. Hypokalemic nephropathy. In: August JR, ed. *Consultations in Feline Internal Medicine* 2. Philadelphia: WB Saunders Co; 1994:322.

POTASSIUM CITRATE

INDICATIONS: Potassium citrate (Urocit-K ★, K-Lyte ✦) is used for the prevention of calcium oxalate urolithiasis. The citrate complexes with calcium and decreases the urinary concentration of calcium oxalate. Potassium citrate also alkalinizes the urine and increases the solubility of calcium oxalate.

ADVERSE AND COMMON SIDE EFFECTS: Studies in dogs have failed to demonstrate serious side effects with use of the drug. In humans, the drug may be associated with mild GI upset, e.g., abdominal discomfort, nausea, vomiting, diarrhea, and loose stools. Reducing the dose or administering the drug with food may alleviate these complaints. If there is evidence of GI upset, the drug should be discontinued. Hyperkalemia may occur and serum electrolytes should be monitored regularly. The drug is contraindicated in animals with hyperkalemia or renal failure. It also is contraindicated in patients with urinary tract infections because the alkaline urinary pH associated with its use may promote further bacterial growth.

DRUG INTERACTIONS: Drugs that decrease GI transit, e.g., anticholinergics, may predispose to gastric irritation induced by potassium citrate. The concurrent use of potassium-sparing agents, e.g., spironolactone and triamterene, predispose to hyperkalemia and should be avoided.

SUPPLIED AS: HUMAN PRODUCTS
Tablets containing 5 mEq (540 mg) and 10 mEq (1,080 mg)
Tablets containing 2.5 g or 25 mmol (mEq) elemental potassium [K-Lyte]

POTASSIUM GLUCONATE

INDICATIONS: Potassium gluconate (Kaon ♣ ★, Tumil-K ★) is indicated in the treatment of hypokalemia in the dog and cat. Potassium gluconate elixir is more palatable and easier to dose for cats than potassium chloride.

ADVERSE AND COMMON SIDE EFFECTS: As for **POTASSIUM CHLORIDE**, except that potassium gluconate is nonacidifying.

DRUG INTERACTIONS: As for **POTASSIUM CHLORIDE**.

SUPPLIED AS: VETERINARY PRODUCTS
Powder containing 468 mg (2 mEq) per 1/4 teaspoon (0.65 g) [Tumil-K]
Tablets containing 468 mg (2 mEq) [Tumil-K]
Gel containing 468 mg (2 mEq) per 1/2 teaspoon (2.34 g) [Tumil-K]
HUMAN PRODUCTS
Elixir containing 20 mEq per 15 mL [Kaon ♣ ★]
Tablets containing 2, 2.3, 2.5, and 5 mEq [generic products ★] and 5 mEq [Kaon ★]

POTASSIUM IODIDE

INDICATIONS: Supersaturated potassium iodide (SSKI ★) has been used for the treatment of sporotrichosis in dogs and cats. Potassium iodide also is used in cats with hyperthyroidism scheduled for thyroidectomy that do not tolerate methimazole well. Iodine decreases the rate of thyroid hormone synthesis and causes a reduction in the size and vascularity of the adenomatous thyroid gland, although the effects are inconsistent and serum T_3 and T_4 may not normalize. In addition, the antithyroid effect may be short-lived, and escape from inhibition generally occurs. This medication should not be used as the sole therapy for cats with hyperthyroid disease but may be used in conjunction with a β-blocking drug or another antithyroid agent.

ADVERSE AND COMMON SIDE EFFECTS: Cats are especially sensitive to iodides. Toxic signs include anorexia, excessive salivation, vomiting, depression, muscle twitching, hypothermia, cardiomyopathy, cardiovascular collapse, and death. Caution is advised in patients with renal impairment, cardiac disease, or hypoadrenocorticism. Safe use during pregnancy and in lactating mothers has not been established.

DRUG INTERACTIONS: Lithium may potentiate the hypothyroid and goitrogenic effects of potassium iodide. The concurrent use of potassium-sparing diuretics or potassium-containing drugs increases the risk of hyperkalemia, cardiac arrhythmias, and cardiac arrest.

SUPPLIED AS: HUMAN PRODUCTS
Tablets containing 130 mg [Thyro-Block ♣]
Oral solution containing 325 mg/5 mL [Pima Syrup ★] and 1 g/mL
[SSKI ★, Potassium Iodide Saturated Solution ★]
Lugol's solution (5 g iodine with 10 g potassium iodide per 100 mL;
solution yields 6.3 mg iodine/drop)

OTHER USES
Cats

HYPERTHYROID DISEASE
30 to 100 mg/day; PO for 1 to 2 weeks prethyroidectomy; combine
with a β-blocker, e.g., propranolol (2.5–5 mg tid; PO)

POTASSIUM PHOSPHATE

INDICATIONS: Potassium phosphate ♣ ★ is indicated in the treatment of hypophosphatemia. In dogs and cats, the most common
cause of hypophosphatemia is diabetic ketoacidosis. It also has been
documented in a cat with hepatic lipidosis.

ADVERSE AND COMMON SIDE EFFECTS: Potassium phosphate
is contraindicated in conditions in which high potassium or phosphate or low calcium are expected. To avoid potassium or phosphate
intoxication, infuse slowly. Infusing high concentrations of phosphate may cause hypocalcemia. In patients with severe renal or
adrenal insufficiency, infusion of the drug may cause hyperkalemia.
High serum potassium concentrations may cause weakness, bradycardia, heart block, hypotension, and cardiac arrest.

DRUG INTERACTIONS: Potassium-containing products should be
used with caution in patients receiving digitalis agents and are contraindicated in these same patients with evidence of heart block.
Captopril and enalapril and potassium-sparing diuretics, e.g.,
spironolactone and triamterene, may predispose to hyperkalemia
with the concurrent use of potassium phosphate.

SUPPLIED AS: HUMAN PRODUCT
For injection providing 3 mmol (285 mg) phosphate and 4.4 mEq
(170 mg) potassium per mL

PRAZIQUANTEL

INDICATIONS: Praziquantel (Droncit ♣ ★) is an anthelmintic used
in dogs and cats to eliminate tapeworms, including *Taenia* spp.,
Dipylidium caninum, Echinococcus granulosus, and *Mesocestoides corti.*
The drug also is effective against *Paragonimus* infections in dogs.
After use of the drug, the parasite loses its ability to resist digestion

by the host, and because of this, it is common to see only disintegrated and partially digested pieces of tapeworm in the stool. Finally, praziquantel has been used to treat *Amphimerus pseudofelineus*, a liver fluke in cats.

ADVERSE AND COMMON SIDE EFFECTS: The drug is very safe but should not be used in puppies or kittens younger than 4 weeks of age. Administration of the drug at dosages of five times the recommended level did not cause signs of toxicity in the dog or cat. Drug overdose may be associated with anorexia, vomiting, salivation, diarrhea, and depression.

DRUG INTERACTIONS: None reported.

SUPPLIED AS: VETERINARY PRODUCTS
For injection containing 56.8 mg/mL
Tablets containing 34 mg (canine formulation) and 23 mg (feline formulation)

OTHER USES
Dogs and Cats
PARAGONIMIASIS
25 mg/kg bid; PO for 2 consecutive days

Cats
AMPHIMERUS PSEUDOFELINEUS
40 mg/kg once daily for 3 days

PRAZOSIN

INDICATIONS: Prazosin (Minipress ✦ ★) is a selective α-adrenergic blocking agent. It causes arterial and venous vasodilation without changes in heart rate or cardiac output and is used to decrease blood pressure in patients with systemic hypertension and decrease pulmonary edema in cases of congestive heart failure.

ADVERSE AND COMMON SIDE EFFECTS: Hypotension and syncope may occur and are most common after administration of the first dose. These problems usually are transient, and repeated doses rarely cause them again. Nausea, vomiting, diarrhea, and constipation also have been reported. Tolerance to the drug has been documented, but temporarily discontinuing the drug, adjusting the dose, or adding an aldosterone antagonist, e.g., spironolactone, to the regimen may alleviate this problem.

DRUG INTERACTIONS: Increased frequency of hypotension may occur with the concurrent use of diuretics and β-adrenergic blocking agents, e.g., propranolol. Highly protein-bound drugs, e.g., pheno-barbital and phenytoin, may potentiate prazosin side effects. Similarly, prazosin may displace or be displaced by the sulfonamides, phenylbutazone, or warfarin.

SUPPLIED AS: HUMAN PRODUCTS
Capsules containing 1, 2, and 5 mg ★
Tablets containing 1, 2, and 5 mg ♣

PREDNISOLONE
PREDNISOLONE SODIUM SUCCINATE
PREDNISONE

INDICATIONS: Prednisolone (Delta-Cortef ★) and prednisone (Deltasone ♣ ★) are intermediate-acting glucocorticoid agents. Prednisone is converted by the liver to prednisolone. Except for cases of liver failure, the drugs essentially can be used interchangeably. Prednisolone also is available in combination with other agents, e.g., salicylate (Pred-C ♣) or antihistamine (Predniderm ♣). Prednisolone is indicated for the treatment of inflammatory conditions of the skin and joints and for supportive care during periods of stress. Prednisolone sodium succinate (Solu-Delta-Cortef ♣ ★) also is beneficial for the treatment of acute hypersensitivity reactions, atopic and contact dermatitis, summer eczema, and conjunctivitis. This drug also is used in animals with severe overwhelming infections with toxicity (in combination with appropriate antibiotic therapy) and for the prevention and treatment of adrenal insufficiency and shock (in conjunction with fluid support). For further information concerning ADVERSE AND COMMON SIDE EFFECTS and DRUG INTERACTIONS, see **GLUCOCORTICOID AGENTS.**

SUPPLIED AS: VETERINARY PRODUCTS

Prednisolone

For injection containing 20 mg/mL as prednisolone sodium phosphate [Cortisate-20 ★]
For injection containing 10 and 50 mg/mL as prednisolone acetate ♣ ★
Tablets containing 5 mg [PrednisTab ★]
For injection containing 10 and 50 mg/mL as prednisolone sodium succinate [Solu-Delta-Cortef ♣ ★]

HUMAN PRODUCTS
Oral syrup containing 15 mg/5 mL [Prelone ★]
Tablets containing 5 mg [generic products ♣]
For injection containing 20 mg/mL as prednisolone sodium phosphate [generic products ♣]

Prednisone

VETERINARY PRODUCTS
Tablets containing 2.5, 5, 10, 20, 25, and 50 mg
For injection containing 10 and 40 mg/mL [Meticorten ★]

HUMAN PRODUCTS
Oral syrup containing 5 mg/mL [Liquid pred ★]
Tablets containing 1, 2.5, 5, 10, 20, 25, and 50 mg ✦ ★

OTHER USES
Dogs

IATROGENIC SECONDARY HYPOADRENOCORTICISM
Administer prednisone or prednisolone at 0.50 mg/kg/day every
other morning
Taper dose gradually and discontinue after 1 month
During periods of severe stress, reinstitute prednisone or pred-
nisolone at 1 to 2 mg/kg/day

IATROGENIC HYPERADRENOCORTICISM
Replace current glucocorticoid with prednisone or prednisolone at
equivalent doses
Taper dose of prednisone or prednisolone to 0.25 mg/kg/day over 1
to 2 months
If the original condition for steroid use recurs before attaining the
0.25 mg/kg/day dose, double the last effective dose and administer
on alternate days
If the 0.25 mg/kg/day dose is reached without recurrence of the
original indication for steroid use, maintain on this dose for 1 month
and then treat for adrenocortical atrophy as outlined above

MAST CELL TUMOR
1 mg/kg; PO

PRIMIDONE

INDICATIONS: Primidone (Mysoline ✦ ★) is an anticonvulsant
agent. In the liver, the drug is metabolized to phenobarbital (contributes approximately 85% of the anticonvulsant activity) and
phenylethylmalonamide (which contributes approximately 15% of
the anticonvulsant activity). Primidone works by raising the seizure
threshold. Serum concentrations are measured just before the next
dose and after steady-state levels have been reached (16 days in the
dog). Effective serum concentrations of phenobarbital are in the
range of 65 to 170 µmol/L (approximately 15 to 40 µg/mL). The use
of primidone for the control of seizures has been discouraged because the drug must be administered three times daily to be effective, absorption is poor, clinically it is no more effective than pheno-

barbital, and finally, primidone is associated with a greater incidence of hepatotoxicity than other anticonvulsant drugs. The drug is not approved for use in cats.

ADVERSE AND COMMON SIDE EFFECTS: Polyuria, polydipsia, and polyphagia are noted during the first few weeks of therapy or when the dose is increased. Sedation and ataxia may occur but tend to resolve with continued treatment. When initiating therapy, transient anxiety and agitation may be observed. Increase in serum liver enzymes and hepatotoxicity is reported, especially with chronic use, e.g., 2 to 3 years.

DRUG INTERACTIONS: Acetazolamide may decrease the absorption of primidone. The combination of primidone and phenytoin potentiates hepatotoxicity. Phenytoin may increase phenobarbital levels by stimulating the conversion of primidone to phenobarbital. The effects of primidone may be enhanced if the drug is used in conjunction with narcotics, phenothiazines, antihistamines, or chloramphenicol. The effects of corticosteroids, β-blockers, quinidine, theophylline, and metronidazole may be decreased if used in conjunction with primidone. Primidone may decrease the absorption of griseofulvin. Patients are predisposed to postural hypotension if the drug is used with furosemide.

SUPPLIED AS: VETERINARY PRODUCT
Tablets containing 250 mg [Neurosyn ★, Mysoline ✦]

HUMAN PRODUCTS
Tablets containing 50, 125, and 250 mg [Mysoline]
Oral suspension containing 50 mg/mL [Mysoline ★]

PROCAINAMIDE

INDICATIONS: Procainamide (Pronestyl ✦ ★, Procan SR ✦ ★) is an antiarrhythmic drug. It is used for the management of ventricular premature contractions and tachycardia and supraventricular tachycardia associated with Wolff–Parkinson–White syndrome with wide QRS complexes. Serum drug concentrations are measured after steady-state levels have been attained (12 hours in the dog) and before the next dose is administered.

ADVERSE AND COMMON SIDE EFFECTS: Weakness, hypotension, decreased myocardial contractility, and vagolytic effects are reported. Procainamide should be avoided in patients with second- or third-degree heart block unless the patient is supported by cardiac pacing. Electrocardiographic changes may include widened QRS complexes and QT intervals, atrioventricular block, and multiform ventricular tachycardia. In addition, anorexia, vomiting, diarrhea, and agranulocytosis have been reported. The drug is contraindicated in patients with myasthenia gravis and in humans with systemic lupus erythematosus (SLE). Procainamide has been associated with causing an SLE syndrome in humans. The drug should be used with caution in patients with significant renal or hepatic dysfunction or those with congestive heart failure.

DRUG INTERACTIONS: Antiarrhythmic effects are increased if procainamide is used with other antiarrhythmic agents. Concurrent use with digoxin should be avoided. Serum levels are increased with cimetidine. Acetazolamide increases the effect of procainamide. Anticholinergic effects are enhanced if procainamide is used with anticholinergic drugs. Procainamide may antagonize the effects of pyridostigmine or neostigmine in patients with myasthenia gravis. The incidence of hypotension is increased if the drug is used with antihypertensive agents. Procainamide may potentiate or prolong the neuromuscular blocking activity of succinylcholine or other drugs, e.g., aminoglycosides.

SUPPLIED AS: HUMAN PRODUCTS
For injection containing 100 and 500 mg/mL
Tablets and capsules containing 250, 375, and 500 mg
Tablets (sustained-release) containing 250, 500, 750, and 1,000 mg

PROCHLORPERAZINE

INDICATIONS: Prochlorperazine (Stemetil ♣, Compazine ★) is a phenothiazine derivative used principally for its antiemetic properties. The drug depresses the chemoreceptor trigger zone.

ADVERSE AND COMMON SIDE EFFECTS: The drug is contraindicated in glaucoma, pyloric obstruction or stenosis, and prostatic hypertrophy.

DRUG INTERACTIONS: Prochlorperazine may prolong the effects of general anesthetics. Phenothiazines should not be given within 1 month of worming with organophosphate medications because their effects may be potentiated. Other CNS depressants enhance hypotension and respiratory depression if used concurrently. The concurrent use of quinidine may cause additive cardiac depression. Antacids and antidiarrheal compounds decrease absorption of oral phenothiazines. Space administration by at least 2 hours. Atropine and other anticholinergics have additive anticholinergic potential and reduce the antipsychotic effect of phenothiazines. Barbiturate drugs increase the metabolism of phenothiazines and may reduce their effects. Barbiturate anesthetics may increase excitation (tremor, involuntary muscle movements) and hypotension. Propranolol may have additive hypotensive effects. Phenothiazines may mask the ototoxic effects of aminoglycoside antibiotics. Phenothiazines inhibit phenytoin metabolism and increase its potential for toxicity. Tricyclic antidepressants, e.g., amitriptyline, may intensify the sedative and anticholinergic effects of phenothiazines.

SUPPLIED AS: HUMAN PRODUCTS
Tablets containing 5, 10, and 25 mg [Compazine]
Capsules containing 10, 15, and 30 mg (sustained-release) [Compazine]
Tablets containing 5 and 10 mg [Stemetil]
Oral syrup containing 1 mg/mL [Compazine, Stemetil]
For injection containing 5 mg/mL [Compazine, Stemetil]

OTHER USES
Dogs
ANTIEMETIC
i)   0.5 mg/kg tid–qid; IM (prochlorperazine)
ii) 0.14 to 0.22 mg/kg bid; SC [Darbazine]

Cats
ANTIEMETIC
i)   0.1 mg/kg qid; IM (prochlorperazine)
ii) 0.5 to 0.8 mg/kg; IM or, bid; SC [Darbazine]

PROPANTHELINE

INDICATIONS: Propantheline bromide (Pro-Banthine ✤ ★) is an anticholinergic agent. It is used in the management of diarrhea, detrusor hyperreflexia, sinus bradycardia, atrioventricular block, and sick sinus syndrome.

ADVERSE AND COMMON SIDE EFFECTS: Tachycardia, weakness, nausea, vomiting, constipation, pupillary dilation, and dryness of the mucous membranes may occur. Signs of drug overdose include urinary retention, excitement, hypotension, respiratory failure, paralysis, and coma.

DRUG INTERACTIONS: Antihistamines, procainamide, quinidine, meperidine, benzodiazepines, and the phenothiazines may enhance the activity of propantheline, and primidone, disopyramide, nitrates, and long-term corticosteroid use may potentiate the adverse effects of the drug. Propantheline may enhance the activity of nitrofurantoin, thiazide diuretics, and sympathomimetic drugs. Propantheline delays the absorption of, but increases serum levels of, ranitidine, and it may decrease the absorption of cimetidine.

SUPPLIED AS: HUMAN PRODUCT
Tablets containing 7.5 and 15 mg

OTHER USES
Dogs
DETRUSOR HYPERREFLEXIA
i) 0.2 mg/kg tid–qid; PO, titrate dose to effect

ii) 5 to 30 mg tid; PO

DIARRHEA/COLITIS/IRRITABLE BOWEL SYNDROME AND
ANTIEMETIC
0.25 mg/kg tid; PO for no longer than 72 hours (diarrhea)

SINUS BRADYCARDIA AND HEART BLOCK
0.5 to 1 mg/kg tid; PO

Cats
DETRUSOR HYPERREFLEXIA
i) 7.5 mg once daily to once every third day; PO, titrate dose to
   effect

ii) 5 to 7.5 mg tid; PO

DIARRHEA AND ANTIEMETIC
0.25 mg/kg tid; PO

CHRONIC COLITIS
0.5 mg/kg bid–tid; PO

SINUS BRADYCARDIA AND HEART BLOCK
i) 0.8 to 1.6 mg/kg tid; PO (the drug generally is ineffective in this
   instance)

ii) 3.75 to 15 mg bid–tid; PO

PROPIONIBACTERIUM ACNES

INDICATIONS: *Propionibacterium acnes* (Immunoregulin ♣ ★) has
nonspecific immunostimulatory properties. It induces macrophage
activation and lymphokine production, enhances cell-mediated immunity, and increases natural killer cell activity that may intensify
antineoplastic, antiviral, and antibacterial activity and stimulate he-
mopoiesis. This agent is marketed as adjunct therapy to antibiotic
treatment for dogs with chronic pyoderma. In uncontrolled studies,
it has been shown to increase survival times in dogs with oral
melanoma and mastocytoma and has been used to treat immunosuppressed cats with rhinotracheitis. *P. acnes* also has been used to
treat cats with clinical signs of FeLV-induced disease. Almost half
the cats improved clinically, and peripheral blood results also improved. Cats may even seroconvert to an FeLV-seronegative status.
Lack of adequate control groups in this study, however, make conclusions difficult to confirm.

ADVERSE AND COMMON SIDE EFFECTS: Occasionally, fever, chills, anorexia, and lethargy are reported shortly after its use. Anaphylaxis may occur, and when it does, the animal should be treated with epinephrine. Extravascular injection may cause tissue inflammation. Safety of the drug has not been evaluated in pregnant animals.

DRUG INTERACTIONS: The beneficial effects of the drug may be negated by the concurrent use of corticosteroids or other immunosuppressive agents. Corticosteroids should be discontinued 1 week before the use of this product.

SUPPLIED AS: VETERINARY PRODUCT
For injection containing 0.4 mg/mL nonviable *Propionibacterium acnes* in 5-mL vials

PROPOFOL

INDICATIONS: Propofol (Rapinovet ♣ ★, Diprivan ♣ ★) is a sedative/hypnotic IV anesthetic agent used for the induction and maintenance of general anesthesia. It is indicated to provide general anesthesia for procedures lasting less than 5 minutes and for induction and maintenance of general anesthesia using incremental doses to effect. It is particularly useful for cases in which a short recovery is desired. Induction, maintenance, and recovery are smooth after single or incremental doses and after IV infusion. Recovery is rapid and occurs partly by redistribution. In unsedated mixed-breed dogs, the recovery time is approximately 15 minutes, and for greyhounds, it is approximately 22 minutes. The drug is rapidly metabolized and noncumulative. It also has been used successfully in young dogs (3 months) and cats (8 months).

ADVERSE AND COMMON SIDE EFFECTS: In dogs, apnea, cyanosis, and pain on injection have been reported. Induction may be associated with a slight bradycardia. Serious cardiac arrhythmias have not been a feature of propofol anesthesia in dogs. Administration (6 mg/kg over 30 seconds) to hypovolemic dogs may cause a profound decrease in arterial blood pressure. Twitching and paddling of the front legs occurs infrequently. Vomiting, retching, and/or salivation may be noted during recovery. With drug overdose, transient apnea and dose-related hypotension or hypertension is reported in cats.

Propofol should not be administered through the same IV catheter with blood or plasma. The drug should be used with caution in patients with a history of epilepsy and disorders of lipid metabolism, e.g., pancreatitis. The drug is supplied in sterile glass ampules and contains no preservatives. Because of the risk of contamination, any unused drug should be discarded.

DRUG INTERACTIONS: Propofol is compatible with a wide range of inhalation anesthetics and premedicant drugs, although dosage requirements are reduced if used concurrently. Propofol enhances the arrhythmogenic effect of epinephrine.

SUPPLIED AS: VETERINARY [Rapinovet] and HUMAN [Diprivan] PRODUCTS
For injection containing 10 mg/mL

OTHER USES
Dogs
BALANCED ANESTHESIA
Premedicate with medetomidine (30 µg/kg; IM) and atropine (0.044 mg/kg; IM); follow with loading dose of propofol (2 mg/kg; IV) and continue with IV infusion at 165 µg/kg/minute

PROPRANOLOL

INDICATIONS: Propranolol (Inderal ♣ ★) is a nonselective β_1- and β_2-blocking agent. It is indicated alone or in conjunction with digoxin in the management of atrial fibrillation. The drug may be of benefit in the treatment of ventricular premature contractions and arrhythmias caused by digitalis toxicity and in the management of systemic hypertension. Propranolol also is useful in the treatment of hypertrophic cardiomyopathy, especially that associated with hyperthyroid disease. Diltiazem may be more effective than propranolol in the treatment of idiopathic hypertrophic cardiomyopathy. The drug also has been recommended for the management of mild fears and anxiety.

ADVERSE AND COMMON SIDE EFFECTS: Drug dosages should be reduced in cats with hyperthyroid disease. Monitoring heart rate is an appropriate method of determining adequate dosage. Propranolol is contraindicated in patients with congestive heart failure unless it is secondary to a tachyarrhythmia responsive to β-blockade. The drug also is contraindicated in those with second- or third-degree heart block and sinus bradycardia and those with bronchoconstrictive lung disease e.g., asthma. Propranolol should not be given to animals with evidence of thromboembolic disease. The drug may cause hypoglycemia and should be used with caution in diabetics. Side effects of propranolol include bronchoconstriction, hypoglycemia, decreased cardiac contractility, hypotension, bradycardia, peripheral vasoconstriction, and diarrhea. Bronchoconstriction can be managed with terbutaline (2–5 mg bid; PO) or oxtriphylline (4–8 mg tid; PO). Drug-induced congestive heart failure can be treated with dobutamine, furosemide, and oxygen therapy. Dextrose can be used to manage the hypoglycemia.

Propranolol should be withdrawn gradually in patients on long-term therapy because of the possibility of sensitizing these animals to the endogenous release of norepinephrine and epinephrine, which may result in tachycardia, arrhythmias, and hypertension.

DRUG INTERACTIONS: Antacids delay GI absorption of propranolol. Antiarrhythmic effects of quinidine, procainamide, and lidocaine are enhanced by propranolol, but toxic effects may be additive. Serum levels of propranolol are increased by cimetidine. The hypotensive effects of propranolol are enhanced by chlorpromazine, cimetidine, furosemide, phenothiazines, and hydralazine. Propranolol increases the serum levels of lidocaine. It also increases the effects of tubocurarine and succinylcholine. The action of terbutaline, epinephrine, and phenylpropanolamine may be antagonized by propranolol. Concurrent use of digitalis may potentiate bradycardia. Concurrent use of salicylates may inhibit the antihypertensive effects of propranolol. The effect of propranolol may be decreased by the concurrent use of thyroid hormone supplementation, and the dose of propranolol may need to be decreased in animals receiving methimazole. The bronchodilatory effects of theophylline may be antagonized by propranolol.

SUPPLIED AS: HUMAN PRODUCTS
Tablets containing 10, 20, 40, 60, 80, 90, and 120 mg
Capsules (extended-release) containing 60, 80, 120, and 160 mg
Oral solution containing 4, 8, and 80 mg/mL [Intensol ★]
For injection containing 1 mg/mL

OTHER USES
Dogs
HYPERTROPHIC CARDIOMYOPATHY
0.3 to 1 mg/kg tid; PO (maximum 120 mg/day)

MILD FEARS and ANXIETY
0.5 to 3 mg/kg bid or PRN; PO

Cats
HYPERTROPHIC CARDIOMYOPATHY
4.5 kg or less; 2.5 mg bid–tid; PO
5 kg or more; 5 mg bid–tid; PO

MILD FEARS and ANXIETY
0.2 to 1 mg/kg tid; PO

PROSTAGLANDIN F$_{2\alpha}$

INDICATIONS: Prostaglandin F$_{2\alpha}$ (Lutalyse ♣ ★) is used in the treatment of pyometra in the dog and cat. The drug causes contraction of the myometrium and relaxation of the cervix. Reduction in uterine size and improvement in clinical signs are not evident for at least 48 hours after the start of therapy. It also has been used alone as an abortifacient in small animals and in combination with intravaginal misoprostol. The latter combination is more expedient (abortion mean—5 days) than $PGF_{2\alpha}$ alone (abortion mean—7 days).

ADVERSE AND COMMON SIDE EFFECTS: Restlessness, vomiting, salivation, diarrhea, tachycardia, fever, pupillary dilation followed by pupillary constriction, and panting occur within the first minute after injection and last approximately 20 to 30 minutes. Walking dogs for 20 to 40 minutes after use of the drug tends to diminish these clinical signs. These signs tend to become less pronounced with subsequent doses and usually are absent by the fifth dose. Death has been reported with use of this product. Additional side effects in cats may include vocalization, restlessness, grooming, tenesmus, salivation, kneading, mydriasis, urination, and lordosis. Reactions in cats may begin as early as 30 seconds after injection and last as long as 1 hour. Normal estrus cycles and normal litters can be expected in most animals after successful therapy. Prostaglandin $F_{2\alpha}$ should be used with caution in animals with closed-cervix pyometra because of the poor therapeutic response, the risk of peritonitis (through retrograde flow of uterine contents via the fallopian tubes), and the risk of uterine rupture (from contraction against a closed cervix).

DRUG INTERACTIONS: The concurrent use of estrogens is not recommended because estrogens enhance the effects of the drug on the uterus.

SUPPLIED AS: VETERINARY PRODUCT
For injection containing 5 mg/mL [Lutalyse] (licensed for use in large animals only)

OTHER USES
Dogs
INDUCTION OF ABORTION
i)   After day 25 of gestation, give 60 µg/kg div. bid or tid; IM for 3 to 6 days (abortion usually occurs in 3–7 days);

ii) In healthy bitches from midgestation to term, give 25 to 250 µg/kg bid; IM; radiography or ultrasound is completed every 3 to 5 days to determine whether abortion is complete;

iii) 30 to 35 days after an unplanned breeding, give 0.1 mg/kg tid; SC, until abortion is complete;

iv) Treatment initiated between days 30 and 43 of gestation; intravaginal misoprostol (1–3 µg/kg) once daily given in conjunction with $PGF_{2\alpha}$ (0.1 mg/kg tid for 48 hours, then 0.2 mg/kg tid to effect; SC).

Cats

INDUCTION OF ABORTION
After day 40 of gestation, give 0.5 to 1 mg/kg; SC, and again in 24 hours (abortion usually occurs in 8–24 hours)

PROTAMINE SULFATE

INDICATIONS: Protamine sulfate ✢ ★ is used as an antidote for heparin intoxication.

ADVERSE AND COMMON SIDE EFFECTS: The drug should be used with caution in patients with a history of cardiovascular disease or a history of allergy to fish. An abrupt decrease in blood pressure, bradycardia, dyspnea, nausea, vomiting, and lassitude are reported. These effects are minimized if the drug is injected slowly (over a 3-minute period). Hypersensitivity also is reported. A rebound effect leading to prolonged bleeding may occur several hours after heparin apparently has been neutralized because of the release of heparin from the heparin–protamine complex or release of additional heparin from extravascular spaces.

DRUG INTERACTIONS: None reported.

SUPPLIED AS: HUMAN PRODUCT
For injection containing 10 mg/mL

PSEUDOEPHEDRINE

INDICATIONS: Pseudoephedrine (Eltor ✢, Sudafed ✢ ★) is a sympathomimetic amine used in dogs in the management of urinary incontinence caused by sphincter incompetence. It has less CNS-stimulating and pressor effects than ephedrine. Patients are started at the lower end of the dose range, increasing if there is no clinical response. The drug is used in humans for its bronchodilatory and nasal decongestant properties.

ADVERSE AND COMMON SIDE EFFECTS: The drug should not be used within 14 days of the use of monoamine inhibitors, e.g., possibly amitraz and selegiline. It is contraindicated in patients with hypertension, glaucoma, and hyperthyroid disease and should be used with caution in those with congestive heart disease and urinary retention. Tachycardia, arrhythmias, nervousness, insomnia, anorexia, nausea, vomiting, and dry mouth are reported.

DRUG INTERACTIONS: The drug should not be used in conjunction with other sympathetic amines because an additive effect and potential toxicity may occur. The activity of β-blocking drugs, e.g., propranolol, may be antagonized by pseudoephedrine.

SUPPLIED AS: HUMAN PRODUCTS
Capsules containing 120 mg
Tablets containing 30 and 60 mg
Syrup containing 30 mg/5 mL

PYRANTEL PAMOATE

INDICATIONS: Pyrantel pamoate (Pyr-A-Pam ♣, Pyran ♣, Nemex ★) is an anthelmintic used to eradicate hookworm (*Ancylostoma caninum, Uncinaria stenocephala*) and roundworm (*Toxocara canis, Toxascaris leonina*) infections in dogs and hookworm (*Ancylostoma* spp.) and roundworm (*Toxocara cati*) infestations in cats. Pyrantel also may be useful in the elimination of *Physaloptera rara* in cats. Nemex is only licensed for use in dogs. Pyrantel is a cholinesterase inhibitor.

ADVERSE AND COMMON SIDE EFFECTS: Cautious use of the drug is advised in patients with liver dysfunction, malnutrition, dehydration, and anemia. Although the drug is considered safe, vomiting may occur.

DRUG INTERACTIONS: The drug should not be used concurrently with levamisole because of similar mechanisms of action and potential toxicity. Adverse effects may be potentiated by the concurrent use of organophosphates or diethylcarbamazine. Piperazine and pyrantel have antagonistic actions and should not be used together.

SUPPLIED AS: VETERINARY PRODUCTS
Tablets containing 35 and 125 mg [Pyr-A-Pam, Pyran]
Tablets containing 22.7 and 113.5 mg (of base) [Nemex]
Oral suspension containing 4.54 mg (of base) per mL of suspension [Nemex]

OTHER USES
Cats

PHYSALOPTERA RARA
5 mg/kg; PO once, repeat in 3 weeks

PYRETHRIN-CONTAINING PRODUCTS

INDICATIONS: Pyrethrin-containing products (Sectrol ♣ ★, Ovitrol ♣ ★, and many others) are naturally occurring insecticides derived from the plant *Chrysanthemum cinerariae-folium*, and commonly are used for flea control. These drugs are gamma-aminobutyric acid (GABA) agonists that stimulate the insect's central nervous system, causing muscular excitation, convulsions, and paralysis. Insect mortality is enhanced when these products are combined with piperonyl butoxide, e.g., Sectrol and Ovitrol. Piperonyl butoxide inhibits pyrethrin metabolism.

ADVERSE AND COMMON SIDE EFFECTS: These products are relatively nontoxic to mammals, and moderate amounts can be ingested without toxic effects. Pyrethrins should not be used in dogs or cats younger than 6 weeks of age. Ingestion of toxic amounts of pyrethrins in mammals causes depression, nausea, vomiting, diarrhea, muscle tremors, convulsions, stupor, pallor, conjunctivitis, respiratory arrest, and death. Hypersalivation is common. Additionally, cats may display ear flicking, paw shaking, and repeated contractions of the superficial cutaneous muscles. Treatment of toxic patients includes cleaning exposed areas of the skin. If ingestion has taken place within the past hour, the induction of emesis (e.g., 1–2 mL/kg of 3% hydrogen peroxide) is indicated. If ingestion has taken place within 3 to 4 hours, gastric lavage and activated charcoal (2 g/kg) then magnesium sulfate or sodium sulfate (0.5 g/kg as a 10% solution) are indicated to limit further absorption. Additionally, fluid therapy, methocarbamol (55–220 mg/kg; IV) to control muscle tremors, and phenobarbital (6 mg/kg; IV) or pentobarbital (4–20 mg/kg; IV) to control seizures may be indicated.

DRUG INTERACTIONS: The use of atropine and diazepam is contraindicated. Atropine decreases acetylcholine levels, which may be undesirable, and diazepam is a GABA agonist. Because pyrethrins cause extrapyramidal stimulation, phenothiazines are contraindicated. Piperonyl butoxide, sesame oil, and isosafrole act synergistically with pyrethrins and commonly are combined with them.

SUPPLIED AS: VETERINARY PRODUCTS
See specific product.

PYRIDOSTIGMINE

INDICATIONS: Pyridostigmine (Mestinon ✤ ★, Regonol ✤ ★) is the anticholinesterase agent most often used in the management of myasthenia gravis because of its long duration of activity and fewer GI side effects.

ADVERSE AND COMMON SIDE EFFECTS: The drug is contraindicated in patients with mechanical obstruction of the GIT or urinary tract, bradycardia, and hypotension. The drug should be used with caution in those with asthma, epilepsy, hyperthyroidism, peptic ulcer, and cardiac arrhythmias. Intravenous injection may cause thrombophlebitis. With drug overdose, nausea, vomiting, diarrhea, miosis, excessive salivation and bronchial secretion, bronchoconstriction, bradycardia, weakness, fasciculation, and hypotension may occur.

DRUG INTERACTIONS: The aminoglycosides may have some neuromuscular blocking effects that may necessitate increased dosage of pyridostigmine. The concurrent use of the following drugs with pyridostigmine may alter neuromuscular transmission and should be avoided: barbiturates, succinylcholine, quinidine, procainamide, potassium-depleting diuretics, and magnesium sulfate. Atropine antagonizes the muscarinic effects of the drug but should be used with caution because atropine may mask the early symptoms of a cholinergic crisis.

SUPPLIED AS: HUMAN PRODUCTS
Tablets containing 60 mg
Tablets (sustained-release) containing 180 mg
Oral syrup containing 60 mg/5 mL
For injection containing 5 mg/mL

PYRIMETHAMINE

INDICATIONS: Pyrimethamine (Daraprim ✦ ★) is used in combination with the sulfonamides, i.e., sulfadiazine, in the treatment of Toxoplasma infections. Pyrimethamine inhibits folic acid metabolism in the parasite and appears to increase the activity of the sulfonamide against toxoplasmosis.

ADVERSE AND COMMON SIDE EFFECTS: Depression, anorexia, vomiting, and reversible bone marrow suppression (anemia, leukopenia, and thrombocytopenia) may occur within 4 to 6 days of initiation of therapy with the pyrimethamine–sulfonamide combination. Cats are especially sensitive to these side effects, and anemia, leukopenia, and thrombocytopenia may develop rapidly. Bone marrow suppression may be mitigated by the addition of folic acid (50 mg/day), baker's yeast (100 mg/kg/day), or folinic acid (1 mg/kg/day) to the diet.

DRUG INTERACTIONS: Pyrimethamine is synergistic with the sulfonamides. The efficacy of pyrimethamine against toxoplasmosis is decreased by folic acid and para-aminobenzoic acid.

SUPPLIED AS: HUMAN PRODUCT
Tablets containing 25 mg

QUINACRINE

INDICATIONS: Quinacrine (Atabrine ★) is used for the eradication of giardiasis and trichomoniasis. In cats, the drug controlled clinical signs of *Giardia* infection but did not stop cyst shedding.

ADVERSE AND COMMON SIDE EFFECTS: Yellowing of the skin, darkening of urine, anorexia, vomiting, nausea, diarrhea, fever, pruritus, and behavioral changes (excessive barking, fly biting) have been reported. The drug should not be given to pregnant animals because it readily crosses the placenta. In humans, hepatotoxicity, agranulocytosis, anemia, and hypersensitivity reactions also have been reported.

DRUG INTERACTIONS: None of significance in small animals.

SUPPLIED AS: HUMAN PRODUCT
Tablets containing 100 mg

QUINIDINE

INDICATIONS: Quinidine gluconate (Duraquin ★, Quinaglute ✦), polygalacturonase (Cardioquin ✦ ★), and sulfate (Quinidex ✦ ★) are used most commonly in the management of ventricular arrhythmias. They also have been used in the treatment of atrial fibrillation. Serum concentrations are measured just before the next dose and after steady-state levels have been attained (28 hours in the dog, 10 hours in the cat). The therapeutic range in dogs is 2.5 to 5 µg/mL.

ADVERSE AND COMMON SIDE EFFECTS: Quinidine is contraindicated in patients with myasthenia gravis, digitalis intoxication, heart block, and escape beats. Anorexia, vomiting, diarrhea, vagolytic response, urine retention, weakness, hypotension, and decreased cardiac contractility are reported. Sinus node suppression, ventricular tachycardia, atrioventricular block, and prolongation of the PR, QRS, and QT intervals also are reported. A paradoxical acceleration in ventricular rate may occur, especially when the drug is used to treat patients with atrial flutter or fibrillation. In these cases, quinidine often is used after patients have first been given a digitalis glycoside. Quinidine intoxication can be antagonized by rapid alkalinization of the blood with sodium bicarbonate. Drug dose should be decreased in cases with liver disease, congestive heart failure, hyperkalemia, or hypoalbuminemia.

DRUG INTERACTIONS: Quinidine increases serum digoxin levels. Cimetidine increases serum quinidine levels. Phenothiazines potentiate the cardiac depressive effects of quinidine. Quinidine potentiates the neuromuscular blocking effects of curariform and depolarizing blocking agents and those induced by neomycin and kanamycin. Anticholinergic drugs have additive vagolytic effects. Phenobarbital and phenytoin decrease the half-life of quinidine, necessitating a readjustment of drug dose. Sodium bicarbonate, antacids, and thiazide diuretics prolong the half-life of quinidine, predisposing to toxicity. Verapamil potentiates hypotension, and nifedipine decreases quinidine serum concentrations, predisposing to breakthrough ventricular tachycardia. Quinidine may enhance the hypotensive effects of β-blocking agents and vasodilators.

SUPPLIED AS: HUMAN PRODUCTS
Tablets and capsules containing 200 mg quinidine sulfate
Tablets (sustained-release) containing 300 mg quinidine sulfate
For injection containing 190 mg/mL quinidine sulfate
Tablets containing 325 mg quinidine gluconate
Tablets (sustained-release) containing 324 mg quinidine gluconate
Tablets containing 275 mg quinidine polygalacturonate (equivalent
to 200 mg quinidine sulfate)

OTHER USES
Dogs and Cats
ATRIAL FIBRILLATION
6 to 8 mg/kg qid; IM

RANITIDINE

INDICATIONS: Ranitidine (Zantac ✤ ★) is a histamine (H_2) antagonist
that is used for the treatment of GI ulceration. It is more potent (5–12
times) in inhibiting gastric acid secretion than cimetidine, but it clinically is no more effective. The drug also has been used to treat gastric
hypersecretion associated with gastrinomas and systemic mastocyto-
sis. H_2 antagonists do not prevent NSAID-induced gastric ulcers, although ranitidine may prevent NSAID-induced duodenal ulceration.
Ranitidine also does not appear to protect the stomach from pred-
nisone-induced gastric hemorrhage. Unlike cimetidine, ranitidine has
less affinity for hepatic cytochrome P-450 enzyme systems, but it still
interferes with the metabolism of drugs removed by this system.

ADVERSE AND COMMON SIDE EFFECTS: Adverse effects in
small animals appear rare. Dogs given dosages greater than 225
mg/kg/day exhibited muscle tremors, vomiting, and rapid respiration. In humans, nausea and bradycardia with IV injection are reported. Pain at the injection site with IM use may occur.

DRUG INTERACTIONS: Propantheline delays absorption and increases peak concentration, thus increasing its bioavailability. Theophylline absorption from controlled-release formulations is decreased by ranitidine-induced achlorhydria. Antacids decrease GI
absorption, and concurrent use should be spaced by at least 2 hours.
Ranitidine may delay the renal clearance of procainamide, the clinical significance of which remains unclear. The drug also decreases
renal clearance of cisplatin in dogs.

SUPPLIED AS: HUMAN PRODUCTS
Tablets containing 150 and 300 mg
Oral syrup containing 15 mg/mL
For injection containing 25 mg/mL

RIFAMPIN

INDICATIONS: Rifampin (Rifadin ✤ ★, Rimactane ✤ ★) is an antibiotic used alone or in combination with other agents in the treatment of actinomycosis, *Coxiella burnetii* (Q Fever), feline leprosy, listeriosis, Rocky Mountain spotted fever, and tuberculosis. It is active against staphylococcus and other intracellular organisms, e.g., Chlamydia. The drug also may be useful in the treatment of chronic staphylococcal infection, e.g., severe pyoderma and chronic osteomyelitis, but it always should be used with another antibiotic because resistance develops rapidly.

ADVERSE AND COMMON SIDE EFFECTS: Hepatopathy and discoloration of the urine are reported. Although rare, anorexia, vomiting, diarrhea, thrombocytopenia, hemolytic anemia, and death have been reported in humans.

DRUG INTERACTIONS: Rifampin induces hepatic microsomal enzyme activity, which may contribute to decreased serum levels of barbiturate drugs, benzodiazepines, chloramphenicol, corticosteroid drugs, dapsone, digitoxin, metoprolol, propranolol, and quinidine. Serum levels of ketoconazole also may be reduced if the drugs are used concurrently.

SUPPLIED AS: HUMAN PRODUCT
Capsules containing 150 and 300 mg

OTHER USES
Dogs
ASPERGILLOSIS AND HISTOPLASMOSIS
10 to 20 mg/kg tid; PO with amphotericin and flucytosine

ACTINOMYCOSIS
10 to 20 mg/kg bid; PO

Cats
ASPERGILLOSIS AND HISTOPLASMOSIS
10 to 20 mg/kg tid; PO with amphotericin and flucytosine

SELEGILINE

INDICATIONS: Selegiline or l-deprenyl (Anipryl ✤, Eldepryl ✤ ★) is a selective, irreversible MAO inhibitor (predominantly type B). It is marketed for the treatment of uncomplicated pituitary-dependent hyperadrenocorticism in dogs. Pituitary-dependent hyperadrenocorticism in dogs may be related to a deficiency of dopamine. In healthy dogs, dopamine serves to inhibit ACTH secretion from the pituitary gland. Anipryl helps restore brain dopamine, facilitates its transmission, increases its synthesis, and inhibits its re-uptake. The drug is started at an oral dose of 1 mg/kg/day and continued for a period of 2 months, during which time response is evaluated on the basis of history and physical examination. If a beneficial response is not seen during this time, the dose is increased to a maximum of 2 mg/kg/day. Beneficial effects generally are noted within the first 2 months of therapy. It also may be used to manage cognitive dysfunction disorders in dogs recognized as various geriatric-onset–related behavioral disorders, e.g., geriatric-onset inappropriate urination. In addition to its effects on dopamine, the drug is known to decrease the production of and increase the clearance of free radicals and exert a protective effect on damaged neurons.

ADVERSE AND COMMON SIDE EFFECTS: In dogs, at doses of 2 mg/kg/day, no untoward clinical effects or laboratory abnormalities were seen over a course of 2 months.

DRUG INTERACTIONS: The concurrent use of meperidine or other opiates should be avoided. Stupor, muscle rigidity, agitation, and increased body temperature have been reported in humans. Fourteen days should be allotted between the discontinuation of Anipryl and the initiation of a tricyclic antidepressant, e.g., amitriptyline or imipramine, and the drug should not be given to animals concurrently receiving MAO inhibitors, e.g., possibly amitraz.

SUPPLIED AS: HUMAN PRODUCT [Eldepryl]
Tablets containing 5 mg
VETERINARY PRODUCT [Anipryl]
Tablets containing 2, 5, and 15 mg

SODIUM BICARBONATE

INDICATIONS: Sodium bicarbonate is indicated for the treatment of metabolic acidosis and the management of hyperkalemia and hypercalcemia.

ADVERSE AND COMMON SIDE EFFECTS: The agent is contraindicated in cases with alkalosis, significant chloride loss associated with vomiting, or with hypocalcemia where infusion of this agent will predispose to hypocalcemic tetany. Sodium bicarbonate should be used with caution in those with potential volume overload, e.g., congestive heart failure and renal disease. Hypercapnia predisposing to ventricular fibrillation may occur in patients during cardiopulmonary resuscitation if adequate ventilatory support is not given.

The use of this drug may cause metabolic alkalosis, hypokalemia, hypocalcemia, hypernatremia, volume overload, and paradoxical CSF acidosis leading to respiratory arrest. Myocardial depression and peripheral vasodilation leading to hypotension, hyperosmolality, CSF acidosis, increased intracranial pressure, and intracranial hemorrhage have been reported. Caution should be used when administering this agent to cats at doses greater than 2 mEq/kg because of the potential for serious acid–base and electrolyte changes.

DRUG INTERACTIONS: If sodium bicarbonate is mixed with calcium-containing fluids, insoluble complexes may form. The action of epinephrine is impaired if it is mixed with sodium bicarbonate. Oral sodium bicarbonate may reduce the absorption of anticholinergic agents, cimetidine, ranitidine, iron products, ketoconazole, and tetracycline antibiotics and reduce the efficacy of sucralfate. Orally administered drugs are best given 2 hours before or after sodium bicarbonate. The alkalinization of urine decreases the urinary excretion of quinidine and ephedrine, whereas the excretion of weakly acidic drugs, e.g., salicylates, is increased.

SUPPLIED AS: VETERINARY PRODUCT
For injection containing 8.4% (1 mEq/mL) ★

HUMAN PRODUCTS
Tablets containing 325 mg (5 gr), 520 mg (8 gr), and 650 mg (10 gr) ★
Tablets containing 500 mg ✦
For injection containing 4.2% (0.5 mEq/mL), 7.5% (0.9 mEq/mL), and 8.4% (1 mEq/mL) ✦ ★

SODIUM CHLORIDE

INDICATIONS: Sodium chloride ✦ ★ is recommended for the treatment of hyponatremia and metabolic alkalosis, the restoration of normovolemia, and the promotion of urinary calcium excretion. It is not recommended for maintenance fluid requirements because of its supraphysiologic levels of sodium and chloride in solution. Hypertonic sodium chloride (3–5%) has been used in cases of sodium depletion associated with a relative increase in body water (syndrome of inappropriate antidiuretic hormone secretion). Isotonic sodium chloride (0.9%) remains in the extracellular space (two thirds in the interstitial space, one third in the intravascular space) after IV injection. Half-strength saline (0.45%) is directed into the intracellular space (one third) and extracellular space (two thirds) after IV administration. Hypertonic saline (7.5%) has been used successfully to reverse the pathologic effects of hemorrhagic/hypovolemic shock in the dog. The effect is almost immediate and of short duration. Plasma volume expansion is negligible in 30 to 60 minutes. Hypertonic saline in conjunction with 6% dextran 70 (5 mL/kg; IV over 5 minutes) is more effective than hypertonic saline used alone in the treatment of hypovolemic shock.

ADVERSE AND COMMON SIDE EFFECTS: Excessive volumes of 0.9% saline may cause hyperchloremic metabolic acidosis and hypokalemia, especially in patients with diarrhea in whom sodium loss is greater than chloride and in those patients in whom the kidney cannot excrete the excess chloride load. Volume overload and pulmonary edema are potential concerns in animals with cardiac or renal insufficiency. Hypernatremia also may occur and lead to irritability, lethargy, weakness, ataxia, stupor, coma, and seizure.

Adverse effects noted with hypertonic saline may include cardiovascular collapse if the product is administered too rapidly, increase in sodium and chloride concentrations, and in osmolality, a decrease in potassium and bicarbonate concentrations, bradyarrhythmias, bronchoconstriction, hemolysis, hemoglobinuria, and signs of pain if the solution is injected into small peripheral veins.

DRUG INTERACTIONS: Glucocorticoids and corticotrophin may predispose to sodium retention and volume overload, especially in patients with congestive heart failure.

SUPPLIED AS: HUMAN and VETERINARY PRODUCTS
For injection containing 0.45% (77 mEq/L) sodium and chloride
For injection containing 0.9% (154 mEq/L) sodium and chloride
For injection containing 3% (513 mEq/L) sodium and chloride
For injection containing 5% (855 mEq/L) sodium and chloride
For injection containing 7% (7 g/100 mL) [HyperSaline-7 ★]
Tablets containing 300 and 600 mg

OTHER USES
Dogs
SHOCK
i) 7.5% saline: 4 to 5 mL/kg slowly over 8 to 10 minutes or longer; IV

Note: 7.5% saline is not available commercially but can be prepared by withdrawing 120 mL of 5% saline and mixing it with 60 mL of 23.4% saline

ii) 7.5% saline in hydroxyethyl starch (Hespan) at 4 mL/kg; IV push, then give additional Hespan at 20 mL/kg; IV push; follow with Plasmalyte, Normosol R, or lactated Ringer's solution; IV to effect

iii) 7% saline in 6% dextran 70 at a dosage of 5 mL/kg given slowly over a 5-minute period; IV, followed by lactated Ringer's solution at a dosage of 20 mL/kg/hour

Cats
SHOCK
7.5% saline alone or in combination with 6% dextran 70; slowly IV at a dose of 3 to 5 mL/kg

Note: Hypertonic saline provokes a rapid improvement in cardiovascular function in cats with hypovolemia; the duration of effect lasts only 15 to 60 minutes. Hypertonic saline combined with dextrose provides a more prolonged effect.

SODIUM IODIDE

INDICATIONS: Sodium iodide ✤ ★ is an antifungal agent used in the treatment of the cutaneous and lymphocutaneous forms of sporotrichosis in small animals.

ADVERSE AND COMMON SIDE EFFECTS: Adverse effects include vomiting, anorexia, lacrimation, depression, cardiomegaly, and cutaneous reactions that generally are reversible when the drug dose is decreased. Nausea can be lessened by mixing the drug with milk before administration. Cats are especially sensitive to iodide toxicosis, necessitating a reduction in drug dosage.

Toxicity in cats is manifested by hypothermia, muscle spasms, depression, vomiting, and diarrhea.

DRUG INTERACTIONS: None reported.

SUPPLIED AS: VETERINARY PRODUCT
For injection containing 200 mg/mL [20%] (large animal product)

SODIUM POLYSTYRENE SULFONATE

INDICATIONS: Sodium polystyrene sulfonate (Kayexalate ✤ ★) is a sulfonic cation-exchange resin. The drug is used to lower serum potassium levels in patients with hyperkalemia by the exchange of sodium for potassium.

ADVERSE AND COMMON SIDE EFFECTS: The drug should be used with caution in patients with renal failure or those who cannot tolerate an increase in serum sodium levels, e.g., patients with congestive heart failure, severe hypertension, or marked edema. Hypokalemia, hypocalcemia, anorexia, nausea, vomiting, diarrhea, and/or constipation have been reported.

DRUG INTERACTIONS: Digitalis toxicity may be potentiated. The efficacy may be reduced by the concurrent use of antacids or laxatives containing magnesium or calcium.

SUPPLIED AS: HUMAN PRODUCT
Oral suspension prepared in the sodium phase with exchange capacity in vitro of approximately 3.1 mmol (in vivo approximately 1 mmol) potassium per g sodium 4.1 mmol (94.3 mg)/g

SPECTINOMYCIN

INDICATIONS: Spectinomycin (Trobicin ✤ ★) is an aminocyclitol broad-spectrum antibiotic effective against gram-negative bacteria including *E. coli, Klebsiella, Salmonella, Proteus,* and *Enterobacter* organisms, as well as gram-positive bacteria, including streptococci and staphylococci. The drug is related structurally to the aminoglycosides, and it shares many similar properties to this group of antibiotics, including minimal protein binding, primary renal excretion, and high water solubility. Spectinomycin, however, is less toxic than the aminoglycosides. It is not ototoxic or nephrotoxic. Penetration into ocular tissue is minimal, and it only enters CSF if active inflammation is present.

ADVERSE AND COMMON SIDE EFFECTS: Neuromuscular blockade is a rare side effect that can be reversed by parenteral calcium administration.

DRUG INTERACTIONS: Antagonism may occur if the drug is used concurrently with chloramphenicol or tetracycline. Spectinomycin is synergistic with lincomycin against mycoplasma organisms.

SUPPLIED AS: HUMAN PRODUCT
For injection containing spectinomycin hydrochloride equivalent to 2 and 4 g spectinomycin base

SPIRONOLACTONE

INDICATIONS: Spironolactone (Aldactone ✤ ★) is a potassium-sparing diuretic agent used alone or in combination with other diuretics in the management of edema unresponsive to other diuretics. The drug inhibits the action of aldosterone in the distal renal tubules. It is indicated when hypokalemia is a concern and diuresis is indicated. Desired clinical response generally takes 2 to 3 days, and clinical effects persist for an additional 2 to 3 days after cessation of drug use.

ADVERSE AND COMMON SIDE EFFECTS: The drug is contraindicated in patients with hyperkalemia, anuria, or renal failure. Hyperkalemia and dehydration may occur. Vomiting, anorexia, lethargy, and ataxia also may occur. Safe use of the drug during pregnancy has not been established, and spironolactone inhibits the synthesis of testosterone.

DRUG INTERACTIONS: Spironolactone increases the half-life of digoxin and may increase or decrease the half-life of digitoxin, necessitating monitoring of serum digitalis levels. Spironolactone may decrease the effects of mitotane. The combination of spironolactone and ammonium chloride may produce systemic acidosis. The di-

uretic action of spironolactone may be antagonized by aspirin and
other salicylates. The concurrent use of other potassium-sparing diuretics, e.g., triamterene, may predispose to hyperkalemia as may
the concurrent use of indomethacin, captopril, and enalapril.

SUPPLIED AS: HUMAN PRODUCT
Tablets containing 25, 50, and 100 mg

STANOZOLOL

INDICATIONS: Stanozolol (Winstrol-V ✤ ★) is an anabolic steroid
with strong anabolic and weak androgenic activity. It is potentially
useful as an adjunct to the management of catabolic disease states.
The drug has been used to stimulate erythropoiesis, arouse appetite,
promote weight gain, and increase strength and vitality. The efficacy
of promoting these positive changes is questionable, and prolonged
treatment (3–6 months) may be required before a response in the
erythron is seen. The drug may be of benefit in animals with chronic
renal failure by stimulating appetite, promoting muscle protein synthesis, reversing catabolism, and enhancing general well-being. It
has been demonstrated to have positive effects on nitrogen balance
and lean body mass in dogs with mild to moderate chronic renal failure. Also see **ANABOLIC STEROIDS.**

ADVERSE AND COMMON SIDE EFFECTS: The drug should be
used with caution in animals with cardiac or renal insufficiency and
in those with hypercalcemia. It may promote sodium and water retention and exacerbate azotemia, and it also may promote hypercalcemia, hyperphosphatemia, and hyperkalemia. It should not be used
in patients with neoplastic disease. The drug is potentially hepatotoxic. Stanozolol should not be used in pregnant animals because of
possible masculinization of the fetus.

DRUG INTERACTIONS: Anabolic agents may potentiate the effect
of anticoagulants. Anabolic agents may decrease blood glucose and
decrease insulin requirements of diabetic patients, and these drugs
may potentiate water retention associated with the use of ACTH or
adrenal steroids.

SUPPLIED AS: VETERINARY PRODUCTS
Tablets containing 2 mg
For injection containing 50 mg/mL

OTHER USES
Dogs
ANEMIA SECONDARY TO CHRONIC RENAL FAILURE
i)   1 to 4 mg once daily; PO
ii) 2 to 10 mg bid; PO

ANABOLIC/APPETITE STIMULANT
i)   1 to 4 mg bid; PO

ii) 25 to 50 mg weekly; IM

Cats

ANEMIA SECONDARY TO CHRONIC RENAL FAILURE
1 to 4 mg once daily; PO

SUCRALFATE

INDICATIONS: Sucralfate (Carafate ★, Sulcrate ♣) accelerates the healing of oral, esophageal, gastric, and duodenal ulcers. It forms a complex with proteinaceous exudates that adheres to the ulcer, providing a protective barrier to the penetration of gastric acid. Sucralfate stimulates prostaglandin production, increases mucus production and mucosal turnover, inactivates pepsin, and absorbs bile acids. Sucralfate may be useful for the prevention of NSAID-induced ulceration. Sucralfate normalizes serum phosphorous levels, which makes it of potential benefit in cases of secondary hyperparathyroidism associated with renal failure.

ADVERSE AND COMMON SIDE EFFECTS: Side effects are rare. Constipation is the only significant problem reported in small animals.

DRUG INTERACTIONS: Antacids and H_2-blocking agents decrease gastric pH and reduce the efficacy of sucralfate and should be spaced apart by at least 1/2 hour. Sucralfate decreases the bioavailability of digoxin, cimetidine, phenytoin, and tetracycline antibiotics. Concurrent oral drug administration should be separated by 2 hours.

SUPPLIED AS: HUMAN PRODUCTS
Tablets containing 1 g
Suspension containing 1 g per 10 mL

SULFADIMETHOXINE

INDICATIONS: Sulfadimethoxine (Albon ★, SULFA 125 and 250 ♣) is a sulfonamide drug used in small animals for the treatment of respiratory, genitourinary, enteric, and soft tissue infections caused by susceptible organisms, including streptococci, staphylococci, *Escherichia, Salmonella, Klebsiella, Proteus,* and *Shigella.* It also is used for the eradication of coccidiosis in dogs, although it is not licensed for this purpose.

ADVERSE AND COMMON SIDE EFFECTS: See SULFONAMIDE ANTIBIOTICS.

DRUG INTERACTIONS: Intramuscular injection is associated with pain and poor blood drug levels and is not recommended. See **SULFONAMIDE ANTIBIOTICS.**

SUPPLIED AS: VETERINARY PRODUCTS
Tablets containing 125, 250, and 500 mg [Albon, SULFA 125 and 250]
Oral suspension containing 50 mg/mL [Albon]
For injection containing 400 mg/mL [Albon]

SULFASALAZINE

INDICATIONS: Sulfasalazine (Azulfidine ★, Salazopyrin ✦) is used in the management of inflammatory bowel disease in the dog and cat. In the colon, bacteria degrade the drug to release aminosalicylic acid and sulfapyridine. The aminosalicylic acid exerts an anti-inflammatory effect by inhibiting prostaglandin synthesis. It also may inhibit the lipoxygenase pathway, and hydroxyeicosatetraenoic and leukotriene synthesis. Sulfasalazine may have immunosuppressive properties, especially on B lymphocytes. Other actions include antibacterial effects, scavenging of reactive oxygen, and inhibition of fibrinolysis.

ADVERSE AND COMMON SIDE EFFECTS: The drug should not be used in animals with sensitivity to salicylates or sulfonamides. It should be used with caution in animals with liver, renal, or hematologic disease. Vomiting, cholestasis, exacerbation of colitis, fever, oligospermia, anemia, leukopenia, allergic dermatitis, and keratoconjunctivitis sicca also have been reported. A baseline Schirmer's tear test is advised before initiation of therapy, and monthly monitoring is recommended. Vomiting and anorexia may develop in cats. The use of enteric-coated tablets may alleviate these signs.

DRUG INTERACTIONS: Antibiotics may alter metabolism of sulfasalazine by altering intestinal flora. Sulfasalazine may displace highly protein-bound drugs, such as methotrexate, phenytoin, phenylbutazone, salicylates, thiazide diuretics, and warfarin. Antacids may decrease absorption. Phenobarbital may decrease the urinary excretion of sulfasalazine. Sulfasalazine may decrease the bioavailability of folic acid and digoxin.

SUPPLIED AS: HUMAN PRODUCTS
Tablets containing 500 mg
Tablets (enteric-coated) containing 500 mg
Oral suspension containing 50 mg/mL [Azulfidine]

SULFONAMIDE ANTIBIOTICS

INDICATIONS: The sulfonamide antibiotics are bacteriostatic drugs that are effective against streptococci, *Bacillus, Corynebac-*

terium, Nocardia, Brucella, Campylobacter, Pasteurella, and *Chlamydia. Pseudomonas, Serratia,* and *Klebsiella* generally are resistant. The sulfonamides readily enter the CSF and are effective in treating meningeal infections. These drugs are ineffective in the presence of pus and necrotic tissue. The combination of a sulfonamide with trimethoprim or pyrimethamine "potentiated sulfonamides," such as trimethoprim–sulfadiazine (Tribrissen), greatly enhances antimicrobial activity. The enhanced spectrum includes *E. coli, Proteus, Salmonella, Staphylococcus, Klebsiella,* and *Streptococcus.* Another example of a potentiated sulfa is the sulfadimethoxine–ormetoprim combination (Primor ★). This agent is indicated in the treatment of skin and soft tissue infections caused by *Staphylococcus aureus* and *E. coli.*

Sulfonamides are classified according to their duration of effect. Short-acting sulfonamides require dosing at 8-hour intervals and include sulfadiazine, sulfamerazine, sulfamethazine, and sulfamethoxazole, and generally are indicated in the treatment of systemic and urinary tract infections; intermediate-acting sulfonamides require dosing every 12 to 24 hours and include sulfisoxazole and sulfadimethoxine, which primarily are indicated in the treatment of urinary tract infections; and long-acting sulfonamides require dosing every few days and includes sulfadoxine which has been used primarily in humans for the treatment of chronic bronchitis and urinary tract infections.

ADVERSE AND COMMON SIDE EFFECTS: Precipitation and crystalluria generally are not a problem in small animals, but sulfonamides should be used with caution in patients with preexisting renal disease, especially if complicated by dehydration or metabolic acidosis. In dogs given high doses of sulfonamides, sulfonamide cystic urolithiasis can develop. Azotemia and renal failure may develop in cats during sulfonamide or trimethoprim–sulfonamide therapy.

Potentially irreversible keratoconjunctivitis sicca (KCS) has been the most common problem with long-term use of these drugs (sulfadiazine, sulfasalazine). Generally, long-term use (3–4 months) of sulfadiazine is necessary before KCS occurs. Pruritus and photosensitization have been reported, and alopecia may occur with long-term use. Other reported conditions associated with the use of these drugs include polyarthritis, urticaria, facial swelling, fever, hemolytic anemia, polydipsia, polyuria, hepatitis, vomiting, diarrhea, anorexia, and seizure. Hypersensitivity, including anaphylaxis, although rare, also has been documented.

Sulfadimethoxine–ormetoprim should not be given to dogs with liver damage or blood dyscrasias, or those with a history of sulfonamide sensitivity. This drug combination should be used with caution in those with thyroid disease. Safety has not been established in pregnant animals. Long-term therapy at recommended doses resulted in elevation in serum cholesterol, increases in thyroid and liver weights, and enlarged basophilic cells in the pituitary. Potentiated sulfonamides may cause iatrogenic hypothyroidism, as noted by low serum thyroxine levels. It is reversible when sulfonamide treatment is discontinued.

DRUG INTERACTIONS: Antacids decrease the absorption of sulfonamides. Methenamine and other acidifying agents increase the risk of sulfonamide crystalliazion in the urine. Para-amenobenzoic acid and local anesthetics may antagonize sulfonamide action. Phenothiazines may increase the toxic effects of sulfonamides.

SUPPLIED AS: VETERINARY PRODUCTS
Tablets containing 100 mg sulfadimethoxine and 20 mg ormetoprim [Primor]
Tablets containing 200 mg sulfadimethoxine and 40 mg ormetoprim [Primor]
Tablets containing 500 mg sulfadimethoxine and 100 mg ormetoprim [Primor]
Tablets containing 1,000 mg sulfadimethoxine and 200 mg ormetoprim [Primor]
For other drugs, see individual product.

OTHER USES
Cats

TOXOPLASMOSIS
15 mg/kg qid; PO (sulfadiazine or sulfamerazine) for at least 2 weeks, along with pyrimethamine at 0.5 to 1 mg/kg daily; PO

SULFUR-CONTAINING SHAMPOOS

INDICATIONS: Sulfur as a topical dermatologic agent is keratolytic, keratoplastic, antibacterial, antifungal, and antiparasitic, and a mild follicular flushing agent. It may be combined with salicylic acid and coal tar (Allerseb T ✚ ★) or with sodium salicylate (Sebbafon ✚ ★). The shampoo is indicated for the treatment of mites, lice, chiggers, some fleas, dermatophytosis, seborrhea, pyoderma, pruritus, crusts, and scales. When salicylic acid is combined with sulfur, a synergistic effect occurs, and the keratolytic effect is enhanced.

ADVERSE AND COMMON SIDE EFFECTS: Sulfur may cause scalding if the product is applied to the skin at concentrations greater than 2%. Coal tar may be especially irritating or even toxic to cats.

DRUG INTERACTIONS: None reported.

TAR-CONTAINING SHAMPOOS

INDICATIONS: Crude coal tars are used in the management of seborrhea, especially the greasy form of the disease. Tars are keratolytic, keratoplastic, antipruritic, and vasoconstrictive. Tar is available in combination with salicylic acid (Allerseb T ✢ ★).

ADVERSE AND COMMON SIDE EFFECTS: Tar shampoos may be drying and irritating to the skin.

DRUG INTERACTIONS: None reported.

TAURINE

INDICATIONS: Taurine is used in conjunction with appropriate supportive therapy in the management of feline-dilated cardiomyopathy. Taurine may contribute to the inotropic, metabolic, and osmotic function of the myocardium. It has been concluded that American cocker spaniels with dilated cardiomyopathy are taurine deficient and are responsive to taurine and carnitine supplementation. Although myocardial function did not return to normal, it improved sufficiently enough to allow discontinuation of cardiovascular drug therapy. Taurine deficiency also has been associated with feline central retinal degeneration and reproductive problems characterized by poor growth, survival, and abnormalities of kittens born to taurine-deficient queens. One investigator has used taurine in conjunction with vitamin B_6 in cats with recurrent seizures. In cases of hepatic lipidosis, supplemental taurine (250–500 mg/day; PO) and l-carnitine (250 mg/day; PO) are given for the first several weeks, with strict attention to caloric intake.

ADVERSE AND COMMON SIDE EFFECTS: No long-term side effects have been reported.

DRUG INTERACTIONS: None reported.

SUPPLIED AS: VETERINARY PRODUCT
Tablets containing 250 mg [Taurine Tablets ✢, Formula V Taurine Tablets ★]

OTHER USES
Cats
SEIZURES
500 mg bid; PO together with vitamin B_6

Dogs
AMERICAN COCKER SPANIEL DILATED CARDIOMYOPATHY
500 mg taurine bid–tid; PO with 1 g carnitine bid–tid; PO

TERBUTALINE

INDICATIONS: Terbutaline (Bricanyl ✣ ★) is a synthetic adrenergic stimulant with selective β-2 and negligible β-1 agonist activity. It is useful as a bronchodilator. The drug also has been used in the management of some cases of first- and second-degree heart block.

ADVERSE AND COMMON SIDE EFFECTS: The drug should not be given to patients with tachycardia associated with digitalis intoxication or glaucoma, nor should it be used within 14 days of the use of an MAO inhibitor, e.g., possibly amitraz and selegiline. The drug should be used with caution in patients with hypertension, diabetes mellitus, thyrotoxicosis, a history of seizure disorders, cardiac arrhythmias, and renal or hepatic dysfunction. Side effects may include tachycardia, hypotension or hypertension, nausea, vomiting, tremor, fatigue, or seizure activity. Treatment of terbutaline toxicosis may include volume expansion to mitigate hypotension and β-blocking agents, e.g., propranolol (dogs: 5–40 mg tid; PO or 0.1–0.3 mg/kg; IV).

DRUG INTERACTIONS: Propranolol antagonizes the bronchodilatory effect of terbutaline. Concurrent use of MAO inhibitors may cause severe hypertension. Use with other sympathetic agents may potentiate the risk of arrhythmias.

SUPPLIED AS: HUMAN PRODUCTS
Tablets containing 2.5 and 5 mg
For injection containing 1 mg/mL ★
Aerosol containing 200 μg per metered spray ★ and 500 μg per metered spray ✣

OTHER USES
Dogs
FIRST- and SECOND-DEGREE HEART BLOCK
2.5 to 5 mg bid–tid; PO

TESTOSTERONE

INDICATIONS: Testosterone is an androgenic steroid used principally in small animals for the management of hormone-responsive urinary incontinence in the neutered male. Veto-Test is marketed in Canada for use in animals with impotence, testicular deficiency, cryptorchidism (in the absence of anatomic defects), and as an aid in the treatment of mammary tumors in bitches. Also see **ANABOLIC STEROIDS.**

ADVERSE AND COMMON SIDE EFFECTS: The drug is contraindicated in patients with prostatic carcinoma. It should be used with caution in those with renal, hepatic, or cardiac disease. Prostatic enlargement and recurrence or exacerbation of perianal adenoma or perianal hernia, as well as behavioral problems, occasionally are reported. Chronic use or high doses may result in oligospermia or infertility in intact males.

DRUG INTERACTIONS: Testosterone may decrease blood glucose concentrations and decrease the requirement for insulin in diabetic patients. The drug may enhance bleeding tendencies in patients taking oral anticoagulants. Androgens may potentiate edema associated with ACTH or adrenal steroid therapy, the significance of which in small animals is unknown.

SUPPLIED AS: VETERINARY PRODUCT
For injection containing 100 mg/mL testosterone [Veto-Test ♣]
HUMAN PRODUCTS
For injection containing 100 and 200 mg/mL testosterone cypionate in oil [Depo-Testosterone ♣ ★]
For injection containing 100 and 200 mg/mL testosterone enanthate in oil [Malogex ♣]
For injection containing 25, 50, and 100 mg/mL testosterone propionate in oil [Malogen ♣, Testex ★]

TETRACYCLINE ANTIBIOTICS

INDICATIONS: The tetracycline antibiotics exert a bacteriostatic effect against many aerobic and anaerobic gram-positive and gram-negative bacteria, spirochetes, mycoplasma, and rickettsiae organisms. These drugs are classified as short-acting/water soluble (tetracycline, oxytetracycline, chlortetracycline), intermediate-acting (demeclocycline), and long-acting/lipid soluble (minocycline, doxycycline). Tetracycline antibiotics are especially useful against *Leptospira, Chlamydia, Brucella, Mycoplasma, Pseudomonas, Rickettsia,* and *Actinomyces* organisms. They also are used in the treatment of protozoan infections. Minocycline is the most effective of this group against *Nocardia* and *Staphylococcus.* Minocycline and doxycycline are second-generation lipid-soluble tetracyclines and are more effective against anaerobes and intracellular bacteria such as *Brucella canis.* These two agents readily diffuse into the eye, brain, CSF, and prostate gland. However, they do not reach sufficient concentrations in the urine to be effective in the treatment of urinary tract infections.

ADVERSE AND COMMON SIDE EFFECTS: Tetracyclines, with the exception of doxycycline, should be avoided in patients with renal failure because of delayed excretion. Tetracyclines, especially chlortetracycline, inhibit protein synthesis. Nausea, vomiting, diarrhea, dose-related renal tubular damage, and metabolic acidosis have been reported. Discoloration of the teeth may occur if these drugs (especially dimethyl chlortetracycline and tetracycline) are given to pregnant bitches in the last 2 to 3 weeks of pregnancy or to puppies in the first 4 weeks after birth. Anaphylaxis associated with the use of parenteral tetracyclines occasionally has been noted in dogs and cats. Hypotension, shock, and urticaria developed in dogs given rapid IV doses of minocycline. Thrombophlebitis frequently occurs after IV injection of tetracycline and is seen more frequently with lipid-soluble tetracyclines. Intramuscular injection is painful and irritating. Intravascular injection of minocycline (10–20 mg/kg daily for 1 month) in dogs has been associated with decreased erythrocyte counts, hemoglobin concentration, and hematocrit and elevations in serum alanine transferase (ALT) activity. Cats are especially sensitive to these drugs. Fever, vomiting, diarrhea, colic, depression, ptyalism, anorexia, and increased serum ALT activity are reported in this species.

DRUG INTERACTIONS: Absorption is decreased by the concurrent use of antacids, antidiarrheal compounds, laxatives, iron, aluminum, or calcium-containing products, including kaolin and pectin or bismuth, and dairy products. Sodium bicarbonate may interfere with absorption of oral tetracyclines by increasing gastric pH. Doxycycline and minocycline are less affected by food or oral products and often are given with food to reduce GI irritation. Tetracyclines potentiate the catabolic effects of glucocorticoids and may contribute to cachexia. In addition, concurrent use of corticosteroids may allow the emergence of resistant organisms during prolonged therapy and may mask clinical signs of infection. Bacteriostatic drugs such as tetracyclines may decrease the bactericidal activity of penicillin, cephalosporin, and aminoglycoside antibiotics. Tetracyclines may increase the bioavailability of digoxin, predisposing to toxicity in a small number of patients, the effects of which can persist for months after discontinuation of the tetracycline. Tetracyclines may potentiate the anticoagulant activity of warfarin, decreasing the dose of the anticoagulant required. Gastrointestinal side effects may be potentiated by theophylline. Tetracyclines may reduce insulin requirements in diabetic patients. Methoxyflurane may contribute to the possibility of nephrotoxicity. Tetracyclines inhibit hepatic microsomal enzymes and may delay the elimination of drugs metabolized by the liver.

SUPPLIED AS: See specific product.

OTHER USES
Dogs
GASTROINTESTINAL BACTERIAL OVERGROWTH
Tetracycline at 10 to 20 mg/kg bid; PO for 1 month

LYME BORRELIOSIS
Tetracycline at 5 mg/kg tid; PO for 10 to 14 days

THEOPHYLLINE

INDICATIONS: Theophylline (Theo-Dur ✿ ★, Theolair ✿ ★, Quibron-T/SR ✿ ★, Slo-Bid ✿ ★) is a bronchodilator indicated for the management of cough due to bronchospasm. It has mild inotropic properties and a mild, transient diuretic activity. Serum levels are measured after steady-state serum levels have been attained (29 hours in the dog, 40 hours in the cat) and just before the next dose. The therapeutic range is 10 to 20 µg/mL (55–110 µmol/L). Toxic blood levels are in excess of 25 µg/mL.

ADVERSE AND COMMON SIDE EFFECTS: The drug should be used with caution in patients with cardiac disease, systemic hypertension, cardiac arrhythmias, GI ulcers, impaired renal or hepatic function, diabetes mellitus, hyperthyroid disease, and glaucoma. Side effects may include nausea, vomiting, anorexia or polyphagia, diarrhea, polydipsia, polyuria, restlessness, muscle twitching, cardiac arrhythmias, tachycardia, hyperglycemia, and nervousness. Seizure activity may occur with marked drug overdose.

DRUG INTERACTIONS: Serum levels may be increased by the concurrent use of thiabendazole, cimetidine, allopurinol, clindamycin, lincomycin, and erythromycin. Phenobarbital and phenytoin decrease the therapeutic effect of the drug. Concurrent use of aluminum or magnesium antacid preparations slows the absorption of theophylline. Propranolol has direct antagonistic effects because propranolol is a β-adrenergic blocking agent and theophylline is a β-adrenergic stimulant. Phenytoin increases theophylline clearance, requiring larger doses of the drug for a clinically beneficial effect. Halothane may increase the incidence of cardiac arrhythmias. Ketamine may cause an increase incidence of seizure activity.

Concurrent use of this drug with allopurinol, cimetidine, furosemide, or epinephrine may cause excessive CNS stimulation.

SUPPLIED AS: HUMAN PRODUCTS
Tablets [Theo-Dur] and capsules [Slo-Bid] (timed-release) containing 50, 100, 200, 300, and 450 mg and additional strengths
Oral liquid containing 80 mg/15 mL [Theolair]

OTHER USES
Cats

SINUS BRADYCARDIA
25 mg/kg once daily in the evening; PO (sustained-release formulation)

THIABENDAZOLE

INDICATIONS: Thiabendazole (Equizole ★, Mintezol ★, Thibenzole ★) is used in the treatment of aspergillosis, and penicilliosis and for the elimination of *Toxocara canis, Toxascaris leonina, Strongyloides stercoralis,* and *Filaroides* infections in dogs. The drug also has been used in the treatment of *Oslerus osleri* infestation in a dog.

ADVERSE AND COMMON SIDE EFFECTS: Initially, anorexia, vomiting, and diarrhea may be noted. If these occur, it is best to discontinue medication for several days and reinstitute the drug at half the dose for 1 week, then gradually increase the dose to the recommended level. The drug should be given with food to enhance absorption and to decrease anorexia. Hair loss also has been reported. Dachshunds may be especially sensitive to the drug.

DRUG INTERACTIONS: Thiabendazole may compete with theophylline and aminophylline for metabolism in the liver, resulting in increased serum levels of the latter two drugs.

SUPPLIED AS: VETERINARY PRODUCTS (large animal products)
Oral suspension containing 4 g/fl oz (135 mg/mL) [Equizole] and 25 g/fl oz (845 mg/mL) [TBZ Cattle Wormer ★]

HUMAN PRODUCTS
Tablets containing 500 mg [Mintezol]
Oral suspension containing 100 mg/mL [Mintezol]

OTHER USES
Dogs
STRONGYLOIDES STERCORALIS
50 to 60 mg/kg; PO

FILAROIDES INFECTIONS
i)   30 to 70 mg/kg div. bid; PO in food for 20 to 45 days

ii) 70 mg/kg bid; PO for 2 days then 35 mg/kg bid; PO for 20 days

ASPERGILLOSIS/PENICILLIOSIS
i)   30 to 70 mg/kg div. bid; PO for 20 to 45 days

ii) 20 mg/kg once daily or div. bid; PO for 6 to 8 weeks

OSLERUS OSLERI
35 mg/kg bid; PO for 5 days, followed by 70 mg/kg bid; PO for 21 days

THIACETARSAMIDE

INDICATIONS: Thiacetarsamide (Caparsolate ♣ ★) is used for the eradication of adult heartworms (*Dirofilaria immitis*). Although not licensed for use in cats, the drug has been used in this species for elimination of adult heartworm and Hemobartonella infections.

ADVERSE AND COMMON SIDE EFFECTS: Animals with significant hepatic, renal, cardiac, or pulmonary disease should not be treated with this drug until the clinical disease has stabilized. The drug should be used with caution in animals with diabetes mellitus and adrenocortical insufficiency. Anorexia, vomiting, depression, icterus, elevation of liver enzymes, azotemia, proteinuria, hematuria, and increased numbers of urinary casts may occur. Thrombocytopenia is common from 5 to 21 days (nadir 10–14 days) after therapy is complete. Thromboembolic disease may accompany use of the drug and generally occurs 1 to 2 weeks after adulticide therapy. Extravascular injection is irritating and can cause skin sloughing. Topical treatment with hot packs and a dimethyl sulfoxide (DMSO)/steroid product (Synotic) or local infiltration of dexamethasone/saline has been suggested to limit irritation.

An idiosyncratic reaction manifested by pulmonary edema and death has been reported in some cats after use of the drug. Other adverse effects may include depression, anorexia, increased respiratory effort, and vomiting. Thiacetarsamide is not recommended by many clinicians for use in asymptomatic cats with heartworm disease.

DRUG INTERACTIONS: Glucocorticoids may have a protective effect on adult heartworms, decreasing the efficacy of thiacetarsamide. In addition, glucocorticoids may cause increased pulmonary vascular intimal proliferation, predisposing to obstruction.

SUPPLIED AS: VETERINARY PRODUCT
For injection containing 10 mg/mL

OTHER USES
Cats
HEMOBARTONELLA FELIS
i) 1 mg/kg once; IV, repeat 2 days later for a total of 2 injections
ii) 0.25 mg/kg once; IV, repeat 2 days later

THIAMINE (B₁)

INDICATIONS: Thiamine (vitamin B_1 ✤ ★) is used in the treatment of thiamine deficiency and occasionally as adjunctive therapy in cases of ethylene glycol toxicity and lead poisoning.

ADVERSE AND COMMON SIDE EFFECTS: The vitamin itself is nontoxic, but IM injection may cause muscle soreness. Deficiency of the vitamin is rare. Cats fed commercial diets or raw fish are predisposed. Clinical signs of vitamin B_1 deficiency may include anorexia, vomiting, weight loss, dehydration, paralysis, gallop heart rhythms in the presence of congestive heart failure, muscle weakness, prostration, abnormal reflexes, convulsions, ventral flexion of the neck, and dilated pupils. Laboratory abnormalities may include mild anemia, hypoproteinemia, hyperglycemia, and increased blood and urine concentrations of pyruvate and lactate.

DRUG INTERACTIONS: Thiamine may potentiate the neuromuscular blocking effect of neuromuscular blocking agents.

SUPPLIED AS: VETERINARY PRODUCT
For injection containing 100, 200, and 500 mg/mL

HUMAN PRODUCTS
Tablets containing 5, 10, 25, 50, 100, 250, and 500 mg
Elixir containing 250 µg/5 mL [Bewon]

OTHER USES
Dogs
ETHYLENE GLYCOL TOXICITY
100 mg/day; PO

THIAMYLAL SODIUM

INDICATIONS: Thiamylal sodium (Anestatal ★) is an ultrashort-acting thiobarbiturate. It is used to induce anesthesia of short duration. Induction is smooth and rapid (1–12 minutes) with minimal excitement. Recovery is dose dependent but generally is complete within 3 hours. Excitement is minimal, and the period of ataxia is short during recovery. It is more potent, has a shorter duration of activity, and is less cumulative than thiopental sodium. Also see **BARBITURATES.**

ADVERSE AND COMMON SIDE EFFECTS: The drug should not be used in animals with severe hepatic or respiratory disturbances. It should be used with caution in animals with cardiac or respiratory disease, including asthma, anemia, metabolic acidosis, ventricular arrhythmias, increased intracranial pressure, myasthenia gravis, and hypovolemia. Liver disease may delay drug detoxification, and azotemia or electrolyte imbalances may prolong anesthesia. Prolonged recovery may occur with hypothermia or cachexia, or after prolonged procedures. The greyhound and other site hound breeds metabolize thiobarbiturates slowly. Methohexital may be a more appropriate choice in these breeds. Extravascular injection is irritating and may cause pain, ulceration, and necrosis of the skin. Intra-arterial injection may cause gangrene of an extremity. The following additional adverse reactions may occur: circulatory depression, thrombophlebitis, pain at the site of injection, respiratory depression and apnea, laryngospasm, bronchospasm, salivation, emergence delirium, urticaria, nausea, and vomiting.

Premature ventricular contractions are common (60–85% of patients) and occur more often than with thiopental sodium. The incidence may be decreased by the preanesthetic use of a phenothiazine. Metabolic acidosis, uremia, and the administration of glucose augment the anesthetic affects of the drug predisposing to toxicity. Also see **BARBITURATES.**

DRUG INTERACTIONS: Death has been reported in a dog receiving Diathal and thiamylal. The incidence of ventricular arrhythmias seen with epinephrine and norepinephrine is increased when used with thiobarbiturates and halothane. Central nervous system and respiratory depression may be potentiated by the concurrent use of narcotics, phenothiazines, and antihistamines. Furosemide may cause or potentiate postural hypotension. Intravenous sulfisoxazole competes with thiopental at plasma protein-binding sites. Other sulfonamides may act similarly. Also see **BARBITURATES.**

SUPPLIED AS: VETERINARY PRODUCT
For injection in 50-mL vials containing 1 g and 250-mL vials containing 5 g

THIOPENTAL SODIUM

INDICATIONS: Thiopental sodium (Veterinary Pentothal kit ★, Pentothal ♣ ★) is an ultrashort-acting thiobarbiturate used for procedures requiring general anesthesia of short duration. Its characteristics include short action, smooth recovery, rapid elimination, and minimal side effects. Also see **THIAMYLAL SODIUM** and **BARBITURATES.**

For additional information concerning ADVERSE AND COMMON SIDE EFFECTS and DRUG INTERACTIONS, see **THIAMYLAL SODIUM** and **BARBITURATES.**

SUPPLIED AS: VETERINARY PRODUCT
For injection containing 5 g (2.5% solution) and 5 g (5% solution) [Veterinary Pentothal Kit ★]

HUMAN PRODUCT
For injection containing 250, 400, and 500 mg and 1, 2.5, 5, and 10 g thiopental base [Pentothal ♣ ★]

TICARCILLIN

INDICATIONS: Ticarcillin (Ticar ♣ ★) is an extended spectrum parenteral penicillin antibiotic with activity similar to, but more potent than, carbenicillin. In humans, the drug is active against gram-negative bacteria, including *Klebsiella pneumoniae, Proteus mirabilis* and *vulgaris, E. coli, Enterobacter aerogenes, Serratia marcescens, Pseudomonas aeruginosa,* and *Bacteroides fragilis,* and gram-positive organisms, including *Staphylococcus aureus,* coagulase-positive staphylococci, enterococci, and streptococcal organisms. Bacterial susceptibility is similar in veterinary medicine. The antibiotic is available in combination with clavulanic acid (Timentin ✦ ★) that is effective against many penicillinase-producing strains of bacteria.

ADVERSE AND COMMON SIDE EFFECTS: Use is contraindicated in animals with hypersensitivity to penicillins or the cephalosporins. Intramuscular injection may cause pain. Also see **PENICILLIN ANTIBIOTICS.**

DRUG INTERACTIONS: Ticarcillin is physically and/or chemically incompatible with aminoglycosides and can inactivate the drug in vitro. Also see **PENICILLIN ANTIBIOTICS.**

SUPPLIED AS: HUMAN PRODUCT
For injection containing 1-, 3-, 6-, 20-, and 30-g vials

TILETAMINE ZOLAZEPAM

INDICATIONS: Tiletamine zolazepam (Telazol ★) is an injectable dissociative anesthetic/tranquilizer useful for sedation and restraint and anesthetic induction or anesthesia of short duration (30 minutes) requiring mild to moderate analgesia.

ADVERSE AND COMMON SIDE EFFECTS: The drug is contraindicated in animals with pancreatic disease and those with significant cardiac, pulmonary, or renal disease. Rapid IM injection is painful. Respiratory depression may occur at higher doses. Other side effects may include salivation, increased bronchial and tracheal secretions (if atropine is not given before its use), increased heart rate and blood pressure, increased cardiac output and myocardial oxygen consumption, and hypertension or hypotension. Vomiting may occur on recovery, and vocalization, hypertonia, muscular twitching, muscle rigidity, erratic and/or prolonged recovery, cyanosis, cardiac arrest, and pulmonary edema also have been reported. The drug should not be used in pregnant animals.

DRUG INTERACTIONS: In cats, anesthesia is prolonged by chloramphenicol by approximately 30 minutes. This does not occur in dogs. Phenothiazines may enhance the cardiac and respiratory depression of the drug. The dose of barbiturate or volatile anesthetic used may need to be reduced. Chemical restraint with this agent will not adversely affect the performance of intradermal skin testing in atopic dogs.

SUPPLIED AS: VETERINARY PRODUCT
For injection containing 250 mg tiletamine and zolazepam, each producing a concentration of 50 mg/mL when reconstituted

TOBRAMYCIN

INDICATIONS: Tobramycin (Nebcin ✦ ★) is an aminoglycoside antibiotic. It is closely related to gentamicin in spectrum, activity, and pharmacologic properties, but it is more active against some strains of *Pseudomonas* that are resistant to gentamicin, and it is less nephrotoxic. Also see **AMINOGLYCOSIDE ANTIBIOTICS.**

ADVERSE AND COMMON SIDE EFFECTS: See AMINOGLYCOSIDE ANTIBIOTICS.

DRUG INTERACTIONS: Tobramycin should not be mixed with other drugs. Also see **AMINOGLYCOSIDE ANTIBIOTICS.**

SUPPLIED AS: HUMAN PRODUCT
For injection containing 10 and 40 mg/mL and in disposable syringes containing 60 mg/1.5 mL and 80 mg/2 mL

TOCAINIDE

INDICATIONS: Tocainide (Tonocard ✦ ★) is an antiarrhythmic agent and analog of lidocaine with similar electrophysiologic and hemodynamic properties. The drug is effective orally. It is used to suppress ventricular premature contractions. Therapeutic plasma levels are quoted as 4 to 10 µg/mL. A positive response to lidocaine appears to be a good predictor of response to tocainide.

ADVERSE AND COMMON SIDE EFFECTS: Tocainide should not be used in patients with second- or third-degree heart block, hypokalemia, myasthenia gravis, and pregnancy. Cautious use is recommended in those with renal or hepatic disease. Reported adverse effects in dogs include anorexia, head trembling, weakness, ataxia, nervousness, and anxiety. Long-term use (greater than 3 months) of the drug appears to predispose to corneal endothelial dystrophy and possibly renal dysfunction.
   In humans, side effects may include urinary retention, polyuria, tremors, dizziness, vertigo, ataxia, agitation, confusion, convulsions, exacerbation of arrhythmias, heart block, bradycardia, hypotension, nausea, vomiting, anorexia, diarrhea, pulmonary edema, dyspnea and leukopenia, anemia, and thrombocytopenia. The drug dose should be reduced or the interval between doses increased in animals with renal disease. Giving the drug with food decreases side effects.

DRUG INTERACTIONS: Tocainide may be combined with other antiarrhythmic agents, e.g., propranolol, quinidine, or disopyramide, to increase effectiveness. Allopurinol increases the serum concentration of tocainide. Metoprolol has additive effects on wedge pressure and cardiac index. In people, the concurrent use of propranolol may lead to paranoia.

SUPPLIED AS: HUMAN PRODUCT
Tablets containing 400 and 600 mg

TRIAMCINOLONE

INDICATIONS: Triamcinolone (Vetalog ♣ ★) is a glucocorticoid. The drug is indicated for the treatment of arthritic disorders and for the treatment of allergic and dermatologic conditions responsive to corticosteroids. Also see **GLUCOCORTICOID AGENTS.**

ADVERSE AND COMMON SIDE EFFECTS: Subconjunctival injection may be associated with granuloma formation requiring surgical excision. Also see **GLUCOCORTICOID AGENTS.**

DRUG INTERACTIONS: See **GLUCOCORTICOID AGENTS.**

SUPPLIED AS: VETERINARY PRODUCTS
For injection containing 2 and 6 mg/mL ♣ ★
Tablets containing 0.5 and 1.5 mg ★

HUMAN PRODUCTS
Tablets containing 1, 2, 4, 8, and 16 mg [Aristocort ♣ ★]
Syrup containing 2 mg/5 mL [Aristocort ♣ ★]

OTHER USES
Dogs and Cats
INFLAMMATORY AND ALLERGIC CONDITIONS
0.11 to 0.22 mg/kg once; IM, SC (remission generally lasts 7–15 days; if signs recur, the dose may be repeated or oral corticosteroid treatment begun)

Cats
PLASMACYTIC PHARYNGITIS
2 to 4 mg once daily to once every 48 hours; PO

POLYMYOPATHY
0.5 to 1 mg/kg once daily; PO

TRIAMTERENE

INDICATIONS: Triamterene (Dyrenium ♣ ★), like spironolactone, has weak diuretic action and a potassium-sparing effect. Unlike spironolactone, triamterene blocks potassium secretion by a direct action on distal renal tubules rather than by inhibiting aldosterone. It may be used in conjunction with other diuretics to promote diuresis in patients refractory to other diuretics.

ADVERSE AND COMMON SIDE EFFECTS: The drug is contraindicated in severe or progressive renal disease, anuria, severe hepatic dysfunction, or elevated serum potassium concentrations. Cautious use is advised in diabetes mellitus or impaired renal or hepatic function. In humans, adverse effects may include diarrhea, nausea, vomiting, dry mouth, pruritus, weakness, hypotension, muscle cramps, hyperkalemia, elevated serum urea and uric acid, hyperchloremic acidosis, granulocytopenia, eosinophilia, and megaloblastic anemia. There is limited information concerning use of the drug in small animals.

DRUG INTERACTIONS: Digitalis effects may be decreased by triamterene. Antihypertensive agents may have an additive hypotensive effect. Lithium clearance is decreased, predisposing to toxicity. Nonsteroidal anti-inflammatory agents can cause a marked decrease in creatinine clearance.

SUPPLIED AS: HUMAN PRODUCTS
Tablets containing 50 and 100 mg ✤
Capsules containing 50 and 100 mg ★

TRIIODOTHYRONINE

See **LIOTHYROXINE** (Cytobin, Cytomel).

TRIMEPRAZINE

INDICATIONS: Trimeprazine (Temaril-P ★, Vanectyl-P ✤) is a phenothiazine antihistamine/corticosteroid used for the relief of pruritus caused by allergy. It also is recommended by the manufacturer as an antitussive agent in dogs.

ADVERSE AND COMMON SIDE EFFECTS: Side effects for trimeprazine include sedation, depression, hypotension, rigidity, tremors, weakness, and restlessness. If the combined veterinary product is used, additional side effects may include polyuria, polydipsia, vomiting, diarrhea, weight loss, elevation in liver enzymes, and iatrogenic Cushing's syndrome. Other side effects may include sodium retention, potassium loss, delayed wound healing, osteoporosis, increased susceptibility to infection, and blood dyscrasias.

DRUG INTERACTIONS: Intensification and prolongation of the action of sedatives, analgesics, and anesthetics may be noted, as well as possible potentiation of organophosphate toxicity and procaine hydrochloride activity. Augmented CNS depression may occur with concomitant use of narcotics, barbiturates, and anesthetics. Quinidine may cause additive cardiac depression. Antacids and antidiarrheal compounds may decrease GI absorption. Concurrent use of propranolol may cause increased serum elevation of both drugs. Phenytoin metabolism may be decreased. Phenothiazines are α-adrenergic blocking agents, and if epinephrine is given, unopposed, β-adrenergic activity leading to vasodilation and an increased heart rate may result. Products containing prednisolone, e.g., Temaril-P, may cause hypokalemia if used concurrently with amphotericin B, furosemide, or the thiazide diuretics. In addition, insulin requirements may increase and serum salicylate levels may decrease. Phenytoin and phenobarbital may increase the metabolism of prednisolone.

SUPPLIED AS: VETERINARY PRODUCTS
Tablets containing 5 mg trimeprazine and 2 mg prednisolone [Temaril-P and Vanectyl-P]

TRIMETHOPRIM–SULFADIAZINE

INDICATIONS: Trimethoprim–sulfadiazine (or sulphadiazine) (Tribrissen ✦ ★) is a bactericidal antibiotic combination recommended for the treatment of alimentary, respiratory, and urinary tract infections and skin and soft tissue infections caused by susceptible organisms, including *E. coli, Enterobacter, Klebsiella, Streptococcus, Staphylococcus, Pasteurella, Clostridia, Salmonella, Shigella, Brucella* spp., *Actinomyces, Corynebacterium* spp., *Bordetella* spp., *Neisseria* spp., *Vibrio* spp., and *Proteus* organisms. It is especially useful for long-term, low-dose treatment of chronic bacterial urinary tract infections. This drug combination also may be used for the eradication of coccidiosis in dogs and cats.

ADVERSE AND COMMON SIDE EFFECTS: The drug should not be used in animals with marked liver disease or blood dyscrasias or in those with sulfonamide sensitivity. A rare idiosyncratic drug reaction leading to fatal hepatic necrosis has been reported.

Anemia, leukopenia, thrombocytopenia, anorexia, and ataxia have been noted at higher doses. Dietary supplementation with folinic acid (leucovorin calcium at 0.5–1 mg/day) may protect the patient against the anemia and leukopenia that accompany the interference of folic acid metabolism. This drug combination has been associated with fever and polyarthritis (Doberman pinschers may be predisposed), cutaneous eruptions, hepatitis, cholestasis, vomiting, anorexia, diarrhea, urticaria, facial swelling, polydipsia, polyuria, kerato conjunctivitis sicca, glomerulonephropathy, and polymyositis. Signs of polyarthritis and fever typically occur 8 to 20 days after the initiation of therapy. Complete recovery of clinical signs is apparent within 1 week after withdrawal of the drug. Skin changes resolve within 3 weeks.

The drug should not be used for more than 14 days in the cat. Excessive salivation may occur in cats given uncoated tablets. In addition, Tribrissen may cause anemia, leukopenia, and anorexia and interfere with thyroid function in cats.

DRUG INTERACTIONS: Antacids may decrease the bioavailability of trimethoprim–sulfadiazine if administered concurrently. Trimethoprim–sulfadiazine may prolong clotting times in patients receiving warfarin and decrease the effect of cyclosporine while increasing the risk of nephrotoxicity of the drug. Sulfonamides may increase the effects of methotrexate, phenylbutazone, phenytoin, salicylates, thiazide diuretics, and probenecid.

SUPPLIED AS: VETERINARY PRODUCTS
For injection containing 40 mg/mL trimethoprim and 200 mg/mL sulfadiazine [Tribrissen 24% ♣ ★]
Tablets containing 5 mg trimethoprim and 25 mg sulfadiazine ♣ ★
Tablets containing 20 mg trimethoprim and 100 mg sulfadiazine ♣ ★
Tablets containing 80 mg trimethoprim and 400 mg sulfadiazine ♣ ★
Tablets containing 160 mg trimethoprim and 800 mg sulfadiazine ★
Oral suspension containing 10 mg trimethoprim and 50 mg sulfadiazine ★

OTHER USES
Dogs
GASTROINTESTINAL BACTERIAL OVERGROWTH
15 mg/kg bid; PO for 1 month

Dogs and Cats
COCCIDIOSIS/TOXOPLASMOSIS
15 to 30 mg/kg bid; PO, SC [Tribrissen]

TYLOSIN

INDICATIONS: Tylosin (Tylan ♣ ★, Tylocine ♣, Tylosin ★) is a macrolide antibiotic. It has activity against gram-negative and gram-positive bacteria, spirochetes, chlamydiae, and mycoplasma organisms. The drug is effective in the treatment of bronchitis, tracheobronchitis, laryngitis, tonsillitis, pneumonia, rhinitis, sinusitis, cellulitis, otitis externa, cystitis, metritis, endometritis, and pyogenic dermatitis caused by susceptible organisms. It also has been used to manage canine and feline colitis.

ADVERSE AND COMMON SIDE EFFECTS: Anorexia, diarrhea, and local pain with IM injection are reported.

DRUG INTERACTIONS: Tylosin may increase serum digitalis levels.

SUPPLIED AS: VETERINARY PRODUCTS
Tablets containing 200 mg ♣
For injection containing 50 and 200 mg/mL ♣ ★ (for swine and cattle)

OTHER USES
Dogs
CHRONIC COLITIS
40 to 80 mg/kg/day in 2 to 3 div. doses; mixed with food or as a bolus with water for 2 weeks, then taper. Some require long-term therapy. May be alternated with sulfasalazine for long-term maintenance.
Note: Tylan Plus Vitamins is no longer marketed. Tylan Soluble Powder contains 3,000 mg/teaspoon (may require dilution for accurate dosing).

CHRONIC INFLAMMATORY BOWEL DISEASE
20 to 40 mg/kg bid; PO

SUSCEPTIBLE INFECTIONS
6.6 to 11 mg/kg once to twice daily; IM

Cats
CHRONIC COLITIS
10 to 20 mg/kg/day in 2 div. doses mixed with food or as a bolus with water. May be alternated with sulfasalazine for long-term maintenance.

CHRONIC INFLAMMATORY BOWEL DISEASE
10 to 20 mg/kg bid; PO

SUSCEPTIBLE INFECTIONS
i) 6.6 to 11 mg/kg once to twice daily; IM

ii) 10 mg/kg bid; IM

URSODIOL

INDICATIONS: Ursodiol, or ursodeoxycholic acid; UDCA (Ursofalk ♣, Actigall ★), is a chloretic agent used to treat chronic inflammatory cholestatic liver disease, bile sludging, dissolution of radiolucent noncalcified gallstones smaller than 20 mm in diameter, primary biliary cirrhosis, chronic persistent hepatitis, cirrhosis, and biliary atresia. The drug promotes biliary flow and has anti-inflammatory properties. Total endogenous bile acids are reduced. It will not dissolve calcified cholesterol or bile pigment gallstones.

ADVERSE AND COMMON SIDE EFFECTS: None have been reported in dogs or cats. In humans, adverse effects may include diar-

rhea, vomiting, constipation, stomatitis, abdominal pain, and flatulence. Mean pre- and postprandial serum bile acid concentrations increased with treatment attributable to the increased UDCA concentration. Thus, serum bile acid concentration may not be an accurate
indication of liver function in animals receiving the drug. The drug
is contraindicated in patients with extrahepatic biliary obstruction.

DRUG INTERACTIONS: Estrogens and clofibrate may increase hepatic cholesterol secretion and predispose to cholesterol gallstone
formation. Aluminum-based antacids absorb bile acids and interfere
with ursodiol by decreasing its absorption. Cholestyramine also
tends to decrease ursodiol's absorption.

SUPPLIED AS: HUMAN PRODUCT
Capsules containing 250 mg [Ursofalk]
Capsules containing 300 mg [Actigall]

VALPROIC ACID

INDICATIONS: Valproic acid (Depakene ✦ ★, Depakote ★, Epival ✦)
is an anticonvulsant drug. It is costly, has a short half-life (2.8 hours)
in the dog, and is potentially hepatotoxic; however, some clinicians
use the drug in combination with phenobarbital in patients not responsive to phenobarbital alone. In humans, target serum concentrations are approximately 50 to 150 µg/mL.

ADVERSE AND COMMON SIDE EFFECTS: The drug is contraindicated in patients with significant hepatic disease. It should be
used with caution in those with thrombocytopenia or impaired
platelet function. The drug is potentially teratogenic and should only
be used in pregnant bitches when the benefits appear to outweigh
the risks. Side effects may include anorexia, vomiting, and diarrhea.
In humans, hepatotoxicity and elevation in liver enzymes occur; this
may be of concern in dogs. Other potential side effects may include
sedation, ataxia, behavioral changes, leukopenia, anemia, pancreatitis,
and edema.

DRUG INTERACTIONS: Valproic acid may increase the serum levels and potentiate the effect of phenobarbital and primidone. Valproic acid may increase or decrease phenytoin levels, predisposing
to seizure activity. Concurrent use of tricyclic antidepressants, e.g.,
amitriptyline, or MAO inhibitors, e.g., possibly amitraz and selegiline, may potentiate CNS depression. Salicylates may increase serum
valproic acid levels. The sedative effects of clonazepam may be increased, but the anticonvulsant activity of both drugs decreased
when used concurrently.

SUPPLIED AS: HUMAN PRODUCTS
Capsules containing 250 mg [Depakene]

Tablets containing 125, 250, and 500 mg [Depakote, Epival]
Oral syrup containing 50 mg/mL [Depakene]

VASOPRESSIN

INDICATIONS: Vasopressin (Pitressin ✚ ★) is a synthetic form of
vasopressin or antidiuretic hormone. It has been used in the diagnosis and management of diabetes insipidus.

ADVERSE AND COMMON SIDE EFFECTS: Abdominal pain,
nausea, vomiting, bronchial constriction, fluid retention, hyponatremia, pain at the site of injection, and the formation of sterile abscesses have been reported. The drug is contraindicated in patients
with cardiorenal disease with hypertension, epilepsy, or hypersensitivity to the drug. The drug should be used with caution in patients
with asthma or heart failure.

DRUG INTERACTIONS: Large doses of epinephrine, heparin, and
demeclocycline may antagonize the effects of Pitressin. Chlorpropamide, carbamazepine, and fludrocortisone may potentiate the
action of Pitressin.

SUPPLIED AS: HUMAN PRODUCT
For injection containing 20 pressor units/mL

VERAPAMIL

INDICATIONS: Verapamil (Isoptin ✚ ★) is a calcium channel-blocking agent. The drug may be useful in the management of atrial flutter, atrial fibrillation, and atrial tachycardia. It is a more potent negative inotropic agent than nifedipine or diltiazem.

ADVERSE AND COMMON SIDE EFFECTS: The drug is contraindicated in sick sinus syndrome, atrioventricular block and myocardial failure (unless tachycardia is contributing to the failure),
shock, hypotension, or digitalis-intoxicated patients. The drug
should be used with caution in those with hepatic or renal impairment and in those with Wolff–Parkinson–White syndrome.
   Adverse effects may include nausea, constipation, fatigue, dizziness, bradycardia, tachycardia, hypotension, exacerbation of congestive heart failure, pulmonary edema, and atrioventricular block.

DRUG INTERACTIONS: Verapamil may increase serum digitalis
and theophylline levels. Epinephrine, isoproterenol, and theophylline may oppose the calcium-blocking action of verapamil. Propranolol and metoprolol may augment the cardiodepressant effect
of verapamil. Calcium salts, vitamin D, and rifampin may decrease

the pharmacologic effects of verapamil. Cimetidine may increase the pharmacologic effects of calcium channel-blocking agents by increasing bioavailability. Highly protein-bound drugs, e.g., oral anticoagulants, salicylates, and sulfonamides, may displace or be displaced by verapamil, predisposing to toxicity. Prazosin and other antihypertensive agents may cause an acute hypotensive effect.

SUPPLIED AS: HUMAN PRODUCTS
Tablets containing 40, 80 and 120 mg
Tablets (sustained-release) containing 120, 180, and 240 mg
For injection containing 2.5 mg/mL

VINBLASTINE

INDICATIONS: Vinblastine (Velban ★, Velbe ✦) has been used in the treatment of lymphomas, carcinomas, mastocytomas, and splenic tumors.

ADVERSE AND COMMON SIDE EFFECTS: Vinblastine is contraindicated in patients with leukopenia, granulocytopenia, or bacterial infection. Side effects of vinblastine may include nausea, vomiting, and myelosuppression. Granulocytic depression occurs within 4 to 9 days of administration, with recovery occurring 7 to 14 days later. Additional side effects may include constipation, stomatitis, ileus, jaw and muscle pain, inappropriate antidiuretic hormone (ADH) secretion, and loss of deep tendon reflexes. Perivascular injection causes severe tissue irritation and necrosis. If this occurs, aspiration of the drug should be attempted and the area infiltrated with sodium bicarbonate (8.4%), dexamethasone or hyaluronidase (150 μg/mL), or topical DMSO. In addition, warm compresses should be applied to the area.

DRUG INTERACTIONS: None of significance in small animals.

SUPPLIED AS: HUMAN PRODUCT
For injection containing 1 mg/mL

VINCRISTINE

INDICATIONS: Vincristine (Oncovin ✦ ★) is a chemotherapeutic agent used in the management of lymphoid and hematopoietic neoplasms, mammary neoplasms in cats, some sarcomas, transmissible venereal tumors in dogs, and immune-mediated thrombocytopenia. The drug often is used in conjunction with other chemotherapeutic agents.

ADVERSE AND COMMON SIDE EFFECTS: The drug should be used with caution in those with liver disease, leukopenia, bacterial infection, or preexisting neuromuscular disease.

Vincristine is less myelosuppressive than vinblastine, causing a mild leukopenia, but it has greater potential to cause peripheral neuropathy (proprioceptive deficits, hyporeflexia, and paralytic ileus and constipation). Perivascular injection causes severe tissue irritation and necrosis. If this occurs, aspiration of the drug should be attempted and the area infiltrated with sodium bicarbonate (8.4%), dexamethasone or hyaluronidase (150 µg/mL), or topical DMSO. In addition, warm compresses should be applied to the area.

Other side effects may include increases in serum liver enzymes, inappropriate ADH secretion, jaw pain, alopecia, stomatitis, and seizure activity.

DRUG INTERACTIONS: Concurrent use of asparaginase may contribute to neurotoxicity, the incidence of which is less common if asparaginase is administered after vincristine.

SUPPLIED AS: HUMAN PRODUCT
For injection containing 1 mg/mL

OTHER USES
Dogs
TRANSMISSIBLE VENEREAL TUMOR
0.025 mg/kg once weekly; IV (maximum 1 mg); usually requires 3 to 6 weeks of therapy

IMMUNE-MEDIATED THROMBOCYTOPENIA
0.01 to 0.025 mg/kg; IV at 7- to 10-day intervals (used alone or in combination with corticosteroids)

VITAMIN E

INDICATIONS: Vitamin E (Aquasol E ✚ ★) is a fat-soluble vitamin. It has been used in the treatment of Scotty cramp and as an anti-inflammatory agent in discoid lupus, pemphigus erythematosus, demodicosis, and acanthosis nigricans. The drug may have a steroid-sparing effect. As an antipruritic agent, it is of limited value and has not been proven efficacious in the treatment of dermatomyositis. In cats, it has been used in the treatment of steatitis. The efficacy of the use of vitamin E in these diseases is unknown.

ADVERSE AND COMMON SIDE EFFECTS: Changes in the hair coat color have been documented in a tricolored collie. Anorexia also may occur. In humans, excessive doses may cause muscle weakness, fatigue, nausea, diarrhea, intestinal cramping, increases in serum cholesterol and triglyceride levels, and decreases in serum thyroxine levels.

DRUG INTERACTIONS: The drug should be given 2 hours before a meal because the inorganic iron present in most commercial diets interferes with its absorption. Concomitant administration of vitamin E may enhance oral anticoagulant activity. Vitamin A absorption, use, and storage may be enhanced by vitamin E. Large doses of vitamin E may delay the hematologic response to iron therapy in those with iron deficiency anemia. Mineral oil may reduce the absorption of oral vitamin E.

SUPPLIED AS: HUMAN PRODUCTS
Capsules containing 100, 200, 400, 500, 600, 800, and 1,000 IU
Drops containing 50 IU/mL

OTHER USES
Dogs
SCOTTY CRAMP
70 IU/kg intermittently; IM (it may reduce the likelihood of recurrences but does not alter severity of an episode)

DISCOID LUPUS
i)   400 IU bid; PO or as a topical ointment may be beneficial

ii) 200 to 800 IU bid; PO with prednisone 1 to 1.5 mg/kg/day; PO eventually tapered to every alternate day

VITAMIN E-DEFICIENT MYOPATHY
400 IU once daily; PO

Cats
STEATITIS
10 to 20 IU/kg bid; PO until clinical signs have resolved

VITAMIN K₁

INDICATIONS: Vitamin K_1 or phytonadione (Aqua-Mephyton ★, Mephyton ★, Konakion ★, Veta-K1 ❦ ★) is used to treat coagulopathy caused by fat-soluble vitamin malabsorption and vitamin K antagonism caused by salicylates, coumarins, and indanediones. It does not correct hypoprothrombinemia due to hepatic disease. Treatment is continued for 5 to 7 days with first-generation toxicants (warfarin, pindone, fumarin, tomarin, isovaleryl indanedione) and for 4 to 6 weeks for second-generation toxicants (brodifacoum, volak, diphacinone, chlorphacinone, bromadiolone).

A lag time of 6 to 12 hours is expected before new clotting factors are synthesized. Vitamin K_3 is less expensive but also is less effective.

ADVERSE AND COMMON SIDE EFFECTS: The drug is contraindicated in patients with severe liver disease. Transient hypotension, dyspnea, and cyanosis are reported rarely. Anaphylaxis has been reported after IV injection of the drug. Intramuscular injection has been associated with acute bleeding from the site of injection during the initial stages of therapy (small-gauge needles are recommended).

DRUG INTERACTIONS: Oral, broad-spectrum antibiotics given long-term potentiate hypoprothrombinemia by suppressing vitamin K-producing intestinal bacteria. Vitamin K antagonizes the effects of anticoagulants. Mineral oil decreases GI absorption of vitamin K. Phenylbutazone, aspirin, chloramphenicol, sulfonamides, diazoxide, allopurinol, cimetidine, metronidazole, anabolic steroids, erythromycin, ketoconazole, propranolol, and thyroid drugs may antagonize the therapeutic effects of phytonadione.

SUPPLIED AS: VETERINARY PRODUCTS
Capsules containing 25 mg [Veta-K1 ★]
For injection containing 10 mg/mL [Veta-K1 ♣ ★]

HUMAN PRODUCTS
For injection containing 2 mg/mL ♣ ★ and 10 mg/mL ♣ ★
Tablets containing 5 mg [Mephyton]
Note: The injectable formulation can be given orally at the same dose (mg/kg basis) when tablets or capsules are not available.

WARFARIN

INDICATIONS: Warfarin (Coumadin ♣ ★) is an anticoagulant. It interferes with clotting by depressing hepatic synthesis of vitamin K-dependent coagulation factors II, VII, IX, and X and anticoagulant proteins C and S. It has no effect on already formed circulating coagulation factors or on circulating thrombi, but it may prevent extension of existing thrombi and prevent new clots from forming. It augments thrombin inactivation and prevents the conversion of fibrinogen to fibrin. Warfarin may be more effective prophylaxis for thromboembolic disease than aspirin in cats with cardiomyopathy.

ADVERSE AND COMMON SIDE EFFECTS: A transient hypercoagulable state occurs when warfarin is introduced. The actual antithrombotic effects are caused by the decrease in factors IX and X, which does not occur for 4 to 6 days in humans. Therefore, for the first 3 to 4 days when anticoagulant protein C levels are low, heparin is used in conjunction with warfarin. The drug is contraindicated in patients with preexisting bleeding tendencies or GI ulceration, or those undergoing surgery. It is embryotoxic and is contraindicated in pregnancy. Clinical signs are due to dose-related hemorrhage and include pale mucous membranes, weakness, dyspnea, prostration, and occasionally hematomas, ecchymosis, epistaxis, hematemesis, hematuria, hematochezia, and death. A single toxic dose is listed as 5 to 50 mg/kg for dogs and cats.

DRUG INTERACTIONS: Drugs that may enhance the anticoagulant effect of warfarin include acetaminophen, allopurinol, alkylating agents, aminoglycosides, amiodarone, anabolic steroids, antimetabolites, aspirin, asparaginase, chloramphenicol, chlorpropamide, cimetidine, danazol, dextran, diazoxide, erythromycin, ethacrynic acid, MAO inhibitors, e.g., possibly amitraz and selegiline, metronidazole, mineral oil, miconazole, nalidixic acid, neomycin, NSAIDs, potassium products, propylthiouracil, quinidine, sulfonamides, tetracyclines, thiazide diuretics, tolbutamide, tricyclic antidepressants, e.g., amitriptyline, thyroid drugs, and vitamin E.

Drugs that may decrease the anticoagulant response include barbiturates, corticosteroids, diuretics, griseofulvin, laxatives, mercaptopurine, rifampin, spironolactone, vitamin C, and dietary vitamin K.

SUPPLIED AS: HUMAN PRODUCTS
Tablets containing 1, 2, 2.5, 4, 5, 7.5, and 10 mg ♣ ★
For injection containing 50 mg/vial ★

OTHER USES
Dogs
THROMBOEMBOLIC DISEASE
0.1 mg/kg once daily; PO (prevention of recurrence)

PULMONARY THROMBOEMBOLIC DISEASE
Heparin started at 200 IU/kg; IV followed by 100 to 200 IU/kg qid; SC or 15 to 20 IU/kg/hour; IV infusion adjusted to prolong activated partial thromboplastin time (APTT) by 1.5 to 2 times baseline values. Warfarin is recommended if anticoagulant therapy is required for longer periods. Warfarin requires 2 to 7 days to become effective. A dose of 0.2 mg/kg, PO, is used initially, followed by 0.05 to 0.10 mg/kg/day to maintain PT time 1.5 to 2 times baseline values. Heparin therapy gradually is tapered and discontinued when desired PT is achieved.

Cats
THROMBOEMBOLIC DISEASE
i) 0.1 to 0.2 mg/kg once daily; PO (prevention of recurrence)
ii) 0.25 to 1.0 mg once daily; PO (prevention of recurrence)

Dogs and Cats
PULMONARY THROMBOEMBOLISM
0.2 mg/kg once daily; PO then 0.05 to 0.1 mg/kg once daily; PO. Adjust dosage to increase prothrombin time (PT) to 1.5 to 2.5 times baseline. If PT exceeds 2.5 times baseline, reduce warfarin dose. If bleeding occurs, discontinue warfarin use and administer blood or phytonadione.

XYLAZINE

INDICATIONS: Xylazine (Anased ♣ ★, Rompun ♣ ★) is an anesthetic agent characterized by a rapid onset, good-to-excellent sedation, excellent analgesia of 15 to 30 minutes duration, and a smooth recovery. Its sedative effects last longer (90–120 minutes). The drug also is used as a diagnostic aid in cases of pituitary hypofunction, e.g., pituitary dwarfism.

ADVERSE AND COMMON SIDE EFFECTS: Use of the drug is contraindicated in animals receiving epinephrine or those with ventricular arrhythmias. It should be used with caution in animals with heart disease, hypotension, shock, respiratory dysfunction, severe hepatic or renal disease, or a history of seizure activity, or those that are severely debilitated. Vomiting 1 to 5 minutes after administration (especially in cats), hypotension, bradycardia, second-degree heart block, polyuria, mild respiratory depression, hyperglycemia, glycosuria, and aggression are reported. Dogs may bloat from aerophagia. In cats, apnea and seizures also have been reported. Bradycardia may be prevented by the administration of atropine or glycopyrrolate. The drug may precipitate early parturition if used in the last trimester of pregnancy.

DRUG INTERACTIONS: Xylazine sensitizes the heart to epinephrine-induced arrhythmias, especially in the face of halothane anesthesia. Other CNS depressants, including barbiturates, narcotics, and phenothiazines, may potentiate CNS depression. Yohimbine (dogs 0.1 mg/kg; IV, cats 0.5 mg/kg; IV) can be used to antagonize the effects of xylazine, shorten recovery times, and reduce anesthetic-related complications.

SUPPLIED AS: VETERINARY PRODUCT
For injection containing 20 and 100 mg/mL

OTHER USES
Dogs
GROWTH   HORMONE   RESPONSE   TEST   FOR HYPOPITUITARISM
300 μg/kg; IV; collect plasma at time 0 and 15, 30, 45, 60, and 90 minutes
Pituitary dwarfs demonstrate little or no response to xylazine stimulation.

ZINC ACETATE

INDICATIONS: Zinc acetate ★ has been used in dogs in the treatment and prophylaxis of hepatic copper toxicosis. The suggested plasma therapeutic concentration is 200 to 500 μg/dL. It appears to take 100 mg of zinc administered twice daily approximately 3 to 6 months to obtain therapeutic serum levels. Zinc cannot be expected to reverse cirrhotic liver changes.

ADVERSE AND COMMON SIDE EFFECTS: Zinc acetate appears to be well tolerated by dogs. Vomiting may occur and may be controlled by giving the drug with a small piece of meat. Note, however, that this drug should not normally be given with food.

DRUG INTERACTIONS: To be effective, zinc must be given separately from food by at least 1 hour.

SUPPLIED AS: HUMAN PRODUCT
Capsules containing 25 and 50 mg [Lemmon Co., Sellersville, PA]

ZINC SULFATE

INDICATIONS: Zinc sulfate (PMS-Egozinc ♣, Orazinc ★) has been used in dogs for the treatment of zinc-responsive dermatoses (especially Siberian huskies and Alaskan malamutes) and as a copper-chelating agent which has been shown in humans to prevent copper reaccumulation in those whose livers already had been depleted of copper with appropriate chelating agents. Therefore, it may have a more important role in preventive copper-associated liver therapy.

ADVERSE AND COMMON SIDE EFFECTS: The product is contraindicated in patients sensitive to zinc. The most common side effects associated with zinc therapy include nausea, anorexia, and vomiting, which can be controlled by dividing the daily dose into two equal portions and administering the drug with food. Zinc gluconate (3 mg/kg/day div. tid; PO) has been suggested as an alternative because it causes less gastric irritation. Toxic zinc levels may result in iron deficiency and hemolytic anemia.

DRUG INTERACTIONS: Excessive zinc will inhibit iron absorption.

SUPPLIED AS: HUMAN PRODUCTS
Capsules and tablets containing 220 mg zinc sulfate (50 mg zinc)
Tablets containing 66 mg (15 mg zinc), 110 mg (25 mg zinc), and 200 mg (45 mg zinc) [Orazinc]

OTHER USES
Dogs
ZINC-RESPONSIVE DERMATOSIS
1 mg/kg/day; PO of elemental zinc; continue treatment for 1 month. If clinical condition does not improve, increase dose by 50%.

Part II

Large Animals

Handbook of Veterinary Drugs, Second Edition, edited by Dana Allen,
Lippincott–Raven Publishers, Philadelphia. © 1998

Section 4

Common Dosages for Large Animals

Race withdrawals are guidelines only, based on detection limits of single doses of drugs. New testing methods, variations from the recommended dose, and individual animal variation may affect detection times. (From the Race Track Division Schedule of Drugs 1994, Agriculture Canada.)

For "Ruminant" listings, most published information deals solely with cattle, and extrapolation to sheep or goats is necessary. Where specific information includes sheep and/or goats, and if it differs from cattle doses, a separate section is included. Further selected drugs (see below) for miniature pigs have been included in the section with horses.

For withdrawal times for milk and meat, ℜ is for label withdrawal at label dose, & is for extralabel withdrawal, and Ψ for products with no known or established withdrawal times. Where there is "0" withdrawal time listed, there is no need to withhold milk or delay slaughter when this product is administered per the label dose and route.

Further information on withdrawal times for extralabel use of drugs can be obtained from the Food Animal Residue Avoidance Databank (FARAD), with regional centers at North Carolina State University (telephone 919-829-4431), the University of Illinois (telephone 217-333-6731), or the University of California (telephone 916-752-7507). The website for primary files is maintained and archived at Oregon State University at: http://www.ace.orst.edu:80/info/farad/. Clinicians are further cautioned that data on withdrawal times are drawn from studies on healthy animals. Disease states may markedly change required withdrawal times.

Drug	Horses (and Miniature Pig Doses, Where Indicated)	Ruminants (Cattle, Sheep, and Goats)
Abamectin	N/A	Label dose: (cattle only) 1 mL (10 mg)/50 kg (200 µg/kg) BW; SC only Withdrawal: Meat: 42 days, nonlactating dairy cattle 2 months prior to calving; not for use in lactating dairy cattle ℞
Acepromazine	Label dose: 60 to 120 mg/454 kg; PO 0.05 mg/kg; IV 0.11 mg/kg; IM 0.165 mg/kg; IP Extralabel dose: 0.02 to 0.05 mg/kg; IV (preanesthetic) 0.4 to 0.1 mg/kg; IV, IM **OR** 2 to 4 mg/45 kg; PO (tranquilization) Race withdrawal: 36 hr Extralabel dose: *Miniature pigs* 0.03 to 0.1 mg/kg; IM (catheter placement) 0.1 to 0.2 mg/kg; IM (calm nursing sow) 0.05 to 0.5 mg/kg; IM (sedation, premedication)	Label dose: 0.05 mg/kg; IV 0.11 to 0.44 mg/kg; IM 0.165 mg/kg; IP 120 mg/454 kg; PO Extralabel dose: 0.5 to 0.1 mg/kg; IM, IV, SC **OR** 60 to 120 mg/454 kg; PO [granules] (sedation in cattle) Similar dose in sheep and goats for use in conjunction with ketamine (2–5 mg/kg; IV) for short-acting anesthesia Withdrawal (label dose, Canada): Meat: 7 days Milk: 48 hr ℞
Acetazolamide (unlicensed for veterinary use)	2.2 mg/kg bid–tid; PO	Cattle: 6 to 8 mg/kg; PO in food or water Withdrawal: Ψ

Drug	Horses (and Miniature Pig Doses, Where Indicated)	Ruminants (Cattle, Sheep, and Goats)
Acetic acid (5% solution) (unlicensed for veterinary use)	250 mL/450 kg; PO daily (enterolith prevention)	Cattle: 2 to 6 L; PO via rumenal intubation, followed with 20 L cold water; PO Sheep and goats: 0.5 to 1 L; PO via rumenal intubation, followed with 2 to 8 L cold water; PO (nonprotein nitrogen induced ammonia toxicosis) Withdrawal: Ψ, but likely none required
Acetylcysteine (10%, in Canada 20% available) (unlicensed for veterinary use)	2 to 5 mL/50 kg bid–tid as an aerosol As enema: 4% solution given 120 to 240 mL per rectum via Foley catheter. Hold in place for 4 to 5 minutes, repeat if necessary in 1 hr. (foal)	Same Withdrawal: Ψ
Albendazole	Extralabel dose: 25 mg/kg bid; PO for 5 days (*D. arnfieldi*) 50 mg/kg bid; PO for 2 days (*S. vulgaris* larvae) 4 to 8 mg/kg bid; PO for 1 month (*Echinococcus* spp)	Label dose: Cattle: 10 mg/kg; PO Withdrawal: Meat: 27 days ℜ Milk: Ψ Extralabel dose: Sheep: 3 mg/kg/day; PO for 35 days (prophylaxis against infective metacercariae of *Fasciola hepatica*) Withdrawal: Ψ
Allopurinol (unlicensed for veterinary use)	5 mg/kg; IV	None

Drug	Horses (and Miniature Pig Doses, Where Indicated)	Ruminants (Cattle, Sheep, and Goats)
Altrenogest: See Progesterone	Label dose: 0.044 mg/kg once daily; PO (1 mL/50 kg) for 15 days (estrus synchronization) Follow with luteolytic dose of prostaglandin $F_{2\alpha}$ Not for use in horses intended for human consumption.	None
Aluminum hydroxide: See Antacids	Extralabel dose: 60 mg/kg; PO	Extralabel dose: Same Withdrawal: Ψ
Amikacin	Label dose: 2 g for 3 days; Intrauterine Extralabel dose: 3.5 to 7.5 mg/kg bid to qid; IM, SC **OR** 7.7 mg/kg once daily; IM, SC Foals: 1 to 10 mg/kg bid; slowly IV or IM Subconjunctival injection: 75 to 100 mg	Not labeled for use in food-producing animals.
Aminocaproic acid (unlicensed for veterinary use)	5 g initially; PO, IV followed by 1 g/hr until bleeding is under control (human dose)	None
Aminophylline	Label dose: 15 to 30 mL bid–qid; PO (1 g = 15 mL, Quiex Forte)	Extralabel dose: 0.5 to 1 g qid; PO per calf (Enzootic pneumonia)

Drug	Horses (and Miniature Pig Doses, Where Indicated)	Ruminants (Cattle, Sheep, and Goats)
Aminophylline (continued)	Extralabel dose: 5 to 10 mg/kg tid; PO Race withdrawal: 96 hr	2 to 9 mg/kg tid; IV (pulmonary dysmaturity) Withdrawal: Ψ
Ammonium chloride	Extralabel dose: 50 g/450 kg once daily; PO (urolithiasis) 132 mg/kg; PO (strychnine intoxication)	Extralabel dose: 0.5% in ration (urolithiasis) 132 mg/kg; PO (strychnine intoxication) 100 g/day; PO administer for 21 days prior to calving. (prevention of parturient paresis in cattle) Withdrawal: Ψ
Amoxicillin	Extralabel dose: 10 to 22 mg/kg tid–qid; IV, IM 20 mg/kg qid; PO Extralabel dose: *Miniature pigs* 10 mg/kg bid; PO	Label dose: 11 mg/kg once daily; IM or SC Withdrawal: Meat: 25 days ℞ Milk: 96 hr & 8.8 mg/kg bid; PO in preruminant calves Withdrawal: Meat: 20 days ℞ 62.5 mg (one tube) per quarter for mastitis Withdrawal: Meat: 12 days ℞ Milk: 60 hr ℞
Amphetamine (unlicensed for veterinary use)	None	0.5 to 4 mg/kg; IV, SC, IP Withdrawal: Ψ

Drug	Horses (and Miniature Pig Doses, Where Indicated)	Ruminants (Cattle, Sheep, and Goats)
Ampicillin	Label dose: 3 mg/lb (6.6 mg/kg) bid; IM or IV (Amp Equine) Extralabel dose: Sodium ampicillin: 25 to 100 mg/kg tid–qid; IV, IM Ampicillin trihydrate: 11 to 22 mg/kg bid–tid; IM Not for use in horses intended for human consumption. Extralabel dose: *Miniature pigs* 4 to 10 mg/kg; IM, IV 10 to 20 mg/kg tid–qid; IM	Label dose: 6 mg/kg once daily; IM (Canada) 2 to 5 mg/lb once daily; IM (US) (Ampicillin trihydrate) Extralabel dose: 5 to 12 mg/kg once daily; IM Withdrawal: (at label dose) Meat: 6 days ℞ Milk: 48 hr ℞ Ampicillin sodium Meat: 14 days &
Amprolium	None Extralabel dose: *Miniature pigs* 100 mg/kg in food or water daily	Label dose: Mix in drinking water at 0.012% amprolium for 5 days. This will give approximately 10 mg/kg/day at normal water consumption. Withdrawal: Meat: 24 hr ℞ (US), 7 days ℞ (Canada) Extralabel dose: 50 to 100 mg/kg daily; PO (prophylaxis against clinical sarcocystosis in lambs) Withdrawal: Ψ

Drug	Horses (and Miniature Pig Doses, Where Indicated)	Ruminants (Cattle, Sheep, and Goats)
Antacids (unlicensed for veterinary use)	Many products; see label for dosage	See package labels
Antihistamines-H$_1$ Blockers	Read package label for individual instruction; doses vary between products	Read package label for individual instruction
Antitussives: See individual products	30 to 60 mL orally q 4 hr or as required for an adult	None
Apramycin	None Extralabel dose: *Miniature pigs* 10 to 20 mg/kg once to twice daily; PO 100 mg/L in drinking water	None
Ascorbic acid	Extralabel dose: 20 g; PO/horse/day	Label dose: 2.2 to 11 mg/kg; IM, IV daily (C-Ject, US) Extralabel dose: 2 g twice weekly; IM Withdrawal: Ψ
Aspirin	Extralabel dose: 15 to 100 mg/kg bid–tid; PO **OR** 30 mg/kg once daily; PO (chronic recurrent uveitis) Extralabel dose: *Miniature pigs* 10 to 20 mg/kg qid; PO **OR** 10 mg/kg bid; PO	Label dose: 1 to 3 boluses bid–tid; PO Powder: 10 to 60 g bid–tid; PO Withdrawal: Ψ
Atracurium (unlicensed for veterinary use)	0.04 to 0.7 mg/kg; IV (foals)	None

Drug	Horses (and Miniature Pig Doses, Where Indicated)	Ruminants (Cattle, Sheep, and Goats)
Atropine	Label dose: 0.4 mg/kg; IV, IM, or SC Extralabel dose: 0.1 to 1.0 mg/kg; IV, IM, SC Extralabel dose: *Miniature pigs* 0.04 mg/kg; IM	Label dose: 0.4 mg/kg; IV, IM, SC Extralabel dose: 0.1 to 1.0 mg/kg; IV, IM, SC Withdrawal: Ψ
Aurothioglucose (unlicensed for veterinary use)	20 mg; IM; 50 mg; IM 1 wk later; then 1 mg/kg; IM at weekly intervals until signs abate and weaning off drug can begin	Goats: 5 mg IM; 10 mg; IM 1 wk later, then 1 mg/kg; IM at weekly intervals until signs abate Withdrawal: Ψ
Azaperone	None Extralabel dose: *Miniature pigs* 0.25 to 0.5 mg/kg; IM (sedation without ataxia) 2.2 mg/kg; IM (calm nursing sow) 2 to 8 mg/kg; IM (sedation; immobilization) Withdrawal: 24 hr for 2.2 mg/kg (label dose)	None
Bacitracin, neomycin, polymixin B sulfate	Extralabel dose: Topically to the cornea or conjunctiva one or more times per day as required	Extralabel dose: Topically to the cornea or conjunctiva one or more times per day as required Withdrawal: Ψ
BAL (Dimercaprol) (unlicensed for veterinary use)	10% solution in oil: give 2.5 to 5 mg/kg q 4 hr; IM for 2 days, then bid for the next 10 days or recovery	4 mg/kg q 4 hr; IM until recovery Withdrawal: Ψ

Drug	Horses (and Miniature Pig Doses, Where Indicated)	Ruminants (Cattle, Sheep, and Goats)
BAL (Dimercaprol) (unlicensed for veterinary use) (continued)	For severe acute poisoning: 5 mg/kg dosage should be given only for the first day	
Beclomethasone (unlicensed for veterinary use)	3,750 μg for an adult horse bid; by inhalation (using Aero-Mask device)	None
Betamethasone	Label dose: 2.5 to 5 mL q 1 to 3 wk; intraarticularly Race withdrawal: 24 hr if given IM	Extralabel dose: 1 to 5 mL; intraarticularly Withdrawal: Ψ
Bethanechol (unlicensed for veterinary use)	0.025 to 0.075 mg/kg tid–qid; SC 0.3 to 0.75 mg/kg tid–qid; PO	None
Bismuth subsalicylate compounds	Label dose: Horses: 6 to 10 oz q 2 to 3 hr; PO Foals: 2 to 4 oz q 2 to 3 hr; PO Extralabel dose: 0.5 to 1 mL/kg q 4 to 6 hr; PO (foals) 1 to 2 L/450 kg bid; PO	Label dose: Cattle: 6 to 10 oz q 2 to 3 hr; PO Calves: 2 to 4 oz q 2 to 3 hr; PO (For bolus products) Generally, one bolus/70 kg calf bid; PO for 2 or 3 days Scour bolus N: 1 bolus/45 kg bid; PO for 2 days Read directions on individual products Withdrawal: Meat: 5 days &
Boldenone undecylenate	Label dose: 0.276 to 1.1 mg/kg; IM repeated at 2- or 3-wk intervals	None

Drug	Horses (and Miniature Pig Doses, Where Indicated)	Ruminants (Cattle, Sheep, and Goats)
Boldenone undecylenate (continued)	Not for use in horses intended for human consumption.	
Botulinum antitoxin (unlicensed for veterinary use)	200 mL; IV, IM (foals) 500 mL; IV, IM (adults)	None
Bupivicaine hydrochloride (unlicensed for veterinary use)	Local infiltration for nerve blocks Race withdrawal: 24 hr for a single 50 mg injection	Local nerve blocks and epidural anesthesia in sheep Withdrawal: Ψ
Butorphanol tartrate	Label dose: 0.1 mg/kg; IV, IM Race withdrawal: 72 hr Not for use in horses intended for human consumption. Extralabel dose: *Miniature pigs* 0.1 to 0.3 mg/kg bid to tid; IM, IV 0.05 to 0.2 mg/kg q 3 to 4 hr; SC, IV	Extralabel dose: 0.01 to 0.1 mg/kg; IV, IM Withdrawal: Meat: 30 days & Milk: 96 hr & (For dose of 0.045 mg/kg IV; Milk: 36 hr)
Calcium borogluconate (23% solution)	Label dose: 250 to 500 mL; IV, SC, IP Extralabel dose: 0.2 to 0.4 mL/kg; slowly IV in 1 to 2 L of D_5W	Label dose: 250 to 500 mL; IV, SC, IP Sheep and swine: 50 to 125 mL; IV, SC, IP Extralabel dose: 1 mL/kg; IV, IM, SC Withdrawal: Ψ
Calcium chloride (unlicensed for veterinary use)	1 to 2 g/450 kg; slowly IV to effect	None
Calcium disodium edetate	Label dose: 1 mL/kg; slowly IV divided 2 to 3 times daily	Extralabel dose: Maximum safe daily dosage is 75 mg/kg; IV drip

Drug	Horses (and Miniature Pig Doses, Where Indicated)	Ruminants (Cattle, Sheep, and Goats)
Calcium disodium edetate (continued)	Extralabel dose: 0.5 mL/kg bid; IV for 3 to 5 days; can be repeated after a 2-day rest period Not for use in horses intended for human consumption.	Withdrawal: Ψ
Captan (unlicensed for veterinary use)	Topical application of a 3% solution	Topical application of a 1% solution W/V in water over the entire body for 3 days; then at weekly intervals until infection resolved Withdrawal: Ψ Use is definitely extralabel.
Carbachol (unlicensed for veterinary use)	2 to 4 mg; SC (adults) 0.5 to 1.0 mg; SC (colts) OR 0.25 to 0.5 mg; SC (foals) Repeat at intervals no shorter than 30 to 60 min, as required.	2 to 4 mg; SC (mature cattle) 0.5 to 2 mg; SC (calves) Withdrawal: Ψ
Carbaryl	Label dose: Dust entire animal with not more than 500 g dust per head; repeat at 14- to 18-day intervals for louse control. OR Apply spray directly to horse's coat not more than twice per week.	Label dose: Dairy cattle: dust top line, sides, and legs; do not apply to underline or udder. Repeat not more than twice per week. OR Mix 1 kg/100 L of water; spray 5 L of the mixture per head of livestock; repeat if necessary.

Drug	Horses (and Miniature Pig Doses, Where Indicated)	Ruminants (Cattle, Sheep, and Goats)
Carbaryl (continued)		Withdrawal: Meat: 1 week ℞
Casein (iodized) (unlicensed for veterinary use)	5 g once daily; PO	None
Cefaclor: See Cephalosporins (unlicensed for veterinary use)	20 to 40 mg/kg tid; PO	None
Cefadroxil: See Cephalo-sporins	Extralabel dose: 22 mg/kg bid; PO	None
Cefamandole: See Cephalosporins (unlicensed for veterinary use)	10 to 30 mg/kg q 4 to 8 hr; IV, IM	None
Cefazolin: See Cephalosporins (unlicensed for veterinary use)	15 mg/kg bid–tid; IV, IM 50 mg subconjuncti-vally	22 mg/kg tid; IM 250 mg; IV regional with tourniquet for treatment of local-ized arthritis Withdrawal: Meat: 30 days &
Cefonicid: See Cephalosporins (unlicensed for veterinary use)	10 to 15 mg/kg once daily; IV, IM	None
Cefoperazone: See Cephalosporins (unlicensed for veterinary use)	30 to 50 mg/kg bid–tid; IV, IM	None
Cefotaxime: See Cephalosporins (unlicensed for veterinary use)	25 to 50 mg/kg bid–tid; IV, IM	None
Cefoxitin: See Cephalosporins (unlicensed for veterinary use)	30 to 40 mg/kg tid–qid; IM	None

Drug	Horses (and Miniature Pig Doses, Where Indicated)	Ruminants (Cattle, Sheep, and Goats)
Ceftazidime: See Cephalosporins (unlicensed for veterinary use)	25 to 50 mg/kg bid; IV, IM	None
Ceftiofur: See Cephalosporins	Label dose: 2 mg/kg once daily; IM Extralabel dose: 2 to 5 mg/kg bid; IV, IM Not for use in horses intended for food. Extralabel dose: *Miniature pigs* 3 to 10 mg/kg once daily; IM 1.1 to 2.2 mg/kg once daily; IM × 7 days (rhinitis)	Label dose: 1 mg/kg once daily; IM for 3 days Withdrawal: Meat: None ℞ Milk: None ℞ (Canada only)
Ceftizoxime: See Cephalosporins (unlicensed for veterinary use)	25 to 50 mg/kg bid–tid; IV, IM	None
Ceftriaxone: See Cephalosporins (unlicensed for veterinary use)	25 to 50 mg/kg bid; IV, IM	None
Cefuroxime axetil: See Cephalosporins (unlicensed for veterinary use)	25 to 50 mg/kg tid; IV, IM 250 to 500 mg/kg bid; PO	None
Cephalexin: See Cephalosporins (unlicensed for veterinary use)	10 to 30 mg/kg tid–qid; PO	None
Cephalothin: See Cephalosporins (unlicensed for veterinary use)	20 to 40 mg/kg tid–qid; IV, IM	None

Drug	Horses (and Miniature Pig Doses, Where Indicated)	Ruminants (Cattle, Sheep, and Goats)
Cephapirin: See Cephalosporins	Extralabel dose: 30 mg/kg q 4 to 6 hr; IV, IM	Label dose: 300 mg in 10 mL mastitis tube. Insert contents of one syringe into each of the four quarters at drying off (benzathine salt [Cefa-Dri, Tomorrow]) Withdrawal: Meat: 42 days ℞ Milk from treated cows must not be used for human consumption during the first 84 hr after calving. ℞ Label dose: Insert contents of one syringe 200 mg/10 mL mastitis syringe (sodium salt [Cefa-Lak, Today]) into affected quarter q 12 hr for 2 treatments. Withdrawal: Meat: 4 days ℞ Milk: 96 hr ℞
Charcoal, activated	Label dose: Toxiban 0.75 to 2 g/kg or 10 to 20 mL/kg; PO Extralabel dose: 1 to 3 g/kg; PO in a slurry (1 g/5 mL water), repeat in 8 to 12 hr if needed	Label dose: Toxiban 0.75 to 2 g/kg or 10 to 20 mL/kg; PO Extralabel dose: 2 to 9 g/kg; PO in a slurry, repeat as needed Withdrawal: Ψ

COMMON DOSAGES FOR LARGE ANIMALS 357

Drug	Horses (and Miniature Pig Doses, Where Indicated)	Ruminants (Cattle, Sheep, and Goats)
Chloral hydrate (unlicensed for veterinary use)	40 to 100 mg/kg; PO (sedation) 60 to 200 mg/kg; IV (foal restraint)	50 to 70 mg/kg; IV (sedation) 10 g/45 kg; PO (acetonemia) Withdrawal: Ψ
Chloramphenicol	Extralabel dose: 25 mg/kg tid–qid; IV, IM [succinate] **OR** 4 to 10 mg/kg tid–qid; PO (foals) 25 to 50 mg/kg tid–qid; PO (adults) [palmitate] Extralabel dose: *Miniature pigs* 10–25 mg/kg bid; IM Prohibited from use in food animals.	Prohibited from use in food animals.
Chlorhexidine	Label strength: 1% topically Extralabel strength: 0.5% to 2% topically	Label strength: 0.35 to 0.55% More concentrated solutions require dilution. Topically as an udder wash or teat dip in cattle Withdrawal: None required Extralabel dose: Udder infusion; 60 mL per infected quarter after milking. Milk out in 24 hours and repeat, leaving second infusion unmilked from quarter.

Drug	Horses (and Miniature Pig Doses, Where Indicated)	Ruminants (Cattle, Sheep, and Goats)
Chlorpromazine hydrochloride (unlicensed for veterinary use)	1 mg/kg; IM Race withdrawal: 96 hr	0.22 to 1.0 mg/kg; IV 1.0 to 4.4 mg/kg; IM Withdrawal: Ψ
Chlortetracycline	None	Label dose: Beef and dairy cattle: 22 mg/kg; PO Calves: 55 mg/kg; PO Lambs: 22 mg/kg; PO Extralabel dose: 10 to 20 mg/kg daily; PO Withdrawal: see individual products as withdrawal varies with product
Chorionic gonadotrophin (HCG)	Label dose: 1,000 U; IV on the first or second day of estrus Service should be permitted 24 or 48 hr later (mares) 1,000 to 2,000 U weekly for 8 injections; IM (stallions) 1,000 U twice weekly for 4- to 6-wk; IM (cryptorchid foals)	Label dose: 1,000 to 2,500 U; IV 10,000 U; IM Repeat in 21 days if necessary (cystic ovaries in cattle) 500 U; IV on days 19 and 20 of the cycle (hasten ovulation) Sheep: 400 to 800 U; IV, IM Goats: 3,000 U; IV Withdrawal: Ψ
Cimetidine (unlicensed for veterinary use)	6.6 mg/kg q 4 to 6 hr; IV, PO **OR** 12 to 16 mg/kg tid; PO 18 mg/kg bid; PO (gastric ulcers) 2.5 mg/kg tid; PO (melanomas)	None

Drug	Horses (and Miniature Pig Doses, Where Indicated)	Ruminants (Cattle, Sheep, and Goats)
Cisapride (unlicensed for veterinary use)	0.1 mg/kg; IM 0.5 to 0.8 mg/kg tid; PO	0.1 mg/kg; IM
Clenbuterol	Label dose: 0.8 µg/kg bid; PO (4 mL [one pump of the metered dose] per 125 kg) 30 µg per 50 kg; slowly IV Extralabel dose: 0.8 µg/kg bid; IM, slowly IV (bronchodilation) 0.8 to 3.2 µg/kg bid; PO 200 mg; IM (uterine relaxation) Race withdrawal: 72 hr	Extralabel dose: 0.8 µg/kg; IM, IV (uterine relaxation) 1.6 µg/kg/day; PO (prevention of abomasal ulceration) 0.2 mg per ewe; PO, IM (controlled parturition) Withdrawal: Ψ
Cloprostenol: See Prostaglandin $F_{2\alpha}$	None	Label dose: 2 mL (0.5 mg); IM (adult cow) 1.5 mL (or 2 mL; IM for animals over 455 kg) (for abortion) Extralabel dose: 100 to 150 mg; IM (pseudopregnancy in goats) Withdrawal: Meat: 2 days ℞ (Canada) Milk: 0 ℞
Clorsulon	None	Label dose: 7 mg/kg; PO Withdrawal: Meat: 8 days ℞ Not for use in lactating dairy cattle.

Drug	Horses (and Miniature Pig Doses, Where Indicated)	Ruminants (Cattle, Sheep, and Goats)
Clorsulon (continued)		Extralabel dose: Goats: 7 to 15 mg/kg; PO
Cloxacillin	None	Label dose: 200 mg/tube of the sodium salt for intramammary infusion Withdrawal: Meat: 10 days ℞ (US) Milk: 48 hr ℞ (US), 60 hr ℞ (Canada) 500 mg/tube of the benzathine salt for dry treatment Withdrawal: Meat and milk: 28 to 30 days (US), 30 days (Canada) ℞
Cobalt	None	Top dress the soil with 100 to 150 g cobalt sulfate/acre, alternatively, mixed with mineral or salt blocks (endemic deficiency areas) **OR** See acetonemia products. See individual product label for dose. Withdrawal: None anticipated
Colistin (unlicensed for veterinary use)	2,500 IU/kg qid; slowly IV	None
Copper, injectable	Label dose: Combination products with copper: 30 mL/450 kg; slowly IV every second day	Label dose: 60 mg; SC (calves) 120 mg; SC (mature cattle) [copper glycinate]

Drug	Horses (and Miniature Pig Doses, Where Indicated)	Ruminants (Cattle, Sheep, and Goats)
Copper, injectable (continued)	Read label for individual product.	Withdrawal: Meat: 30 days ℞, see individual products.
Copper naphthenate	Label dose: External use only; remove necrotic tissue, cleanse area, and apply.	Label dose: External use only; remove necrotic tissue, cleanse area, and apply. Not to be used on the teats of lactating dairy cattle.
Copper sulfate	Label dose: Apply the powder freely to wounds twice daily. Repeat as indicated.	Extralabel dose: 5% solution for footbaths **OR** 2 to 4 L as a 0.4% solution; PO (phosphorus toxicity) **OR** 1 g/adult cow daily; PO (copper deficiency) 35 mg/head/day; PO (swayback prevention in lambs) Withdrawal: Ψ
Corticotropin	Label dose: 200 IU; IM, SC Repeat 3 to 7 days as required (adult horse)	Extralabel dose: 200 IU; IM daily (mature cow) Withdrawal: Ψ
Coumaphos	Label dose: 1% dust topically 3% spray topically or according to labeled instructions for concentrated products	Label dose: 1% dust topically, 55 g/head 3% spray (KRS) Withdrawal: Meat: 7 days ℞ Concentrated products: Mix according to label instructions.

Drug	Horses (and Miniature Pig Doses, Where Indicated)	Ruminants (Cattle, Sheep, and Goats)
Coumaphos (continued)		Directions may vary for lactating and nonlactating cattle. Withdrawal: Milk: 14 days ℞ Sheep and goats Withdrawal: Meat: 15 days (Co-Ral 25% Wettable Powder) ℞
Cromolyn sodium (unlicensed for veterinary use)	80 mg; nebulized once daily **OR** 200 to 300 mg nebulized per horse	None
Dantrolene (unlicensed for veterinary use)	Extralabel dose: 9 mg/kg; PO presurgically (postanesthetic myopathy prevention) 2.0 mg/kg; slowly IV in saline (acute myopathy) Race withdrawal: 36 hr Extralabel dose: *Miniature pigs* 2 to 5 mg/kg tid; PO, IV (malignant hyperthermia)	None
Decoquinate	None	Label dose: 0.5 mg/kg body weight per day Mix according to package directions. Withdrawal: Meat: 0 ℞ Not for use in lactating dairy cattle.
Dembrexine	Label dose: 0.33 mg/kg bid; PO for 10 days Race withdrawal: 72 hr	None

Drug	Horses (and Miniature Pig Doses, Where Indicated)	Ruminants (Cattle, Sheep, and Goats)
Detomidine	Label dose: 0.2 to 0.04 mg/kg; IV, IM Extralabel dose: 0.01 to 0.02 mg/kg; IV followed by butorphanol (0.044–0.066 mg/kg; IV), or ketamine (2.2 mg/kg; IV)	None
Dexamethasone	Label dose: 2 to 5 mg; IV, IM 5 to 10 mg; PO daily Extralabel dose: 0.02 to 0.2 mg/kg; IV, IM, PO 0.5 to 2 mg/kg; IV (shock) 0.1% suspension every 3 to 8 hr applied to eyes Race withdrawal: 24 hr	Label dose: 5 to 20 mg; IM, IV 5 to 10 mg; PO (anti-inflammatory for adult cattle) Extralabel dose: 20 mg; IM (parturition induction in cattle) 8 to 16 mg; IM (parturition induction in sheep past 138 days' gestation) 10 mg; IM (parturition induction in goats past 135 days' gestation) 20 mg; IM combined with luteolytic dose of prostaglandin $F_{2\alpha}$ (for abortion after 150 days' gestation) Withdrawal: Meat and milk: 0 & Most products are not intended for use in food-producing animals (US).

Drug	Horses (and Miniature Pig Doses, Where Indicated)	Ruminants (Cattle, Sheep, and Goats)
Dextran 70 (unlicensed for veterinary use)	500 mL of 32% dextran 70 into abdominal cavity during surgery (intestinal adhesion prevention)	None
Diazepam (unlicensed for veterinary use)	Extralabel dose: 0.03 to 0.5 mg/kg; slowly IV, repeat in 30 min if needed Extralabel dose: *Miniature pigs* 0.5 to 3.0 mg/kg; IM (tranquilization) 5.5 mg/kg; IM (sedation)	Extralabel dose: 0.5 to 1.5 mg/kg; IV, IM Withdrawal: 30 days for the 0.1 mg/kg; IV &
Dichlorvos	Label dose: 1 packet (78 g) per 901 to 1200 lb (400–533 kg); PO Extralabel dose: 35 mg/kg; PO **OR** 0.93% solution topically Extralabel dose: *Miniature pigs* 20 mg/kg; PO	Label dose: Cattle: 30 to 60 mL; PO per animal Withdrawal: 0 days ℞
Diethylcarbamazine	Extralabel dose: 1 mg/kg once daily; PO for 21 days (onchocerciasis) 50 mg/kg; PO for 10 days (verminous myelitis)	None
Digoxin	Extralabel dose: IV priming dose: 12 to 14 mg/kg; IV Oral priming dose: 34 to 70 mg/kg; PO	Extralabel dose: Priming dose: 22 mg/kg; IV Maintenance dose: follow loading dose

Drug	Horses (and Miniature Pig Doses, Where Indicated)	Ruminants (Cattle, Sheep, and Goats)
Digoxin (continued)	IV maintenance dose: 6 to 7 mg/kg/day; IV Oral maintenance dose: 17 to 35 mg/kg/day; PO	by infusion of 0.86 mg/kg/hr; IV **OR** 11 mg/kg tid; IV Withdrawal: Ψ
Dihydrostreptomycin	Extralabel dose: 11 mg/kg bid; IM, SC	Label dose: Calves (pneumonia): 2 mL bid to tid; IM for 4 to 5 days Cattle: 1 mL/20 kg; IM once (leptospirosis) 2 to 4 mL/100 kg once or twice daily; IM (coliform mastitis) Withdrawal: Meat: 30 days ℞ Milk: 96 hr ℞ Extralabel dose: 25 mg/kg once daily; IM **OR** 12.5 mg/kg bid; IM (leptospirosis)
Dimethyl glycine (unlicensed for veterinary use)	1 to 1.6 mg/kg once daily; PO	None
Dimethyl sulfoxide	Label dose: Gel: topical use 2 to 3 times daily Solution: topical use 2 to 3 times daily Not to exceed 100 g or 100 mL per day Extralabel dose: 0.5 to 4 g/kg bid; IV	Extralabel dose: Topical use only. If used IV; 0.5 to 4 g/kg bid; IV IV solution should be diluted to 20% concentration (approximately five-fold dilution) in saline or D_5W Withdrawal: Milk: 48 hr & Meat: 96 hr & (topical use)

Drug	Horses (and Miniature Pig Doses, Where Indicated)	Ruminants (Cattle, Sheep, and Goats)
Dimethyl sulfoxide (continued)	IV solution should be diluted to 20% concentration (approximately five-fold dilution) in saline or D_5W Race withdrawal (as topical): 36 hr	Meat: 20 days & Milk: 72 hr & (IV use)
Dioctyl sodium sulphosuccinate (docusate sodium)	Label dose: Orally: 8 oz/gal water Enema: 4 to 6 oz/gal water Extralabel dose: 17 to 66 mg/kg q 48 hr; PO (intestinal impaction) **OR** 10 mL per rectum in warm water (meconium impaction)	Label dose: 300 mL; PO (adult cattle) 50 mL; PO (sheep and goats), repeat as required (frothy bloat) Withdrawal: Ψ Extralabel dose: 50 mg/kg/day; PO (abomasal impaction)
Dipyrone	Label dose: 10 to 20 mL; IV, IM, SC or 20 to 60 mL; IV, IM (4 mL/45 kg) Extralabel dose: 44 to 66 mg/kg; IV, IM, SC. Injections can be repeated 2 or 3 times daily. Injections should be given slowly. Race withdrawal: 36 hr for single dose and 120 hr for 5-day treatment	Extralabel dose: 50 mg/kg; IV, IM, SC Withdrawal: Meat: 35 days & Milk: 7 days &
Dobutamine (unlicensed for veterinary use)	1 to 10 μg/kg/min; IV (250 mg in 500 mL saline infused at 0.45 mL/kg/hr)	None

Drug	Horses (and Miniature Pig Doses, Where Indicated)	Ruminants (Cattle, Sheep, and Goats)
Dopamine (unlicensed for veterinary use)	2 to 5 µg/kg/min; IV	2 to 5 µg/kg/min; IV
Doxapram	Label dose: 0.44 to 0.55 mg/kg; IV Extralabel dose: 0.5 to 1.0 mg/kg q 5 min; IV Do not exceed 2 mg/kg in foals **OR** 0.02 to 0.05 mg/kg/min; IV (resuscitation in neonatal foals)	Extralabel dose: 5 to 10 mg/kg; IV (treatment of poisoning) Withdrawal: Ψ
Echothiopate iodide (unlicensed for veterinary use)	0.03% bid; applied to eyes	None
Enilconazole	Topically through endoscopic flushing 33.3 mg/mL solution. 60 mL once daily (gutteral pouch mycosis)	None
Enrofloxacin	Extralabel dose: 2.5 to 5 mg/kg bid; PO 5.0 mg/kg once daily; IV, IM Extralabel dose: *Miniature pigs* 2.5 to 5 mg/kg once daily; IM	Extralabel dose: 2.5 to 5 mg/kg once daily; PO in calves, otherwise, IM Not to be used in growing animals. Withdrawal: Ψ 28 days at 2.5 to 5 mg/kg bid; PO Milk: 96 hr (Note: Fluoroquinolones are banned for extralabel use in food-producing animals in the US.)

Drug	Horses (and Miniature Pig Doses, Where Indicated)	Ruminants (Cattle, Sheep, and Goats)
Ephedrine (unlicensed for veterinary use)	0.7 mg/kg bid; PO	None
Epinephrine	Label dose: 1 mL/45 kg; IV, IM, SC, or 3 to 8 mL; IM, SC Use IV route only for emergencies such as anaphylaxis.	Label dose: 1 mL/45 kg; IV, IM, SC **OR** 3 to 8 mL; IM, SC Extralabel dose: Sheep: 1 to 3 mL; IM, SC Use IV route only for emergencies such as anaphylaxis. Withdrawal: Ψ
Ergonovine	Label dose: 1 to 4 mg; IM, IV (mare)	Label dose: 1 to 4 mg; IM, IV (cow) Extralabel dose: 0.4 to 1 mg; IM, IV (ewe and doe) Withdrawal: Ψ
Erythromycin	Extralabel dose: 2.5 to 5 mg/kg tid–qid; IV [lactobionate] **OR** 25 mg/kg tid–qid; or 37.5 mg/kg bid; PO [base or estolate] combined with rifampin at 10 mg/kg bid; PO (*R. equi* pneumonia) Therapy must often be prolonged (4–20 wk)	Label dose: 2.2 to 4.4 mg/kg once daily; IM (cattle) 11 mg/kg once daily; IM (lambs >4.5 kg) 2.2 mg/kg; IM (older sheep) Withdrawal: Meat: 14 days for cattle & 3 days for sheep ℜ Milk: 72 hr ℜ Note: Withdrawal times may vary with product. Consult individual product.

Drug	Horses (and Miniature Pig Doses, Where Indicated)	Ruminants (Cattle, Sheep, and Goats)
Erythromycin (continued)		**OR** 300 mg per quarter (mastitis × 3 treatments) Withdrawal: 　Meat: 14 days ℞ 　Milk: 36 hr ℞ **OR** 600 mg per quarter (dry treatment) Withdrawal: 　Meat: 14 days ℞ 　Milk: 72 hr (Canada) ℞, 96 hr (US) ℞, after calving
Estradiol	Extralabel dose: 　5 to 10 mg; IM (anestrus) 　0.004 to 0.008 mg/kg q 2 days; IM (urinary incontinence)	Label dose: 　3 to 5 mg; IM (anestrus in cows) 　10 mg; IM (pyometra, retained placenta, mummified fetus; cows) 　4 mg; IM (persistent corpus luteum, cow) 　3 mg; IM (anestrus, heifers) Extralabel dose: 　0.05 mg/kg; IM with 0.125 mg/kg progesterone bid; IM for 7 days (lactation induction in cattle) Withdrawal: Ψ
Ethyl alcohol (50%) (unlicensed for veterinary use)	5 to 10 mL/50 kg as an aerosol (respiratory therapy) 4.4 mL/kg of a 25% solution; IV	Same

Drug	Horses (and Miniature Pig Doses, Where Indicated)	Ruminants (Cattle, Sheep, and Goats)
Ethyl alcohol (50%) (continued)	followed by 2 mL/kg q 4 hr; IV for 4 days (methanol or ethylene glycol toxicity)	
Ethylenediamine dihydroiodide	Label dose: 7.5 to 15 g bid; PO for 7 days	Label dose: 7.5 to 15 g bid; PO for 7 days (cattle) Withdrawal: Ψ
Famotidine (unlicensed for veterinary use)	Extralabel dose: 0.2 mg/kg tid; IV 1 to 2 mg/kg tid; PO	None
Febantel	Label dose: 6 mg/kg; PO	Extralabel dose: Sheep: 5 mg/kg; PO Withdrawal: Ψ
Fenbendazole	Label dose: 5 mg/kg; PO (Strongyles, pinworms) **OR** 10 mg/kg; PO (Ascarids) Extralabel dose: 50 mg/kg; PO (*S. westeri*) Extralabel dose: *Miniature pigs* 10 mg/kg once daily; PO for 3 days (whipworms)	Label dose: 5 mg/kg; PO **OR** 10 mg/kg; PO for *Moniezia benedeni* and arrested 4th stage larvae of *Ostertagia ostertagi* Withdrawal: Meat: 8 days (US), 10 days (Canada) & Milk: 96 hr & **OR** 10 mg/kg; PO (*Moniezia* spp and arrested 4th stage larvae of *O. ostertagi*) Extralabel dose: Goats: 25 mg/kg; PO Withdrawal: Ψ

Drug	Horses (and Miniature Pig Doses, Where Indicated)	Ruminants (Cattle, Sheep, and Goats)
Fenoterol (unlicensed for veterinary use)	5 puffs per adult horse by face mask	None
Fenprostalene: See Prostaglandin F$_{2\alpha}$	Extralabel dose: 0.5 mg/450 kg; SC	Label dose: 1 mg; SC (cow) Withdrawal: Meat: 24 hours (Canada ℜ) Milk: 0 ℜ
Fentanyl/droperidol	None Extralabel dose: *Miniature pigs* 1 mL/12 to 25 kg; IM (minor procedures) 1 mL/9 to 14 kg; IM (sedation)	None
Florfenicol	None	Label dose: 20 mg/kg; 2 doses separated by 48 hr; IM Withdrawal: 36 days; not for use in dairy cattle
Floxacillin: See Cloxacillin (unlicensed for veterinary use)	10 mg/kg qid; IM	None
Flumethasone	Label dose: 1.25 to 2.5 mg/450 kg once daily; IM, IV or IA Race withdrawal: 24 hr	Extralabel dose: 1.25 to 5 mg/500 kg/day; IV, IM (cow) Withdrawal: Meat: 4 days & Milk: Ψ
Flunixin meglumine	Label dose: 1.1 mg/kg once daily; PO, IM, IV	Extralabel dose: 1.1 mg/kg once daily to tid; IV, IM **OR**

Drug	Horses (and Miniature Pig Doses, Where Indicated)	Ruminants (Cattle, Sheep, and Goats)
Flunixin meglumine (continued)	Extralabel dose: 1.1 mg/kg once daily to tid; PO, IM, IV 0.25 mg/kg tid; IM, IV (endotoxemia) Race withdrawal: 48 hr for oral dose and 72 hr for IM or IV Extralabel dose: *Miniature pigs* 0.5 to 1.0 mg/kg once to twice daily; SC, IV	0.5 to 1.1 mg/kg once or twice daily; IM, IV (viral pneumonia or acute respiratory distress) 2.2 mg/kg bid–tid; IM (secretory diarrhea) Withdrawal: Meat: 14 days & Milk: 96 hr &
Fluprostenol: See Prostaglandin $F_{2\alpha}$	Label dose: 250 mg/450 kg; IM	None
Flurbiprofen (unlicensed for veterinary use)	Apply to eyes tid to qid	None
Folic acid (unlicensed for veterinary use)	75 mg; IM (foal) **OR** 75 mg; IM q 3 days (during anti-protozoal therapy for protozoal myelitis)	None
Follicle-stimulating hormone (FSH)	Label dose: 10 to 50 mg/450 kg; IV, IM, SC (FSH-P) 7 to 35 mg/450 kg; IM (Ovaset)	Label dose: (FSH-P) 10 to 50 mg; IM, IV, SC (cattle) 5 to 25 mg; IM, IV, SC (sheep) (Ovaset) 7 to 35 mg; IM (cattle) 3.5 to 17.5 mg IM (sheep) (Superovulation) Day 1: a.m. and p.m., 11.3 mg; IM Day 2: a.m. and p.m., 9.8 mg; IM Day 3: a.m. and p.m., 9.0 mg; IM

Drug	Horses (and Miniature Pig Doses, Where Indicated)	Ruminants (Cattle, Sheep, and Goats)
Follicle-stimulating hormone (FSH) (continued)		Day 4: a.m. and p.m., 7.5 mg; IM (cattle) (Folltropin-V) Withdrawal: Meat: 10 days (Canada) ℜ Milk: Ψ
Formaldehyde solution	None	Extralabel dose: 2% to 5% as a foot bath for treatment and prevention of foot rot in cattle and sheep
Furazolidone: See Nitrofurans	Label dose: Topically; spray lightly once or twice daily	Banned for use in food-producing animals
Furosemide	Label dose: 0.5 to 1.0 mg/kg; IM or IV **OR** 500 mg/454 kg; IM, IV once daily, **OR** 250 mg/454 kg; IM, IV twice daily for 3 days Extralabel dose: 1 to 3 mg/kg bid; IM, IV **OR** 1 mg/kg; IV or by aerosol (bronchodilation) Race withdrawal: 24 hr; IM or IV and 36 hr; PO Note: Some regions allow the use of furosemide prerace for documented bleeders.	Label dose: 0.5 to 1.0 mg/kg; IM, IV **OR** 500 mg/kg; IM, IV once daily, **OR** 250 mg; IM, IV twice daily per 454 kg × 3 days Extralabel dose: 2.2 to 4.4 mg/kg bid; IV, IM Withdrawal at label dose: Meat: 2 days ℜ Milk: 48 hr ℜ

Drug	Horses (and Miniature Pig Doses, Where Indicated)	Ruminants (Cattle, Sheep, and Goats)
Gentamicin	Label dose: 2 to 2.5 g diluted with 200 to 500 mL saline intrauterine once daily for 3 to 5 days during estrus Extralabel dose: 2 to 4 mg/kg bid; IM, IV, SC **OR** 6.6 mg/kg; IV once daily 10 to 40 mg; subconjunctivally 0.2 to 2.0 g; intrauterine 150 mg (buffered); intra-articular Extralabel dose: *Miniature pigs* 2 to 4 mg/kg bid–tid; IM	Label dose: 200 mg diluted in 16 mL saline; intrauterine one time only; or 200 mg/20 mL intra-uterine syringe Withdrawal: Meat: 30 days (Canada ℞) **OR** Extralabel dose: 2.2 mg/kg tid; IV, IM (coliform mastitis) Withdrawal: Meat: 18 months & Milk: 5 days &, 10 days if infused into udder
Glucocorticoids: See individual products	See individual products	See individual products
Glycerol (unlicensed for veterinary use)	1 g/kg; PO (CNS trauma) **OR** 5% as an aerosol (respiratory therapy)	Same Withdrawal: Ψ
Glycopyrrolate	Extralabel dose: 0.01 mg/kg; IV (facilitate rectal exam) 1 mg; by nebuliza-tion or SC (obstructive lung disease) Extralabel dose: *Miniature pigs* 0.01 mg/kg; IM (preanesthetic)	None

Drug	Horses (and Miniature Pig Doses, Where Indicated)	Ruminants (Cattle, Sheep, and Goats)
Gonadorelin (GnRH)	Extralabel dose: 50 mg; SC, 2 and 0.5 hr before breeding (low libido) **OR** 40 mg; IM, 6 hr before breeding (induce ovulation)	Label dose: 100 mg; IM per cow Withdrawal: Meat and Milk: 0 ℞ (US) Meat: 7 days ℞ Milk: 12 hr ℞ (Canada)
Griseofulvin	Label dose: 2.5 g/450 kg; PO once daily for 10 days to 3 weeks Extralabel dose: 10 g/450 kg once daily; PO for 2 weeks, then 5 g/450 kg once daily; PO for 7 weeks	Extralabel dose: 20 mg/kg once daily; PO (in milk or feed) for 14 to 50 days Withdrawal: Ψ
Guaifenesin (glyceryl guaiacolate)	Label dose: 110 mg/kg; slowly IV to effect (anesthetic induction) Extralabel dose: 110 mg/kg; IV (convulsions) 0.1 to 0.2 g/50 kg qid; PO (expectorant) Race withdrawal: 24 hr	Extralabel dose: 110 mg/kg; IV Withdrawal: Ψ
Halothane	Label dose: Induction: 2% to 2.5% Maintenance: 0.5% to 2% Extralabel dose: Induction: 3% to 5% Maintenance: 1% to 3%	Same Withdrawal: Ψ

Drug	Horses (and Miniature Pig Doses, Where Indicated)	Ruminants (Cattle, Sheep, and Goats)
Heparin (unlicensed for veterinary use)	10 IU/kg; IV (loading dose) 15 IU/kg/hr; IV (maintenance) 40 to 100 IU/kg bid to qid; SC (acute laminitis) 40 to 80 IU/kg bid; IV, SC (adhesion prevention)	None
Hyaluronic acid	Label dose: 40 mg; IV 10 to 100 mg intra-articularly Extralabel dose: 20 to 120 mg around inflamed tendon	Extralabel dose: Same Withdrawal: Ψ
Hydralazine (unlicensed for veterinary use)	0.5 mg/kg; IV	None
Hydrochlorothiazide	Extralabel dose: 0.5 mg/kg bid; PO Race withdrawal: 60 hr	Label dose: 125 to 250 mg/cow once or twice daily; IV, IM Withdrawal: Milk: 3 days ℞
Hydrocortisone sodium succinate (unlicensed for veterinary use)	1 to 4 mg/kg; IV drip	Same Withdrawal: Ψ
Hydroxyzine (unlicensed for veterinary use)	0.5 to 1.0 mg/kg tid; IM, PO	Same Withdrawal: Ψ
Imipramine (unlicensed for veterinary use)	100 to 600 mg/450 kg bid; PO for 2 weeks (improve ejaculation) 0.55 mg/kg tid; IM, IV 1.5 mg/kg tid; PO (narcolepsy)	0.55 mg/kg tid; IM, IV 1.5 mg/kg tid; PO (narcolepsy) Withdrawal: Ψ

Drug	Horses (and Miniature Pig Doses, Where Indicated)	Ruminants (Cattle, Sheep, and Goats)
Insulin	Extralabel dose: 0.15 U/kg bid; IM, SC **OR** 0.1 to 0.2 U regular insulin/kg; SC, IV with simultaneous D₅W at 0.1 to 0.2 mL/kg/min.; IV (hyperkalemia)	Extralabel dose: 200 U long-acting insulin/450 kg bid; SC along with IV glucose drip (hepatic lipidosis) **OR** 200 U long-acting/450 kg q 48 hr; SC along with dextrose; IV (ketosis) Withdrawal: Ψ
Iodochlorhydroxyquin	Label dose: 10 g/450 kg; PO daily Extralabel dose: 15 g/450 kg; PO daily until feces become firm, then reduce dose gradually if response obtained	None
Ipratromium bromide (unlicensed for veterinary use)	2 to 3 µg/kg as respiratory aerosol by ultrasonic nebulization (4–6 hours bronchodilation)	None
Iron dextran	Extralabel dose: 400 to 600 mg/450 kg; IM (split dose in 2 sites) Extralabel dose: *Miniature pigs* 50 mg/animal; IM, repeat in 2 to 3 wk	None
Isoflupredone	Label dose: 5 to 20 mg; IM or intrasynovially/ intra-articularly Race withdrawal: 48 hr	Label dose: 10 to 20 mg; IM May repeat in 12 to 24 hr Withdrawal: Meat: 5 days ℞ (Canada)

Drug	Horses (and Miniature Pig Doses, Where Indicated)	Ruminants (Cattle, Sheep, and Goats)
Isoflupredone (continued)		7 days ℞ (US) Milk: 72 hr ℞ (Canada), Ψ (US)
Isoflurane	Label dose: Induction: 3% to 5% Maintenance: 1.5% to 1.8% Extralabel dose: Maintenance: 1% to 3.5%	Extralabel dose: Same Withdrawal: Ψ
Isoniazid (unlicensed for veterinary use)	5 to 15 mg/kg bid; PO	10 mg/kg/day; PO for 1 month (actinomycosis) Withdrawal: Milk: 100 days &
Isoproterenol (unlicensed for veterinary use)	0.4 µg/kg; by slow infusion IV (discontinue when heart rate doubles) 0.05 to 1.0 µg/kg; IV (foal resuscitation) 5 to 10 mL of 0.05% solution qid; as an aerosol	None
Isoxsuprine (unlicensed for veterinary use)	0.6 to 1.8 mg/kg bid; PO Race withdrawal: 36 hr	0.66 mg/kg; PO once, for pulmonary dysmaturity Withdrawal: Ψ
Itraconazole (unlicensed for veterinary use)	3 mg/kg bid; PO for up to 3 months.	None
Ivermectin	Label dose: 0.2 mg/kg; PO Extralabel dose: *Miniature pigs* 0.3 mg/kg; PO, SC, IM (Repeat in 14 days for sarcoptes)	Label dose: 0.2 mg/kg; SC Withdrawal: Meat: 35 days ℞ Not for use in lactating cattle Sheep drench: 0.2 mg/kg; PO

Drug	Horses (and Miniature Pig Doses, Where Indicated)	Ruminants (Cattle, Sheep, and Goats)
Ivermectin (continued)		Withdrawal: Meat: 14 days ℞ (Canada), 11 days ℞ (US) Cattle pour-on: 0.5 mg/kg; topically Withdrawal: Meat: 49 days ℞ (Canada), 48 days ℞ (US) Not for use in dairy cattle. Minor Use: Reindeer (Warbles): 0.2 mg/kg; SC Withdrawal: Meat: 56 days ℞ Calves: One sustained-release bolus (1.72 g) per calf weighing at least 100 kg and not more than 300 kg. BW. Withdrawal: Meat: 184 days ℞
Kanamycin	Extralabel dose: 7.5 mg/kg tid; IV, IM	Extralabel dose: 6 mg/kg bid; IM **OR** 10 to 20 mg; sub-conjunctivally Withdrawal: Ψ
Kaolin-pectin	Label dose: Adult: 15 to 30 mL/45 kg; PO q 2 to 3 hr Foal: 15 mL/10 kg; PO q 2 to 3 hr Extralabel dose: 2 to 4 L/450 kg; PO	Label dose: 15 to 30 mL/45 kg; PO q 2 to 3 hr Calves: 15 mL/10 kg; PO q 2 to 3 hr Extralabel dose: 180 to 300 mL/adult Cow: q 3 to 6 hr; PO Withdrawal: Ψ

Drug	Horses (and Miniature Pig Doses, Where Indicated)	Ruminants (Cattle, Sheep, and Goats)
Ketamine	Extralabel dose: 1.5 to 2.0 mg/kg; IV Must be preceded with a sedative/hypnotic (see xylazine, diazepam, detomidine), or muscle relaxants (see guaifenesin) Race withdrawal: 96 hr Extralabel dose: *Miniature pigs* Sedation 5 to 20 mg/kg; IM Immobilization 20 to 30 mg/kg; IM Sedation, premedication; with diazepam, 1 to 2 mg/kg; IM followed by 12 to 20 mg/kg; IM ketamine With xylazine, 2.2 mg/kg; IM, followed by 12 to 20 mg/kg; IM ketamine	Extralabel dose: 2.0 mg/kg; IV (following initial sedative agent) Withdrawal: Meat: 5 days & Milk: 72 hr &
Ketoconazole (unlicensed for veterinary use)	30 mg/kg once or twice daily; PO (dissolve in 0.2 N HCl)	None
Ketoprofen	Label dose: 2 to 2.2 mg/kg once daily; IV, IM for up to 5 days (musculoskeletal pain) Extralabel dose: 0.5 mg/kg; IV q 6 hr (endotoxemia)	None

Drug	Horses (and Miniature Pig Doses, Where Indicated)	Ruminants (Cattle, Sheep, and Goats)
Lactulose (unlicensed for veterinary use)	150 to 200 mL qid; PO per adult horse	None
Lasalocid	None: Toxic	Label dose: 250 mg/head/day; PO for cattle 200 to 299 kg, and 350 mg/head/day; PO for cattle >300 kg (feed additive) Withdrawal: 0 ℞ Extralabel dose: Sheep: 0.5 to 2 mg/kg; PO (30 g/ton of feed)
Levamisole	Extralabel dose: 8 mg/kg; PO Extralabel dose: *Miniature pigs* 10 mg/kg; PO	Label dose: (Injectable) Cattle: 6.0 mg/kg; SC Sheep and goats: 8.0 mg/kg; SC (Canada) Withdrawal: Meat: 7 days ℞ Milk: (Canada) 48 hr ℞ Extralabel dose: 3.3 to 8.0 mg/kg; SC Label dose: (Oral) 5.4 to 11 mg/kg; as drench or bolus Withdrawal: Meat: 2 days (cattle), 3 days (sheep, US) to 10 days ℞; see individual product

Drug	Horses (and Miniature Pig Doses, Where Indicated)	Ruminants (Cattle, Sheep, and Goats)
Levamisole (continued)		Pour-on: 2.5 mL/50 kg; topically Withdrawal: Meat: 10 days ℞ Milk: (Canada) 72 hr ℞ Pellets: 100 g/100 kg feed Withdrawal: Meat: 10 days Milk: (Canada) 60 hr ℞ Not for use in lactating dairy cattle (US)
Levothyroxine	Label dose: 35 to 100 mg/450 kg once daily; PO Extralabel dose: 10 mg/450 kg once daily; PO in 70 mL corn syrup	None
Lidocaine	Label dose: 2 to 50 mL local infiltration to effect (local anesthetic) Extralabel dose: 0.5 mg/kg; as bolus IV q 5 min until 2 to 4 mg/kg total (antiarrhythmic) Race withdrawal: infiltration 24 hr; topical (with DMSO) 36 hr	Label dose: 5 to 100 mL (cattle), 3 to 10 mL (sheep) local infiltration to effect (local anesthetic) Withdrawal: Meat: 5 days Milk: 96 hr ℞
Lincomycin	None; can induce fatal colitis in horses Extralabel dose: *Miniature pigs* 11 mg/kg once daily; IM	None; can cause fatalities if given to cattle
Loperamide (unlicensed for veterinary use)	0.1 to 0.2 mg/kg bid–tid; PO	None

Drug	Horses (and Miniature Pig Doses, Where Indicated)	Ruminants (Cattle, Sheep, and Goats)
Luteinizing hormone (LH)	Label dose: 25 mg; IV, SC (mare)	Label dose: 25 mg; IV, SC (cows) 2.5 mg; IV, SC (sheep and goats) Withdrawal: Ψ
Magnesium hydroxide	Extralabel dose: 200 to 250 mL (Milk of Magnesia) tid; PO (adult)	Label dose: 1 to 6 bolets; PO (1 bolus per 27 kg) Withdrawal: Milk: 12 to 24 hr (see individual products) **OR** 361 g (in 454 g powder) in 3.8 L water. Give 10 mL/kg orally by stomach tube. Gel: mature cattle 108 g; PO per animal Withdrawal: Meat: Ψ Milk: 12 to 24 hr ℜ (see individual product)
Magnesium sulfate (unlicensed for veterinary use)	0.2 to 0.4 g/kg dissolved in 4 L warm water, once daily; PO	0.44 mg/kg of a 20% solution; IV, SC (grass tetany) 1 to 2 g/kg; PO (cathartic) 2.5 g/kg/day; PO (abomasal impaction) Withdrawal: Ψ
Mannitol	Label dose: 1.65 to 2.2 g/kg; IV Extralabel dose: 0.25 to 2.0 g/kg; slowly IV	Label dose: 1.65 to 2.2 g/kg; IV Extralabel dose: 1 to 2 g/kg; IV Withdrawal: Ψ

Drug	Horses (and Miniature Pig Doses, Where Indicated)	Ruminants (Cattle, Sheep, and Goats)
Mebendazole	Label dose: 8.8 mg/kg; PO Extralabel dose: 20 mg/kg; PO (*D. arnfieldi*)	Extralabel dose: 10 mg/kg; PO (sheep) Withdrawal: Ψ
Meclofenamic acid	Label dose: 2.2 mg/kg/day; PO for 5 to 7 days Race withdrawal: 48 hr (single dose, detectable in urine for 96 hours following 7 daily doses)	Extralabel dose: 2.2 mg/kg/day; PO Withdrawal: Ψ
Megestrol acetate	Extralabel dose: 65 to 85 mg/kg once daily; PO	None
Melengestrol acetate	None	Label dose: 0.25 to 0.5 mg/head/day in feed Withdrawal: Meat: 48 hr (Canada), 3 to 5 days (US) ℞
Menadione sodium bisulphite (vitamin K₃)	Label dose: 50 to 100 mg/450 kg once daily; IV (prevention) 100 to 200 mg/450 kg once daily; IV (treatment) Use is not recommended: Nephrotoxic	Extralabel dose: 0.4 mg/kg; PO daily Withdrawal: Ψ
Meperidine (unlicensed for veterinary use)	1 to 2 mg/kg; IM, IV Up to 4 mg/kg; IM, SC *Miniature pigs* 2 to 10 mg/kg; IM q 4 hr	1 mg/kg; IV (cattle) Up to 2.5 mg/kg; IV (ewes) Withdrawal: Ψ

Drug	Horses (and Miniature Pig Doses, Where Indicated)	Ruminants (Cattle, Sheep, and Goats)
Mepivicaine hydrochloride	Label dose: Infiltration: 200 mL/500 kg 25 to 40 mL topically for ventriculectomy 3 to 15 mL; nerve block 5 to 20 mL; epidurally 10 to 15 mL; intra-articularly Race withdrawal: 48 hr	Extralabel dose: Local infiltration Withdrawal: Ψ
Methionine	Label dose: 5 to 15 g/454 kg daily; in feed Extralabel dose: 20 to 50 mg/kg; PO	None
Methocarbamol	Label dose: 4.4 to 22 mg/kg; IV **OR** 22 to 55 mg/kg; IV (severe muscle spasms) Extralabel dose: 110 mg/kg; IV (convulsions) Race withdrawal: 24 hr	Extralabel dose: 110 mg/kg; IV Withdrawal: Ψ
Methylcellulose flakes (unlicensed for veterinary use)	0.25 to 0.5 kg/450 kg in 10 L water; PO **OR** 125 to 175 g daily in feed	None
Methylene blue (unlicensed for veterinary use)	4 to 9 mg/kg; slowly IV	4.4 to 8.8 mg/kg; IV drip Withdrawal: Ψ
Methylprednisolone acetate	Label dose: 200 mg; IM 80 to 400 mg; intratendinous	Extralabel dose: 20 to 240 mg; intra-articularly Withdrawal: Ψ

Drug	Horses (and Miniature Pig Doses, Where Indicated)	Ruminants (Cattle, Sheep, and Goats)
Methylprednisolone acetate (continued)	40 to 240 mg; intra-articularly Extralabel dose: 2 to 4 mg/kg; IM Race withdrawal: 96 hr	
Methylsulfonomethane	Label dose: 10 g bid; PO for 4 days, then once daily Extralabel dose: 0.5 to 1.0 g/450 kg once daily; PO	None
Metoclopramide (unlicensed for veterinary use)	0.25 mg/kg tid to qid; SC, IV 0.6 mg/kg q 4 hr; PO	0.3 mg/kg q 4 to 6 hr; SC Withdrawal: Ψ
Metronidazole (unlicensed for veterinary use)	15 mg/kg qid; IV, PO **OR** 20 mg/kg bid; IV, PO *Miniature pigs* 66 mg/kg once daily; PO	75 mg/kg; IV 3 times over 12-hr intervals Topical as 5% ointment plus urethral douche of 30 mL of a 1% solution (bovine trichomoniasis) Withdrawal: 100 days & Note: This is banned for use in food-producing animals in the US.
Miconazole (unlicensed for veterinary use)	1% solution; apply to eyes qid	Same Withdrawal: Ψ
Mineral oil	Label dose: 225 to 3785 mL/day; PO Extralabel dose: 10 mL/kg; PO	Label dose: 225 to 3785 mL/day; PO (cattle) 57 to 227 mL/day; PO (sheep and goats) Extralabel dose: 1 to 4 L; PO (cattle) 100 to 500 mL; PO (sheep and goats)

Drug	Horses (and Miniature Pig Doses, Where Indicated)	Ruminants (Cattle, Sheep, and Goats)
Monensin	None: Toxic	Label dose: 5 to 33 g/ton feed (feed efficiency) 22 g/ton feed (coccidiosis) (cattle) One capsule for cattle 200 to 350 kg 20 g/ton feed (goats, coccidiosis) Withdrawal: 0 ℞ Extralabel dose: 30 to 40 g/ton dry roughage (legume bloat) 200 mg/head/day (dairy cattle, sub-clinical ketosis) 0.75% in salt mixture (sheep, coccidiosis) Withdrawal: Meat: 0 & No restriction for lactating cattle in Canada but restricted from feeding to lactating dairy cattle in the US.
Morantel tartrate	None	Label dose: Pellets (US): 49 g pellets per 1000 kg body weight in feed. (Canada): 1 kg pellets per 1000 kg body weight in feed. Repeat at 2- to 3-wk intervals for larval forms that may have survived first dose (cattle and goats).

Drug	Horses (and Miniature Pig Doses, Where Indicated)	Ruminants (Cattle, Sheep, and Goats)
Morantel tartrate (continued)		Premix: (Canada) Dilute to 10.0 g/kg and feed 100 g/100 kg. Bolus: 1 bolus/250 kg body weight Withdrawal: Meat: 30 days ℞ (Canada), 14 days ℞ (US) Milk: 0 ℞ (US) Extralabel dose: 10 mg/kg; PO (sheep) Withdrawal: Ψ
Morphine (unlicensed for veterinary use)	0.02 to 0.04 mg/kg; IV 0.2 to 0.4 mg/kg; IM 0.05 to 0.1 mg/kg; epidurally (analgesia) *Miniature pigs* 0.2 mg/kg; IM q 4 hr (<20 mg total dose)	0.05 to 0.1 mg/kg; epidurally (analgesia) Withdrawal: Ψ
Moxalactam: See Cephalosporins (unlicensed for veterinary use)	50 mg/kg tid; IV, IM	None
Moxidectin	None	Label dose: 1.0 mL/50 kg; SC, maximum of 10 mL per site Withdrawal: Meat: 36 days ℞ Not for use in lactating dairy cattle
Nafcillin (unlicensed for veterinary use)	10 mg/kg qid; IM	None

Drug	Horses (and Miniature Pig Doses, Where Indicated)	Ruminants (Cattle, Sheep, and Goats)
Naloxone	Extralabel dose: 0.01 to 0.02 mg/kg; IV	None
Naltrexone (unlicensed for veterinary use)	0.4 mg/kg; IV (prevents cribbing for 6 hr)	None
Naproxen (unlicensed for veterinary use)	10 mg/kg bid; PO up to 14 consecutive days Race withdrawal: 96 hr single dose and 120 hr for 5-day regimen	None
Naquasone	Label dose: 1.1 mL/100 kg bid; IM for the first day, then once daily for 2 additional days Race withdrawal: 24 hr oral dose and 36 hr; IM	Label dose: 1 to 2 boluses initially followed by ½ to 1 bolus a day to effect; PO (adult cattle) 20 mL; IM prior to, at the time of, or immediately following parturition. Follow-up with bolus form in 12 to 36 hr. Withdrawal: Meat: 21 days ℞ (Canada), Ψ (US) Milk: 48 hr ℞ (Canada), 72 hr ℞ (US)
Natamycin (unlicensed for veterinary use)	Apply to eyes q 2 to 4 hr	None
Neomycin	Label dose: 7 mg/kg daily; PO for 3 to 5 days (Canada)	Label dose: 7 mg/kg daily for 3 to 5 days; PO (Canada),

Drug	Horses (and Miniature Pig Doses, Where Indicated)	Ruminants (Cattle, Sheep, and Goats)
Neomycin (continued)	Extralabel dose: 1 g/450 kg qid; PO **OR** 2 g/450 kg bid; PO **OR** 1.5 g bid; PO (foal) *Miniature pigs* 7 to 12 mg/kg bid; PO, **OR** 10 mg/kg qid; PO	22 mg/kg in divided daily doses for a maximum of 14 days; PO (US) Withdrawal: Meat: 14 to 30 days. Appears to vary with product; check individual label. Extralabel dose: 7 to 12 mg/kg bid; PO Avoid use in dairies.
Neostigmine	Label dose: 0.02 mg/kg; SC	Label dose: 0.02 to 0.03 mg/kg; SC Extralabel dose: 1.1 to 2.2 mg/50kg; SC, IV Withdrawal: Meat: 7 days & Milk: 48 hr &
Netilmicin (unlicensed for veterinary use)	2 mg/kg bid–tid; IM, IV	None
Niacin (nicotinic acid)	None	Label dose: 6 g/head bid; PO (cattle)
Nitrofurazone: See Nitrofurans	Label dose: Intrauterine use (solution); 30 to 100 mL IU every day to every second day. Topical ointment, solution, and powder; apply once to several times per day for 5 to 7 days.	Banned in food-producing animals

Drug	Horses (and Miniature Pig Doses, Where Indicated)	Ruminants (Cattle, Sheep, and Goats)
Nizatidine (unlicensed for veterinary use)	6.6 mg/kg tid; PO	None
Norepinephrine bitartrate (unlicensed for veterinary use)	0.01 mg/kg; IM	Same Withdrawal: Ψ
Novobiocin	None	Label dose: Novobiocin alone, 150 mg or 400 mg intramammary infusion per quarter (dry treatment) Withdrawal: Meat: 30 days ℜ Milk: 72 hr after calving ℜ (Canada) Combination products: 150 mg and 400 mg; intramammary infusion Withdrawal: See individual products.
Omeprazole (unlicensed for veterinary use)	0.5 to 2.0 mg/kg once or twice daily; IV 0.7 mg/kg once daily; PO (clinical ulceration)	None
Orgotein	Label dose: 5 mg; deep IM daily or qod for 14 days, then twice weekly for 2 or 3 weeks Extralabel dose: 5 mg; intra-articularly 1 to 4 times in a 7-day period	None

Drug	Horses (and Miniature Pig Doses, Where Indicated)	Ruminants (Cattle, Sheep, and Goats)
Oxfendazole	Label dose: 10 mg/kg; PO. May be repeated in 24 to 48 hours for early and late 4th stage larvae.	Label dose: 4.5 mg/kg; PO Withdrawal: Meat: 7 days ℞ (Paste formulation) Meat: 11 days ℞ (cattle) Not approved for use in lactating cattle. Extralabel dose: 5 mg/kg; PO (sheep, *Moniezia* spp) Withdrawal: Ψ
Oxibendazole	Label dose: 10 to 15 mg/kg; PO 15 mg/kg; PO (*S. westeri*)	None
Oxymorphone hydrochloride	Extralabel dose: 0.02 to 0.03 mg/kg; IM, IV	None
Oxytetracycline	Extralabel dose: 10 to 20 mg/kg once daily; IV Extralabel dose: *Miniature pigs* 6 to 11 mg/kg; IM, IV **OR** 10 to 20 mg/kg qid; PO	Label dose: 6 to 11 mg/kg once daily; IV, IM 5 to 22 mg/kg once daily to q 12 hr; PO Withdrawal: Oral products: Meat: 4 to 10 days ℞ Milk: 60 to 96 hr ℞ Injectables: Meat: 18 to 22 days ℞ Milk: (Canada) 60 to 72 hr ℞ (check individual products for specific requirements)

Drug	Horses (and Miniature Pig Doses, Where Indicated)	Ruminants (Cattle, Sheep, and Goats)
Oxytetracycline (continued)		Label dose: Long-acting product: 20 mg/kg once; IM, IV, SC Maximum dose at one site 20 mL Not approved for use in lactating dairy cattle. Withdrawal: Meat: (IM; IV) 21 to 28 days ℞ 48 days (SC) (Canada), 36 days (US) ℞ Mastitis infusions Withdrawal: Milk: 60 to 72 hr ℞ Check individual product label.
Oxytocin	Label dose: Obstetrics: 50 to 100 U; IV, IM, SC Milk letdown: 10 to 20 U; IV, IM, SC Extralabel dose: 2.5 to 5 U/450 kg q 20 min; IV as a bolus **OR** 80 to 100 U; IV in 500 mL saline as a drip (induction of parturition) 1 to 3 U/450 kg; IM (milk letdown) *Miniature pigs* 10 to 20 U; IM per animal	Label dose: Obstetrics: 50 to 100 U; IV, IM, SC (cattle) 30 to 50 U; IV, IM, SC (sheep) 10 to 20 U; IV, IM, SC (milk letdown, cattle) 5 to 20 U; IV, IM, SC (milk letdown, sheep) 20 to 40 U; IV, IM, SC (mastitis) Withdrawal: Meat: 3 days ℞ (Canada), Ψ (US) Milk: 24 hr ℞ (Canada), Ψ (US)
Pancuronium (unlicensed for veterinary use)	0.04 to 0.066 mg/kg; IV	None

Drug	Horses (and Miniature Pig Doses, Where Indicated)	Ruminants (Cattle, Sheep, and Goats)
Paregoric (unlicensed for veterinary use)	0.25 to 0.5 mL/kg tid–qid; PO **OR** 15 to 30 mL tid–qid; PO (foals)	15 to 30 mL tid–qid; PO (calves) Withdrawal: Ψ
Paromomycin (unlicensed for veterinary use)	None	50 mg/kg bid; PO (calves, crypto-sporidiosis)
Penicillamine (unlicensed for veterinary use)	3 to 4 mg/kg qid; PO for 10 days	12 to 25 mg/kg bid; PO Withdrawal: Ψ
Penicillin benzathine combined with procaine penicillin	Label dose: 4286 to 13,333 U/kg; IM of each of both types of peni-cillin. Repeat in 2 to 5 days 10,000 to 40,000 IU/kg q 48 to 72 hr; IM	Label dose: 4286 to 13,333 U/kg; SC of each of both types of peni-cillin. Repeat in 2 to 5 days. Limit to 2 doses in beef cattle. Withdrawal: Meat: 14 days (Canada), 30 days (US) ℞ Extralabel dose: 40,000 IU/kg q 48 to 72 hr; IM Withdrawal: Ψ See penicillin G procaine
Penicillin G, potassium or sodium salt (unlicensed for veterinary use)	10,000 to 50,000 IU/kg qid; IM, IV	Same Withdrawal: Ψ See penicillin G procaine
Penicillin G procaine	Label dose: 2610 to 7500 IU/kg/day; IM Race withdrawal: 48 hr Extralabel dose: 20,000 to 50,000 IU/kg bid to tid; IM *Miniature pigs* 22,000 to 45,000 IU/kg once daily; IM	Label dose: 6666 to 7500 IU/kg/day; IM Withdrawal: Meat: 5 days (Canada) ℞, 4 to 10 days (US) ℞ Milk: 72 hr (Canada) ℞, 48 hr (US) ℞

Drug	Horses (and Miniature Pig Doses, Where Indicated)	Ruminants (Cattle, Sheep, and Goats)
Penicillin G procaine (continued)		Extralabel dose: 20,000 to 54,000 IU/kg once or twice daily; IM, SC
		Note: Clinically effective doses of penicillin far exceed most label doses. Withdrawal times correspondingly increase, i.e., at 27,000 IU/kg once daily; IM
		Withdrawal: Meat: 16 days & Milk: 5 days &
		Increased IM dose Withdrawal: Meat: 21 days &
		Increased dose and volume at injection site Withdrawal: Meat: 40 days &
		Increased SC dose Withdrawal: Meat: 42 days &
		Intrauterine infusion: 1 dose Withdrawal: Meat: 14 days Milk: 3 days &
Penicillin V (unlicensed for veterinary use)	110,000 mg/kg bid–qid; PO	None
Pentazocine (unlicensed for veterinary use)	0.66 mg/kg; IV, IM Race withdrawal: 72 hr *Miniature pigs* 2 mg/kg q 4 hr; IM	None

Drug	Horses (and Miniature Pig Doses, Where Indicated)	Ruminants (Cattle, Sheep, and Goats)
Pentobarbital	Label dose: 87 to 108 mg/kg; IV, IP or intracardiac (euthanasia) Extralabel dose: 2 to 20 mg/kg tid; IV (convulsion control)	Label dose: 87 to 108 mg/kg; IV, IP or intra-cardiac (euthanasia) Extralabel dose: 20 to 30 mg/kg to effect; IV (anesthesia) 2 mg/kg; IV (standing sedation) Withdrawal: Ψ
Pentoxifylline	Label dose: 2 g/454 kg tid; PO for 6 wk Race withdrawal: 48 hr Extralabel dose: 7 mg/kg once daily; PO **OR** 8.5 mg/kg bid; PO	None
Pentylenetetrazol (unlicensed for veterinary use)	6 to 10 mg/kg; IV	6 to 10 mg/kg; IV **OR** 10 to 20mg/kg; IV (bar-biturate toxicity) Withdrawal: Ψ
Phenobarbital (unlicensed for veterinary use)	20 mg/kg; IV (loading dose), 2.2 mg/kg; IV (maintenance) (cerebrocortical dis-ease) 5 to 25 mg/kg; IV over 30 min (foals)	Same for mature ruminants Withdrawal: Ψ
Phenoxybenzamine (unlicensed for veterinary use)	For acute laminitis, diarrhea: 0.7 to 1.0 mg/kg; IV in 500 mL saline twice at 12-hr intervals Urethral tone reduction: 0.7 mg/kg; PO q 6 hr	None
Phenylbutazone	Label dose: 2 to 4.4 mg/kg once daily; slowly IV	Extralabel dose: 9 mg/kg; PO, IV (loading dose)

Drug	Horses (and Miniature Pig Doses, Where Indicated)	Ruminants (Cattle, Sheep, and Goats)
Phenylbutazone (continued)	4.4 to 8.8 mg/kg/day divided bid–tid; PO Race withdrawal: 96 hr Extralabel dose: *Miniature pigs* 4 to 8 mg/kg bid; PO	2 to 5 mg/kg; PO, IV (maintenance, given every other day) Withdrawal: Meat: 30 days Milk: 5 days Two injections: Meat: 35 days Milk: 7 days Three injections: Meat: 40 to 45 days &
Phenylephrine (unlicensed for veterinary use)	10% ophthalmic solution applied to eyes	Same Withdrawal: Ψ
Phenytoin (unlicensed for veterinary use)	5 to 10 mg/kg; IV (convulsing foals) 1 to 5 mg/kg q 4 hr; IM, IV, PO (maintenance) 10 to 22 mg/kg bid; PO (digoxin-induced arrhythmias) 10 to 15 mg/kg/day; PO (Australian Stringhalt) 8 to 6 mg/kg tid; PO (convulsions of viral meningitis)	5 to 10 mg/kg; IV (acute convulsions) 1 to 5 mg/kg q 4 hr; IM, IV, PO (maintenance) Withdrawal: Ψ
Pilocarpine (unlicensed for veterinary use)	Ophthalmic gel; 4% applied to eyes bid–tid	Same Withdrawal: Ψ
Piperazine	Label dose: 104 to 112 mg/kg; PO Extralabel dose: *Miniature pigs* 200 mg/kg; PO	None

Drug	Horses (and Miniature Pig Doses, Where Indicated)	Ruminants (Cattle, Sheep, and Goats)
Pipercillin (unlicensed for veterinary use)	15 to 50 mg/kg bid–tid; IV, IM	None
Poloxalene	None	Label dose: Liquid: 110 mg/kg daily; PO 1 g/45 kg/day as a top dressing or in feed Double dose for severe bloat conditions. Withdrawal: 0 ℜ
Polymixin B (unlicensed for veterinary use)	10,000 U/kg qid; PO	4000 U/kg; IV (coliform mastitis) Withdrawal: Milk: 120 hr & Meat: Ψ
Polysulfated glycosaminoglycan	Label dose: 250 mg intra-articularly once weekly for up to 5 wk **OR** 500 mg q 4 days; IM for 7 treatments	Extralabel dose: 250 mg intra-articularly once weekly for up to 5 wk **OR** 500 mg q 4 days; IM for 7 treatments Withdrawal: Ψ
Potassium chloride	Extralabel dose: 5 to 20 g; PO in divided doses (digitalis toxicity) 0.5 mEq/kg/hr; IV Not to exceed 3 mEq/kg/day (hypokalemia)	Extralabel dose: 50 g/450 kg/day; PO 0.5 mEq/kg/hr; IV Not to exceed 3 mEq/kg/day
Pralidoxime (PAM) (unlicensed for veterinary use)	10 to 40 mg/kg; slowly IV, may be repeated. Use in conjunction with atropine.	10 to 40 mg/kg; slowly IV, may be repeated. Use in conjunction with atropine Withdrawal: Ψ

Drug	Horses (and Miniature Pig Doses, Where Indicated)	Ruminants (Cattle, Sheep, and Goats)
Prednisolone	Label dose: 0.1 to 0.2 mg/kg at 12-, 24-, or 48-hr intervals; IM or IV **OR** 0.2 to 0.8 mg/kg; IM (suspension) Extralabel dose: 0.2 to 3.0 mg/kg; once or twice daily; PO, IM 2 to 5 mg/kg; IV (septic shock) Race withdrawal: 24 hr	Label dose: 100 to 200 mg; IM Withdrawal: Meat: 5 days Milk: 72 hr (Canada) ℞ Extralabel dose: 0.2 to 1.0 mg/kg; IV, IM Withdrawal: Ψ
Prednisone	Extralabel dose: 0.02 to 1.0 mg/kg bid; IM, PO Race withdrawal: 24 hr	None
Pregnant mare's serum gonadotrophin (PMSG)	Extralabel dose: 1,000 U; SC, IM, IV	Label dose: 1,000 to 1,250 U; IM, IV, SC (cattle) 300 to 1,000 U; IM, IV, SC (sheep) Withdrawal: Meat: 7 days ℞ Milk: Ψ Extralabel dose: 1,500 to 3,000 U; IM between day 8 and 13 of the cycle (superovulation in cattle) 500 to 1,000 U; IM (anestrus in cattle) 400 to 700 U; IM following vaginal progestagen sponge removal (estrus synchronization in sheep)
Primidone	Extralabel dose: 1 to 2 mg bid–qid; PO (foal)	None

Drug	Horses (and Miniature Pig Doses, Where Indicated)	Ruminants (Cattle, Sheep, and Goats)

Progesterone	Label dose:
	    50 to 100 mg/454 kg; IM
	Extralabel dose:
	    150 mg/450 kg once daily; IM (suppress estrus)
	    300 mg/450 kg once daily; IM (maintain pregnancy)
	Repositol: 1,000 mg/450 kg; IM (abortion prevention)
		Label dose:
		    50 to 300 mg/450 kg; IM (cattle)
		    10 to 15 mg/animal daily; IM (sheep and goats)
		Extralabel dose:
		    0.125 mg/kg bid; SC in combination with estrogen (17-ß estradiol) at 0.05 mg/kg bid; SC for 7 days (lactation induction in cattle)
		Withdrawal:
		    See individual products

Promazine	Label dose:
	    1 to 2 mg/kg; PO
	Extralabel dose:
	    0.5 mg/kg; IV
	Race withdrawal: 96 hr
		Extralabel dose:
		    0.44 to 1.0 mg/kg; IV, IM
		Withdrawal: Ψ, zero tolerance

Propantheline (unlicensed for veterinary use)	30 to 45 mg; IV (adult horse)	None
Proparacaine (unlicensed for veterinary use)	0.5% ophthalmic solution	Same Withdrawal: Ψ

Propofol	Extralabel dose:
	    After premedication with xylazine (0.5 mg/kg; IV), give 2.4 mg/kg; IV for induction.
	    Maintenance at 0.3 mg/kg/min; IV
		None

Propranolol (unlicensed for veterinary use)	0.38 to 0.78 mg/kg tid; PO 0.05 to 0.16 mg/kg bid; IV	None

Drug	Horses (and Miniature Pig Doses, Where Indicated)	Ruminants (Cattle, Sheep, and Goats)
Propylene glycol: See also cobalt-containing products	Extralabel dose: 3 mL/50 kg as an aerosol (5%)	For combination products see label instructions
Prostaglandin F$_{2\alpha}$	Label dose: 5 mg/450 kg; SC (Canada) (dinoprost tromethamine) Extralabel dose: *Miniature pigs* 5 mg; IM	Label dose: 25 mg; IM (cattle) (dinoprost tromethamine) Withdrawal: Meat: 2 days (Canada) ℞, 0 days (US) ℞ Milk: 0 ℞ **OR** 30 mg, combined with dexamethasone at 20 mg; IM if pregnancy is beyond 150 days (abortifacient in cattle) Goats: 2 to 3 mg; IM (pseudopregnancy) **OR** 8 to 10 mg; IM (sheep and goats) Withdrawal: Ψ
Protamine sulfate (unlicensed for veterinary use)	1% solution; administer 1 mg by slow IV injection to antagonize each 100 U of heparin remaining in the patient; hence, the dose should be reduced as time between heparin administration and start of treatment increases (i.e., after 30 min give only 0.5 mg	100 mg/adult cow; IV in a 1% solution (bracken fern toxicosis) Withdrawal: Ψ

Drug	Horses (and Miniature Pig Doses, Where Indicated)	Ruminants (Cattle, Sheep, and Goats)
Protamine sulfate (continued)	for q 100 U heparin) (heparin-induced hemorrhages).	None
Psyllium mucilloid	Label dose: 120 to 180 g/454 kg daily; PO Extralabel dose: 1 g/kg 1 to 4 times daily; PO	
Pyrantel	Label dose: 6.6 mg/kg; PO Extralabel dose: 13.2 mg/kg; PO (tapeworms) Extralabel dose: *Miniature pigs* 6.6 mg/kg; PO	Extralabel dose: 25 mg/kg; PO Withdrawal: Ψ
Pyrilamine maleate: See Antihistamines	Label dose: 88 to 132 mg/454 kg; IM, IV, SC Extralabel dose: 1 mg/kg; IV, IM, SC	Extralabel dose: 1 mg/kg; IV, IM, SC Withdrawal: Ψ
Pyrimethamine	Extralabel dose: 1.0 mg/kg once daily; PO for a minimum of 3 months, in combination with a sulfonamide (equine protozoal myelitis)	None
Quinidine (unlicensed for veterinary use)	1.5 to 2 mg/kg q 20 min; IV until conversion or desired effect [Gluconate] Total dose not to exceed 6 mg/kg **OR** 22 mg/kg q 2 hr; PO until conversion or desired effect [Sulfate] Not to exceed 132 mg/kg total dose	48 mg/kg; IV over a 4-hr period [Sulfate] Withdrawal: Ψ 15 mg/kg; IV

Drug	Horses (and Miniature Pig Doses, Where Indicated)	Ruminants (Cattle, Sheep, and Goats)
Ranitidine (unlicensed for veterinary use)	0.9 mg/kg tid; IV **OR** 0.7 mg/kg qid; IV 6.6 to 11 mg/kg bid; PO *Miniature pigs* 150 mg/animal bid; PO	45 mg/kg; PO (sheep) Withdrawal: Ψ
Reserpine (unlicensed for veterinary use)	1 to 2 mg/kg; IV every other day	None
Rifampin (unlicensed for veterinary use)	5 to 10 mg/kg bid; PO (*R. equi* pneumonia, in combination with erythromycin) Therapy must often be prolonged (4–20 weeks) 5 mg/kg bid; PO (bacterial endocarditis) 2.5 to 5 mg/kg bid; PO (internal or recurrent abscesses)	2.5 to 5 mg/kg; PO Withdrawal: Ψ
Romifidine	Label dose: 0.04 to 0.1 mg/kg; IV Extralabel dose: 28 to 51 µg/kg; IV, followed by butorphanol 4 minutes later at 8 to 22.5 µg/kg IV **OR** Administer in the same syringe 34 to 71 µg/kg romifidine with 10 to 25 µ/kg butorphanol; IV.	None
Sodium bicarbonate	Label dose: Emergency use: 200 to 300 mL; IV by rapid infusion.	Label dose: Emergency use: 200 to 300 mL; IV by rapid infusion. For less urgent

Drug	Horses (and Miniature Pig Doses, Where Indicated)	Ruminants (Cattle, Sheep, and Goats)
Sodium bicarbonate (continued)	For less urgent metabolic acidosis: 2 to 5 mEq/kg over 4 to 8 hours; IV Extralabel dose: Replace 2/3 of estimated base deficit; IV over 4 hr (severe metabolic acidosis) 30 g bid; PO (acidosis in chronic renal failure)	metabolic acidosis: 2 to 5 mEq/kg over 4 to 8 hours; IV Extralabel dose: Replace 2/3 of estimated base deficit; IV over 4 hr Withdrawal: Ψ
Sodium chloride	Extralabel dose: Isotonic (0.9%): 40 mL/kg/day; IV (maintenance) 40 to 100 mL/kg/hr; IV (shock; if the higher dose is used central venous pressure should be monitored) **OR** Hypertonic (7.5%) saline: 4 to 5 mL/kg over 10 min; IV (hemorrhagic shock) Can also be applied topically to eyes for corneal ulcer treatment	Label dose: Isotonic (0.9%): 40 mL/kg/day; IV (maintenance) 40 to 100 mL/kg/hr; IV (shock; if the higher dose is used central venous pressure should be monitored) Label dose: Hypertonic (7.5%) saline: 50 to 100 mL/45 kg IV. Can repeat in 12 hr Withdrawal: 0 ℞ Extralabel dose: 4 to 5 mL/kg over 10 min; IV (hemorrhagic shock, abomasal disease) Feed to 4% in ration (urolithiasis prevention) None
Sodium cromoglycate (unlicensed for veterinary use)	200 mg bid; aerosol by jet nebulizer	Label dose:

Drug	Horses (and Miniature Pig Doses, Where Indicated)	Ruminants (Cattle, Sheep, and Goats)
Sodium iodide	Label dose: 10 to 40 mL; IV as a mucolytic Extralabel dose: 20 to 40 mg/kg once daily; PO for several weeks	66 to 222 mg/kg IV **OR** 10 to 40 mL; IV (cattle), 5 to 20 mL; IV (sheep) as a mucolytic Withdrawal: Meat: 7 days & Not for use in lactating dairy cattle Extralabel dose: 80 mg/kg; IV (10% solution for sheep, 20% solution for cattle) at weekly intervals (*Actinobacillus*) Withdrawal: Ψ
Sodium sulfate (unlicensed for veterinary use)	12 g/kg dissolved in warm water; PO	1 to 3 g/kg; PO (cathartic) 1 g/day for 4 wk; PO (sheep, mobilize excessive hepatic copper) Withdrawal: Ψ
Sodium thiosulfate (unlicensed for veterinary use)	20 to 40 mL/kg; slowly IV (20% solution)	30 to 40 mg/kg; IV, PO **OR** 5 g/day; PO (copper poisoning in cattle) Withdrawal: Ψ
Spectinomycin	Extralabel dose: 20 mg/kg tid; IM Extralabel dose: *Miniature pigs* 25 to 50 mg/kg once daily; PO	Extralabel dose: 1 g; intrauterine (ureaplasma infection) 12 mg/kg once daily; IM Withdrawal: Meat: 30 days & Milk: 96 hr & None

Drug	Horses (and Miniature Pig Doses, Where Indicated)	Ruminants (Cattle, Sheep, and Goats)
Stanozolol	Label dose: 0.55 mg/kg; IM up to 4 doses once weekly	None
Sucralfate (unlicensed for veterinary use)	2 to 4 g/450 kg bid–qid; PO	
Sulbactam benzathine and ampicillin (Synergistin)	6.6 mg/kg once daily; IM	5.5 mL/100 kg once daily; IM for 3 days Withdrawal: Meat: 14 days ℞ Not for use in lactating dairy cattle. Milk: 72 hr at labeled IM dose, 84 hr if infused into the udder &
Sulfadiazine-trimethoprim: See Sulfonamides; Potentiated	Label dose: 30 mg/kg once daily; PO 24 mg/kg daily; IM, IV Extralabel dose: 30 mg/kg bid–tid; PO 15 mg/kg bid; IV 2.5 to 3 g; intrauterine Extralabel dose: *Miniature pigs* 25 to 50 mg/kg once daily; PO	Label dose: 30 mg/kg once daily; PO Withdrawal: Meat: 10 days ℞
Sulfadimethoxine	Extralabel dose: 25 mg/kg; IV, IM, SC the first day, followed by 12.5 mg/kg; IV, IM, SC per day for 3 to 6 days Extralabel dose: *Miniature pigs* 25 mg/kg; PO	Label dose: 55 mg/kg once daily; PO (initial dose), followed by 27.5 mg/kg once daily. PO on 4 subsequent days Withdrawal: Meat: 5 to 7 days Milk: 60 hr ℞ **OR** 137.5 g/kg (SR bo-

Drug	Horses (and Miniature Pig Doses, Where Indicated)	Ruminants (Cattle, Sheep, and Goats)
Sulfadimethoxine (continued)		luses) daily; PO Withdrawal: Meat: 21 days Extralabel dose: 25 mg/kg IV, IM, SC the first day, followed by 12.5 mg/kg; IV, IM, SC per day for 3 to 6 days. Withdrawal: Meat: 5 to 7 days & Milk: 56 hr & See individual products.
Sulfadoxine-trimethoprim: See Sulfonamides; Potentiated	None	Label dose: 3 mL/45 kg once daily; IM, IV Withdrawal: Meat: 10 days ℞ (Canada) Milk: 96 hr ℞ (Canada)
Sulfamethazine	Label dose: 225 mg/kg on day one; PO, followed by 112.5 mg/kg; PO on subsequent days.	Label dose: 150.5 to 247.5 mg/kg; PO on day 1, then 78 to 123 mg/kg; PO on subsequent days Withdrawal: Meat: 10 to 12 days ℞ Milk: 96 hr ℞ (Canada) Sustained-release bolus: 250 to 500 mg/kg once; PO Withdrawal: Meat: 28 days ℞ See individual products. See individual products.

Drug	Horses (and Miniature Pig Doses, Where Indicated)	Ruminants (Cattle, Sheep, and Goats)
Sulfonamides	Extralabel dose: 100 to 200 mg/kg; IV, IM, SC on day 1, then 50 to 100 mg/kg; IV, IM, SC on subsequent days. Check individual labels.	None
Terbutaline (unlicensed for veterinary use)	0.02 to 0.06 mg/kg bid; IV 1:1,000 to 1:100,000,000; Intradermally (anhidrosis testing)	
Testosterone	Label dose: Proprionate or aqueous suspension; 300 to 500 mg/450 kg once weekly; IM for 3 to 5 wk For maintenance, repeat every 3 to 6 wk	Label dose: Aqueous suspension: 50 mg/day or 100 mg/wk; IM (cattle) 10 to 25 mg once a day; IM (sheep) Withdrawal: Ψ
Testosterone and estradiol	Label dose: 2.5 mL; IM once a week for 3 wk Maintenance: 2.5 mL; IM q 4 to 8 wk (Anadiol) 2.5 to 5 mL; IM once a week for 4 wk (Uni-Bol), thereafter 2.5 to 5 mL; IM once every 4 wk (maintenance)	Label dose: One implant (200 mg testosterone propionate, 20 mg estradiol benzoate) inserted under the skin of the ear in the center one third of the ear (cattle) Withdrawal: Meat: 60 days & Label dose:

Drug	Horses (and Miniature Pig Doses, Where Indicated)	Ruminants (Cattle, Sheep, and Goats)
Tetanus antitoxin	Label dose: 1500 U; IV, IM, SC, IP; can be repeated in 7 days (prevention) 30,000 to 100,000 U (treatment) (Note: label dose will vary with product)	(prophylaxis) 1,500 U; IM, SC Can be repeated in 7 days (cattle) 500 U; IM, SC (sheep, calves, and swine) 200 U; IM, SC (lambs) Withdrawal: Meat: 21 days ℞ Label dose: (treatment) 10,000 to 50,000 U; IM (cattle) 3,000 to 15,000 U; IM (sheep and swine) Withdrawal: Meat: 21 days ℞ (Canada)
Tetracycline hydrochloride	Label dose: Insert 1 bolus (4 g) into uterus. Repeat after 2 days if needed.	Label dose: 5 to 10 mg/kg bid; PO for 3 to 5 days in feed (calves) Cows: 1 bolus (4 g) into uterus; repeat after 2 days if needed. 10 mg/kg bid; PO for 3–5 days (lambs and sheep) Withdrawal: Meat: 4 days Milk: 96 hr (Canada) ℞ (Check individual products for specific dose and withdrawal requirements; vari-

Drug	Horses (and Miniature Pig Doses, Where Indicated)	Ruminants (Cattle, Sheep, and Goats)
Tetracycline hydrochloride (continued)		ation can be expected among products.)
Theophylline: See Aminophylline (unlicensed for veterinary use)	1 mg/kg qid; PO	28 mg/kg once daily; PO 20 mg/kg bid; PO Caution: Therapeutic drug monitoring is essential to prevent toxicity. Withdrawal: Ψ
Thiabendazole (unlicensed for veterinary use)	44 mg/kg; PO **OR** 88 mg/kg; PO (*P. equorum*) 440 mg/kg; PO (verminous arteritis)	75 mg/kg; PO Withdrawal: Meat: 3 days (cattle), 30 days (sheep and goats) Milk: 96 hr Note: The withdrawal times are from previously labeled dose when the product was still available for veterinary use.
Thiamine (Vitamin B₁)	Label dose: 250 to 750 mg daily; PO **OR** 500 mg/450 kg twice weekly; PO (powder) 1 to 2 g daily; PO (liquid) 100 mg; IM or SC 50 to 300 mg/45 kg; IM, IV Extralabel dose: 0.5 to 5 mg/kg; IM	Label dose: 100 mg; IM, SC **OR** 100mg/100kg; IM (cows) 10 mg; IM, SC (calves) **OR** 100 to 300 mg/45 kg; IM, IV Extralabel dose: 10 to 20 mg/kg diluted in D₅W; slowly IV, then once daily; IM, SC for 3 to 5 days (polioencephalomalacia) 20 mg/kg daily; SC

Drug	Horses (and Miniature Pig Doses, Where Indicated)	Ruminants (Cattle, Sheep, and Goats)
Thiamine (Vitamin B₁) (continued)		for 15 days (acute lead toxicity) Withdrawal: Ψ
Thiopental: See Thiobarbiturates	Label dose: (with preanesthetic) 6 to 13 mg/kg (average 8.25 mg/kg); IV (without preanesthetic) 9 to 15.5 mg/kg (Pentothal) **OR** 4.4 to 10 mg/kg (Induthol); IV, up to 12.5 mg/kg for small ponies Maximum 9 mg/kg; IV in horses >545 kg Extralabel dose: 10 to 15 mg/kg; IV (maintenance) *Miniature pigs* 10 mg/kg; IV (to effect)	Label dose: (with premedication, bovine over 136 kg) 8.2 to 10 mg/kg; IV Dose range 8.2 to 15.4 mg/kg; IV, not to exceed 22 mg/kg total dose 6.6 mg/kg; IV (unweaned calves) 10 to 14 mg/kg; IV (sheep) Extralabel dose: Induction: 3 to 5 mg/kg; IV (with preanesthetic) Maintenance: 15 to 22 mg/kg; IV over 4 to 5 min (calves) Maintenance: 20 to 22 mg/kg; IV over 4 to 5 min (goats) Withdrawal: Ψ None
Ticarcillin	Label dose: 6 g intrauterine; daily for 3 to 5 days Extralabel dose: 40 to 80 mg/kg tid; IV, IM	
Tilmicosin	None	Label dose: 10 mg/kg once; SC Withdrawal: Meat: 28 days ℜ Not for use in lactating dairy cattle

Drug	Horses (and Miniature Pig Doses, Where Indicated)	Ruminants (Cattle, Sheep, and Goats)
Tobramycin (unlicensed for veterinary use)	1 to 1.7 mg/kg tid; IV, IM	None
Tolazoline	Label dose: 4 mg/kg; slowly IV Extralabel dose: 7.5 mg/kg; IV for countering 1 mg/kg; IV xylazine (plus a slow infusion)	Extralabel dose: 0.3 mg/kg; IV given 8 min after caudal epidural xylazine Withdrawal: Ψ
Triamcinolone (unlicensed for veterinary use)	0.02 to 0.1 mg/kg; IM, SC 6 to 18 mg; intra-articularly or intra-synovially 0.02 to 0.1 mg/kg; IM 10 mg; subconjuncti-vally q 2 to 4 days Race withdrawal: 24 hr	0.02 to 0.04 mg/kg; IM 6 to 18 mg; intra-articularly Withdrawal: Ψ
Trichlorfon	Extralabel dose: 40 mg/kg; PO (nematodes and bots) 20 mg/kg; PO (ascarids and bots) 10 mg/kg; PO (bots only)	Label dose: Pour-on: 32.5 mL of 8% solution per 100 kg (cattle) Withdrawal: Meat: 21 days ℞ Extralabel dose: 44 to 110 mg/kg; PO (cattle and sheep) Withdrawal: Ψ
Trifluridine (unlicensed for veterinary use)	Ophthalmic; apply q 2 to 3 hr	Same Withdrawal: Ψ
Tripelennamine: See Antihistamines	Label dose: 0.4 to 1.1 mg/kg; IM, IV Extralabel dose: 1 mg/kg bid–tid; IM, IV	Label dose: 0.4 to 1.1 mg/kg; IM, IV Withdrawal: Meat: 3 days (Canada); 4 days (US) ℞

Drug	Horses (and Miniature Pig Doses, Where Indicated)	Ruminants (Cattle, Sheep, and Goats)
Tripelennamine: See Antihistamines (continued)		Milk: 36 hr (Canada); 24 hr (US) ℞
Tropicamide (unlicensed for veterinary use)	0.5% to 1% ophthalmic drops; apply once to eyes	Same Withdrawal: Ψ
Tylosin	None: Injection has been fatal Extralabel dose: *Miniature pigs* 5 to 8.8 mg/kg; IM	Label dose: 17.6 mg/kg once daily; IM Withdrawal: Meat: 21 days ℞ Not for use in lactating cattle Extralabel dose: 6.6 mg/kg once daily; IM (goats) 400 mg once daily; IM for 2 days (sheep, chlamydial abortion) Withdrawal: Ψ
Vancomycin (unlicensed for veterinary use)	20 to 40 mg/kg bid–qid; IV, PO	None
Vasopressin injectable (pitressin, ADH) (unlicensed for veterinary use)	40 IU once daily; IM	0.25 IU/kg; IV (closure of the esophageal groove) (goats) Withdrawal: Ψ
Vitamin A	Label dose: 1,000 IU/kg in feed Extralabel dose: 2,000 IU/kg in feed (growth)	Label dose: 1,000 IU/kg feed Extralabel dose: 2 million IU per cow; IM (vitamin A deficiency) 2,200 IU/kg feed (growth in cattle) 400 IU/kg feed (growth in sheep) 3,200 to 3,800 IU/kg feed (lactating cattle)

Drug	Horses (and Miniature Pig Doses, Where Indicated)	Ruminants (Cattle, Sheep, and Goats)
Vitamin A (continued)		750 IU/kg feed (pregnant sheep) Withdrawal: Meat: 60 days ℜ Milk: Ψ
Vitamin D₃	None	Label dose: 10 million IU/adult cow; IM during the period from the 2nd to the 8th day preceding calving. When calving is delayed, a second dose can be given 8 days after the initial injection (prevention of parturient paresis in cows). Withdrawal: Ψ Note: If using products containing vitamin A, a 60-day meat withdrawal is suggested.
Vitamin E-Selenium	Label dose: 1 mL E-Se (2.5 mg selenium) per 45 kg; by deep IM injection, may be repeated at 5- to 10-day intervals 30 g Vetre-Sel-E mixed in ration per day, ½ to 1½ tsp Equ-SeE per 4.5 kg daily in feed	Label dose: (Alphasel Powder) Calves: 30 g on day 1 followed by 15 g daily; PO **OR** 30 g; PO at day 2 of age. Repeat in 1 wk **OR** 15 g/wk; PO Lambs: ½ calf dose Withdrawal: Meat: 21 days ℜ Bo-Se: 2.5 to 3.75 mL/45 kg; SC, IM (calves)

Drug	Horses (and Miniature Pig Doses, Where Indicated)	Ruminants (Cattle, Sheep, and Goats)
Vitamin E-Selenium (continued)		Withdrawal: 　Meat: 30 days ℞ 　2.5 mL/45 kg (ewes) 　1 mL/18 kg; SC, IM (lambs over 2 wk) Withdrawal: 　Meat: 14 days ℞ Dystosel: preventive dose 　1 mL/45 kg (calves & prenatal cows & ewes) 　0.25 mL per animal; IM (newborn lambs) 　0.5 mL per animal; SC, IM (2–8 wk) Treatment: 　Calves: 2 mL/45 kg; SC, IM 　Lambs: 0.5 mL; SC, IM Withdrawal: 　Meat: 21 days ℞ Not for use in lactating dairy cattle. See individual products for further information.
Vitamin K$_1$	Label dose: 　0.5 to 2.5 mg/kg; slowly IV, diluted in D$_5$W or 0.9% saline (acute hypoprothrominemia with severe hemorrhage) Not to exceed 10 mg/min in mature animals or 5 mg/min in newborn animals	Label dose: 　0.5 to 2.5 mg/kg; slowly IV, diluted in D$_5$W or 0.9% saline (acute hypoprothrominemia with severe hemorrhage) Not to exceed 10 mg/min in mature animals or 5 mg/min in newborn animals

Drug	Horses (and Miniature Pig Doses, Where Indicated)	Ruminants (Cattle, Sheep, and Goats)
Vitamin K₁ (continued)	0.5 to 2.5 mg/kg; SC, IM (nonacute hypo-prothrominemia) Extralabel dose: 0.5 to 1.0 mg/kg q 4 to 6 hr; SC (warfarin toxicosis) 1 to 2 mg/kg; SC divided at several sites (sweet clover poisoning)	0.5 to 2.5 mg/kg; SC, IM (nonacute hypo-prothrominemia) Withdrawal: Ψ
Warfarin (unlicensed for veterinary use)	Begin with 0.018 mg/kg once daily; PO, increasing by 20% weekly until the one-stage pro-thrombin time is increased by 2 to 4 seconds.	None
Xylazine	Label dose: 1.1 mg/kg; IV 2.2 mg/kg; IM 0.3 to 0.6 mg/kg IV prior to sodium pentobarbital, sodium thiopental, nitrous oxide, ether, halothane, or glyceryl guaiacolate Extralabel dose: 0.2 to 1.1 mg/kg; IV **OR** 0.33 mg/kg; IV followed by 0.033 to 0.066 mg/kg; IV butorphanol **OR** 1.1 mg/kg; IV followed by 1.76 to 2.2 mg/kg; IV ketamine **OR**	Label dose: 0.11 to 0.33 mg/kg IM (cattle) Withdrawal: Meat: 3 days Milk: 48 hr ℜ (Canada) Extralabel dose: 0.05 to 0.33 mg/kg; IM (cattle) 0.01 to 0.22 mg/kg; IM (sheep and goats) Use extreme caution with xylazine ad-ministration to small ruminants 0.05 mg/kg diluted into 5 mL saline; epidurally.

Drug	Horses (and Miniature Pig Doses, Where Indicated)	Ruminants (Cattle, Sheep, and Goats)
Xylazine (continued)	0.6 mg/kg; IV with 0.02 mg/kg acepromazine; IV **OR** 0.17 to 0.22 mg/kg diluted into 10 mL saline, epidurally Race withdrawal: 24 hr *Miniature pigs* 0.5 to 3.0 mg/kg; IM	Withdrawal: Meat: 7 days (US) & Milk: 72 hr (US) &
Yohimbine	Extralabel dose: 0.12 mg/kg; slowly IV (antagonism of detomidine or xylazine) 0.75 mg/kg; IV (restore intestinal motility) *Miniature pigs* 0.125 mg/kg; IV (xylazine reversal)	Dose not established; use to effect. Withdrawal: Meat and milk: 7 days &
Zeranol	None	36- or 72-mg implants; SC (cattle, in the ear only) Withdrawal: Meat: 65 days & 12 mg; SC (lambs, in the ear only) Withdrawal: Meat: 40 days ℞

Handbook of Veterinary Drugs, Second Edition, edited by Dana Allen,
Lippincott–Raven Publishers, Philadelphia. © 1998

Section 5

Antiparasitic, Anthelmintic, and Antimicrobial Agents in Large Animals

TABLE 1. **Antimicrobial Agents in Large Animals Pending Culture**[a]

Organism	Drugs of Choice	Alternative Drugs
Actinobacillus lignieresii	Sodium iodide and sulfas	Sodium iodide and tetracyclines
Actinobacillus equuli, A. suis	Gentamicin	Cephalothin, chloramphenicol (E), trimethoprim-sulfa
Actinomyces	Penicillin G	Tetracyclines
Anaerobic organisms	Penicillin G	Metronidazole
Bacillus anthracis	Penicillin G	Tetracyclines, dihydrostreptomycin
Bacteroides spp	Penicillin G	Ampicillin, chloramphenicol (E), metronidazole
Bacteroides spp (penicillinase-producing)	Metronidazole	Chloramphenicol (E)
Bordetella bronchiseptica	Gentamicin	Tetracycline (R), chloramphenicol (E), trimethoprim-sulfa

TABLE 1. **(Continued)**

Organism	Drugs of Choice	Alternative Drugs
Brucella abortus	Tetracyclines	Tetracyclines with dihydrostreptomycin
Campylobacter (abortions)	Penicillin/ dihydrostreptomycin	Tetracyclines
Chlamydia psittaci	Tetracyclines	Erythromycin
Clostridia spp	Penicillin G	Tetracyclines, erythromycin
Coccidia	Sulfonamides	Amprolium (R; TOXIC to Equidae)
Dermatophilus	Tetracyclines	Penicillin/ dihydrostreptomycin
Ehrlichia	Tetracyclines	
Enterobacter	Gentamicin	Kanamycin, chloramphenicol (E)
Escherichia coli	Gentamicin	Amikacin, trimethoprim-sulfa, chloramphenicol (E)
Fusobacterium necrophorum	Tetracyclines	Penicillin, sulfonamides
Haemophilus spp	Tetracyclines	Penicillin, sulfonamides
Hemolytic Streptococcus	Penicillin G	Erythromycin, ampicillin, chloramphenicol (E), cephalothin
Klebsiella	Amikacin	Trimethoprim-sulfa, gentamicin, kanamycin
Leptospira spp	Tetracyclines	Dihydrostreptomycin, erythromycin
Listeria monocytogenes	Tetracyclines	Penicillin
Mycoplasma spp (treatment is seldom successful)	Tetracyclines	Tylosin
Nonhemolytic Streptococcus	Chloramphenicol (E)	Erythromycin, ampicillin
Pasteurella hemolytica, P. multocida	Gentamicin (E), ceftiofur, trimethoprim-sulfa	Tetracyclines, tilmicosin (R), flor-fenicol penicillin G

TABLE 1. (Continued)

Organism	Drugs of Choice	Alternative Drugs
Proteus mirabilis	Gentamicin	Chloramphenicol (E), kanamycin
Pseudomonas spp	Gentamicin	Amikacin, trimethoprim-sulfa, polymixin B
Rhodococcus equi	Erythromycin and rifampin	Trimethroprim-sulfa, chloramphenicol (E), gentamicin
Salmonella spp	Trimethoprim-sulfa	Gentamicin, amikacin, ampicillin, chloramphenicol (E)
Sarcocystis (ruminants)	Monensin (ruminants only, TOXIC to Equidae)	Salinomycin
Sarcocystis falcatula (horses)	Trimethoprim-sulfa and pyrimethamine	N/A
Staphylococcus aureus	Penicillin G sensitive: Penicillin G Penicillin G resistant: Erythromycin	Ampicillin, lincomycin

E, equine; R, ruminant.
[a] With modifications with permission, from Brumbaugh GW. Rational selection of antimicrobial drugs for treatment of infections in horses. *Vet Clin North Am: Equine Practice* 1987;3:191–220.

TABLE 2. **Anthelmintics in Horses**

Drug	Indications	Larvacidal
Albendazole (Extralabel)	*Dictyocaulus arnfieldi, Strongylus vulgaris, Echinococcus* spp	+ at 50 mg/kg bid; PO for 2 days
Dichlorovos	*Parascaris* spp	–
	Large and small strongyles (at 35 mg/kg; PO)	–
	Bots	–
	Oxyuris spp	N/A
Diethylcarbamazine (Extralabel)	*Onchocerca*	+
	Ascarids	
Febantel	Large and small strongyles	+ for 4th stage *Oxyuris*
	Parascaris spp	
	Oxyuris spp	
Fenbendazole	*Parascaris* spp	
	Large and small strongyles	– at label dose, + at 10 mg/kg; PO for 5 days, 50 mg/kg for 3 days
	Oxyuris spp	
Ivermectin	*Parascaris* spp	
	Large and small strongyles	+
	Onchocerca	
	Habronema	+
	Draschia (summer sores)	
	Bots	
	Lice	
Levamisole (Extralabel)	Large and small strongyles	–
		–
Mebendazole	Large and small strongyles	+
	Parascaris spp	
	Oxyuris spp	
Oxfendazole	*Parascaris* spp	+ 4th stage *Oxyuris equi*
	Large and small strongyles	
	Oxyuris spp	

TABLE 2. (Continued)

Drug	Indications	Larvacidal
Oxibendazole	*Parascaris* spp	−
	Large and small strongyles, threadworms	−
	Oxyuris spp	−
Piperazine	*Parascaris* spp	+
	Large and small strongyles	−
	Oxyuris spp	
Thiabendazole	Large and small strongyles	+ at 440 mg/kg; PO
	Parascaris spp	
	Oxyuris spp	
Trichlorfon	Bots	N/A
	Parascaris spp	
	Oxyuris spp	

TABLE 3. Anthelmintics in Ruminants[a]

Drug	Indications	Larvacidal
Albendazole	*Fasciola* spp	+ L4
	Gastrointestinal nematodes	(*Dictyocaulus, Ostertagia, Trichostrongylus*)
	Tapeworms	
	Lungworms	
Clorsulon	*Fasciola* spp	+
Febantel (Extralabel)	(Sheep)	
	All gastrointestinal nematodes (except *Trichuris*)	
	Strongyloides	
	Lungworms	
	Tapeworms	
Fenbendazole	All gastrointestinal nematodes (including *Trichuris* and lungworms)	±
	Tapeworms (*Moniezia*)	

TABLE 3. **(Continued)**

Drug	Indications	Larvacidal
Ivermectin	All gastrointestinal nematodes (except *Trichuris* and *Nematodirus*) *Dictyocaulus*, *Hypoderma* spp Lice, mites, *Oestrus ovis*	+
Levamisole	Most gastrointestinal nematodes Lungworms	± variable
Mebendazole (Extralabel)	(Sheep) All gastrointestinal nematodes (except *Trichuris*) Lungworms Tapeworms	–
Pyrantel (Extralabel)	*Hemonchus*	–
Thiabendazole	Most gastrointestinal nematodes (except *Trichuris*)	–
Trichlorfon (Pour-on)	Cattle grubs and lice	N/A

^aIndications may include drugs not approved for horses or ruminants. Where ruminants are indicated, many products are not approved for sheep or goats. Large strongyles include *Strongylus vulgaris, Strongylus edentatus,* and *Strongylus equinum.* Threadworm includes *Strongyloides* spp. Extralabel use may be based on anecdotal reports rather than on controlled clinical studies. The species the drug is indicated in is not listed here. The reader is directed to the section on drug descriptions.

Section 6

Description of Drugs for Large Animals

ABAMECTIN

INDICATIONS: Abamectin (Endecto♣★) is one of the series of antiparasitic agents derived from the avermectin family of compounds. It is used for treatment of parasitic infestations in cattle due to gastrointestinal round worms, the lungworm *Dictyocaulus viviparus* (adult and 4th stage larvae), grubs (*Hypoderma bovis* and *H. lineatum*), sucking lice (*Linognathus vituli* and *Haematopinus eurysternus*), and mange mites (*Sarcoptes scabiei var bovis* and *Psoroptes ovis*). Abamectin stimulates the release of γ-aminobutyric acid (GABA) from nerve endings in parasites, which results in paralysis and death of the parasite, acting in a similar fashion to ivermectin. As such, abamectin does not have any measurable effect against flukes or tapeworms, presumably because they do not have GABA as a nerve impulse transmitter. Further, abamectin does not affect mammals because it does not penetrate their central nervous system, where GABA acts as a neurotransmitter.

ADVERSE AND COMMON SIDE EFFECTS: Transitory discomfort has been observed in some animals, as well as a low incidence of transitory soft tissue swelling following SC administration. The swelling disappears without treatment and can be minimized by dividing doses greater than 10 mL into two separate sites of injection. When used for treatment of *Hypoderma* spp, proper timing must be adhered to because destruction of the larvae during the periods when they are in the vertebral canal or esophagus can lead to staggering, or paralysis in the case of *H. bovis*, or bloat in the case of *H. lineatum*. These reactions are not specific for abamectin. This drug should not be administered to calves less than 16 weeks old. Caution is to be used if administering this drug to severely stressed or debilitated animals. It is not to be used in any other species because this product has been specifically formulated for use in cattle.

DRUG INTERACTIONS: None reported.

SUPPLIED AS: VETERINARY PRODUCT
For injection containing abamectin 10 mg/mL in 200 mL and 500 mL collapsible packs

ACEPROMAZINE

INDICATIONS: Acepromazine [formerly acetylpromazine] (Ace-project★, Acepro♣★, Acevet♣, AC Promazine♣, Ace♣, Atravet♣, Atravet Soluble Granules♣, Promace★, Promazine★, Tranquazine★) is a phenothiazine drug approved for use as a sedative in horses to ease handling or trailering. Used as a preanesthetic, it markedly potentiates barbiturates. It also has antispasmodic effects through its partial blockade of α-adrenergic receptors and has been used in spasmodic colic. It is used in cases of clinical tetanus to reduce muscle spasms. Additionally, the drug is used to cause relaxation and protrusion of the penis for catheterization in the stallion or gelding, and to calm nervous cattle (used in conjunction with local anesthetics) for surgical procedures. Acepromazine is not to be used in horses intended for human consumption and has not been approved in food-producing animals (in US, approved in Canada) because of the potential risk of drug residues in meat and meat products.

ADVERSE AND COMMON SIDE EFFECTS: Tranquilization of dangerous animals may lead to a false sense of security; painful procedures should be avoided because there is little analgesic effect. Horses may react to sudden noises or movements despite appearing somnolent. Even at high therapeutic doses, recumbency is unusual and the risk of the horse stepping or falling on attending personnel is minimal. An adequate blood volume and arterial blood pressure are necessary for the use of acepromazine because of its marked arterial hypotensive effects; use of acepromazine in colic other than that due to spasmodic colic is contraindicated. The drug is extensively bound to plasma proteins (> 99%). A reduced dose is advised in the horse in low-protein states such as protein-losing enteropathy.

Acepromazine temporarily lowers the hematocrit of a horse by 25% and up to 50% in a dose-dependent manner via splenic sequestration. Penile protrusion occurs within 30 minutes following administration and can last for 100 minutes; the extent and duration of penile protrusion are dose related. Priapism can occur in the horse, more commonly in stallions or recently castrated geldings, or in combination with etorphine. Thus, its use in stallions should be avoided. In cattle, acepromazine may induce only mild sedation or be ineffective in unmanageable or hyperexcited cattle. When used as a premedicant in cattle, recovery from general anesthesia may not be as smooth as when not given. Death has occurred in cattle injected with acepromazine after prolonged transport. Results are unpredictable in diseases associated with shock, such as colic. The central nervous system seizure threshold is decreased with phenothiazines and should not be used in susceptible animals such as foals with neonatal maladjustment or as a premedicant for myelograms. The tranquilizing effect may last longer than the label indication of 8 hours.

DRUG INTERACTIONS: Toxicity of carbamates and organophosphates, e.g., physostigmine and trichlorfon, may be enhanced by the administration of phenothiazines; concurrent use is contraindicated. Benztropine mesylate (8 mg; IV for an adult horse) may reverse acepromazine-induced penile prolapse. Do not mix acepromazine in the same syringe with glycopyrrolate or diazepam.

SUPPLIED AS: VETERINARY PRODUCTS
For injection containing 10 and 25 mg/mL
Tablets containing 10 and 25 mg
For oral use as soluble granules 1.25 g/225 g

OTHER USES
Horses
STANDING CHEMICAL RESTRAINT
Acepromazine is often combined with sedatives (0.02 mg/kg acepromazine, 0.66 mg/kg xylazine; IV) or opioids (acepromazine 0.04 mg/kg; IV with 0.6 mg/kg; IV meperidine or 0.02 mg/kg; IV butorphanol or 0.4 mg/kg; IV pentazocine).

ACUTE LAMINITIS
Acepromazine (0.044 mg/kg bid; IM) is also used for 4 to 5 days for α-adrenergic blockade against presumed arterial hypertension during acute laminitis.

Ruminants
GENERAL ANESTHESIA
For procedures requiring short-acting general anesthesia, administer 0.05 to 0.1 mg/kg; IM or IV, followed by ketamine at 2 to 5 mg/kg; IV.

ACETAZOLAMIDE

INDICATIONS: Acetazolamide (AK-Zol★, Apo-Acetazolamide♣, Diamox♣★) is a carbonic anhydrase inhibitor that increases the urinary excretion of bicarbonate and decreases extracellular potassium, reduces intraocular pressure, and reduces the rate of formation of cerebrospinal fluid, but transiently causes an increase in cerebrospinal fluid pressure. It is most commonly used to reduce intraocular pressure in glaucoma, a disease not common in large animals. Acetazolamide has been advocated as maintenance treatment to prevent periodic paralysis in horses, but it is yet to be proven effective.

ADVERSE AND COMMON SIDE EFFECTS: In humans, acetazolamide can cause somnolence, behavioral changes, and paresthesia. Hypersensitivity reactions are rare, manifesting as fever, skin rash, and bone marrow suppression. The drug depresses uptake of iodine by the thyroid gland. Teratogenic effects have been reported and the drug should not be used in pregnant animals.

DRUG INTERACTIONS: Acetazolamide has been associated with drug-induced osteomalacia when used in conjunction with phenytoin.

SUPPLIED AS: HUMAN PRODUCTS
Capsules (extended release) containing 500 mg
Tablets containing 125 mg and 250 mg

OTHER USES
Horses
PERIODIC PARALYSIS
2 to 4 mg/kg bid–qid; PO

ACETIC ACID (5%)

INDICATIONS: Acetic acid (vinegar) is used to treat nonprotein nitrogen-induced ammonia toxicosis in ruminants. The acetic acid administered lowers rumen pH, which favors the shift in uncharged ammonia to the charged ammonium ion, which reduces absorption of ammonia. Cold water is also administered to reduce the rumen temperature and hence the formation of ammonia. Acetic acid is also suggested as a drug useful for the prevention of enterolith formation in horses, where it may act by altering colonic pH.

ADVERSE AND COMMON SIDE EFFECTS: Acetic acid is irritating to mucous membranes and should be administered through a stomach tube.

DRUG INTERACTIONS: Unknown.

SUPPLIED AS: Commercially available as a liquid.

OTHER USES Acetic acid is also used in solutions for udder washes and in proprietary preparations as a poultice.

ACETYLCYSTEINE

INDICATIONS: Acetylcysteine (Mucomyst♣★, Mucosil★,Parvolex♣★) is a mucolytic agent that breaks disulfide bonds in mucus, helping liquefy excessively viscous or inspissated mucous secretions of the respiratory tract. It is used in chronic bronchitis in foals and horses. Acetylcysteine can be administered through a bronchoscope and followed by immediate suction of secretions. Mild exercise and coughing following use may aid movement of secretion from the lungs.

Acetylcysteine has also been used with some success in persistent meconium retention in foals. It has the reported advantage over other preparations for its success in breaking the disulfide bond of the mucoproteins in the meconium plug of newborns.

ADVERSE AND COMMON SIDE EFFECTS: When nebulized, acetylcysteine can cause bronchospasm; pretreatment with a β_2 bronchodilator may prevent this. Dilution to less than 10% solution will reduce the activity of acetylcysteine.

DRUG INTERACTIONS: Acetylcysteine inactivates ampicillin, amphotericin B, erythromycin lactobionate, and tetracycline antibiotics if used together as an aerosol.

SUPPLIED AS: HUMAN PRODUCTS
For oral inhalation or intratracheal instillation containing a 10% or 20% sterile solution
Parvolex is also labeled for IV and oral use.

OTHER USES
Horses
MECONIUM IMPACTION
As an enema for foals with meconium impaction, 120 to 240 mL of a 4% solution is administered via a 30 F Foley catheter and retained in place for 4 to 5 minutes. Repeat in 1 hour and with a slightly higher volume if necessary. The solution is made by mixing in 8 g acetylcysteine powder and 20 g sodium bicarbonate (baking soda; to bring the pH to 7.6) in sufficient water to make 200 mL.

ALBENDAZOLE

INDICATIONS: Albendazole (Valbazen♣★) is a broad-spectrum anthelmintic recommended for the treatment of internal parasites of cattle, including liver flukes (adult stage of *Fasciola hepatica*, *Fascioloides magna*), tapeworms (adult *Moniezia benedeni*), gastric worms (adult *Haemonchus placei*, *Trichostrongylus axei*, adult, 4th larval, and inhibited 4th larval stage of *Ostertagia ostertagi*), intestinal worms (adult stages of *Trichostrongylus colubriformis*, *Bunosto-*

mum phlebotomum, Nematodirus helvetianus, and *Oesophagostomum redietum*), and lungworms (adult and 4th larval stages of *Dictyocaulus viviparus*). Albendazole is also used in sheep for most adult gastrointestinal nem-atodes and lungworms. Albendazole is the only broad-spectrum anthelmintic effective against adult liver flukes (*F. hepatica*) in sheep.

ADVERSE AND COMMON SIDE EFFECTS: The drug should not be used in female cattle in the first 45 days of pregnancy (21 days, Canada) or within 45 days (21 days, Canada) of removing bulls from the herd.

DRUG INTERACTIONS: None listed.

SUPPLIED AS: VETERINARY PRODUCTS
As a suspension containing 113.6 mg/mL
As a 3% paste

OTHER USES
Sheep
MONIEZIA
3 to 8 mg/kg; PO is said to be 100% effective.

FLUKES
10 to 20 mg/kg; PO

ALLOPURINOL

INDICATIONS: Allopurinol (Apo-allopurinol✦, Lopurin★, Zyloprim✦★) is a xanthine oxidase inhibitor used in humans for the treatment of gout. Allopurinol has been suggested for use in horses as a preventive agent for reperfusion injury of colic.

ADVERSE AND COMMON SIDE EFFECTS: The most common adverse effects in humans are hypersensitivity reactions. Information regarding adverse effects in horses is not available.

DRUG INTERACTIONS: Allopurinol may interfere with hepatic inactivation of other drugs, and with oral dicoumarol. Concomitant use with theophylline leads to an increase of the active metabolite of theophylline. Administration of iron during allopurinol medication is not recommended. Concurrent administration of co-trimoxazole has been associated with thrombocytopenia in a few patients.

SUPPLIED AS: HUMAN PRODUCT
Tablets containing 100, 200 and 300 mg

ALTRENOGEST

INDICATIONS: Altrenogest (Regu-Mate♥★) is a progestin used to suppress estrus in mares for a predictable occurrence of estrus following drug withdrawal. Suppression of estrus will encourage regular cycles following winter anestrus, facilitate scheduled breeding, and help manage mares exhibiting prolonged estrus. Ovulation will occur 5 to 7 days following the onset of estrus. Use of prostaglandin $F_{2\alpha}$ or a synthetic analogue immediately following an 8- to 12-day course of altrenogest (label indication is 15 days) will induce estrus.

ADVERSE AND COMMON SIDE EFFECTS: Altrenogest is contraindicated in pregnant mares because higher doses have caused fetal abnormalities in laboratory animals. Pregnant women and women in childbearing years should use extreme caution handling the product because accidental absorption could lead to disruption of the menstrual cycle or prolongation of pregnancy.

DRUG INTERACTIONS: None listed.

SUPPLIED AS: VETERINARY PRODUCTS
For oral administration, altrenogest solution containing 2.2 mg/mL and gel containing 2.15 mg/g syringe

AMIKACIN

INDICATIONS: Amikacin (Amiglyde-V♥★, Amikacin sulfate★, Amikin♥★) is a bactericidal aminoglycoside antibiotic effective against many aminoglycoside-resistant bacteria. The drug resists degradation by aminoglycoside-inactivating enzymes known to affect gentamicin, tobramycin, and kanamycin, including *Escherichia coli, Pseudomonas, Staphylococcus,* and *Proteus.* It is used in the intrauterine treatment of genital tract infections such as endometritis, metritis, and pyometra in mares. Indications for parenteral use include bacteremia or septicemia in neonatal foals and skin and soft tissue infections caused by *E. coli, Proteus, Pseudomonas,* or *Klebsiella.* Serum levels peak 15 minutes following IV injection and 1 hour following IM injection. Serum levels should be monitored. The trough is variable and occurs just before the next dose. Peak levels from 15 to 20 µg/mL and trough levels of less than 5 µg/mL are desirable.

ADVERSE AND COMMON SIDE EFFECTS: Amikacin should be used with caution in animals with compromised kidney function and is contraindicated in cases of severe renal impairment. Toxic levels can cause renal tubular damage, which may be reversible once the drug is discontinued. Concurrent use with other aminoglycosides should be avoided because of potential toxic additive effects.

Amikacin causes transient pain on injection. Ototoxicity can occur but is difficult to detect clinically. Weakness from neuromuscular blockade may also occur. Cost and potential drug residues preclude its use in food-producing animals. See also **AMINOGLYCOSIDE ANTIBIOTICS**.

DRUG INTERACTIONS: See **AMINOGLYCOSIDE ANTIBIOTICS**.

SUPPLIED AS: VETERINARY PRODUCTS
For injection containing 50 mg/mL
Solution for intrauterine infusion containing 250 mg/mL

HUMAN PRODUCT
For injection containing 50 and 250 mg/mL

AMINOCAPROIC ACID

INDICATIONS: Aminocaproic acid (Amicar♥★) is a human drug used to treat systemic hyperfibrinolysis that occurs in diseases such as surgical complications, hematologic disorders, or neoplastic disease. It has been used in horses as a treatment for exercise-induced pulmonary hemorrhage. There is, however, no evidence to support such use.

ADVERSE AND COMMON SIDE EFFECTS: Rapid IV injections of aminocaproic acid may result in hypotension, bradycardia, or other arrhythmias. Aminocaproic acid has a narrow margin of safety in humans.

DRUG INTERACTIONS: None listed.

SUPPLIED AS: HUMAN PRODUCTS
For injection containing 250 mg/mL
Syrup containing 250 mg/mL
Tablets containing 500 mg

AMINOGLYCOSIDE ANTIBIOTICS

INDICATIONS: The aminoglycoside antibiotics, including amikacin, dihydrostreptomycin, gentamicin, kanamycin, neomycin, streptomycin, and tobramycin, are indicated in the treatment of certain gram-negative, gram-positive, and mycobacterial infections. They are primarily effective against aerobic gram-negative bacteria such as *E. coli, Klebsiella, Proteus,* and *Enterobacter,* and some are also effective against *Pseudomonas* infections. Gentamicin is more effective than kanamycin but less effective than tobramycin against *Pseudomonas aeruginosa.* Amikacin sulfate injection is especially useful against *Pseudomonas* and *Klebsiella* spp, which are resistant to gentamicin. To establish optimum dosing levels, it is desirable to take samples at peak and trough times.

ADVERSE AND COMMON SIDE EFFECTS: Nephrotoxicity, deafness, vestibular toxicity, respiratory paralysis, and cardiovascular depression have been reported with the use of these drugs. Endotoxemia predisposes to cardiovascular-induced depression. These drugs should be used with caution or avoided entirely in food-producing animals because they can persist for long periods of time as tissue residues. Neomycin is the most nephrotoxic aminoglycoside, followed in decreasing order of nephrotoxicity by gentamicin, tobramycin, kanamycin, amikacin, and streptomycin. Monitoring the urine for the appearance of casts, which in this case is a more sensitive indicator of impending renal dysfunction than serum urea or creatinine levels, is recommended.

DRUG INTERACTIONS: Aminoglycoside antibiotics can potentiate the action of neuromuscular blocking agents leading to respiratory depression, apnea, or muscle weakness, especially in animals with renal insufficiency. The neuromuscular blocking activity can be reversed with calcium. Furosemide may enhance the ototoxicity and nephrotoxicity of the aminoglycosides. Gentamicin, dihydrostreptomycin, kanamycin, neomycin, and streptomycin may decrease cardiac output and produce hypotension and bradycardia and should be avoided in animals in shock or with serious cardiac insufficiency. IV calcium gluconate should be used to reverse myocardial depression and restore blood pressure. Prolonged high oral doses of neomycin may cause diarrhea and malabsorption due to selective overgrowth of resistant indigenous intestinal flora. Aminoglycosides may cross the placental barrier and produce fetal intoxication and should not be given to pregnant animals. Penicillins should not be mixed with aminoglycosides before injection because inactivation of the aminoglycoside may occur.

SUPPLIED AS: See individual drug.

AMINOPHYLLINE

INDICATIONS: Aminophylline (theophylline ethylenediamine) (Aminophylline♥★, Lufyllin★, Dilor★, Dyflex★, Neothylline★, Phyllocontin♥★) is one of the more soluble forms of theophylline, an adenosine antagonist. Pharmacologic effects of aminophylline include brief but potent diuresis, increased mechanical efficiency of the heart, and bronchodilation. Aminophylline is used primarily in horses to treat bronchospasm of small-airway disease, but its narrow therapeutic range limits its safe use. Aminophylline can be used to accelerate recovery from benzodiazepine sedatives because it is an effective respiratory stimulant. Aminophylline also has mast cell stabilizing properties.

Theophylline has been used as an adjunctive treatment for undifferentiated bovine respiratory disease. Because of the increased mortality and the need for therapeutic drug monitoring, this drug should be considered for treating bovine respiratory disease only where no effective alternative drug is available and the desired effects of theophylline are essential for animal recovery.

ADVERSE AND COMMON SIDE EFFECTS: Rapid IV administration of aminophylline can result in life-threatening cardiac arrhythmias. Signs of aminophylline toxicity include sweating, restlessness, and tachycardia. Monitoring blood levels may help reduce the risk.

DRUG INTERACTIONS: The combination of reduced doses of aminophylline with a β_2-adrenergic agonist may achieve effective bronchodilation with reduced risk of toxicity. Clearance of theophylline (active form of aminophylline) is increased twofold during administration of phenytoin and also is increased when given with rifampin. Clearance of theophylline is delayed, increasing the risk of toxic signs, in animals receiving cimetidine, enrofloxacin, propranolol, or certain macrolide antibiotics, such as erythromycin. Synergistic toxicity is seen in combination with cardiac glycosides or sympathomimetics.

SUPPLIED AS: HUMAN PRODUCTS
For injection containing 25, 50, and 250 mg/mL
Tablets containing 100, 200, 225, 350, and 400 mg

AMMONIUM CHLORIDE

INDICATIONS: Ammonium chloride (Ammonium Chloride Enseals★, MEq-AC★, Urigard-AC Solution★, Uroeze★) is used as a urinary acidifier and as an expectorant. In ruminants, ammonium chloride is used to acidify urine for the prevention of urolithiasis caused by phosphate crystals. Because of its effect of urinary acidification, ammonium chloride can hasten urinary excretion of strychnine in cases of strychnine toxicity. Ammonium chloride can also be used for correction of metabolic alkalosis in edematous patients requiring sodium restriction. However, this is rarely of practical consideration in large animal practice. Ammonium chloride is reported to prevent parturient paresis. The mechanism is proposed to be the dietary acidification causing increased intestinal calcium absorption and enhanced calcium resorption from bone.

ADVERSE AND COMMON SIDE EFFECTS: The ammonium ion is toxic at high concentrations. Acidosis can result from its administration. The drug is not to be used in animals with severe hepatic disease. High doses in sheep have been associated with increased coughing and associated rectal prolapse.

DRUG INTERACTIONS: Animals with large doses of salicylates (e.g., acetylsalicylic acid) may develop increased serum salicylate levels.

SUPPLIED AS: VETERINARY PRODUCTS

Small Animal Products

Tablets containing 357 mg
Granules containing 535 mg/teaspoon (3.35 g)
Tablets containing 200 mg in a protein base (Uroese)
Powder containing 200 and 400 mg/0.65 g in a protein base (Uroese)
Solution: each 0.5 mL contains 100 mg ammonium chloride in palatable base containing DL-methionine and vitamin B complex

Large Animal Product

Feed additive containing 99% ammonium chloride

HUMAN PRODUCT
Tablets containing 500 mg

OTHER USES
Cattle

PARTURIENT PARESIS
100 g/day; PO for 21 days prior to calving

Horses

URINARY ACIDIFICATION
Ammonium sulfate (99% ammonium sulfate, bulk chemical form), instead of the chloride salt, can be used to acidify urine. Dose is 175 mg/kg bid; PO.

AMOXICILLIN

INDICATIONS: Amoxicillin (Amoxi-Bol★, Amoxi-Drop★, Amoxi-Inject★, Amoxi-Mast★, Amoxi-Tabs★, Amoxil✦, Biomox★, Robamox★, Moxilean✦) is an aminopenicillin chemically similar to penicillin G but with activity against some gram-negative bacteria, and it resists acid hydrolysis in the stomach. Amoxicillin has similar antimicrobial activity to ampicillin but is apparently more completely absorbed following oral administration. Amoxicillin is not resistant to bacterial penicillinase. It is useful for treating soft tissue, respiratory, urinary tract, and intestinal infections caused by susceptible bacteria. It has been used successfully to treat experimental *Salmonella dublin* infections in 1-month-old calves. Amoxicillin is available in the United States for parenteral treatment of bovine pneumonia and foot rot, as an oral antibiotic for neonatal calf scours, and for intramammary treatment of mastitis in cattle.

ADVERSE AND COMMON SIDE EFFECTS: Abdominal discomfort and diarrhea can occur with oral medication. Intramuscular injection should be as a 10% suspension. Effectiveness may be limited by the relatively large injection volume and discomfort associated with administration. As with other penicillins, there is a potential for hypersensitivity reactions.

DRUG INTERACTIONS: None listed.

SUPPLIED AS: VETERINARY PRODUCTS
Oral suspension containing 50 mg/mL
Suspension for injection containing 250 mg/mL (25 g/vial)
Tablets containing 50, 100, 200, and 400 mg
Boluses containing 400 mg
Mastitis suspension containing 62.5 mg per disposable syringe

AMPHETAMINE

INDICATIONS: Dextro-Amphetamine (Dexedrine♥★) is a powerful central nervous system stimulant that has been used for heroic measures in treatment of "downer" cows. It is also of use for treating narcolepsy in large animals.

ADVERSE AND COMMON SIDE EFFECTS: Potential for drug abuse by humans exists when this product is kept in a veterinary pharmacy.

DRUG INTERACTIONS: None listed.

SUPPLIED AS: HUMAN PRODUCTS
Tablets containing 5 and 10 mg
Capsules containing 5, 10, and 15 mg

AMPICILLIN

INDICATIONS: Ampicillin (ampicillin sodium [Amp-Equine★, Ampicin♥, Omnipen-N★, Penbritin♥, Polycillin-N★, Totacillin-N★], ampicillin trihydrate [Polyflex♥★]) is a broad-spectrum penicillin with bactericidal activity against a wide range of gram-positive and gram-negative bacteria. Ampicillin is useful for treating bacterial pneumonia, soft tissue and postsurgical infections, and mastitis caused by bacteria susceptible to ampicillin. Ampicillin does not resist penicillinase. The drug is approved for treatment of pneumonia in cattle but may be ineffective at the label dose. Because the trihydrate salts will achieve serum levels only approximately one half that of the sodium salt, they should not be used where higher minimal inhibitory concentrations (MIC) are required.

ADVERSE AND COMMON SIDE EFFECTS: A risk of allergic reaction is present; prior hypersensitivity to another penicillin increases the risk of a reaction. The drug causes minimal direct toxicity. Bacterial resistance to ampicillin is increasingly common. Some authors have suggested that ampicillin can induce diarrhea in horses, but recent literature suggests this is not the case.

DRUG INTERACTIONS: Use of ampicillin and allopurinol concurrently will increase the risk of skin rash.

SUPPLIED AS: VETERINARY PRODUCTS
For injection in the trihydrate form in 10- and 25-g vials
For injection in the sodium salt form in 1- and 3-g vials

HUMAN PRODUCT
For injection (sodium salt) in 125-, 250-, and 500-mg, and 1-, 2-, and 10-g vials

AMPROLIUM

INDICATIONS: Amprolium (Amprol♣, Corid★) is a coccidiostatic drug active against first-generation schizonts of developing coccidia. It is used in calves as an aid for treatment of coccidiosis caused by *Eimeria bovis* and *Eimeria zuernii*.

ADVERSE AND COMMON SIDE EFFECTS: Amprolium is a thiamine antagonist and high doses (321 to 880 mg/kg daily; PO) can cause polioencephalomalacia in calves and sheep.

DRUG INTERACTIONS: Amprolium is a thiamine analogue. Concurrent administration of thiamine can antagonize anticoccidial activity of amprolium.

SUPPLIED AS: VETERINARY PRODUCTS
Oral solution containing 96 mg/mL (9.6%)
Soluble powder containing 20%
Feed mix containing 25%
Feed additive crumbles containing 1.25%

OTHER USES
Sheep
SARCOCYSTOSIS
50 to 100 mg/kg daily; PO for prophylaxis against morbidity and mortality associated with *Sarcocystis* spp in lambs

ANTACIDS

INDICATIONS: Antacids containing aluminum and magnesium oxides and hydroxides, including Stat Plus Electrolytes♣, Maalox ♣★, Oxamin Bolus♣, and Oxamin Powder♣, are used to neutralize stomach acid. Combinations of the varying compounds are used to provide both a fast-acting and a persistent acid-neutralizing effect. Antacids are used to treat stomach ulcers in horses, abomasal ulcers in cattle, and simple indigestion or grain overload in cattle. These products may also be ruminatoric.

ADVERSE AND COMMON SIDE EFFECTS: Some antacid products can cause systemic alkalosis. Aluminum-containing antacids can cause ileus, whereas magnesium-containing products may cause loose feces or diarrhea.

DRUG INTERACTIONS: Antacids can chelate and decrease bioavailability of iron and tetracyclines. Aluminum-containing antacid compounds decrease bioavailability of phenothiazines, digoxin, prednisone, prednisolone, ranitidine, and, possibly, cimetidine. Antacid-induced change in urine pH increases urinary excretion and decreases blood concentrations of salicylates.

SUPPLIED AS: VETERINARY PRODUCT
See individual products.

ANTIHISTAMINES

INDICATIONS: Antihistamines [H₁] (Antihist Solution♣, Antihistamine Injection♣★, Antihistamine Oral♣, Antihistamine Powder♣, Histavet-P★, Pyrahist-10♣, Pyrilamine Maleate Injection★, Re-Covr★, Ved-Hist★, Vetastim♣) act as competitive antagonists for specific type-1 histamine receptors. They are more effective in preventing the actions of histamine than reversing them. Oral antihistamines are used for treatment of allergic and anaphylactic conditions in large animals. The powder form is used orally in horses for the relief of urticaria due to allergy and difficulty breathing due to inhaled allergens. Treatment of allergic reactions in large animals may be disappointing due to the influence of other mediators in addition to histamine. Injectable antihistamines (e.g., Re-Covr★, Vetastim♣) have also been advocated as adjunctive therapy along with IV calcium for milk fever in cattle.

ADVERSE AND COMMON SIDE EFFECTS: At low doses antihistamines can cause sedation. Higher doses of antihistamines may cause central nervous system (CNS) excitement, hyperpyrexia, and even death. Prolonged administration of oral antihistamines can cause constipation or diarrhea. Antihistamines should be used with caution in the pregnant animal because certain agents have teratogenic potential.

DRUG INTERACTIONS: Severe CNS depression can occur with concomitant use of barbiturates or chlorpromazine.

SUPPLIED AS: VETERINARY PRODUCTS
For injection containing 25 mg pyrilamine maleate and 10 mg ephedrine/mL
For injection containing 20 mg/mL pyrilamine maleate
For injection containing tripelennamine hydrochloride 20 mg/mL
Powder containing 50 mg pyrilamine maleate with 20 mg DL-ephedrine

OTHER USES: Antihistamines are also found in combination with antibiotics and corticosteroid products [Azimycin♣★, Dexamycin♣].

ANTITUSSIVES

INDICATIONS: Antitussives should only be used in animals with a severe, nonproductive cough that deters eating or drinking or results in physical exhaustion, because the cough is a necessary defense mechanism. Proprietary products include Cough Aid♣, Equintussi Cough Syrup♣, Expectorant Compound II★, Glytussin★, and Heave Aid♣. Most of the proprietary products act mainly as expectorants, some of the antihistamines being directly antitussive. Opioid analgesics (see **BUTORPHANOL, MORPHINE, MEPERIDINE**) also have potent antitussive properties.

ADVERSE AND COMMON SIDE EFFECTS: If productive coughing is suppressed, recovery from lower respiratory tract disease can be prevented or delayed.

DRUG INTERACTIONS: See individual products. Little information is available.

SUPPLIED AS: VETERINARY PRODUCTS
Syrup containing ammonium bicarbonate, ammonium chloride, chloroform, and menthol [Cough Aid, Equintussi Cough Syrup, Cough Aid]
Oral Powder containing ammonium chloride, camphor, menthol, and ammonium bicarbonate [Heave Aid]
Oral powder containing ammonium chloride, guaifenesin, and potassium iodide [Expectorant Compound II, Glytussin]

APRAMYCIN

INDICATIONS: Apramycin (Apralan♣, Apralan 75★) is an amino-cyclitol antibiotic used for the treatment of bacterial enteritis caused by E. coli in piglets. Oral absorption decreases markedly with increasing age of the piglets. Single oral doses of 10, 30, and 100 mg/kg give peak blood levels at 1 to 4 hours, with detectable serum levels at 12 to 24 hours.

ADVERSE AND COMMON SIDE EFFECTS: None listed.

DRUG INTERACTIONS: None listed.

SUPPLIED AS: VETERINARY PRODUCTS
Soluble powder, 50-g activity container (containing 1.5 g/measure; Apralan)
Feed additive, 50 lb (containing 75 g/lb; Apralan 75)

ASCORBIC ACID

INDICATIONS: Vitamin C [ascorbic acid] (Apo-C♣, Ascobicap♣, Cetane★, Centravite-C♣, C-Ject 250★, Redoxon♣★, Sodium Ascorbate★, Vitamin C Injectable♣, Vitamin C Injection★, and others) is a water-soluble vitamin that has been advocated for periods of high-stress training in horses in which there is some suggestion that the body becomes depleted of the vitamin. Vitamin C has also been used for adjunctive treatment of exercise-induced pulmonary hemorrhage in horses and bronchopneumonia in cattle, but such use has yet to be shown of benefit. Vitamin C has been used at high doses to treat red maple toxicity in horses. The proposed beneficial effect is the reduction of methemoglobin to hemoglobin. Vitamin C has poor oral bioavailability.

ADVERSE AND COMMON SIDE EFFECTS: None listed. Some animals will have local inflammatory reactions to SC or IM injections.

DRUG INTERACTIONS: None listed.

SUPPLIED AS: VETERINARY PRODUCTS
For injection containing 250 mg/mL★
Powder containing 99 g/100 g (500-g pouch)

HUMAN PRODUCTS
Tablets containing 50, 100, 200, 250, 500, 1,000, and 1,500 mg
Liquid containing 1,000 mg/5 mL
Liquid containing 60 and 100 mg/mL

OTHER USES
Horses
RED MAPLE TOXICITY
30 to 50 mg/kg bid; IV or SC

ASPIRIN

INDICATIONS: Aspirin or acetylsalicylic acid (ASA Bolus♣, Acetylsalicylic Acid Tablets♣, Asen 60♣, Aspirin 60 Grain★, Aspirin 240 Grain Boluses★, Aspirin Bolus ★, Aspirin Boluses★, Aspirin Powder★, Aspirin Tablets ★, Bexprin♣, Centra ASA 60♣, Centra ASA 240♣, LA Aspirin Boluses★) is classified as a nonsteroidal anti-inflammatory drug (NSAID) and has three basic properties: anti-inflammatory, antipyretic, and analgesic. Acetylsalicylic acid (ASA) acts by inhibition of the formation of prostaglandins, uncoupling oxidative phosphorylation, and inhibiting other chemical mediators of inflammation and the local release of bradykinin. ASA also inhibits platelet aggregation by selectively favoring prostacyclin (PGI_2) production. ASA is used as an antipyretic in horses and cattle and for minor pain relief, particularly musculoskeletal. Less than the maximum dose in cattle is likely to be subtherapeutic. There are currently no FDA-approved large animal aspirin boluses.

ADVERSE AND COMMON SIDE EFFECTS: ASA can cause, or exacerbate, gastric ulceration, which may be due to inhibition of prostaglandins. At toxic doses ASA can cause combined respiratory and metabolic acidosis.

DRUG INTERACTIONS: ASA competes for protein-binding sites with drugs such as penicillin, thiopental, and phenytoin.

SUPPLIED AS: VETERINARY PRODUCTS
As bolus containing 15.5 or 15.6 g/bolus (240 gr)
Tablets containing 3.9 g (60 gr)
Oral granules containing 14.5 g/20 g (Asen) or 5 g/15 g (Bexprin)

OTHER USES
Horses
UVEITIS
ASA is useful as an anti-inflammatory agent for chronic, recurrent uveitis at 25 mg/kg bid; PO for 3 to 5 days, then 30 mg/kg once daily; PO for as long as needed.

ATRACURIUM

INDICATIONS: Atracurium (Tracrium♣★) is a neuromuscular blocking agent used as an adjunct for surgical anesthesia. It is recommended for chemical restraint during mechanical ventilation in neonatal intensive care of foals, but its high cost may preclude such use.

ADVERSE AND COMMON SIDE EFFECTS: Atracurium should only be used in settings with facilities for assisted ventilation, and by highly trained personnel. Atracurium has no analgesic properties. If given rapidly, the drug can induce urticaria in humans by causing histamine release.

DRUG INTERACTIONS: Edrophonium or neostigmine can be used to reverse and decrease the duration of neuromuscular blockade. Inhalation anesthetics act synergistically with atracurium, allowing decreased doses of atracurium. Concomitant use of aminoglycosides, tetracyclines, polymixins, and colistin will potentiate neuromuscular blockade by atracurium.

SUPPLIED AS: HUMAN PRODUCT
For injection containing 10 mg/mL

ATROPINE

INDICATIONS: Atropine (Atropine Sulfate Injectable♣, Atropine Sulphate Injection★, Atropine Sulphate ♣★, and others) is an alkaloid of belladonna, classified as an anticholinergic, antispasmodic, and mydriatic. Atropine inhibits structures innervated by the postganglionic parasympathetic nervous system. It decreases spasms of hyperperistalsis of diarrhea and inhibits salivary and respiratory secretions. Atropine blocks vagal-induced bradycardia and bronchospasm induced by parasympathetic stimulation as found in organophosphate poisoning. It is used as a mydriatic in uveitis and for fundoscopic examination. Atropine is also used as an antidote in organophosphate poisoning. Atropine is not used frequently as a preanesthetic in horses because they only infrequently develop bradycardia and do not salivate excessively.

ADVERSE AND COMMON SIDE EFFECTS: Atropine should be used with caution in horses as it can cause potentially fatal intestinal ileus, even if applied topically to the conjunctiva. Excessive doses of atropine can cause central nervous system stimulation and excitement.

DRUG INTERACTIONS: None applicable in large animals.

SUPPLIED AS: VETERINARY PRODUCT
For injection containing 0.5, 0.54, and 15 mg/mL

AUROTHIOGLUCOSE

INDICATIONS: Aurothioglucose (Solganal♣★) is a gold compound that is used in animals to treat pemphigus foliaceus. It is used in humans for the treatment of rheumatoid arthritis. Although its anti-inflammatory mechanism of action is not well understood, it appears to decrease synovial inflammation and retard cartilage and bone destruction. It has been used experimentally, with some success, in treatment of pemphigus foliaceus in horses that is poorly or nonresponsive to glucocorticoid therapy. It has also been effective in causing remission of signs of pemphigus foliaceus in a goat.

ADVERSE AND COMMON SIDE EFFECTS: Effects that may occur immediately after injection include anaphylaxis, syncope, bradycardia, difficulty swallowing or breathing, and angioneurotic edema. It should be used with caution in patients with skin rash, hypersensitivity to other medications, or hepatic or renal disease, if there is evidence of cardiovascular compromise. Overdose through increasing the dose too rapidly will result in signs of renal damage, including hematuria, proteinuria, and hematologic effects, including thrombocytopenia and granulocytopenia. Although these precautions are specified for humans, it is reasonable to take similar precautions when using this drug in animals. For large doses it is advisable to divide the injections into several injection sites.

DRUG INTERACTIONS: Aurothioglucose should not be used with penicillamine or antimalarials.

SUPPLIED AS: HUMAN PRODUCT
Suspension for injection containing 50 mg/mL in 10-mL multidose vials

AZAPERONE

INDICATIONS: Azaperone (Stresnil♣★) is a potent sedative/tranquilizer for use in pigs. It has a rapid onset of action of approximately 5 to 10 minutes following IM injection, with a peak effect after 15 to 30 minutes and a duration of action from 1 to 6 hours. During this time the animal remains conscious but indifferent to the environment. Its main uses are to reduce aggression and fighting during weaning and mixing of pigs. Injections should be deep IM behind the neck or in the rump, after which the animals should not be disturbed for 20 minutes.

ADVERSE AND COMMON SIDE EFFECTS: It is not to be used for castration because the period of hemorrhaging may be extended. The effects on breeding stock have not been determined. Do not inject the drug SC.

DRUG INTERACTIONS: None listed.

SUPPLIED AS: VETERINARY PRODUCT
For injection containing 40 mg/mL, in 50-mL vial

BACITRACIN, NEOMYCIN, POLYMIXIN B SULFATE

INDICATIONS: Bacitracin zinc, neomycin, polymixin B sulfate combinations (BNP Ointment♣, Mycitracin★, Neobacimyx★, Trioptic-P★, Triple Antibiotic Ointment★, Vetropolycin★) is a petroleum-based antibiotic ointment for the broad-spectrum treatment of superficial bacterial infections of the conjunctiva and cornea. This antibiotic combination should not be relied on as the sole therapy for deep ocular infections. The combination product is also available with hydrocortisone (BNP-H Ointment♣, Neobacimyx-H★, Trioptic-S★, Vetropolycin-HC♣). Polymixin B alone has been used by some clinicians for treatment of endotoxemia of coliform mastitis in cattle and bacitracin for acute colitis in horses. Neither of these clinical uses have been evaluated by clinical trials for safety or efficacy.

ADVERSE AND COMMON SIDE EFFECTS: Sensitivity to this combination is rare but may manifest as itching, burning, or inflammation at the site of medication.

DRUG INTERACTIONS: None listed.

SUPPLIED AS: VETERINARY PRODUCTS
Ointment; each gram contains 400 or 500 U bacitracin, 3.5 mg neomycin, and 5,000 U polymixin B sulfate or 10,000 U polymixin B sulfate [Trioptic-P], hydrocortisone at 1% if present.
Feed additive of bacitracin containing 30 g/454 g [Moorman's BMD 30] and 110 mg/kg in soya meal base [Rhone Poulenc]

OTHER USES
POLYMIXIN B
Cattle

ENDOTOXEMIA
Acute coliform mastitis; 6000 U/kg in 10 mL 0.9% saline; IV over 1 minute

BACITRACIN
Horses

ACUTE DIARRHEA
Bacitracin alone has been used experimentally with some success to treat acute diarrhea. Doses used were 22 mg/kg bid; PO for 2 days followed by 22 mg/kg daily; PO for 3 days.

BAL (DIMERCAPROL)

INDICATIONS: BAL or dimercaprol [British Anti-Lewisite] (BAL: Dimercaprol in Oil♦★) is a chelator used to treat toxicity due to arsenic or other heavy metals.

ADVERSE AND COMMON SIDE EFFECTS: Administration of dimercaprol causes a rise in systolic and diastolic arterial blood pressure accompanied by tachycardia. Conjunctivitis, blepharospasm, lacrimation, rhinorrhea, salivation, and abdominal pain have been noted in people receiving dimercaprol. Sterile abscesses at the site of injection occasionally occur. A transient reduction of polymorphonuclear leukocytes may also be observed. The drug is contraindicated in cases of hepatic insufficiency, except when the result of arsenic toxicity.

DRUG INTERACTIONS: Do not administer dimercaprol within 24 hours of iron or selenium compounds. Dimercaprol can form toxic complexes with iron and selenium.

SUPPLIED AS: HUMAN PRODUCT
For IM injection containing 100 mg/mL

BECLOMETHASONE

INDICATIONS: Beclomethasone (Beclovent♦★) is a potent anti-inflammatory corticosteroid with strong topical and weak systemic activity. When administered by aerosol it has direct anti-inflammatory action on the bronchial mucosa. Because at therapeutic doses for aerosol therapy there is little systemic effect, beclomethasone can replace oral steroid administration for airway inflammation and eliminate untoward systemic side effects. Aerosol beclomethasone has been effective in treating horses for recurrent airway obstruction (heaves or chronic obstructive pulmonary disease).

ADVERSE AND COMMON SIDE EFFECTS: As with all inhalation therapy, a potential exists for paradoxic bronchospasm. In humans with long-term use overgrowth of yeast (*Candida* spp) has occurred.

DRUG INTERACTIONS: None listed.

SUPPLIED AS: HUMAN PRODUCT
For aerosol administration containing 250 µg in a metered dose container

BETAMETHASONE

INDICATIONS: Betamethasone (Betasone♦★, Betavet Soluspan★, B-S-P★, Celestone Soluspan♦★, Cel-U-Jec★, Celestone Phosphate★, Selectoject★) is a potent glucocorticoid used for treating nonseptic inflammatory joint disease in horses and cattle. Its action is prolonged and injection can be repeated at 3-week intervals if clinical signs persist.

ADVERSE AND COMMON SIDE EFFECTS: Betamethasone is not to be used in animals with acute or chronic bacterial infections unless therapeutic doses of antibacterial agents are also used. Betamethasone should not be used in pregnant cattle. See **GLUCOCORTICOID AGENTS** for further information on adverse effects and drug interactions.

SUPPLIED AS: VETERINARY PRODUCTS
For injection containing 12 mg/mL betamethasone acetate with 3.9 mg/mL betamethasone sodium phosphate [Betavet Soluspan], or 5 mg/mL betamethasone diproprionate and 2 mg/mL betamethasone sodium phosphate [Betasone]

HUMAN PRODUCT
For injection containing 3 mg/mL betamethasone acetate with 3 mg/mL betamethasone sodium phosphate

BETHANECHOL

INDICATIONS: Bethanechol (Duvoid♣★, Bethanechol Chloride♣★, Myotonachol♣★, Urabeth★, Urecholine♣★) is a synthetic acetylcholine derivative used to stimulate gastrointestinal motility in postoperative gastrointestinal ileus and to stimulate urinary bladder contraction. Bethanechol has also been used to enhance gastric emptying and minimize gastroesophageal reflux for foals with gastric ulceration. Its use has also been advocated for stimulation of detrusor muscle activity to aid in bladder emptying in horses with urinary incontinence. Because the treatment produces varying results, clinicians should start with the lowest dose.

ADVERSE AND COMMON SIDE EFFECTS: The drug should not be administered by the IM or IV routes because the incidence of serious toxic side effects, such as bronchoconstriction, colic, and hypotension, is greatly increased. Use of bethanecol in cases of obstruction of the urinary tract or intestinal tract is not advised.

DRUG INTERACTIONS: Do not administer bethanechol with other cholinergic or anticholinesterase agents (e.g., neostigmine) because of additive effects and toxicity. Administration with ganglionic blocking agents will produce a critical fall in blood pressure. Atropine, epinephrine, quinidine, and procainamide antagonize the effects of bethanechol.

SUPPLIED AS: HUMAN PRODUCTS
For injection containing 5 mg/mL
Tablets containing 10, 25, and 50 mg

OTHER USES
Horses

Bethanecol has been used to treat urospermia in stallions, but without much success.

BISMUTH SUBSALICYLATE

INDICATIONS: Bismuth subsalicylate (Pepto-Bismol♥★, Bismo-Kote★, Bismu-Kote★, Bismusal Suspension★, Gastro-Cote★, PMS-Bismuth Subsalicylate Liquid♣) is a demulcent and gut protectant. Bismuth subsalicylate is reported to be a gut protectant, but its efficacy in this regard is questionable.

ADVERSE AND COMMON SIDE EFFECTS: Chronic use of bismuth salts can cause encephalopathy and osteodystrophy.

DRUG INTERACTIONS: None listed.

SUPPLIED AS: VETERINARY PRODUCT
Oral liquid containing 17.5 mg/mL bismuth subsalicylate

HUMAN PRODUCTS
Liquid containing 17.47 mg/mL bismuth subsalicylate
Liquid containing 35 mg/mL bismuth subsalicylate

BOLDENONE UNDECYLENATE

INDICATIONS: Boldenone undecylenate (Equipoise♥★) is a long-acting anabolic agent for horses used for treating debilitated animals and improving appetite, weight gain, and physical condition. Boldenone undecylenate is a steroid ester with marked anabolic properties and only small amounts of androgenic properties. The drug is not a substitute for a balanced diet.

ADVERSE AND COMMON SIDE EFFECTS: Treatment may result in undesirable androgenic effects (masculinization, behavioral change), particularly in the case of overdose. Boldenone is not to be used in immature colts and fillies, stallions, pregnant mares, or brood mares in the breeding season.

DRUG INTERACTIONS: None listed.

SUPPLIED AS: VETERINARY PRODUCT
For injection containing 25 and 50 mg/mL

BOTULINUM ANTITOXIN

INDICATIONS: Botulinum antitoxin [polyvalent] is used for the early treatment of clinical cases of botulism in foals and horses. Once the toxin has entered the synaptic terminals and clinical signs are present, the antitoxin is ineffective; it will, however, neutralize toxin not yet taken up at the nerve terminal.

ADVERSE AND COMMON SIDE EFFECTS: None listed.

DRUG INTERACTIONS: None indicated.

SUPPLIED AS: VETERINARY PRODUCT
For injection containing antiserum 100 to 150 IU/mL
Sources: (a) New Bolton Center, Pennsylvania 1-610-444-5800 ext 2321; (b) Veterinary Dynamics, California 1-800-654-9743

BUPIVICAINE HYDROCHLORIDE

INDICATIONS: Bupivicaine hydrochloride (Marcaine♥★, Sensorcaine♥★) is a long-acting local anesthetic that is two to four times more potent than lidocaine and is used for local nerve blocks and epidural anesthesia. It has been used for prolonged regional analgesia in horses with diseases such as laminitis and experimentally in sheep for epidural anesthesia.

ADVERSE AND COMMON SIDE EFFECTS: As for most local anesthetics, the central nervous system (CNS) may be stimulated, producing restlessness and tremor that may proceed to clonic convulsions. Certain local anesthetics may also cause sedation or behavioral changes. At high levels, which affect the CNS, the cardiovascular system is also affected by decreasing electrical excitability, conduction rate, and force of contraction of the myocardium. Hypersensitivity to local anesthetics can occur but is rare. The 0.75% solution should not be used for obstetric anesthesia. Bupivicaine is more cardiotoxic than lidocaine and the toxicity seems to be aggravated by hypoxemia and acidemia. Hepatic disease may increase the potential for toxicity of local anesthetics.

DRUG INTERACTIONS: The addition of epinephrine to local anesthetics greatly prolongs and intensifies their action.

SUPPLIED AS: HUMAN PRODUCT
For injection containing 0.25%, 0.5%, and 0.75% with or without epinephrine

BUTORPHANOL TARTRATE

INDICATIONS: Butorphanol Tartrate (Torbugesic♥★, Torbutrol♥★) is a centrally-acting narcotic agonist-antagonist analgesic with potent antitussive properties. Butorphanol has a ceiling effect above which dose (0.11 mg/kg) there is no increase in analgesia or side effects. It is used in horses for the relief of abdominal pain of colic. Analgesia lasts approximately 4 hours. Butorphanol is also used in combination with sedatives (xylazine 0.6 mg/kg; IV or acepromazine 0.04 mg/kg; IV with butorphanol 0.03 mg/kg; IV) for standing chemical restraint in horses and as an adjunct for sedation in cattle. Unlike classical narcotic agonists, butorphanol does not cause histamine release. Studies of milk residues in dairy cattle after a single IV injection of 0.045 mg/kg showed that trace quantities may be detected up to 36 hours after the injection.

ADVERSE AND COMMON SIDE EFFECTS: Butorphanol should be used with caution with other sedative or analgesic agents because the effects are likely additive. Because there are no well-controlled studies in breeding horses, weanlings, and foals, butorphanol should be used with discretion in these animals. There may be variable degrees of response to the same dose between individual animals and differing breeds of horses. Ataxia after administration is usually mild and temporary, lasting 3 to 10 minutes. Rapid IV injection of high doses (20 times recommended dose) can result in a short period of inability to stand, muscle fasciculations, or a brief convulsive seizure. Administration of 10 times the recommended dose may cause muscle fasciculations about the head and neck, ataxia, salivation, and nystagmus. Repeat administration at that dose may result in constipation. Butorphanol is a controlled substance, but it is not included in the narcotics schedule.

DRUG INTERACTIONS: Opioids may prolong or worsen antibiotic-induced colitis.

SUPPLIED AS: VETERINARY PRODUCTS
For injection containing 0.5 mg/mL and 10.0 mg/mL
Tablets containing 1, 5, and 10 mg

OTHER USES
Butorphanol has potent antitussive properties but is seldom indicated for such use in large animals.

CALCIUM BOROGLUGONATE

INDICATIONS: Calcium borogluconate (Cal Aqua 25.75%✤, Cal-Nate 23% Solution✤, Cal-Nate 1069★, Cal-MPK 1234★, Cal-MP 1700★, Calciphos★, Calcium 23% Solution★, Calcium Gluconate✤★, Calcium Borogluconate✤, Calcium Borogluconate 23%✤, Calcium Gluconate 23%✤, Cal-Glu-Sol✤, Cal Mag-K✤, Cal Mag D Solution #2✤, Cal Mag Phos✤, Mag Cal✤, Cal Plus✤, Calcium Magnesium Dextrose✤, Maglucal Plus✤, Cal-Dextro Solution No 2✤, Cal-

Dextro♣★, Norcalciphos♣★, Calphos♣, Supercal♣, and others) is used for the treatment of hypocalcemia in cattle, sheep, and horses. Products containing magnesium are also indicated for treatment of hypomagnesemic tetany (grass tetany) and transport tetany. Certain of the calcium products also contain phosphorus or potassium for treatment of related deficiencies or diseases complicated by hypokalemia. During administration there is usually a positive inotropic effect. IV atropine has been used to abolish cardiac arrhythmias associated with calcium administration.

ADVERSE AND COMMON SIDE EFFECTS: IV administration should be slow to prevent heart block. Administration should be stopped if severe arrhythmias or bradycardia occur. Animals with hypocalcemia and endotoxemia, such as cows with acute coliform mastitis, are especially prone to cardiac arrhythmias caused by IV calcium therapy.

DRUG INTERACTIONS: Magnesium antagonizes the cardioexcitatory effects of calcium. Calcium borogluconate is incompatible if mixed with cephalothin, prednisolone phosphate, tetracyclines, sodium bicarbonate, phenylbutazone, and sulfonamides.

SUPPLIED AS: VETERINARY PRODUCTS
For injection containing a 23% solution (W/V) of calcium borogluconate equivalent to 19.78 mg/mL calcium or 25.75% equivalent to 21.42 mg/mL calcium; alone or combined with dextrose, magnesium, phosphorus, and/or potassium compounds (see individual products)

CALCIUM CHLORIDE

INDICATIONS: Calcium chloride♣★ in solution is used as one form of calcium replacement therapy for treatment of hypocalcemic tetany in mares. The salt is usually given in a 10% solution. A moderate fall in blood pressure due to peripheral vasodilation may occur with administration.

ADVERSE AND COMMON SIDE EFFECTS: Calcium chloride should not be injected into tissues. It is irritating to the gastrointestinal tract if given orally.

DRUG INTERACTIONS: Calcium chloride is incompatible if mixed before administration with cephalothin, chlorpheniramine, hydrocortisone, prednisolone phosphate, kanamycin sulfate, tetracyclines, or sodium bicarbonate.

SUPPLIED AS: HUMAN PRODUCT
For injection containing 100 mg/mL

CALCIUM DISODIUM EDETATE

INDICATIONS: Calcium disodium edetate (CaNa$_2$EDTA) (Leadidate✚, Calcium Disodium Versenate✚★) is a chelating agent used to treat lead poisoning in horses and cattle. It removes free lead from bone and also from blood and soft tissues by forming lead chelate that is excreted by the kidneys.

ADVERSE AND COMMON SIDE EFFECTS: Administer CaNa$_2$EDTA slowly to prevent tachycardia, dyspnea, and body tremors. Renal toxicity can occur. Adequate hydration should be ensured when using EDTA. Dilution in D$_5$W or 0.9% saline will reduce the potential for thrombophlebitis.

DRUG INTERACTIONS: Avoid administering the drug simultaneously with barbiturates and sulfonamides.

SUPPLIED AS: VETERINARY PRODUCT
For injection containing a 6.6% solution

HUMAN PRODUCT
For injection containing 200 mg/mL

CAPTAN

INDICATIONS: Captan (Orthocide✚★, Captan 10✚) is a plant fungicide available at garden supply centers or nurseries that is commonly used, albeit extralabel, to treat dermatophytosis (ringworm) in horses and cattle.

ADVERSE AND COMMON SIDE EFFECTS: Captan can cause skin sensitization in some horses.

DRUG INTERACTIONS: None listed.

SUPPLIED AS: GARDEN SUPPLY OUTLETS
Powder containing 50% captan

CARBACHOL

INDICATIONS: Carbachol (carbamylcholine chloride) (Carbachol✚★) is an acetylcholine derivative that produces similar physiologic effects to acetylcholine but is more stable in the body. Carbachol is used to treat colic in horses caused by impactions, rumen atony and impaction in cattle, and to stimulate uterine contractions for obstetric procedures and treatment of retained placenta.

ADVERSE AND COMMON SIDE EFFECTS: IV or IM injection may increase the risk of untoward effects. Carbachol may produce bronchoconstriction and hypotension. Profuse sweating may occur in the horse. It is contraindicated in old or cachectic animals and pregnant animals, in mechanical obstruction of the intestinal tract, and in respiratory and cardiac disease. Carbachol is a very potent drug. Excessive peristaltic movements in animals with severe intestinal obstruction can cause rupture or intussusception. High doses in cattle (> 4 mg/454 kg) may actually inhibit ruminoreticular activity.

DRUG INTERACTIONS: The prior administration of oils and saline cathartics is recommended if the drug is used for equine colic due to impaction or intestinal atony. Atropine is antidotal.

SUPPLIED AS: HUMAN PRODUCTS
For injection containing 0.25 mg/mL
Ophthalmic drops containing 0.75%, 1.5%, 2.25%, or 3% carbachol [Isopto Carbachol]
Ophthalmic injection for intraocular use only 0.01% [Miostat]

OTHER USES
OPHTHALMIC
Carbachol is used for its brief miotic effects in cataract extractions and other anterior chamber procedures. It will also reduce intraocular pressure in animals that have become resistant to pilocarpine or physostigmine.

CARBARYL

INDICATIONS: Carbaryl (Dusting Powder♣, Equi-Shield Fly Repellent Spray★, Sevin♣, and other combination products) is a moderate, reversible carbamate cholinesterase inhibitor. It is used to control external parasites of horses and cattle.

ADVERSE AND COMMON SIDE EFFECTS: Toxic effects are unlikely but may include bronchoconstriction, colic, salivation, and diarrhea. DO NOT apply before milking; only immediately after milking. Wash udder thoroughly before milking.

DRUG INTERACTIONS: Atropine is antidotal.

SUPPLIED AS: VETERINARY PRODUCT
Powder or spray of varying concentrations (see individual products)

CARBENICILLIN

INDICATIONS: Carbenicillin (Geocillin★) is a synthetic penicillin with a broad range of antibacterial activity particularly for infections caused by *Pseudomonas aeruginosa, Proteus,* and certain strains of *Escherichia coli,* but is ineffective against most strains of *Staphylococcus aureus.* Carbenicillin does not resist penicillinase and must be administered parenterally. Carbenicillin may also be used subconjunctivally for corneal ulcers infected with *Pseudomonas* spp.

ADVERSE AND COMMON SIDE EFFECTS: Carbenicillin appears to be similar to other penicillins regarding adverse effects, especially hypersensitivity. Additionally, hypokalemia and platelet-associated bleeding problems have been reported.

DRUG INTERACTIONS: None listed.

SUPPLIED AS: HUMAN PRODUCT
Tablets containing 382 mg

CEPHALOSPORINS

INDICATIONS: Cephalosporins (Cefa-Dri♥★, Cefa-Lak♥★, Cefa-Tabs♥★, Cefa-Drops♥★, Excenel♥, Naxcel★, and many human preparations) are antibiotics similar to penicillin in that their structure includes a β-lactam ring and they inhibit bacterial cell wall synthesis similarly to the penicillins. Although widely used, cephalosporins tend to be expensive and should be reserved for diseases that require alternatives to penicillins. Cephalosporins are divided into first-, second-, and third-generation drugs. First-generation cephalosporins (cephalothin, cephapirin, cefazolin, cephalexin, cefadroxil) have good activity against gram-positive bacteria and modest activity against gram-negative bacteria. Second-generation cephalosporins (cefamandole, cefoxitin, cefaclor, cefuroxime axetil, cefonicid) have somewhat increased activity against gram-negative organisms, but less than third-generation cephalosporins (cefotaxime, moxalactam, ceftazidime, ceftizoxime, ceftiofur, ceftriaxone, cefoperazone), which are more active against the Enterobacteriaceae, including β-lactamase–producing strains. However, third-generation cephalosporins are generally less active against gram-positive bacteria than first-generation agents. Various diseases have specific cephalosporins as drugs of choice, e.g., cephalothin for β-lactamase–producing staphylococcal infections, cefoxitin for treatment of aerobic and mixed aerobic-anaerobic infections such as lung abscesses, and cefotaxime for gram-negative meningitis. Absorption, body distribution, and half-lives vary greatly among the cephalosporins. Large animal veterinary products are used for treatment of mastitis (Cefa-Lak♥★, Today★), dry treatment of the mammary gland (Cefa-Dri♥★, Tomorrow★), and for bacterial pneumonia (Excenel 0, Naxel★) in cattle. Presently, ceftiofur is the only parenteral cephalosporin approved for use in cattle and horses. Although effective against many gram-negative bacteria, ceftiofur has no activity against *Pseudomonas* spp and has limited activity against gram-positive and anaerobic bacteria. Ceftiofur is approved for treatment of adult horses with respiratory disease caused by *Streptococcus zooepidemicus*. However, its expense does not warrant its use in such penicillin-responsive diseases.

Cefazolin has been used as a regional IV injection to increase therapeutic levels in synovial fluid. The dose was 250 mg in mature cattle. This may provide an alternate means to systemic injection to provide adequate concentrations in a localized area, with therapeutic levels persisting for approximately 4 hours if the tourniquet is left in place for 2 hours.

(Refer to the individual product for further information.)

ADVERSE AND COMMON SIDE EFFECTS: Hypersensitivity reactions similar to those caused by penicillins are the most common side effects. Because of the structural similarity of cephalosporins and penicillins, allergic reaction to one increases the risk of a similar reaction to the other. Certain cephalosporins, such as cephalothin and cephaloridine, can be nephrotoxic at high doses.

DRUG INTERACTIONS: Concurrent use with aminoglycosides may potentiate aminoglycoside-induced nephrotoxicity. Cephalosporin nephrotoxicity may be increased with concurrent use of furosemide or ethacrynic acid. Probenecid slows tubular secretion of most cephalosporins. Recent evidence shows in vitro antagonism between cephalosporins and chloramphenicol.

SUPPLIED AS: VETERINARY PRODUCTS
Intramammary products containing 300 mg cephapirin benzathine [Cefa-Dri♣★, Tomorrow★] or 200 mg cephapirin sodium [Cefa-Lak♣★, Today★]
For injection containing 50 mg/mL ceftiofur
Tablets (cefadroxil) containing 50, 100, and 200 mg;1 g
Drops (cefadroxil) containing 50 mg/mL

CHARCOAL, ACTIVATED

INDICATIONS: Activated charcoal (Activated Charcoal Liquid★, Actidote★, Acta-Char★, Acta-Char Liquid★, Charcodote♣★, Charcodote Aqueous♣★, Charcodote TFS♣★, Charcocaps★, Liqui-Char★, SuperChar★, Toxiban★) is an adsorbent for use in toxicities caused by ingested poisons, such as organophosphates. Activated charcoal may also adsorb free endotoxin in the lumen of the intestinal tract in salmonellosis. Activated charcoal is neither metabolized nor absorbed by the intestine.

ADVERSE AND COMMON SIDE EFFECTS: None listed.

DRUG INTERACTIONS: None listed.

SUPPLIED AS: VETERINARY PRODUCTS
Granules containing 47.5 charcoal and 10.0 g kaolin per 100 g
Suspension containing 10.4% charcoal and 6.25% kaolin
Suspension containing 10.4% charcoal and 6.25% kaolin and 10% sorbitol

HUMAN PRODUCTS
Suspension containing 50 g/250 mL, 30 g/240 mL, 30 g/120 mL, and others
Suspension (micronized) containing 200 mg/mL
Capsules containing 260 mg
Tablets containing 325 mg

CHLORAL HYDRATE

INDICATIONS: Chloral hydrate (Noctec✦★, Novo-Chlorhydrate✦) was one of the first central nervous system depressants to be used in veterinary surgery. Although still a valuable hypnotic for use in large animals, it is not a satisfactory anesthetic when used alone because it has low pain-relieving powers. Anesthetic doses severely depress the respiratory and vasomotor centers, approaching the LD_{50} for the drug. It is best used for its hypnotic effect in combination with local anesthetics, but the wide availability of potent tranquilizing agents has reduced its use in North America. There appears to be a latent period of action in which further depression occurs 10 to 15 minutes after injection of the drug.

ADVERSE AND COMMON SIDE EFFECTS: Perivascular injection can cause severe pain, tissue swelling, and destruction of the jugular vein and sloughing of adjacent tissues. Chloral hydrate is irritating to the stomach, especially when empty.

DRUG INTERACTIONS: Chloral hydrate can be used in combination with magnesium sulfate and pentobarbital as a sedative or anesthetic agent for large animals.

SUPPLIED AS: HUMAN PRODUCTS
Capsules containing 500 mg
Syrup containing 250 mg or 500 mg/5 mL
Rectal suppositories containing 325, 500, or 650 mg

OTHER USES
Cattle

Chloral hydrate can also be used in cattle to depress nervous excitement that may accompany acetonemia. Given orally it increases the breakdown of starch in the rumen and influences rumen production of propionate; hence, it may also help correct the metabolic disturbance in ketosis.

CHLORAMPHENICOL

INDICATIONS: Chloramphenicol (Amphicol Film Coated Tablets★, Azramycine S125♣, Azramycine S250♣, Bemachol★, Chlor 125 Palm♣, Chlor Palm 250♣, Chlor Tablets♣, Choralean Drops♣, Chloramphenicol 1%♣★, Chlorasone★, Chlorbiotic★, Chloricol♣★, Karomycin Palmitate 125♣, Karomycin Palmitate 250♣, Medichol★, Vedichol★, Viceton★, and others) is a broad-spectrum antibiotic with activity against gram-positive and gram-negative bacteria, as well as rickettsia and the psittacosis-lymphogranuloma group. It diffuses readily into all body cavities. Highest concentrations are found in the liver and kidney. The lungs, heart, spleen, and skeletal muscle contain concentrations similar to that of blood. Chloramphenicol attains approximately 75% of blood levels in milk, pleural and ascitic fluid, and the placenta. It also diffuses readily into the cerebrospinal fluid, reaching 50% of serum levels within 3 to 4 hours of administration. Its use in bacterial meningitis has been seriously questioned because bactericidal drugs are considered necessary for combating bacterial infections of the central nervous system. Chloramphenicol palmitate is administered orally and the succinate form parenterally. Ophthalmic preparations are available for bacterial infections of the eyes. Chloramphenicol is used in horses with mixed bacterial infections, such as can occur in pleuritis. Its short half-life in horses limits its practical use. Any product containing chloramphenicol must not be used in food-producing animals.

ADVERSE AND COMMON SIDE EFFECTS: Chloramphenicol is not to be administered to breeding animals, even though there were no reported associated problems during prior widespread use in food animals. The drug is prohibited from use in food-producing animals because of the potential for induction of fatal aplastic anemia and granulocytopenia that may occur in humans consuming meat products containing the drug. Prolonged use in animals may produce hematologic disturbances. Allergic reactions are infrequently observed.

DRUG INTERACTIONS: Chloramphenicol inhibits biotransformation of phenytoin and dicumarol and may lower prothrombin levels. It also prolongs metabolism of local anesthetics. Chloramphenicol should not be administered in conjunction with or within 2 hours of pentobarbital anesthesia because it prolongs recovery time. Chloramphenicol antagonizes the actions of penicillins and cephalosporins on bacteria in vitro but is synergistic with tetracyclines. Chloramphenicol may delay response to iron preparations.

SUPPLIED AS: VETERINARY PRODUCTS
Tablets containing 50, 100, 250, and 500 mg; 1 and 2.5 g
Capsules containing 100, 250, and 500 mg
Suspension containing 25, 50, 125, and 250 mg/mL
Ophthalmic preparations in solution containing 4 mg/mL
Ointment containing 10 mg/g

HUMAN PRODUCTS
Capsules containing 250 mg
Suspension containing 50 mg/mL (palmitate)
For injection containing 1 g (sodium succinate)

CHLORHEXIDINE

INDICATIONS: Chlorhexidine is a topical antiseptic used for surgical scrubs and for teat washing and dips in cattle (Bou-Matic Super
Udder Wash♣, Chlorasan★, Della-Prep♣, Dihexamin Udder Wash♣,
Hibitane Udder Wash♣, Monarch Prep Udder Wash♣, Nolvasan★,
Sani-Wash♣, Virosan Solution★, and many others). Used as a teat
dip it controls and prevents the spread of mastitis-causing organisms. It is also included in ointment (Chlorasan Antiseptic Oint-
ment★, Hibitane Veterinary Ointment♣), in a powder for treatment
of eye and wound infections (Eye and Wound Powder♣), and to dis-
infect inanimate objects to prevent the spread of infectious disease in
the veterinary clinic (ChlorHex Surgical Scrub★, Hibitane Disinfec-
tant♣). Chlorhexidine is rapidly bactericidal to both gram-positive
and most gram-negative bacilli. It is not virucidal. Chlorhexidine is
effective in the presence of soaps, blood, and pus, although activity
may be reduced. Chlorhexidine has a residual effect with up to 26%
of the active ingredient remaining on the skin after 29 hours.

ADVERSE AND COMMON SIDE EFFECTS: Under ordinary use,
chlorhexidine causes no adverse effects, but prolonged repetitive use
may result in contact dermatitis and photosensitivity.

DRUG INTERACTIONS: Alcohols enhance the efficacy of chlorhexidine.

SUPPLIED AS: VETERINARY AND HUMAN PRODUCTS
See individual product.

OTHER USES
Cattle
Chlorhexidine has been used for an udder infusion to permanently
dry off chronic mastitic quarters in dairy cattle.
Dose: 60 mL chlorhexidine diacetate is infused into quarter after
milking, milked out for subsequent milking, then an additional
60 mL is infused and the quarter is left unmilked.

CHLORPROMAZINE

INDICATIONS: Chlorpromazine (Apo-Chlorpromazine♣, Chlor-prom♣, Chlorpromanyl♣, Largactil♣★, Novo-Chlorpromazine♣★, Ormazine★, Thorazine★) is a phenothiazine used for sedation and tranquilization in large animals but has produced undesirable effects in horses such that it is not advocated for general use in equine practice. In fact, its use alone in horses is contraindicated. It is indicated for treatment of amphetamine toxicosis and has been considered by some as the neuroleptic drug of choice in cattle as a preanesthetic. Clinical effects are prominent for 4 to 5 hours but total effects may last 24 hours. Chlorpromazine is also indicated to treat clinical signs of tetanus in sheep and goats. Lack of a ready veterinary formulation and availability of other phenothiazines limits this drug's use in large animal practice.

ADVERSE AND COMMON SIDE EFFECTS: Tranquilization of dangerous animals with chlorpromazine may lead to a false sense of security. Painful procedures should be avoided because there is little analgesic effect. Horses may have episodes of violent excitement and incoordination following drug administration. An adequate blood volume and arterial blood pressure is necessary for the use of chlorpromazine because of its marked arterial hypotensive effects. Use in combination with epidural anesthesia is contraindicated because of potentiation of arterial hypotension. Teratogenic effects have been found in laboratory animals, but there are no reports of teratogenic effects in domestic animals.

DRUG INTERACTIONS: Toxicity of carbamates and organophosphates may be enhanced by administration of phenothiazines. Concurrent use is contraindicated. Chlorpromazine potentiates the toxicity of the herbicide paraquat.

SUPPLIED AS: HUMAN PRODUCTS
Capsules containing 30, 75, and 150 mg
Tablets containing 10, 25, 50, 100, and 200 mg
Oral liquid containing 5 or 20 mg/mL
For injection containing 25 mg/mL
Suppositories containing 25 and 100 mg

CHORIONIC GONADOTROPHIN

INDICATIONS: Chorionic gonadotrophin [human chorionic gonadotrophin, HCG] (A.P.L.♣, Chorionad♣, Chorionic Gonado-tropin★, Chorulon♣★, Follutein★, Progon 10,000♣) is a gonadal-stimulating hormone obtained from the urine of pregnant women. It is capable of supplementing or substituting for luteinizing hormone secreted by the anterior pituitary gland to promote follicle maturation and ovulation, and for the formation of the corpus luteum. In the male, chorionic gonadotrophin stimulates the interstitial cells to produce testosterone. It is used for the treatment of cystic ovaries, nymphomania, impotence, and hypogenitalism due to pituitary hypofunction, and to hasten ovulation, particularly in the mare. IV administration is satisfactory for a prompt effect, such as ovulation, but the IM route is more desirable when a prolonged effect such as Leydig cell stimulation is desired. For ovarian stimulation, other products (e.g., PMSG) are more effective.

ADVERSE AND COMMON SIDE EFFECTS: Chorionic gonadotrophin is a foreign protein and can cause anaphylaxis when administered parenterally. Continued administration may result in antihormone antibody production, and the product may become ineffective in such animals.

DRUG INTERACTIONS: None listed.

SUPPLIED AS: VETERINARY PRODUCT
For injection containing 5,000 and 10,000 U

OTHER USES
Horses and Cattle

Cryptorchidism may respond to early injections of chorionic gonadotrophin therapy, providing the inguinal canal is patent. Cryptorchid animals should not be used for breeding because cryptorchidism is a genetically influenced condition.

CIMETIDINE

INDICATIONS: Cimetidine (Apo-Cimetidine♣, Novo-Cimetidine♣, Nu-Cimet♣, Peptol♣, Tagamet♣★) is an H_2-receptor antagonist that reduces gastric acid secretion in a dose-dependent competitive manner, by blocking histamine-induced gastric acid secretion. The H_2 blockers are highly selective in action and virtually without effect on H_1 receptors. Although the H_2 receptors are widely distributed throughout the body, the extragastric receptors appear to be of only minor physiologic importance. The H_2 blockers also inhibit, at least partially, gastric secretion elicited by muscarinic agonists, or gastrin. Cimetidine is used in horses to treat gastric ulcers and as a preventive measure for foals considered in high-risk environments for the development of gastric ulcers, such as hospitalized neonates. Cimetidine has been used experimentally in ruminants but only affected abomasal pH at extreme doses and by direct instillation into the abomasum. Recently, cimetidine has been used with some success to treat melanomas in horses. The mechanism of action is thought to be the resulting augmentation of cell-mediated and humoral immunity by cimetidine's blocking of histamine-induced suppressor T-cell activation.

ADVERSE AND COMMON SIDE EFFECTS: Adverse reactions are low in incidence and relatively minor and include skin rash, diarrhea, constipation, and loss of libido. Rapid IV injection may cause profound bradycardia. Cimetidine may increase serum creatinine, through competition for sites of renal secretion.

DRUG INTERACTIONS: Cimetidine binds to androgen receptors and may cause sexual dysfunction such as impotence or gynecomastia. Because ranitidine lacks antiandrogenic activity, it can substitute for cimetidine. Concurrent use of cimetidine with warfarin, phenytoin, theophylline, phenobarbital, diazepam, propranolol, and imipramine may result in the accumulation of the latter drugs through impairment of hepatic microsomal metabolism.

SUPPLIED AS: HUMAN PRODUCTS
Tablets containing 200, 300, 400, 600, and 800 mg
Syrup containing 60 mg/mL
For injection containing 150 mg/mL

OTHER USES
Horses
MELANOMAS
2.5 mg/kg tid; PO for 4 to 12 months or as required by the persistence of the melanomas. Regrowth may occur once treatment is discontinued.

CISAPRIDE

INDICATIONS: Cisapride (Prepulsid♣, Propulsid★) is used to stimulate intestinal activity in horses. Cisapride exerts its effects primarily by stimulating the release of acetylcholine from myenteric plexus, possibly mediated by serotonin. It is 100 times more potent than metoclopramide but is free of dopamine receptor-blocking activity. Through this action it appears to stimulate intestinal activity along the entire intestinal tract, at least in humans and small animals.

Administered at 0.1 mg/kg IM, it decreased the incidence of postoperative ileus in cases of simple or strangulated obstructions of the small intestine. Bioavailability in horses is not known nor is its efficacy in promoting gastrointestinal activity when administered orally.

ADVERSE AND COMMON SIDE EFFECTS: Cisapride should not be used when there is gastrointestinal hemorrhage or blockage. The most frequent side effects are gastrointestinal in nature, with diarrhea and abdominal discomfort. For these effects the dose should be reduced. Central nervous system effects have also been reported in people, with reports of headache, sedation, and sleep disorders. Use in animals could result in similar adverse reactions.

DRUG INTERACTIONS: Concomitant administration of oral ketoconazole or itraconazole is contraindicated because these can inhibit metabolism of cisapride, resulting in an increase in cisapride concentration.

SUPPLIED AS: HUMAN PRODUCTS
Tablets containing 5, 10, and 20 mg
Suspension containing 1 mg/mL, 200 mL

CISPLATIN

INDICATIONS: Cisplatin (Platinol♣★) is an active cytotoxic drug with a narrow therapeutic range, and its usefulness as a systemic agent is limited by substantial neurotoxicity, nephrotoxicity, and toxicity to the gastrointestinal tract. It has been used intralesionally in horses with surface tumors, including equine sarcoids, squamous cell carcinomas, and squamous cell papillomas. A mean relapse-free interval of 21.6 months for sarcoids and 14 months for the carcinoma/papillomas has been reported. Treatment consisted of a total of four sessions at 2-week intervals. A dose of 0.97 mg/cm^3 of tumor tissue, for tumor volumes ranging from 10 to 20 cm^3 was used. Cisplatin was mixed with sterile, medical grade sesame oil, at 10 mg cisplatin to 1 mL water and 2 mL oil. Because the powdered cisplatin was discontinued, this regimen has been modified by using 1 mg/mL (no oil) injected intralesionally.

ADVERSE AND COMMON SIDE EFFECTS: Local toxicosis was reported to be minimal when used intralesionally in horses. In humans even a single systemic dose can cause nephrotoxicity and ototoxicity. Nausea and vomiting are also common side effects.

DRUG INTERACTIONS: Cisplatin should not be used with other platinum-containing compounds.

SUPPLIED AS: HUMAN PRODUCT
For injection containing 0.5 and 1 mg/mL

CLENBUTEROL

INDICATIONS: Clenbuterol (Ventipulmin♣) is a sympathomimetic amine with a high degree of selectivity for β_2 sites in the body, with minimal β_1 (cardiac) activity. Stimulation of β_2 sites causes relaxation of the smooth muscle of bronchi and the uterus. Clenbuterol is used for the treatment of respiratory disease in horses with bronchospasm. It has also been used in cattle to induce uterine relaxation in obstetric procedures, such as prolapsed uterus, correction of dystocias, and Cesarean section of cattle and sheep. Clenbuterol has been used successfully to delay lambing in term ewes for a 10-hour period overnight. No effect on perinatal mortality, clinical condition of the ewe, or postparturient behavior was observed.

Although recommended by some authors for facilitating obstetric manipulation in mares, strong abdominal contractions may negate any advantage gained through the effects of uterine relaxation.

ADVERSE AND COMMON SIDE EFFECTS: Infrequently, transient sweating, muscle tremors, and tachycardia may occur with IV administration. Clenbuterol should be discontinued in pregnant mares at the time of expected foaling because it can abolish uterine contractions.

DRUG INTERACTIONS: Clenbuterol antagonizes the effects of oxytocin and $PGF_{2\alpha}$.

SUPPLIED AS: VETERINARY PRODUCTS (not yet available in the US)
Syrup containing 0.025 mg/mL
For injection containing 0.03 mg/mL

OTHER USES
Cattle
Clenbuterol has also been suggested as a preventive of abomasal ulceration in veal calves at a dose of 1.6 µg/kg/day; PO. Clenbuterol has also been used illicitly as a repartitioning agent in veal calves.

Sheep
CONTROL PARTURITION
0.2 mg per ewe; IM, PO will delay the onset of labor overnight (8–10 hours) in ewes with signs of impending parturition, which include filling of the teats, warmth in the udder, and swelling of the vulva. Higher doses may decrease lamb viability.

CLORSULON

INDICATIONS: Clorsulon (Curatrem★) is a parasiticide used in cattle, sheep, and goats for the treatment and control of the liver fluke *Fasciola hepatica*. The drug is effective against both immature and adult flukes and has a 10-fold dose margin of safety.

ADVERSE AND COMMON SIDE EFFECTS: None listed.

DRUG INTERACTIONS: None listed.

SUPPLIED AS: VETERINARY PRODUCT
Oral liquid containing 85 mg/mL

CLOXACILLIN

INDICATIONS: Cloxacillin (Dariclox★, Dry-Clox❖★, Orbenin Quick Release❖, Orbenin-DC★) is used for the treatment of mastitis in cattle caused by *Streptococcus agalactiae* and *Staphylococcus aureus* sensitive to penicillin, including penicillin-resistant strains. Cloxacillin is not destroyed by penicillinase produced by certain strains of *S. aureus*. Its antibacterial properties against nonpenicillinase-producing organisms are similar but less effective than penicillin G. Cloxacillin has been suggested for use in horses for respiratory infections caused by penicillinase-producing gram-positive organisms.

ADVERSE AND COMMON SIDE EFFECTS: As for other penicillins, allergic reactions can occur with cloxacillin. See **PENICILLINS**.

DRUG INTERACTIONS: See **PENICILLINS** for further information.

SUPPLIED AS: VETERINARY PRODUCTS
Intramammary preparations containing 500 mg benzathine cloxacillin per 10-mL unit [Dry-Clox❖★, Orbenin-DC★]
Intramammary preparations containing 200 mg cloxacillin sodium per 10-mL unit [Dariclox★, Orbenin Quick Release❖]

COBALT

INDICATIONS: Cobalt❖★ is a component of vitamin B_{12}. Deficient animals show reduced milk production with severe deficiency causing emaciation, progressive inappetence, and anemia. Regions around the Great Lakes, as well as New England and Florida, are cobalt-deficient areas in North America. Australia, New Zealand, Great Britain, and portions of Africa are also cobalt-deficient areas. Cobalt sulfate or chloride is part of patent medicines in Canada (Ketamalt❖, Ketol❖, and others) used for the treatment and prevention of ketosis (acetonemia) in cows and sheep (pregnancy toxemia).

ADVERSE AND COMMON SIDE EFFECTS: Cobalt is relatively nontoxic.

DRUG INTERACTIONS: None listed.

SUPPLIED AS: VETERINARY PRODUCTS
Feed additive: in mineral or salt blocks, or as top dressing on pasture
Cobalt-containing acetonemia products (Canada only)
Liquid containing: cobalt chloride with choline chloride, ethylenedi-
amine dihydroiodide, propylene glycol, and other compounds. See
individual products.

COLISTIN

INDICATIONS: Colistin (polymixin E, colistimethate sodium)
(Coly-Mycin M Parenteral♥★) is a polymixin antibiotic used to treat
gram-negative infections caused by *Escherichia coli, Pseudomonas
aeruginosa, Salmonella,* and *Proteus.* The drug is poorly absorbed from
the digestive tract and if used orally for treatment of enteric infections is relatively free of side effects. Gentamicin or carbenicillin are
preferred drugs for systemic treatment of *Pseudomonas* infections.
Colistin has been suggested as a component of treatment for coliform mastitis in cows, but the merit of any antibiotic treatment for
this disease is disputed.

ADVERSE AND COMMON SIDE EFFECTS: Colistin is both neurotoxic and nephrotoxic, especially at high doses, which has limited
its clinical use. If used systemically in animals with renal impairment, the dose should be reduced. Absorption of topical preparations containing polymixins can lead to hypersensitization.

DRUG INTERACTIONS: When used with other neuromuscular
agents, polymixins may infrequently be associated with muscular
weakness, paresis, or complete paralysis leading to respiratory arrest.

SUPPLIED AS: HUMAN PRODUCT
For injection containing 75 mg/mL

COPPER, INJECTABLE

INDICATIONS: Injectable copper (Caco Injection♥, Caco Iron Cop-
per♥, Caco-Iron-Copper Solution♥, Centra Copper Injection♥,
Molycu★) is used as a hematinic for horses recovering from debili-
tating diseases, and for copper deficiency in large animals.

ADVERSE AND COMMON SIDE EFFECTS: Sheep are highly susceptible to copper toxicity. Administration of twice the recommended levels of soluble preparations can cause heavy mortalities in
sheep and calves. Administration to cattle with liver disease or grazing plants containing toxic alkaloids that can induce liver damage,
such as Tansy Ragwort, is contraindicated.

DRUG INTERACTIONS: None listed.

SUPPLIED AS: VETERINARY PRODUCTS
For injection containing 60 mg/mL [Molycu★]
For injection as copper gluconate (195 and 200 mg/mL) in combination with sodium cacodylate (6.4 and 6.5 mg/mL) and ferric chloride (1 and 1.13 mg/mL).
See individual product.

COPPER NAPHTHENATE

INDICATIONS: Copper naphthenate (Coppercure♣, Copperox♣, Coppersept♣, Kopper Kare♣, Koppersol♣, Kopertox♣★) is a topical antifungal, antiseptic, and astringent, used for treating thrush, hoof punctures, cracked hooves, foot rot in cattle and sheep, and ringworm. It is also suggested for treating wounds after dehorning.

ADVERSE AND COMMON SIDE EFFECTS: Avoid direct contact with mucous membranes or the eyes. Do not apply to the teats of lactating animals.

DRUG INTERACTIONS: None listed.

SUPPLIED AS: VETERINARY PRODUCT
Solution containing copper naphthenate 37.5% W/V

COPPER SULFATE

INDICATIONS: Copper sulfate (Acidified Copper Sulfate★, Caustic Dressing Powder★, Caustic Powder★, Copper Sulfate-S♣, Equi-Phar Caustic Powder★, Proudsoff★, Vinco Acidified Copper Sulfate★) is used as a caustic dressing for debridement and coagulation of wounds and in foot baths for the treatment of foot rot in cattle and sheep. Copper sulfate is also used in feeds or salt mixtures to prevent copper deficiency in cattle and sheep. Copper sulfate is included in topical preparations for treating ulcerative posthitis in sheep. Oral solutions of copper sulfate are reported to induce closure of the esophageal groove in ruminants.

ADVERSE AND COMMON SIDE EFFECTS: If the product is used in sheep as a foot bath, it may stain the wool. Sheep are highly susceptible to copper toxicity. Supplementation of copper in sheep diets should only be done where deficiency is known to exist.

DRUG INTERACTIONS: None listed.

SUPPLIED AS: VETERINARY PRODUCTS
Powder containing copper sulfate 50% [Caustic Powder★] or 51.5% [Caustic Dressing Powder★]

Powder containing 510 mg/g [Copper Sulfate-S♥]
Granules containing copper sulfate 99%
Chemical grade copper sulfate

CORTICOTROPIN

INDICATIONS: Corticotropin (ACTH♥, A.C.T.H.♥, A.C.T.H. 40♥, A.C.T.H. 40 I.U.♥, ACTH Gel★), also known as adrenocorticotropin, stimulates the adrenal cortex to secrete cortisol, corticosterone, aldosterone, and a number of weakly androgenic substances. ACTH is used in horses as a long-acting preparation for the treatment of musculoskeletal stiffness and arthritic conditions. ACTH is also used for bovine ketosis.

ADVERSE AND COMMON SIDE EFFECTS: Hypersensitivity may occur with repeated injections.

DRUG INTERACTIONS: Concurrent use of ketoconazole blunts the response of cortisol to the administration of ACTH.

SUPPLIED AS: VETERINARY PRODUCT
For injection containing 40 and 80 IU/mL in a repository preparation

OTHER USES
Horses

The ACTH stimulation test is used in horses suspected of having functional pituitary adenoma and ACTH is given at 1 IU/kg ACTH gel; IM or, 100 IU of synthetic ACTH; IV.

COUMAPHOS

INDICATIONS: Coumaphos (Co-Ral Dust Insecticide★, Co-Ral Animal Insecticide 1% Dust★, Co-Ral♥★, Co-Ral 1% Dust★, Co-Ral Livestock Insecticide Spray★, Co-Ral 25% Wettable Powder★, KRS Spray♥, and others) is an organophosphate used mainly to treat external parasites of livestock but has been used more recently as a feed additive anthelmintic for cattle. One advantage over other anthelmintics has been that it can be used in lactating animals without discarding milk. Coumaphos is effective against various species of adult *Haemonchus, Ostertagia, Trichostrongylus, Cooperia,* and *Trichuris* of sheep and cattle.

ADVERSE AND COMMON SIDE EFFECTS: Coumaphos has a narrow range of safety if administered as a drench at higher doses (20–30 mg/kg). As for other organophosphates, atropine is antidotal. For further information and drug interactions, see **ORGANOPHOS-**

PHATES in Description of Drugs for Small Animals. For topical products, treat lactating dairy cattle only after milking.

SUPPLIED AS: VETERINARY PRODUCTS
Topical powder containing 1% and wettable powder containing 25% coumaphos
Spray containing 3% coumaphos
Concentrated liquids containing 11.6% and 42% coumaphos

CROMOLYN SODIUM

INDICATIONS: Cromolyn sodium [sodium cromoglycate] (Gastrocrom★, Nalcrom♣, Novo-Cromolyn♣, Nasalcrom★, Intal Nebulizer Solution♣★, Intal Spincaps ♣★, Intal Inhaler♣, Intal Syncroner♣, Opticrom♣★, PMS-Sodium Cromoglycate♣, Vistacrom♣) is used for the treatment of horses with allergic respiratory disease. It inhibits the release of histamine from pulmonary mast cells and other mediators (including leukotrienes) from the lung during allergic responses mediated by IgE. As such, it must be administered by inhalation and in advance of exposure to the allergen. Because cromolyn sodium has no inherent activity to relax bronchial smooth muscle, it has no place in the treatment of acute bronchospasm in horses. Recent Canadian regulatory information has incriminated sodium cromoglycate as a major reason for a positive urine test for prohibited substances in race horses.

ADVERSE AND COMMON SIDE EFFECTS: Rare but serious effects may include hypersensitivity to the drug, manifested by laryngeal edema, angioedema, urticaria, or anaphylaxis. When using a nebulizer to administer the drug, strict attention to cleanliness of the nebulizer is required to avoid bacterial contamination of the nebulized aerosol. This product should not be given by injection.

DRUG INTERACTIONS: None listed.

SUPPLIED AS: HUMAN PRODUCTS
Dry powder for inhalation containing 20 mg
Solution for nebulization containing 10 mg/mL
Pressurized metered-dose inhaler containing 1 mg/puff (Canada), and 800 µg/puff (US)
Nasal solution containing 20 or 40 mg/mL
Oral capsules containing 100 mg
Ophthalmic solution containing 2% or 4%

DANTROLENE

INDICATIONS: Dantrolene (Dantrium♣★) is a skeletal muscle relaxant used in the prevention and treatment of malignant hyperthermia. Dantrolene has been advocated for use in preventing anesthetic-associated and exertional myopathy in horses but has not proven to be efficacious. Draft breeds may require lower than the recommended dose.

ADVERSE AND COMMON SIDE EFFECTS: Sedation, nausea, vomiting, constipation, and, possibly, hypotension occur. Drug overdose may cause generalized muscle weakness. Hepatotoxicity has been documented in humans following long-term drug therapy.

DRUG INTERACTIONS: Concurrent use of other central nervous system (CNS) depressants may cause additive CNS depression.

SUPPLIED AS: HUMAN PRODUCTS
Capsules containing 25, 50, and 100 mg
For injection containing 20 mg

DECOQUINATE

INDICATIONS: Decoquinate (Deccox Premix✤, Deccox★, Deccox Plus✤) is a feed additive coccidiostat for chickens and is used for the prevention of coccidiosis caused by *Eimeria bovis* and *Eimeria zurnii* in cattle. Decoquinate acts by preventing the sporozoite stage from developing once it has penetrated the host intestinal cell. It is to be fed for at least 28 days when coccidiosis is considered to be a hazard. Decoquinate is not effective for treating clinical coccidiosis.

ADVERSE AND COMMON SIDE EFFECTS: The drug should not be fed to animals of breeding age nor to lactating cattle.

DRUG INTERACTIONS: None listed.

SUPPLIED AS: VETERINARY PRODUCTS
Powder containing 60 g/kg
Pellets containing 0.25 g/kg in calf starter-grower

DEMBREXINE

INDICATIONS: Dembrexine (Sputolysin Powder✤) is a secretolytic with expectorant and secondary antitussive effects. It acts by altering the viscosity of respiratory mucus and improves the efficiency of respiratory tract clearance. Because of the effect on mucous production, there may be an initial increase in visible nasal discharge or cough before clinical improvement. It is reported to increase the concentrations of antibiotics in lung secretions. Dembrexine is used in horses with respiratory diseases such as chronic bronchitis or small airway disease in combination with other specific drugs for the underlying disease.

ADVERSE AND COMMON SIDE EFFECTS: None noted. The effect on fertility in breeding stock has not been determined. This drug should not be used in horses intended for food.

DRUG INTERACTIONS: None listed.

SUPPLIED AS: VETERINARY PRODUCT
Powder containing 5 mg/g

DETOMIDINE

INDICATIONS: Detomidine (Dormosedan♥★) is a synthetic α_2-adrenoceptor agonist with potent sedative and analgesic properties. It is used in horses for chemical restraint of particularly fractious animals for procedures such as nasogastric intubation, bronchoscopy, and for pain relief for minor surgical procedures and colic. Detomidine produces profound lethargy, reduced sensitivity to environmental stimuli (sight, sound), and, after a short period of incoordination, a fixed, base-wide stance during the period of sedation. Its sedative and analgesic effects depend on the dose and route of administration and will last from 30 minutes to 2 hours. Sensitivity to touch is little affected and in some cases may be enhanced, in which case some horses that appear deeply sedated may respond excessively to sudden external stimuli.

ADVERSE AND COMMON SIDE EFFECTS: The heart rate is markedly decreased and partial atrioventricular block may occur. A diuretic effect may be observed within 45 to 60 minutes of treatment. The respiratory rate slows initially but returns to normal within 5 minutes. Piloerection, sweating, salivation, and partial, transient penile prolapse may be seen. This drug should not be used in horses with preexisting atrioventricular or sinoatrial block or in horses with severe cardiac insufficiency, cerebrovascular disease, respiratory disease, or chronic renal failure. The safety of detomidine has not been established in breeding animals.

DRUG INTERACTIONS: Atropine (0.02 mg/kg; IV) will prevent the occurrence of the cardiac arrhythmias. Reversal of sedation can be accomplished with α_2-blocking agents, such as yohimbine. Use the drug with caution if combining it with other sedatives. There are recent reports of the occurrence of fatal arrhythmias when detomidine has been administered to horses that were under treatment with trimethoprim/sulfa drugs. Because little is known of the predisposing conditions in these cases, an alternative sedative should be chosen if possible when trimethoprim/sulfas have been given to the horse.

SUPPLIED AS: VETERINARY PRODUCT
For injection containing 10 mg/mL

DEXAMETHASONE

INDICATIONS: Dexamethasone (Azium Solution♥★, Azium Powder♥★, Dexamethasone★, Dexamethasone Injection♥★, Dexamethasone Powder♥, Dexamethasone Tablets★, Dexamethasone 21 Phosphate Injection♥, Dexamethasone Sodium Phosphate Injection★, Dexaject♥, Dexaject SP★, Dexamethasone 2♥, Dexamethasone 2.0 Injection★, Dexamethasone 5♥, Dexameth-A-Vet★, Dexamone 2♥, Dexasone★, DexAVet★, Dexone♥, Dextab♥, Dixazone♥, Hostadex♥, and others) is a potent anti-inflammatory corticosteroid, with 25 times the potency of cortisone and a long duration of action. All corticosteroids have similar modes of action and effects, the difference being mainly in anti-inflammatory potency and duration of action. Corticosteroids have numerous and widespread actions, influencing carbohydrate, lipid, and protein metabolism. The most important factor in their anti-inflammatory action is to inhibit the recruitment of neutrophils and monocyte-macrophages into affected tissues. Local heat, redness, and swelling is prevented or suppressed, but the underlying cause of disease remains. Anti-inflammatory effects of dexamethasone are beneficial in arthritis and inflammatory conditions in musculoskeletal injuries, and in immunologic diseases, such as purpura hemorrhagica, allergic rhinitis, and urticaria. Dexamethasone is also useful for the treatment of primary ketosis in cattle, the principal mechanism being mainly the reduction of milk production. Dexamethasone is advocated for treatment of shock, but the doses required for large animals are often impractical, and the beneficial effects have been seriously questioned in controlled clinical studies in human shock patients. Dexamethasone is used for treating cerebral edema, but its efficacy has been questioned. Ophthalmologic preparations are used to reduce uveal tract inflammation in diseases such as equine recurrent uveitis. Dexamethasone can induce premature parturition in cattle, sheep, and goats. It will also induce abortion in cattle when combined with prostaglandin $F_{2\alpha}$ in the last trimester of gestation.

ADVERSE AND COMMON SIDE EFFECTS: High, continued doses can cause suppression of adrenocortical function. Use of dexamethasone in horses under certain conditions has been associated with the occurrence of laminitis, possibly due to increased vascular reactivity to biogenic amines. Corticosteroids should not be used in bacterial, viral, or parasitic infections unless concurrent anti-infective agents are used. Clinical signs may abate with their use, but with their sole use the underlying disease remains active. Topical use of corticosteroids on the eye is contraindicated if corneal ulceration is present. If long-term therapy is undertaken, withdrawal should be gradual to avoid problems of iatrogenic adrenal suppression. Corticosteroids given to animals in the last trimester of pregnancy can induce premature parturition and predispose to retained placenta and metritis.

Dexamethasone may delay wound healing. See also **GLUCOCOR-TICOID AGENTS**.

DRUG INTERACTIONS: Corticosteroid actions are potentiated by erythromycin, possibly by interference with metabolism of the corticosteroids. See also **GLUCOCORTICOID AGENTS**.

SUPPLIED AS: VETERINARY PRODUCTS
For injection containing 2, 4, and 5 mg/mL [sodium phosphate]
Oral powder in packets containing 10 mg
Tablets containing 0.25 mg
In combination with other medications [Azimycin♣★, Naquasone♣★, Dexamycin♣, Tresaderm♣★]
See package label for specific details.

OTHER USES
Horses

PURPURA HEMORRHAGICA AND GLOMERULONEPHRITIS
0.044 to 0.1 mg/kg; IM for 10 to 14 days, then weaned off over 3 to 4 weeks by reducing doses by half each week

DEXTRAN

INDICATIONS: Dextran (Gentran♣★, Macrodex♣★, Rheomacrodex♣★) is a complex carbohydrate in solution used for plasma volume expansion. A key role for its use in large animals is as a peritoneal lavage solution to prevent formation of adhesion in horses undergoing abdominal surgery. The proposed mechanism of this adhesion prevention is to increase surface separation of serosal surfaces.

ADVERSE AND COMMON SIDE EFFECTS: Administration should be avoided in horses with excessive contamination or leakage of bacteria during surgery because it increases the prevalence of peritonitis under these conditions. Thus, if the horse has evidence of moderate to severe serosal inflammation on the intestine, if any devitalized intestine appears present, or an enterotomy or anastomosis was performed, use of dextrans in the lavage fluid is contraindicated.

DRUG INTERACTIONS: None listed.

SUPPLIED AS: HUMAN PRODUCTS
For infusion containing 0.8 mmol dextran or 10 g dextran/mL in 5% dextrose or 0.9% NaCl

DIAZEPAM

INDICATIONS: Diazepam (Apo-Diazepam♣, Diazepam Solution★, E Pam♣, Meral♣, Novo-Dipam♣, PMS-Diazepam♣, Zetram★, Valium★) is a muscle relaxant, sedative, and anticonvulsive drug. Diazepam is used as a premedicant for general anesthesia to ensure smooth induction and recovery, particularly for foals and small ruminants, and for treating clinical tetanus. Diazepam is also indicated to treat novice stallions that appear anxious or fearful, or that pay more attention to the handler than the mare.

ADVERSE AND COMMON SIDE EFFECTS: IV injection can be irritating. Teratogenic effects have been reported in humans.

DRUG INTERACTIONS: Metabolism may be decreased and excessive sedation may occur if diazepam is given with cimetidine, erythromycin, ketoconazole, or propranolol. Additive central nervous system effects may be anticipated if diazepam is given along with barbiturates, narcotics, or anesthetics. Antacids may slow the rate of drug absorption. The pharmacologic effects of digoxin may be potentiated. Rifampin may induce hepatic microenzymal activity and decrease the efficacy of diazepam. An increase in the duration and intensity of respiratory depression may occur if diazepam is used with pancuronium or succinylcholine. Diazepam should not be mixed with other drugs without consulting references. Absorption to plastics may occur.

SUPPLIED AS: HUMAN PRODUCTS
Tablets containing 2, 5, and 10 mg
For injection containing 5 mg/mL

OTHER USES
Diazepam may be used in feed to sedate particularly fractious animals.

DICHLORVOS

INDICATIONS: Dichlorvos (Atgard C Swine Wormer♣★, Cutter Dichlorvos Horse Wormer★, Disvap Livestock Spray and Fogging Solution♣, Vapona Concentrate★) is a cholinesterase inhibitor used as an anthelmintic feed additive in swine against *Trichuris*, *Oesophagostomum*, and *Ascaris* spp, and in horses to treat migrating and sessile bot infestation, *Strongylus vulgaris*, *S. equinum*, *Parascaris equorum*, and the pinworms *Oxyuris equi* and *Probstmayria vivipara*. The pellets slowly release the drug, adding a safety factor as it is absorbed over a 2- to 3-day period. Used as a fogging solution, it can be applied to premises or directly to dairy and beef cattle, and horses, to reduce the population of stable flies, horn flies, and house flies. Spray lightly on areas of the animal on which flies congregate.

ADVERSE AND COMMON SIDE EFFECTS: Toxicity can cause colic, excess salivation, diarrhea, bradycardia, and respiratory distress. Do not use in the milk room. The margin of safety is generally less than other broad-spectrum anthelmintics.

DRUG INTERACTIONS: Atropine is antidotal. Praladoxime will reactivate cholinesterase if given shortly after exposure.

SUPPLIED AS: VETERINARY PRODUCTS
Resin pellets containing 9.6% in packets of 4 kg
Powder in packets containing 78 g
Solution containing 0.9%
Liquid concentrate containing 40.2% for treatment of environment

DIETHYLCARBAMAZINE

INDICATIONS: Diethylcarbamazine (Carbam★, Decacide Tabs♥★, Diethylcarbamazine Citrate★, Filaribits♥★, Nemacinde★) is an antifilarial compound that causes immobilization of the parasite and alters the surface membrane of the parasite, rendering it more susceptible to destruction by host defenses. It is used in horses for the treatment of verminous myelitis and onchocerciasis.

ADVERSE AND COMMON SIDE EFFECTS: In humans, there may be mild, temporary malaise, weakness, and anorexia, or intense itching or skin rash in heavy *Onchocerca* infections. Similar effects may occur in horses.

DRUG INTERACTIONS: Pretreatment with corticosteroids may be undertaken to minimize adverse reactions.

SUPPLIED AS: VETERINARY PRODUCTS (Small-Animal Products Only)
Syrup containing 60 mg/mL
Tablets containing 50, 60, 100, 180, 200, 300, and 400 mg

DIGOXIN

INDICATIONS: Digoxin (Lanoxin♥★, Cardoxin♥★, Cardoxin LS★, Lanoxicaps★, Novo-Digoxin♥) is a cardiac glycoside that has positive inotropic and negative chronotropic actions. It is used in large animals in the treatment of congestive heart failure and for assisting the treatment of supraventricular tachycardia or arrhythmias, such as atrial fibrillation in horses, and for dilated cardiomyopathy in cattle. Digoxin is used before quinidine in atrial fibrillation in horses and cattle with fast heart rates (>60 and 100 beats/min, respectively). Side effects of quinidine treatment may be decreased in animals pretreated with digoxin. Therapeutic drug monitoring can assist in initial therapy to optimize effect and to minimize toxicity.

Peak concentrations should not exceed 2.5 ng/mL. Low oral bioavailability in cattle limits its use to intravenous treatment.

ADVERSE AND COMMON SIDE EFFECTS: Frequent electrocardiographic monitoring is indicated during digitalis administration. Signs of toxicity include depression, ataxia, and gastrointestinal upset, including diarrhea, weakness, and cardiac arrhythmias. Digoxin is contraindicated in ventricular arrhythmias and second- and third-degree heart block. Digitalis has no direct positive inotropic effect on the normal heart and may actually decrease cardiac output in such use.

DRUG INTERACTIONS: Concurrent use with quinidine may increase plasma concentrations of digoxin, possibly by displacement of digoxin from binding sites in tissues. Phenylbutazone, phenobarbital, phenytoin, and rifampin may speed the metabolism of digoxin. Diuretics that deplete potassium (e.g., furosemide) should be withheld when using digoxin.

SUPPLIED AS: VETERINARY PRODUCTS
Elixir containing 0.05 and 0.15 mg/mL

HUMAN PRODUCTS
Capsules containing 0.05, 0.1, and 0.2 mg
Tablets containing 0.0625, 0.125, 0.25, and 0.5 mg
Elixir containing 0.05 mg/mL
For injection containing 0.05, 0.1, and 0.25 mg/mL

DIHYDROSTREPTOMYCIN

INDICATIONS: Dihydrostreptomycin (Ethamycin♣) is an aminoglycoside antibiotic similar to streptomycin, which was produced initially for treatment of tuberculosis in humans. Resistance to this form of aminoglycoside has become widespread, but it remains useful for treating leptospirosis and actinomycosis. It is a suggested treatment for tuberculosis in the horse, although this disease is extremely rare in North America. The drug is also used in combination with long-acting tetracyclines for brucellosis in countries that have no eradication program. It is present in a number of combined products with other antibiotics, particularly penicillin G (Combisec♣, D.P. Booster♣, Quartermaster★, Special Formula 17900-Forte Suspension♣). Its presence in these combined products limits extralabel use of penicillin as it greatly increases the risk of toxicity and residues due to the presence of dihydrostreptomycin.

ADVERSE AND COMMON SIDE EFFECTS: Toxic levels can cause renal tubular damage, which may be reversible once the drug is discontinued. Avoid use with other aminoglycosides because of potential additive toxic effects. The drug causes transient pain on injection. Ototoxicity can occur but is difficult to detect clinically. Dihydrostreptomycin has much higher ototoxic potential than streptomycin. Weakness from neuromuscular blockade can also occur. See also **AMINOGLYCOSIDE ANTIBIOTICS**.

DRUG INTERACTIONS: Concurrent use of furosemide can increase the ototoxic potential and predispose to renal tubular damage. See also **AMINOGLYCOSIDE ANTIBIOTICS**.

SUPPLIED AS: VETERINARY PRODUCTS
For injection containing 500 mg/mL
Mastitis tubes containing 100 mg combined with 100,000 U penicillin G procaine, 150 mg novobiocin, 50,000 U polymixin B, 20 mg hydrocortisone, and 12.5 mg hydrocortisone sodium succinate
Mastitis tubes containing 1 g combined with 1,000,000 U procaine penicillin G
Powder containing 72,000 mg combined with potassium penicillin G 31,500,000 IU and assorted vitamins/400 g

DIMETHYL GLYCINE

INDICATIONS: Dimethyl glycine♥★ is a nutritional supplement used in athletes in the hope that it delays fatigue or reduces lactate accumulation. Some studies suggest improvement in time trials for racing greyhounds over longer distances, but controlled crossover trials in exercising horses failed to identify beneficial effects on performance or in a number of related physiologic parameters. Unpublished reports also make claims that dimethyl glycine may reduce the incidence of repeated bouts of exertional rhabdomyolysis.

ADVERSE AND COMMON SIDE EFFECTS: None listed.

DRUG INTERACTIONS: None listed.

SUPPLIED AS: CHEMICAL PRODUCT
As a powder containing free base dimethyl glycine

DIMETHYL SULFOXIDE

INDICATIONS: Dimethyl sulfoxide (Domoso Gel♥★, Domoso Solution♥★) is a potent solvent with a wide range of actions and proposed uses. It may increase the penetration of low molecular weight compounds through intact skin. It also has anti-inflammatory actions, analgesic properties, scavenges free radicals, interferes with neutrophil chemotaxis, and is a potent diuretic. It has been used topically to decrease inflammation in musculoskeletal injuries and for soft tissue inflammation such as may occur with thrombophlebitis. It has been proposed as a treatment for cerebral edema and acute central nervous system injury, such as spinal or head trauma, or neonatal maladjustment syndrome of foals. However, the available literature concerning efficacy is conflicting. The IV route for therapy is common but remains extralabel.

ADVERSE AND COMMON SIDE EFFECTS: The drug is not to be used in horses with ocular disease, liver or kidney problems, or animals with a history of allergy. Topical treatment may occasionally cause transient erythema and associated irritation of the area, possibly due to mast cell degranulation. Dryness of the skin and oyster-like breath odor have also been reported. Do not use more than 100 g or 100 mL daily or for longer than 30 days in the horse. It is not to be used in pregnant mares or mares intended for breeding. SC injection results in a marked local necrotizing reaction. IV injection of undiluted solution can cause hemoglobinuria. IV administration may also cause muscle fasciculations, sweating, intravascular hemolysis, and hemoglobinuria. Wear rubber gloves when handling because contact of dimethyl sulfoxide with human skin will result in malodorous breath and systemic side effects. It should be used in well ventilated areas as 70% of the product is excreted through the respiratory tract.

DRUG INTERACTIONS: Topical application may facilitate absorption of undesirable medications (such as mercury blisters) previously applied to the skin.

SUPPLIED AS: VETERINARY PRODUCTS
Topical gel preparation containing 90% dimethyl sulfoxide
Solution containing 90% medical grade dimethyl sulfoxide

DIOCTYL SODIUM SULFOSUCCINATE

INDICATIONS: Docusate sodium [dioctyl sodium sulfosuccinate, DSS, DOS] (Anti-Gaz Emulsion♣, Anti-Bloat♣, Bloat-Aid♣, Bloat-Go♣, Bloat Remedy★, Bloat Treatment★, Bloban♣, Dioctate♣, Dioctol♣, Dioctynate★, Disposable Enema Syringe★, Docusate Solution★, Docu-Soft Enema★, Enema DSS★, Enema SA★, Pet Enema★, Tympanex Suspension♣, Veterinary Surfactant★) is a surface-acting anionic surfactant used as an aid in the treatment of frothy bloat in ruminants and for the treatment of large colon or gastric impactions in horses. At recommended dosages docusates have minimal laxative effects. The clinical usefulness is to hydrate intestinal contents by emulsifying feces, water, and fat in the intestinal lumen.

ADVERSE AND COMMON SIDE EFFECTS: Toxicity can occur at three to five times the recommended dose in horses; therefore, do not exceed a total dose of 200 mg/kg. Signs of toxicity include increased heart rate, respiratory rate, and intestinal sounds and severe watery diarrhea followed by dehydration, recumbency, and death.

DRUG INTERACTIONS: Docusates increase intestinal absorption of other drugs administered concurrently and may increase their toxicity.

SUPPLIED AS: VETERINARY PRODUCTS
Suspension containing 2.0 to 8.5 mg/mL in emulsified soybean oil
Enema solution containing 5%
Premeasured enema syringe containing 250 mg/12 mL

OTHER USES
Sheep

This agent has been used in abomasal emptying defects in sheep, but only with limited success.

DIPYRONE

INDICATIONS: Dipyrone (Dipyrone 50% Injection★, Dipyrone 50%♣, Dipyrone Injection★) is an analgesic, antipyretic, anti-inflammatory, and antispasmodic used in large animals as a smooth muscle antispasmodic and analgesic, particularly in horses. It is indicated in conditions where pain is caused by hyperperistalsis, spasmodic colic, or esophageal contraction in choke. Its efficacy for analgesia in cases of colic has been questioned.

ADVERSE AND COMMON SIDE EFFECTS: Overdosage can cause convulsions. Prolonged use can cause agranulocytosis and leukopenia. SC injection can cause irritation at the injection site.

DRUG INTERACTIONS: Dipyrone is contraindicated for use in conjunction with phenylbutazone or barbiturates because of drug interactions involving the microsomal enzyme system. Dipyrone can interfere with or mask the presence of prohibited drugs in racehorses for up to 5 days. Use with chlorpromazine hydrochloride can result in clinically serious hypothermia.

SUPPLIED AS: VETERINARY PRODUCT
For injection containing 500 mg/mL

DOBUTAMINE

INDICATIONS: Dobutamine (Dobutrex♥★, Dobutamine Hydrochloride Injection♥★) is a positive cardiac inotrope similar in nature and action to dopamine used to improve peripheral perfusion.

It has been advocated for neonatal foals suffering from asphyxia, for horses with circulatory shock caused by endotoxemia, and for severe hypotension that may occur in foals due to snake bite. Although some authors suggest using dobutamine for treating foals with oliguric renal failure, it has no effect on the dopaminergic receptors of the renal vasculature.

ADVERSE AND COMMON SIDE EFFECTS: Before dobutamine is administered, the animal must have hypovolemia corrected by appropriate fluid therapy. Tachycardia and arrhythmias may occur during infusion.

DRUG INTERACTIONS: Propranolol may negate the effects of dobutamine. Halothane may increase the likelihood of arrhythmias.

SUPPLIED AS: HUMAN PRODUCT
For injection containing 12.5 mg/mL

DOPAMINE

INDICATIONS: Dopamine (Intropin♥★, Dopamine Hydrochloride and 5% Dextrose Injection♥★) is the immediate metabolic precursor of norepinephrine and epinephrine. Its positive cardiac inotropic effects are used to improve peripheral perfusion. Its use has been advocated in neonatal foals suffering from asphyxia, horses with circulatory shock caused by endotoxemia, and for severe hypotension due to snake bite. It is also used in oliguric renal failure of foals as it can increase glomerular filtration rate via specific dopaminergic receptors in the kidney.

ADVERSE AND COMMON SIDE EFFECTS: Before dopamine is administered, the animal must have hypovolemia corrected by appropriate fluid therapy. Tachycardia and arrhythmias may occur during infusion. Extravasation of large amounts of dopamine during infusion can result in ischemic necrosis of the area.

DRUG INTERACTIONS: Phenytoin may decrease the effects of dopamine, leading to hypotension and bradycardia.

SUPPLIED AS: HUMAN PRODUCTS
For injection containing 40 mg/mL
For infusion containing 0.8, 1.6, or 3.2 mg/mL in 5% dextrose

DOXAPRAM

INDICATIONS: Doxapram (Dopram-V Injectable♥★) is a central respiratory stimulant used for hastening recovery from anesthesia, such as with pentobarbital and/or chloral hydrate, and for stimulating respiratory centers of neonatal animals following Cesarean section or dystocia. Onset of action is rapid and the dose should be adjusted according to clinical response. A patent airway should be ensured. Doxapram can also be administered SC or sublingually in the neonate if the IV route is not available. Doxapram is indicated for treatment of poisonings in which there is depression of the respiratory center.

ADVERSE AND COMMON SIDE EFFECTS: Excessive doses can cause respiratory alkalosis. High doses can cause convulsions.

DRUG INTERACTIONS: Do not mix with alkaline solutions. Doxapram-stimulated respiration is severely depressed by morphine or meperidine.

SUPPLIED AS: VETERINARY PRODUCT
For injection containing 20 mg/mL

OTHER USES
Horses

Doxapram is also used as a respiratory stimulant to facilitate endoscopic examination of laryngeal motion in the horse.

ECHOTHIOPHATE IODIDE

INDICATIONS: Echothiophate iodide (Phospholine Iodide♥★) is a long-acting anticholinesterase agent used for the treatment of glaucoma when other agents such as timolol or physostigmine are not effective. It is suggested for treatment of glaucoma in the horse, but this is not commonly diagnosed in large animals.

ADVERSE AND COMMON SIDE EFFECTS: Long-term use of echothiophate carries the risk in humans for the development of cataracts. Humans may have allergic reactions to the drug, or more rarely, retinal detachment.

DRUG INTERACTIONS: None listed.

SUPPLIED AS: HUMAN PRODUCT
Ophthalmic drops containing 0.06%, 0.125%, and 0.25%

ENILCONAZOLE

INDICATIONS: Enilconazole (Imaverol♥, Clinafarm EC 13.8%★) is a benzimidazole that inhibits fungal growth with potent antifungal action against dermatophytes. It has been used in a horse to treat guttural pouch mycosis as an adjunct to other systemic treatment (itraconazole). In its diluted form it is nonirritating.

ADVERSE AND COMMON SIDE EFFECTS: The concentrated solution is irritating to the skin and eyes, but these are no longer problems if the solution is properly diluted.

DRUG INTERACTIONS: None listed.

SUPPLIED AS: VETERINARY PRODUCTS
Solution in concentrate at 100 mg/mL✤
Chemical grade 13.8% W/W★

ENROFLOXACIN

INDICATIONS: Enrofloxacin (Baytril✤★) is a synthetic fluoroquin-olone. Enrofloxacin is effective in small animals against a broad range of microbes, including gram-positive and gram-negative bacteria, and some mycoplasmas. Enrofloxacin has been used to treat calves with salmonellosis, coliform diarrhea or septicemia, and cattle with pneumonic pasteurellosis, but data on safety or efficacy in large animals are scant. Parenteral (IM, SC) applications and oral routes have similar kinetics in preruminant cattle. Oral administration in calves has produced effective blood levels both from direct administration into the buccal cavity or when mixed with milk or milk substitutes. Two-week-old calves treated at 15 mg/kg PO for 14 days and 30 mg/kg for 1 week suffered no ill effects. Treatment of sheep with mycoplasma-associated balanoposthitis or vulvovaginitis has been disappointing despite suggested effectiveness in vitro. IV and IM administration in horses suggests it may provide effective serum concentrations at once daily dosing, but the IM route was found to result in excessive irritation.

Enrofloxacin is supposed to be tightly bound to calcium and organic materials. It is unlikely to receive approval in the US for food-producing animals (laying hens) because of binding to the shell. Enrofloxacin also is thought to bind to hay and bedding.

ADVERSE AND COMMON SIDE EFFECTS: Enrofloxacin should not be used in young growing animals because it causes cartilaginous damage. Irritation may occur at the site of injection.

DRUG INTERACTIONS: Absorption is hindered by antacid preparations as well as sucralfate. Nitrofurantoin may antagonize the effects of enrofloxacin. See **FLUOROQUINOLONE ANTIBIOTICS** in the Description of Drugs for Small Animals.

SUPPLIED AS: VETERINARY PRODUCTS
Tablets containing 5.7, 22.7, and 68 mg

For injection containing 22.7 and 50 mg/mL
Solution (turkey egg dip) containing 32.3 mg/mL

EPHEDRINE

INDICATIONS: Ephedrine✦★ is a sympathomimetic that acts by direct activation of adrenergic receptors, similar to epinephrine. Although weaker, ephedrine differs from epinephrine in that it has a longer duration of action and can be given orally. If given over time the effects diminish as stores of norepinephrine are eventually depleted. The main indication for the drug in veterinary medicine is in the reduction of allergic responses and vasoconstriction and decongestion of congested mucous membranes (if applied topically).

ADVERSE AND COMMON SIDE EFFECTS: Central nervous system (CNS) excitement, tachycardia, and muscle tremors may occur.

DRUG INTERACTIONS: Sodium bicarbonate may increase the pharmacologic effects of ephedrine with excessive CNS stimulation and cardiovascular effects.

SUPPLIED AS: HUMAN PRODUCTS
Tablets containing 15 and 30 mg ephedrine✦
Capsules containing 25 mg★
For injection containing 50 mg/mL

EPINEPHRINE

INDICATIONS: Epinephrine (Epichlor✦, Epinject★, Adrenalin✦★) is an endogenous catecholamine with a wide variety of effects on organs innervated by the sympathetic nervous system, including positive inotropic and chronotropic effects, vasoconstriction or vasodilation of blood vessels (depending on organ location), bronchodilation, mydriasis, and decrease in the frequency and amplitude of intestinal peristalsis. Epinephrine is not absorbed to any extent by the oral route and has a very short half-life in the body. It is used alone as an emergency drug for treatment of anaphylaxis, hypotension, and cardiac arrest. Epinephrine is also used as a local hemostatic for superficial mucosal bleeding and in combination with local anesthetics to localize their action and delay their absorption.

ADVERSE AND COMMON SIDE EFFECTS: Cardiac arrhythmias, including tachycardia and fatal ventricular fibrillation, can occur following inadvertent overdosage.

DRUG INTERACTIONS: Thyroid therapy, digitalis therapy, halogenated hydrocarbon anesthetics, and thiobarbiturates predispose to myocardial toxicity of catecholamines.

SUPPLIED AS: VETERINARY PRODUCT
For injection containing 1.0 mg/mL (1:1,000) epinephrine

HUMAN PRODUCT
For injection containing 0.1 mg/mL (1:10,000)

ERGONOVINE

INDICATIONS: Ergonovine (Ergonovine Maleate Solution♣) is an ergot alkaloid with potent stimulatory activity on myometrial contraction in the periparturient animal. It is used mainly in the postpartum animal to favor uterine contraction and involution, in prolapsed uterus, post-Cesarean section, and uterine hemorrhage. Following IM injection, clinical effects begin within 15 minutes and last 2 to 4 hours.

ADVERSE AND COMMON SIDE EFFECTS: Ergonovine should not be used prepartum because oxytocin is a superior myometrial stimulant for obstetrics. Prolonged or excessive use may cause dry gangrene, vascular damage, hypotension, and depression of the respiratory rate and volume.

DRUG INTERACTIONS: Ergonovine should not be mixed with any other medications.

SUPPLIED AS: VETERINARY PRODUCT (Canada only)
For injection containing 0.2 mg/mL

ERYTHROMYCIN

INDICATIONS: Erythromycin (Alto-Erythromycin♣, Apo-Erythro Base♣, Erythro-36♣★, Erythro-100★, Erythro-200♣★, Erythro-Dry★, Erythro-Dry Cow♣, Gallimycin-36♣★, Gallimycin♣, Gallimycin-50♣, Gallimycin 200♣, Gallimycin-Dry Cow★, Ilosone♣★, Ilotycin♣★, Novo-Rythro Estolate♣, Uddermate★, and others) is a macrolide antibiotic with bacteriostatic activity primarily against gram-positive bacteria and some strains of *Listeria*. Erythromycin diffuses well through most tissues and is useful for treating staphylococcal infections resistant to penicillin and for treating intracellular organisms, such as *Rhodococcus equi* in foals. Erythromycin is also used in mastitis preparations for intramammary use. The estolate form of erythromycin is less susceptible to stomach acid than the base or stearate and is better absorbed through the gastrointestinal tract. Recent work in the horse suggests twice daily treatment with oral products provides sufficiently effective blood levels, and that the salt forms (phosphate and stearate) may in fact be better absorbed than the estolate form because of higher variability in gastric pH in horses than in humans, and hence less inactivation of the salts and the base by a low gastric pH. Until further work is done, caution is advised against using this regimen, as the horses were adult, and hence not on a diet that would stimulate low gastric pH, and the safety at the higher level was not established beyond three doses.

ADVERSE AND COMMON SIDE EFFECTS: Oral administration can result in diarrhea. The incidence is low and it is unclear whether this is due to microflora alteration or irritation of the gastrointestinal tract by the drug. It is felt that many gastrointestinal problems caused by erythromycin in humans are associated with gastric acid degradation of erythromycin to its metabolites, which act as motilin antagonists. Temporary withdrawal of the medication usually is sufficient treatment. The estolate salt is more palatable than the uncoated base. Erythromycin is a potential hepatotoxin and has been incriminated in immune-mediated thrombocytopenia. Swedish and Dutch workers, however, have found that low doses can induce fatal colitis in adult horses. This may be a geographic problem associated with differences in feeds or gut flora, but has yet to be clarified.

A syndrome of hyperthermia in foals treated with erythromycin has been reported in Kentucky, with foals outside in high environmental temperatures and suffering from respiratory disease. Treatment was symptomatic, and until more information is available, it is advised that foals under medication and in hot, humid environmental conditions may be at risk.

DRUG INTERACTIONS: Erythromycin may delay the hepatic breakdown of theophyllines, corticosteroids, and digoxin. Theophylline toxicity readily occurs with concurrent administration of erythromycin. Kaolin will impair absorption of orally administered erythromycin. Erythromycin should not be used with chloramphenicol or lincomycin because these drugs have the same or anatomically proximate sites of action. At low doses, erythromycin may antagonize the antimicrobial action of the penicillins. Erythromycin lactobionate is incompatible if mixed with aminophylline, multiple vitamins, cephalothin, pentobarbital, sodium iodide, heparin, penicillin G, and tetracyclines. There is the possibility of increased digitalis effect in humans using both drugs. The occurrence in large animals is unknown. Erythromycin may cause prolongation of bleeding times in those receiving warfarin therapy.

SUPPLIED AS: VETERINARY PRODUCTS
For injection containing 100 and 200 mg/mL
Mastitis products containing 50 mg/mL
Tablets containing enteric-coated particles 33 and 500 mg
Feed additive containing 110 g/kg

HUMAN PRODUCTS
Tablets (enteric coated) containing 250, 333, and 500 mg (base)
Tablets containing 600 mg (ethylsuccinate salt)
Tablets (film coated) containing 250, 333, and 500 mg
Oral syrup containing erythromycin estolate 25 and 50 mg/mL
Oral liquid containing 200 mg/5 mL or 400 mg/5 mL (ethylsuccinate)
For injection containing 1,000 mg (gluceptate salt)
For injection containing 500 and 1,000 mg

OTHER USES
Horses
POSTOPERATIVE ILEUS
As little as 100 g/kg/hr to 0.5–1.0 mg/kg may increase gastrointestinal motility by mimicking the effects of the endogenous hormone motilin. Higher doses may cause inhibition through downregulation of motilin. Clinicians should be cautioned that even very low doses of erythromycin given orally to adult horses can in some regions be associated with fatal colitis.

ESTRADIOL

INDICATIONS: Estradiol (estradiol cypionate, ECP✤★) is a synthetic estrogen that acts to stimulate and maintain normal physiologic processes of the female reproductive tract. Synthetic estrogens are more prolonged in action. Estrogen therapy in mares and cows may be used in uterine infections, atony, or poor uterine drainage, in combination with appropriate antimicrobial therapy. Estradiol cypionate has been used as an abortifacient for cows and mares in the first half of pregnancy, but prostaglandins are a more rational choice.

ADVERSE AND COMMON SIDE EFFECTS: Estradiol may cause prolonged estrus, precocious development, genital irritation, and reduction of milk yield. Large doses of estrogens can cause postparturient straining in the cow with vaginal or uterine prolapse. Administration of estrogens to pregnant cows can induce abortion. Prolonged or excessive administration leads to ovarian suppression and hypoplasia, followed by ovarian cysts.

DRUG INTERACTIONS: None listed.

SUPPLIED AS: VETERINARY PRODUCT
For injection containing 1✤ and 2★ mg/mL

OTHER USES
Horses
URINARY INCONTINENCE
Urinary incontinence of non-neurogenic origin in aged mares at 0.004 to 0.008 mg/kg; IM every other day

Cattle

Estradiol therapy with progesterone has been used to induce lactation in sterile heifers and dry cows at a dose of 0.05 mg/kg; IM with 0.125 mg/kg; IM progesterone, bid for 7 days. Addition of 5 mg/cow reserpine and 20 mg/cow dexamethasone; SC on days 17, 18, and 19 to this regimen will increase milk yield. Estradiol is also used alone as an implant (Compudose♣★) or in the benzoate form in combination with testosterone (Implus H♣★, Synovex-H♣★) or progesterone (Calf-oid♣★, Implus-S♣★, Synovex-C♣★, Synovex-S♣★) as anabolic agents or growth promoters.

ETHYL ALCOHOL

INDICATIONS: Ethyl alcohol when used as an aerosol is a mucokinetic agent in the horse useful for rehydrating and emulsifying mucus and frothy secretions, particularly in clinically severe small airway disease. It is also used systemically to treat toxicity due to ingested methanol or ethylene glycol, but such toxicity is usually restricted to small animals.

ADVERSE AND COMMON SIDE EFFECTS: Ethyl alcohol given by aerosol can cause airway irritation and bronchoconstriction.

DRUG INTERACTIONS: None listed.

SUPPLIED AS: Commercially available from chemical supply companies.

ETHYLENEDIAMINE DIHYDROIODIDE

INDICATIONS: Ethylenediamine dihydroiodide (EDDI Organic Iodide★, EDDI-40♣, Edd-Iodine-42♣, Ethyodide★, Ethyl Dihydro♣, Iodexine 42♣, Organic Iodide★, Organic Iodide 20★, Organic Iodide 40★, Organic Iodine★, Organic Iodine 20★, Organic Iodine 40 Saline Base★) is an oral iodine supplement used as an aid for treating iodine deficiencies, bovine foot rot and infertility, and as an expectorant for respiratory disease.

ADVERSE AND COMMON SIDE EFFECTS: Signs of iodism, such as increased salivation, sneezing, eyelid swelling, and eye irritation, indicate the need for withdrawal of the supplement, after which clinical signs abate.

DRUG INTERACTIONS: None listed.

SUPPLIED AS: VETERINARY PRODUCT
As a powder to be mixed in feed or drinking water. See individual products for concentration and mixing instructions.

FAMOTIDINE

INDICATIONS: Famotidine (Apo-Famotidine♣, Gen-Famotidine♣, Novo-Famotidine♣, Nu Famotidine♣, Pepcid♣★) is a histamine (H₂)-receptor antagonist. Although it is more potent than cimetidine, no studies indicate that it is actually more efficacious than cimetidine or ranitidine in the management of gastric hyperacidity and gastrointestinal ulcer. A dose has been suggested for the horse, but its effectiveness has not been demonstrated.

ADVERSE AND COMMON SIDE EFFECTS: In humans depression, anxiety, insomnia, conjunctival infection, nausea, vomiting, anorexia, dry mouth, diarrhea, arthralgia, bronchospasm, pruritus, fever, and thrombocytopenia have been reported. There is little experience with use of the drug in horses. Famotidine has a large volume of distribution in horses and will accumulate in very sick animals. Colic has been observed with use of higher doses. Famotidine is contraindicated in animals with cardiovascular disease.

DRUG INTERACTIONS: None listed.

SUPPLIED AS: HUMAN PRODUCTS
Tablets containing 10, 20, and 40 mg
For injection containing 10 mg/mL
Suspension containing 8 mg/mL

FEBANTEL

INDICATIONS: Febantel (Cutter Paste Wormer♣★, Rintal Suspension★) is a broad-spectrum anthelmintic used for control of internal parasites, such as large strongyles, ascarids, pinworms, and the various small strongyles in horses of all ages and ponies. Febantel is also combined with trichlorfon as an equine anthelmintic (Negabot-Plus Paste♣) to include mouth and stomach stages of bots in the spectrum of activity. Febantel is safe for breeding mares and stallions. The drug is also effective in sheep for control of lungworms, tapeworms, and most gastrointestinal nematodes, with the exception of *Trichuris* and *Strongyloides*.

ADVERSE AND COMMON SIDE EFFECTS: Repeat doses of febantel at eight times the therapeutic dose produces a self-limiting diarrhea. Trichlorfon is a cholinesterase inhibitor. See **TRICHLORFON** for adverse reactions to Negabot-Plus Paste♣. Febantel is not to be administered to horses intended for slaughter.

DRUG INTERACTIONS: None listed.

SUPPLIED AS: VETERINARY PRODUCTS
Oral paste containing 2.73 g febantel/6 g syringes
Suspension containing 2.75 g/fluid ounce
Combination products contain 2.73 g febantel and 16 g trichlorfon
per syringe.

OTHER USES
Horses
STRONGYLOIDES WESTERI
50 mg/kg; PO

Sheep
GASTROINTESTINAL NEMATODES
5 mg/kg; PO

FENBENDAZOLE

INDICATIONS: Fenbendazole (Moorman's Moorguard Swine De-
wormer★, Panacur♣★, Safe-Guard♣★, in many formulations) is a
broad-spectrum anthelmintic of the benzimidazole group used in
horses for large strongyles, small strongyles, pinworms, and ascarids and for treating cattle parasitized by adult and 4th stage
larvae of lungworm (*Dictyocaulus viviparus*), stomach worms
(*Haemonchus contortus, Ostertagia ostertagi*), intestinal worms (*Cooperia* spp, *Trichostrongylus colubriformis, Nematodirus helvetianus, Bunos-
tomum phlebotomum, Oesophagostomum radiatum, Monezia benedeni*),
arrested 4th stage larvae of *Ostertagia ostertagi,* and the adult stomach worm *Trichostrongylus axei.* Fenbendazole is compatible with
trichlorfon, which can be used concurrently for stomach bots in
horses.

ADVERSE AND COMMON SIDE EFFECTS: At high doses a local
or systemic hypersensitivity reaction may result from the release of
dying parasite antigens.

DRUG INTERACTIONS: None listed.

SUPPLIED AS: VETERINARY PRODUCTS
Oral paste containing 100 mg/g
Granules containing 222 mg/g for use in horses
Suspension containing 100 mg/mL for use in horses and cattle

OTHER USES
Cattle
OSTERTAGIASIS
Fenbendazole is especially efficacious in its activity against tissue
stages of *Ostertagia.*

FENOTEROL

INDICATIONS: Fenoterol (Berotec✚, Berotec Forte✚) is a β_2 agonist with bronchodilatory properties that has been used for treatment of allergic airway disease in horses. It is available in metered-dose inhalers and when used in conjunction with specially equipped face masks (Aeromask) has been shown to produce effective bronchodilation in horses.

ADVERSE AND COMMON SIDE EFFECTS: Adverse side effects can include tachycardia, nervousness, excitability, muscle tremor, or colic, but when used as an aerosol no such signs were observed.

DRUG INTERACTIONS: None listed.

SUPPLIED AS: HUMAN PRODUCTS
Metered-dose aerosol systems containing 100 or 200 µg per actuation
Inhalation solution containing 0.25, 0.625, or 1.0 mg/mL

FENTANYL/DROPERIDOL

See **INNOVAR-VET** Description of Drugs for Small Animals.

FLORFENICOL

INDICATIONS: Florfenicol (Nuflor✚★) is a synthetic, broad-spectrum, long-acting antibiotic for use in bovine respiratory complex, or shipping fever. It is related to chloramphenicol but because of differing chemical structure is reported to be free of associated risk of adverse effects on human health. A key advantage of this drug is that treatment involves only two IM injections, spaced 48 hours apart, which reduces animal handling. However, at current pricing it may not be cost effective in all situations of shipping fever.

ADVERSE AND COMMON SIDE EFFECTS: No adverse reactions were encountered during the clinical evaluation of this drug. However, transient diarrhea or inappetence may be noted with its use. These signs should abate within a few days after the end of treatment. The drug should not be used in breeding animals because this has not been assessed for safety. Do not inject more than 10 mL at each site. Administer only in the neck musculature.

DRUG INTERACTIONS: None listed.

SUPPLIED AS: VETERINARY PRODUCT
For injection containing 300 mg/mL in 100-, 250-, and 500-mL bottles

FLUMETHASONE

INDICATIONS: Flumethasone (Flucort Solution♥★) is a long-acting glucocorticoid used in horses to treat musculoskeletal injuries and ketosis in cattle. Flumethasone is a modification of prednisolone and is possibly the most potent corticosteroid. Flumethasone has 60 to 80 times the anti-inflammatory and gluconeogenic effects of prednisone, and 4 times that of dexamethasone. Anti-inflammatory effects of flumethasone are beneficial in arthritis and inflammatory conditions in musculoskeletal injuries and in immunologic diseases, such as purpura hemorrhagica, allergic rhinitis, and urticaria. Flumethasone is also useful in the treatment of primary ketosis in cattle. Ophthalmologic preparations are used to reduce uveal tract inflammation (Anaprime♥★). For more information see **GLUCO-CORTICOID AGENTS**.

ADVERSE AND COMMON SIDE EFFECTS: High, continued doses of flumethasone can cause suppression of adrenocortical function. Corticosteroids should not be used in bacterial, viral, or parasitic infections unless concurrent anti-infective agents are used. Clinical signs may abate with their use but the underlying disease remains active. Topical use of corticosteroids on the eye is contraindicated if corneal ulceration is present. If long-term therapy is undertaken, withdrawal should be gradual to avoid problems of iatrogenic adrenal suppression. Corticosteroids given to animals in the last trimester of pregnancy can induce premature parturition and predispose to retained placenta and metritis. Corticosteroids may delay wound healing. See also **GLUCOCORTICOID AGENTS**.

DRUG INTERACTIONS: Corticosteroid actions are potentiated by erythromycin, possibly by interfering with metabolism of the corticosteroids. See also **GLUCOCORTICOID AGENTS**.

SUPPLIED AS: VETERINARY PRODUCTS
For injection containing 0.5 mg/mL
Ophthalmic gel containing 0.10 mg/mL with 5 mg neomycin sulfate and 10,000 IU polymixin B

FLUNIXIN MEGLUMINE

INDICATIONS: Flunixin meglumine (Banamine♥★, Citation★, Cronyxin♥, Equileve★, Equi-Phar Equigesic★, Flumeglumine★, Meflosyl Solution★, Suppressor★) is a nonsteroidal anti-inflammatory drug (NSAID) with analgesic and antipyretic properties similar to those of phenylbutazone. Flunixin meglumine has potent analgesic properties in the horse and may be used to manage the visceral pain of colic. Flunixin is also advocated as a component of therapy for endotoxemic shock of equine colic or coliform mastitis in cattle, where its actions may prevent thromboxane-associated fluid shifts from the general circulation. Flunixin meglumine has been found to reduce lung consolidation in experimentally induced viral pneumonia in calves. Parenteral flunixin is the NSAID of choice for managing inflammation in the equine eye, such as equine recurrent uveitis. This drug is also being used in postoperative abdominal surgery in horses to prevent the occurrence of adhesions. The evidence appears to be based on experimental laboratory data using ibuprofen, with laboratory animals as models. Therefore, the application to horses remains only theoretical.

ADVERSE AND COMMON SIDE EFFECTS: The analgesic properties of flunixin meglumine have been implicated in masking diagnostic signs of profound pain of colic or pleuritis. High doses can cause gastrointestinal ulceration, particularly in hypovolemic animals. Inadvertent intra-arterial injection may cause temporary ataxia, hysteria, hyperventilation, and muscle weakness. The effect of flunixin meglumine on reproduction in horses has not been determined.

DRUG INTERACTIONS: None established.

SUPPLIED AS: VETERINARY PRODUCTS
Granules containing 25 mg/g
Paste containing 50 mg/g
For injection containing 50 mg/mL (equivalent to 83 mg/mL flunixin)

OTHER USES
Horses
ENDOTOXEMIA
For prevention of fluid shifts and vascular damage during endotoxemia at a dose of 0.25 mg/kg qid; IV is suggested.

Cattle
NEONATAL DIARRHEA
2.2 mg/kg bid–tid; IM has been reported to reduce fecal output in calves with secretory diarrhea. However, other treatments for calfhood diarrhea, such as fluid therapy, are far more essential to the survival of the calf.

FLURBIPROFEN

INDICATIONS: Flurbiprofen sodium (Ocufen♣★) is a propionic acid derivative similar to ibuprofen. These compounds are aspirin-like drugs that act to inhibit cyclo-oxygenase but are better tolerated by the patient. Flurbiprofen is used as an ophthalmic medication to decrease ocular inflammation in the horse.

ADVERSE AND COMMON SIDE EFFECTS: Flurbiprofen may induce hypersensitivity and delay wound healing.

DRUG INTERACTIONS: Concurrent ophthalmic use with carbachol negates the desired actions of carbachol. Concurrent administration with some local anesthetics produces greater miotic inhibition.

SUPPLIED AS: HUMAN PRODUCT
Ophthalmic solution containing 0.03%

FOLIC ACID

INDICATIONS: Folic acid (Apo-Folic♣★, Folvite ♣★, Folic Acid Injection★, Foldine♣, Novo-Folacid ♣) is a member of the vitamin B complex group essential for the maintenance of normal erythropoiesis. Folic acid deficiency may occur due to blood loss, prolonged malabsorption, or sulfonamide administration. It may be indicated in cases where pyrimethamine is used on a long-term basis, such as in equine protozoal myelitis. Dietary deficiencies in large animals are rare but there is a suggestion that it may occur in horses fed rations lacking grass.

ADVERSE AND COMMON SIDE EFFECTS: The drug is reportedly nontoxic.

DRUG INTERACTIONS: Chloramphenicol may antagonize the hematologic response.

SUPPLIED AS: HUMAN PRODUCTS
Tablets containing 0.4, 0.8, 1, and 5 mg
For injection containing 5 and 10 mg/mL

FOLLICLE-STIMULATING HORMONE

INDICATIONS: Follicle-stimulating hormone (FSH-P♣★, Folltropin-V♣, Lutropin-V♣, Ovaset♣, Super-OV♣) is a purified pituitary extract with follicle-stimulating hormone (FSH) activity and luteinizing hormone (LH) activity. It is used primarily in sexually mature heifers and cows to induce superovulation. It is also used in mares, cows, sheep, and goats to assist ovulation.

ADVERSE AND COMMON SIDE EFFECTS: None listed.

DRUG INTERACTIONS: None listed.

SUPPLIED AS: VETERINARY PRODUCT
For injection containing 1, 5, 7.5, and 20 mg/mL

FORMALDEHYDE SOLUTION

INDICATIONS: Formaldehyde solution is a bactericidal solution of formaldehyde gas. The solution will kill most bacterial spores, animal viruses, and *Mycobacterium tuberculosis* and as such is used as a reliable disinfectant and fumigant. It will also destroy superficial tissue and has been used for treatment of infections about the hoof corium and between the claws, as occurs in foot rot.

ADVERSE AND COMMON SIDE EFFECTS: Formaldehyde solution is corrosive when applied to normal tissue and gives off a penetrating and irritating gas.

DRUG INTERACTIONS: None listed.

SUPPLIED AS: VETERINARY PRODUCT
Poulty House Fumigator formaldehyde gas at 37% by weight
Also commercially available from chemical supply houses

OTHER USES
Cattle
CHRONIC MASTITIS
Formaldehyde can be administered intramammary to destroy chronically infected quarters in cattle. An intense acute inflammatory reaction is to be expected.

FUROSEMIDE

INDICATIONS: Furosemide (Disal★, Diuride★, Equi-Phar Furosemide Injection★, Furoject★, Furotabs★, Furos-A-Vet★, Furosemide Injection 5%★, Lasix♣★) is a potent loop diuretic that acts to prevent chloride reabsorption in the ascending loop of Henle. Furosemide is used for udder edema in cattle, edema of congestive heart failure, and edema of "stocking up" in horses. It is widely used in the race horse industry to prevent exercise-induced pulmonary hemorrhage, but its efficacy in prevention of such pulmonary hemorrhage remains to be established. However, one of its effects in addition to diuresis, is bronchodilation. Furosemide is also indicated in oliguric renal failure because it is postulated to block the metabolic activity of tubular cells, thereby sparing the metabolic demands of the cells. Furosemide may also enhance renal blood flow.

ADVERSE AND COMMON SIDE EFFECTS: Metabolic alkalosis can occur from contraction of the extracellular fluid volume. It may cause electrolyte disturbances if used more than 48 hours in cattle. Hypokalemia or hyponatremia may occur if used over prolonged periods. Furosemide may lower serum calcium.

DRUG INTERACTIONS: None applicable to large animals.

SUPPLIED AS: VETERINARY PRODUCTS
For injection containing 50 mg/mL
As a bolus containing 2 g
Tablets containing 12.5 and 50 mg

HUMAN PRODUCTS
Tablets containing 20, 40, and 80 mg
Oral solution containing 8 and 10 mg/mL
For injection containing 10 mg/mL

GENTAMICIN

INDICATIONS: Gentamicin (Garacin★, Garasol Pig Pump ♣, Garasol Solution Injectable♣, Gen-Gard★, Gentaglyde Solution★, Gentaject★, Genta Ved 100★, Gentamicin Sulfate Injection★, Gentasul 50♣, Gentasul 100♣, Gentocin I.U.♣★, Gentocin Ophthalmic♣★, Gentocin Solution♣★, Gentocin Spray♣★, Tamycin★) is an aminoglycoside antibiotic effective against predominately gram-negative bacterial infections such as *Escherichia coli* and *Pseudomonas*. It is used for soft tissue infections, endometritis, metritis, and pyometra. It is also used in the treatment of bacteremia or septicemia in neonatal foals caused by *E. coli*, *Proteus*, *Pseudomonas*, or *Klebsiella*. Most anaerobes are resistant to gentamicin. Gentamicin has been used in cattle for treating acute coliform mastitis, but the need for any antibiotic treatment in this disease has been questioned. If serum level monitoring is available, the peak should be 10 μg/mL and the trough less than 1.0 μg/mL. See also **AMINOGLYCOSIDE ANTIBIOTICS**.

ADVERSE AND COMMON SIDE EFFECTS: Gentamicin should be used with caution in animals with compromised kidney function. It is contraindicated in cases of severe renal impairment. Toxic levels can cause renal tubular damage, which may be reversible once the drug is discontinued. Avoid concurrent use with other aminoglycosides because of the potential additive toxic effects. The drug causes transient pain on injection. Ototoxicity can occur but is difficult to detect clinically. Weakness from neuromuscular blockade can occur at high doses. Recent evidence suggests that renal toxicity may be lessened by once daily administration of the total dose.

DRUG INTERACTIONS: Concurrent use of furosemide can increase the ototoxic potential. Dehydration can predispose to renal tubular damage. Gentamicin is not to be mixed with any other product.

SUPPLIED AS: VETERINARY PRODUCTS
For injection containing 5, 50, and 100 mg/mL
Oral solution containing 4.35 mg/mL

Intrauterine solution containing 10 mg/mL
Ophthalmic solution containing 3 mg/mL or spray containing 1 mg/mL
Soluble powder containing 5 g/75 g, 6 g/18 g, and 2 g/30 g

OTHER USES
Gentocin is also contained in combination with corticosteroids for use as in ophthalmic (Gentocin Durafilm♣) and topical (Otomax Ointment♣, Topagen Ointment♣, Topagen Spray♣) preparations. Injectable products have been used subconjunctivally for the treatment of corneal ulcers when topical ointments or drops are not practical.

GLUCOCORTICOID AGENTS

INDICATIONS: Glucocorticoid agents are recommended for the treatment of allergic and immune-mediated diseases, cardiogenic and septic shock, and trauma and edema of the central nervous system and spinal cord. Beneficial effects include stabilization of lysosomal and capillary membranes, decrease in activation of the complement and clotting cascades, binding of endotoxin, positive inotropic effect, dilation of precapillary sphincters, prevention of gastrointestinal mucosal ischemia associated with shock, increase in glucogenesis, inhibition of the formation of vasoactive substances (kinins, prostaglandins), decrease in collagen and scar formation, and decrease in the accumulation of phagocytes at areas of inflammation. Analgesic activity is only related to prostaglandin inhibition. These agents do not possess direct analgesic activity.

The glucocorticoids are classified according to their duration of action. As biologic half-life increases, anti-inflammatory potency increases and mineralocorticoid potency decreases. Short-acting drugs (<12 hours) include hydrocortisone and cortisone acetate. Intermediate-acting drugs (12–36 hours) include prednisone, prednisolone, methylprednisolone, and triamcinolone. The long-acting steroids (>48 hours) include paramethasone, flumethasone, betamethasone, and dexamethasone. Topical corticosteroids are used for their local anti-inflammatory, antipruritic, and vasoconstrictive effects.

ADVERSE AND COMMON SIDE EFFECTS: Polyuria, polydipsia, polyphagia, panting, lethargy, weakness, and bilateral symmetrical alopecia are the most common clinical signs of glucocorticoid excess. Weight loss, anorexia, and diarrhea may also follow use of these drugs. Hemorrhagic gastroenteritis, pancreatitis, and hepatopathy have been reported with the use of corticosteroids. Glucocorticoid drugs suppress inflammation, reduce fever, increase protein catabolism and their conversion to carbohydrates leading to a negative nitrogen balance, promote sodium retention and potassium diuresis, retard wound healing, lower resistance to infection, and cause a reduction in the number of circulating lymphocytes. Iatrogenic hyperadrenocorticism may follow prolonged use of parenteral as well as topical glucocorticoid agents. Glucocorticoids are contraindicated in animals with acute or chronic bacterial infections unless therapeutic doses of an effective bactericidal agent are used concurrently. Corticosteroids may mask signs of infection such as elevation in body temperature. These drugs should be used with caution in animals with congestive heart failure, diabetes mellitus, and renal disease. Their use during the healing phase of bone fractures is not recommended. Corticosteroids have been associated with increased incidence of cleft palate and other congenital malformations. In addition, their use may be associated with the induction of the first stage of parturition when administered during the last trimester of pregnancy and may precipitate premature parturition followed by dystocia, fetal death, retained placenta, and metritis.

DRUG INTERACTIONS: Glucocorticoids may decrease the efficacy of bacteriostatic antibiotics by decreasing the inflammatory response and diminishing the phagocytic activity of leukocytes. Amphotericin B, furosemide, and the thiazide diuretics may potentiate hypokalemia. Hypokalemia may predispose to digitalis toxicity. Glucocorticoids may reduce serum salicylate levels. Phenytoin, phenobarbital, and rifampin may increase the metabolism of glucocorticoids, and insulin requirements of diabetic patients may increase. Hepatic metabolism of methylprednisolone may be inhibited by erythromycin. The concomitant use of glucocorticoids and cyclosporine may lead to increases in serum levels of both drugs. Live attenuated-virus vaccines should generally not be given to animals receiving glucocorticoid drugs. Concurrent use of nonsteroidal anti-inflammatory drugs may increase the potential for gastrointestinal ulceration. Estrogens may potentiate the effects of hydrocortisone and other glucocorticoids.

SUPPLIED AS: See specific product.

GLYCEROL

INDICATIONS: Glycerol [glycerin] (Glycerol♥★) is an inert substance used to soothe and relieve inflammation primarily involving mucous membranes. In the horse, its anhydrous form has been advocated for oral use in the treatment of central nervous system trauma to manage cerebral edema. Glycerol is also nebulized into the respiratory tract to rehydrate and emulsify secretions. Glycerol [glycerin] is also used in many topical medications as a vehicle.

ADVERSE AND COMMON SIDE EFFECTS: At high concentrations glycerin will absorb water and is irritating and dehydrating to exposed tissue. If used as an aerosol, glycerol is irritating and can cause bronchoconstriction.

DRUG INTERACTIONS: None listed.

SUPPLIED AS: CHEMICAL PRODUCT
Anhydrous glycerin containing 99.95% glycerol

GLYCOPYRROLATE

INDICATIONS: Glycopyrrolate (Glycopyrrolate Injection★, Robinul♣★, Robinul-V♣★, Robinul Forte♣★) is an anticholinergic drug similar in action to atropine. Relative to atropine, glycopyrrolate has more effective antisialogue effects and is less likely to cause significant tachycardia while being more effective at blocking bradyarrhythmias. Glycopyrrolate is also more effective than atropine at blocking gastric acid secretion. Glycopyrrolate has been used in the horse to block intestinal peristalsis while performing rectal palpation.

ADVERSE AND COMMON SIDE EFFECTS: Mydriasis and xerostomia may be noted with its use. Excretion of the drug may be prolonged in animals with impaired renal or gastrointestinal function. It should not be given to pregnant animals. Refer also to Adverse and Common Side Effects of **ATROPINE**, which would be expected to be similar.

DRUG INTERACTIONS: As for **ATROPINE**, which include enhancement of activity if used with antihistamines, procainamide, quinidine, meperidine, benzodiazepines, and phenothiazines. Adverse effects may be potentiated by primidone and long-term corticosteroid use (via increasing intraocular pressure). Glycopyrrolate may enhance the actions of nitrofurantoin, thiazide diuretics, and sympathomimetic agents. The drug may antagonize the activity of metoclopramide.

SUPPLIED AS: VETERINARY PRODUCT
For injection containing 0.2 mg/mL ★

HUMAN PRODUCTS
Tablets containing 1 and 2 mg
For injection containing 0.2 mg/mL

OTHER USES
Horses
RESPIRATORY DISEASE
Recently, glycopyrrolate has been used in aerosol form for treatment of chronic obstructive lung disease.

GONADORELIN

INDICATIONS: Gonadorelin [GnRH] (Cystorelin♥★, Factrel♥★, Fertiline♥, Fertagyl♣) is a decapeptide hypothalamic-releasing factor responsible for stimulating the release of follicle-stimulating hormone and luteinizing hormone from the anterior pituitary gland. Gonadorelin is used to treat ovarian follicular cysts (cystic ovaries) in cattle with incomplete luteinization. Most cysts on the ovaries will clear within 3 days of injection.

ADVERSE AND COMMON SIDE EFFECTS: None have been reported at 10 times the recommended dose.

DRUG INTERACTIONS: None reported.

SUPPLIED AS: VETERINARY PRODUCT
For injection containing 50 and 100 µg/mL

OTHER USES
Horses and Cattle

Gonadorelin has also been used empirically to induce ovulation at the time of breeding in both cattle and horses. It has also been advocated for treatment of stallions with lowered libido.

GRISEOFULVIN

INDICATIONS: Griseofulvin (Fulvicin U/F♥★, Fulvicin U/F Powder♥★, Griseofulvin P/G♣, Grisovin FP♣, Grifulvin V★, Grisactin★, Gris-PEG★, Grivate★) is an oral fungistatic antibiotic used in the treatment of infections by dermatophytic fungi of the skin, hair, and claws. Griseofulvin inhibits the growth of various species of *Microsporum, Epidermophyton,* and *Trichophyton* and is used primarily to treat ringworm in horses and calves. It is ineffective against other fungi, including *Candida*. On oral administration, griseofulvin is deposited in new epithelial cells that make up the skin, hair, and claws and prevents fungal infection of the newly formed tissues. The microsize formulation has a fine particle size with a greater surface area for absorption, resulting in higher blood levels in human studies.

ADVERSE AND COMMON SIDE EFFECTS: Griseofulvin may interfere with spermatogenesis. Although teratogenic effects have been seen in cats, griseofulvin has been fed to mares for alternate 30-day periods with no abnormal effects. The manufacturer, however, suggests it not be given to pregnant mares or breeding stock. Hepatotoxicity and photosensitization have also been reported but are rare. The drug is not to be used in horses intended for food.

DRUG INTERACTIONS: Phenobarbital decreases absorption of the drug. Coumarin anticoagulant activity may be reduced by griseofulvin. Vaccination or viral infection induces interferon synthesis, which in turn inhibits hepatic enzyme systems and may prolong the elimination of griseofulvin.

SUPPLIED AS: VETERINARY PRODUCTS
Tablets (microsize) containing 250 and 500 mg★
Powder containing 2.5 g/15-g packet

HUMAN PRODUCTS
Tablets (microsize or ultramicrosize) containing 125, 165, 250, 333, and 500 mg
Capsules containing 250 mg
Suspension containing 125 mg/5 mL

OTHER USES
Horses

Griseofulvin can also be used for the treatment of equine sporotrichosis.

GUAIFENESIN

INDICATIONS: Guaifenesin [formerly glyceryl guaiacolate] (Guailaxin★) is a centrally acting muscle relaxant with sedative and analgesic effects. It is used in large animals to treat convulsions, and for induction of general anesthesia, usually in combination with an ultrashort-acting barbiturate. The duration of action is brief, with a single muscle relaxant dose lasting 15 to 40 minutes. The primary disadvantage of guaifenesin is the large volume of parenteral solution required to produce sedation. Guaifenesin also has expectorant properties. It reduces the stickiness of mucus in chronic bronchitis and accelerates airway particle clearance.

ADVERSE AND COMMON SIDE EFFECTS: Inadvertent perivascular injection can result in tissue sloughing. If used at higher than recommended parenteral doses, guaifenesin can cause respiratory paralysis. Concentrations greater than 5% can cause hemolysis. Females may have more rapid elimination of guaifenesin and require more frequent dosing to maintain effects.

DRUG INTERACTIONS: Physostigmine and other cholinesterase agents (e.g., neostigmine, pyridostigmine, and edrophonium) are contraindicated with its use.

SUPPLIED AS: VETERINARY PRODUCT
For injection containing 50 g/1,000 mL (reconstitute 50 g with 954 mL sterile water)

OTHER USES
Horses and Cattle

Guaifenesin is also found in combination expectorant products (Guaitex♣) for use in large animals as an aid to liquefy respiratory secretions.

HALOTHANE

INDICATIONS: Halothane (Fluothane♣★, Halothane BP♣) is an inhalant drug used for the induction of general anesthesia. It is a fast, potent anesthetic that allows for smooth induction without excitement and a quick, uneventful recovery.

ADVERSE AND COMMON SIDE EFFECTS: Dose-dependent hypotension has been documented. Hepatic necrosis, although rare, may occur with the use of halothane, the incidence of which increases with each use of this agent. Should unexplained fever, jaundice, or other signs of liver dysfunction occur, its subsequent use in that animal is contraindicated. High doses of halothane may cause uterine atony and postpartum bleeding, and it is generally not recommended for obstetrical procedures unless uterine relaxation is required. Goats may be especially sensitive to halothane-induced liver disease, but this remains poorly documented.

DRUG INTERACTIONS: The drug is potentially arrhythmogenic, especially in the presence of epinephrine and the thiobarbiturates. Use with D-tubocurare can cause a reduction in blood pressure.

SUPPLIED AS: HUMAN AND VETERINARY PRODUCT
Halothane is supplied in 250 mL bottles

HEPARIN

INDICATIONS: Heparin (Calcilean♣, Calciparin★, Heparin Sodium Injection★, Hep-Lock★, Hepalean-Lok♣, Hepalean♣, Heparin Leo♣, Liquaemin Sodium★) is a potent endogenous anticoagulant. It is used in horses at risk for thrombosis, such as in endotoxemia and animals at risk for developing disseminated intravascular coagulation (DIC). Heparin is also used empirically in acute laminitis because one proposed pathogenesis of the disease includes microthrombi formation in the vessels of the hoof. In the case of burn victims, heparin has been used to increase the effectiveness of repair mechanisms, to decrease thrombosis and the development of gangrene, and to protect against the development of DIC. In studies on an ischemic bowel model in horses, heparin has been shown to reduce abdominal adhesion formation. The mechanism is presumed to be interfering with the formation of thrombin, thus preventing conversion of fibrinogen to fibrin.

ADVERSE AND COMMON SIDE EFFECTS: Bleeding and thrombocytopenia are the most common adverse effects of the drug, leading to prolonged activated partial thromboplastin time. Horses develop a temporary anemia, which is thought to occur from enhanced phagocytosis of red blood cells by the reticuloendothelial system. Protamine zinc may be used to reverse the adverse effects of bleeding. IM injection can result in hematoma formation, and SC injection may result in edema at the injection site. Other side effects reported have included osteoporosis with long-term use, diminished renal function following long-term, high-dose therapy, rebound hyperlipidemia, hyperkalemia, alopecia, suppressed aldosterone synthesis, and priapism.

DRUG INTERACTIONS: Heparin may antagonize the action of corticosteroids, insulin, and corticotropin and increase serum levels of diazepam. Antihistamines, IV nitroglycerin, digoxin, and tetracyclines may antagonize the effects of heparin. Heparin should be used with caution with other drugs that may adversely affect coagulation, such as aspirin, phenylbutazone, dextran, dipyridamole, and warfarin.

SUPPLIED AS: HUMAN PRODUCTS
Sodium Salt
For injection containing 2, 10, 40, 50, 100, 1,000, 2,000, 2,500, 5,000, 7,500, 10,000, 20,000, 25,000, and 40,000 U/mL
Calcium Salt
For injection containing 25,000 U/mL

OTHER USES
Horses
ACUTE LAMINITIS
40 to 100 IU/kg; SC, IV

HYPERLIPEMIA
100 to 250 IU/kg; IV for use in ponies and horses with hyperlipemia to stimulate lipoprotein lipase. Lower doses of 40 IU/kg; IV have been beneficial and lessen the risk of inducing blood clotting problems.

ABDOMINAL ADHESION PREVENTION
40 IU/kg at surgery and 40 to 80 IU bid for 48 hours; IV for the first dose, then SC

HYALURONIC ACID

INDICATIONS: Hyaluronic acid [sodium hyaluronidase] (Equron★, Equiflex★, HY50★, Hy-50Hylan♣, Hyalovet 20♣★, Hyalovet Syringe Vials★, Hylartil Vet♣, Hylartin-V★, Hyonate♣, Hyvisc★, Legend Injectable Solution★, Synacid♣★) is a naturally occurring substance present in connective tissue that functions within joints to act as a lubricant and shock absorber. Hyaluronic acid may also provide nourishment to articular cartilage and has anti-inflammatory properties. Hyaluronic acid is used intra-articularly or injected into peritendinous areas for treatment of noninfectious degenerative joint disease or tendinous/ligamentous injuries. Injections may be repeated, but no more frequently than at 2-week intervals.

ADVERSE AND COMMON SIDE EFFECTS: Transient heat or swelling may occur following intra-articular injection but should resolve spontaneously without treatment within 96 hours.

DRUG INTERACTIONS: None listed.

SUPPLIED AS: VETERINARY PRODUCT
For injection containing 5, 10, and 17 mg/mL

HYDRALAZINE

INDICATIONS: Hydralazine (Apresoline♥★, Apo-Hydralazine♥, Novo-Hydralazin♥, Nu-Hydral♥, Hydralazine Hydrochloride Injection★) is an arterial vasodilator. It helps increase cardiac output and decrease mitral regurgitation and left atrial size. Data are only available for its use in healthy horses and at this time its place for treating cardiac problems in horses is not established.

ADVERSE AND COMMON SIDE EFFECTS and **DRUG INTERACTIONS:** None yet described for large animals. See **HYDRALAZINE** in Description of Drugs for Small Animals.

SUPPLIED AS: HUMAN PRODUCTS
Tablets containing 10, 25, 50, and 100 mg
For injection containing 20 mg/mL

HYDROCHLOROTHIAZIDE

INDICATIONS: Hydrochlorothiazide (Aquazide-H★, Apo-Hydro♥, Diaqua★, Diuchlor H♥, Esidrex★, Hydro-D★, HydroDiuril♥★, Hydrozide Injection★, Mictrin★, Neo-Codema♥, Novo-Hydrazide♥, Oretic★, Urozide♥) is a diuretic suggested for use as maintenance therapy for periodic paralysis in horses.

ADVERSE AND COMMON SIDE EFFECTS: Hypokalemia, hypochloremic alkalosis, dilutional hyponatremia, and loss of water-soluble vitamins may occur with chronic use. Other side effects may include diarrhea, polyuria, hyperglycemia, hyperlipidemia, hypotension, and hypersensitivity/dermatologic reactions.

DRUG INTERACTIONS: Concurrent use with corticosteroids, corticotropin, or amphotericin B may predispose to hypokalemia. Thiazide hypokalemia, hypomagnesemia, or hypocalcemia predisposes to digitalis toxicity and hydrochlorothiazide may prolong the half-life of quinidine due to alkalinization of the urine. Sulfonamides may potentiate the action of hydrochlorothiazide. Diuretics may increase the risk of nonsteroidal anti-inflammatory drug-induced renal failure secondary to decreased renal blood flow.

SUPPLIED AS: VETERINARY PRODUCT
For injection containing 25 mg/mL

HUMAN PRODUCTS
Tablets containing 25, 50, and 100 mg
Oral solution containing 10 mg/mL

HYDROCORTISONE SODIUM SUCCINATE

INDICATIONS: Hydrocortisone sodium succinate (Solu-Cortef♣★, A-Hydrocort★★) is a glucocorticoid primarily used in cases of allergic reactions or shock or in animals suffering venomous snake bite. Use of this specific glucocorticoid drug for large animals is seldom essential and can be prohibitively expensive. For information concerning adverse and common side effects and drug interactions, see **GLUCOCORTICOID AGENTS**.

SUPPLIED AS: HUMAN PRODUCT
For injection containing 100, 250, 500, and 1,000 mg/vial

HYDROXYZINE

INDICATIONS: Hydroxyzine (Anxanil★, Apo-Hydroxyzine♣, Atarax♣★, E-Vista★, Hydroxacen★, Hyzine-50★, Hy-Pan★, Multipox♣, Neucalm★, Novo-Hydroxyzin♣, Nu-Hydroxyzin♣, PMS-Hydroxyzine♣, Quiess★, Vistaject-25★, Vistaril★, Vistacon 50★, Vistaject-50★, Vistazine★) is an anxiolytic, antihistaminic agent. The drug also has anticholinergic, antiemetic, and bronchodilator effects. It has been used in horses and ruminants for the treatment of urticaria.

ADVERSE AND COMMON SIDE EFFECTS: Transitory drowsiness is the most common side effect.

DRUG INTERACTIONS: Barbiturates and other sedatives may potentiate central nervous system depression. Hydroxyzine inhibits and reverses the vasopressor effect of epinephrine.

SUPPLIED AS: HUMAN PRODUCTS
Tablets and capsules containing 10, 25, 50, and 100 mg (Hydrochloride and Pamoate Salts)
Syrup containing 10 mg/5 mL
For injection containing 25 and 50 mg/mL

IMIPRAMINE

INDICATIONS: Imipramine (Apo-Imipramine♣, Impril♣, Janimine★, Norfranil★, Novo-Pramine♣, PMS-Imipramine♣, Tipramine★, Tofranil♣★, Tofranil-PM★) is a tricyclic antidepressant structurally related to phenothiazines and is used in horses for the treatment of narcolepsy. It has also been used to treat ejaculatory dysfunction in stallions.

ADVERSE AND COMMON SIDE EFFECTS: In humans, hypotension, tachycardia, arrhythmias, anxiety, ataxia, seizure, constipation, mydriasis, urinary retention, pruritus, anorexia, vomiting, diarrhea, jaundice, and bone marrow suppression leading to granulocytopenia and thrombocytopenia have been documented. Experience with the drug in horses is minimal.

DRUG INTERACTIONS: Barbiturates potentiate adverse effects of imipramine but decrease serum levels of the drug. Cimetidine increases serum imipramine levels. Phenothiazines may enhance the drug's effects.

SUPPLIED AS: HUMAN PRODUCTS
Tablets containing 10, 25, 50, and 75 mg (hydrochloride and pamoate salts)
Injection containing 12.5 mg/mL

INSULIN

INDICATIONS: Insulin (Purified Pork Regular Insulin★, Regular Iletin II Pork, 500 Units★, Novolin R★, Iletin Regular♣, Humulin-R♣★, Velosulin BR Human★ [short-acting], Caninsulin♣, Iletin NPH♣, Novolin-N★, Humulin-N♣★, Purified Pork Lente Insulin★, Iletin II Pork Lente♣★, Iletin Lente♣, Iletin I Lente★, Iletin II★ [intermediate-acting] and Novolin-Ultralente♣, Humulin-U♣★ [long-acting] and many others) are used in the management of ketosis and hepatic lipidosis in cattle and hyperlipemia in horses and ponies. Insulin is also indicated for emergency treatment of hyperkalemia-associated electrocardiographic abnormalities that occur in foals with ruptured bladders. Most current large animal veterinary literature refers to use of protamine zinc insulin, a long-acting formulation that, unfortunately, is no longer available.

ADVERSE AND COMMON SIDE EFFECTS: Overdose may cause hypoglycemia leading to disorientation, weakness, hunger, seizure, coma, and death. If overdose occurs, the animal should be fed sugar with water or food. If seizures occur, dextrose solutions should be given IV until seizure activity stops.

DRUG INTERACTIONS: Information regarding drug interactions with use of insulin in large animals is sparse. See **INSULIN** in Description of Drugs for Small Animals.

SUPPLIED AS: HUMAN PRODUCTS
For injection containing 100 U/mL
Available in short-acting (regular), intermediate-acting, and long-acting formulations
Human semisynthetic and recombinant DNA origin, pork, and beef and pork formulations

VETERINARY PRODUCT
For injection containing 40 U/ mL (Caninsulin✤)

OTHER USES
Horses
HYPERLIPEMIA (PONIES)
30 U long-acting insulin/200 kg bid; IM with 100 g glucose bid; PO on the first and succeeding odd days. 15 U long-acting insulin/200 kg bid with 100 g galactose daily; PO on even days.

IODOCHLORHYDROXYQUIN

INDICATIONS: Iodochlorhydroxyquin [clioquinol] (Rheaform★) is used empirically in horses for treatment of chronic diarrhea. It is thought to work by altering colonic microbial flora. It may provide temporary cessation of clinical signs.

ADVERSE AND COMMON SIDE EFFECTS: In humans, iodochlorhydroxyquin administered at high doses or for prolonged periods of time has been associated with a toxic neuropathy, with optic neuropathy, and with a permanent loss of vision. There are no such reports in the horse.

DRUG INTERACTIONS: None listed.

SUPPLIED AS: VETERINARY PRODUCT
Boluses containing 10 g

IPATROMIUM BROMIDE

INDICATIONS: Ipatromium bromide (Atrovent✤) is an anticholinergic agent that when administered by aerosol causes bronchodilation by blockade of M_3-muscarinic receptors on smooth muscle. The compound's quaternary structure discourages systemic absorption from the respiratory tract. Additionally, unlike other parasympatholytic agents, ipatromium bromide does not inhibit mucociliary clearance. It has been used for its bronchodilating effects in horses with recurrent airway obstruction (heaves or chronic obstructive pulmonary disease). Its onset of action is slower than after β_2-adrenoceptor agonists, but the effects tend to be longer lasting, at 4 to 6 hours.

ADVERSE AND COMMON SIDE EFFECTS: Ipatromium bromide should not be used for the abatement of acute bronchospasm because of its relatively slow onset of action. If ipatromium reaches the eye, there can be ocular complications of mydriasis, increased intraocular pressure, glaucoma, and eye pain.

DRUG INTERACTIONS: In humans the bronchodilative effect is additive to theophylline and β-adrenoceptor agonists. Ipatromium should be used with caution in patients receiving other anticholinergic drugs because of possible additive effects.

SUPPLIED AS: HUMAN PRODUCT
Solution; each mL contains ipratropium 0.25% in isotonic solution
Aerosol containing 20 µg/actuation

IRON DEXTRAN

INDICATIONS: Iron dextran (Actoferon✚, APA FER-100✚, Co-op Injectable Iron✚, Dexafer✚, Injectable Iron✚★, Injectable Iron Dextran★, Injectable Iron 10%★, and others) is indicated for the treatment of iron deficiency anemia.

ADVERSE AND COMMON SIDE EFFECTS: IM injection can be irritating. Allergic reactions and anaphylaxis have occasionally been reported in people.

DRUG INTERACTIONS: Clinical response may be delayed in patients concurrently receiving chloramphenicol.

SUPPLIED AS: VETERINARY PRODUCTS
For injection containing 100 and 200 mg elemental iron/mL

ISOFLUPREDONE

INDICATIONS: Isoflupredone (Predef 2X Sterile Aqueous Suspension✚★) is a potent corticosteroid used for treatment of bovine ketosis. Isoflupredone has glycogen deposition activity and is 10 times more potent than prednisone for gluconeogenic activity. Administration to ketotic cows causes blood glucose levels to return to normal levels, followed by a reduction in blood and urine ketones. Generally, there is a concomitant increase in appetite and rise in milk production to previous levels within 3 to 5 days following injection.

Isoflupredone is also indicated for musculoskeletal injuries in cattle and horses and for treatment of allergic reactions. Although it has been suggested for use as an adjunctive treatment of overwhelming sepsis, the dose required based on extrapolation from human data is highly impractical, and the efficacy of corticosteroid treatment in such circumstances is highly debatable.

ADVERSE AND COMMON SIDE EFFECTS: Isoflupredone should not be given for ketosis secondary to pneumonia, mastitis, or metritis unless accompanied by appropriate antibiotic treatment. As for most glucocorticoids, suppression of signs of inflammation may mask signs of infection.

DRUG INTERACTIONS: See GLUCOCORTICOID AGENTS.

SUPPLIED AS: VETERINARY PRODUCT
For injection containing 2 mg/mL

OTHER USES
Horses
MUSCULOSKELETAL INFLAMMATION
5 to 20 mg; IM
5 to 20 mg; intra-articularly or into synovial sheaths

ISOFLURANE

INDICATIONS: Isoflurane (Aerrane♥★, Forane♥★, IsoFlo♥★, Iso-Thesia★) is an inhalant anesthetic agent. It is especially useful in horses because induction and recovery times are more rapid with isoflurane than with halothane. Cardiovascular status is better maintained with isoflurane, and isoflurane does not sensitize the heart to epinephrine-induced cardiac arrhythmias as does halothane.

ADVERSE AND COMMON SIDE EFFECTS: Dose-dependent cardiac and respiratory depression occurs. Hypotension, respiratory depression, arrhythmias, nausea, and postoperative ileus have been reported. Studies in ponies suggest that isoflurane may be more likely than halothane to produce anesthetic-associated myopathy even when arterial blood pressure is maintained above 60 mm Hg.

DRUG INTERACTIONS: Isoflurane potentiates the effects of muscle relaxants.

SUPPLIED AS: HUMAN AND VETERINARY PRODUCT
Supplied in 100-mL bottle

ISONIAZID

INDICATIONS: Isoniazid (Dom-Isoniazid♣, Isotamine ♣★, Isoniazid♣★, Nydrazid★, Laniazid★, PMS-Isoniazid♣) is used to treat actinomycosis of the mandible in cattle and, in combination with rifampin, tuberculosis in horses. It is inexpensive and readily consumed in small amounts of grain.

ADVERSE AND COMMON SIDE EFFECTS: Isoniazid appears nontoxic at the recommended dosage but may cause abortion and thus should not be used in pregnant cattle. In humans, isoniazid can cause severe liver damage. Peripheral neuritis is the most common side effect in humans.

DRUG INTERACTIONS: Isoniazid inhibits the breakdown of phenytoin if both drugs are administered concurrently. Aluminum hydroxide gel decreases gastrointestinal absorption of isoniazid and if used concurrently should be administered at least 1 hour after isoniazid.

SUPPLIED AS: HUMAN PRODUCTS
Tablets containing 50, 100, and 300 mg
Syrup containing 10 mg/mL
Injection containing 100 mg/mL

ISOPROTERENOL

INDICATIONS: Isoproterenol (Isuprel♣★) is a β-adrenergic agent used for the short-term management of incomplete heart block, sinus bradycardia, and sick sinus syndrome, but is seldom used for these problems in large animals. It also is used to promote bronchodilation, but other more selective drugs are available.

ADVERSE AND COMMON SIDE EFFECTS: Nervous excitation, weakness, tachycardia, and ectopic beat formation are reported. The drug is considered more arrhythmogenic than dopamine or dobutamine, so it is rarely used in the treatment of heart failure or shock.

DRUG INTERACTIONS: Digitalis may have additive effects and lead to arrhythmias if used with isoproterenol. If used with theophylline or epinephrine, there is a possibility of increased cardiotoxic effects. Its effects are antagonized by propranolol.

SUPPLIED AS: HUMAN PRODUCTS
For injection containing 0.02 and 0.2 mg/mL
For inhalation delivering 125 (♣) and 131 µg/dose (★) and also as a 1:100 or 1:200 solution
Sublingual tablets containing 10 mg

ISOXSUPRINE

INDICATIONS: Isoxsuprine (Vasodilan★) is a β_2-adrenergic agent that relaxes myometrial and vascular smooth muscle. It is used in horses to treat navicular disease. Isoxsuprine has also been used empirically in acute laminitis to increase blood flow to the hooves. However, as one of the main proposed pathophysiologic mechanisms involves intense α-adrenergic vasoconstriction, specific α-blockers would be more logical treatment (see **PHENOXYBENZAMINE**).

ADVERSE AND COMMON SIDE EFFECTS: Side effects in humans include tachycardia, hypotension, abdominal distress, and severe rash.

DRUG INTERACTIONS: None listed.

SUPPLIED AS: HUMAN PRODUCTS
Tablets containing 10 and 20 mg
(no longer commercially available in Canada as of 1994, but can be obtained as powder)

ITRACONAZOLE

INDICATIONS: Itraconazole (Sporanox✦★) is an imidazole derivative similar to ketoconazole used for treating superficial and systemic fungal infections. The primary effect of imidazoles on fungi is their ability to alter membrane permeability by blocking synthesis of cellular sterols. Equine sporotrichosis and osteomyelitis associated with *Coccidioides immitis* have been successfully treated with this product. Additionally, mycotic nasal granulomas were eliminated in two horses with *Aspergillus* infections, but itraconazole was not successful in *Conidiobolus coronatus* rhinitis in another horse.

ADVERSE AND COMMON SIDE EFFECTS: Specific data are not available. In a recent report, three horses given 3 mg/kg bid; PO for 3 to 4.5 months showed no adverse side effects. See also **KETO-CONAZOLE**.

DRUG INTERACTIONS: Unknown.

SUPPLIED AS: HUMAN PRODUCT
Capsules containing 100 mg

IVERMECTIN

INDICATIONS: Ivermectin (Heartgard✦★, Ivomec ✦★, Eqvalan✦★) is a broad-spectrum antiparasitic agent. It is used in large animals for the eradication of adult and most larval stages of most gastrointestinal roundworms and lungworm of the *Dictyocaulus* spp, and ectoparasites, such as lice, mites, and certain insect larva, including cattle grub (*Hypoderma bovis, Hypoderma lineatum*), nasal bot (*Oestrus ovis*) of sheep, and nasal bots (*Gasterophilus intestinalis, Gasterophilus nasalis*) in horses. Ivermectin has no activity against flukes or tapeworms. In small ruminants ivermectin has close to 100% efficacy against gastrointestinal nematodes and certain lungworms and is effective treatment against mange mites. It is not effective against *Mullerius capillarius, Trichuris* spp, or *Nematodirus* spp. Recent evidence suggests resistance to ivermectin is developing in some intestinal parasites affecting small ruminants. Ivermectin use in dairy cows at therapeutic doses may result in detectable levels of ivermectin in the plasma for more than 3 months after injection.

ADVERSE AND COMMON SIDE EFFECTS: Ivermectin has a wide margin of safety. IM injection in horses has been associated with death in rare instances, presumably due to clostridial myositis at the site of injection. Horses will occasionally develop transitory ventral edema due to death of microfilaria of *Onchocerca*. No treatment is usually required.

DRUG INTERACTIONS: None listed.

SUPPLIED AS: VETERINARY PRODUCTS
For injection containing 1% (for use in cattle, swine, and sheep; NOT for use in horses)
Premix for swine containing 0.6%
Drench for sheep containing 0.08%
Pour-on 0.5% (for use in cattle)
Oral paste 1.87% (for use in horse) containing 120 mg/6.42g
Oral liquid 1% (10 mg/mL)
Sustained-release bolus containing 1.72 g
Tablets containing 68, 136, and 272 µg

OTHER USES
Horses

AORTOILIAC THROMBOSIS
Ivermectin is used in South America at high doses for treatment of aortoiliac thrombosis. This disease is considered to be reasonably common and the treatment, though empirical, is said to be effective.

KANAMYCIN

INDICATIONS: Kanamycin (Kantrim★) is an aminoglycoside antibiotic with activity against *Staphylococcus aureus* and *albus, Klebsiella pneumonia, Salmonella* spp, *Enterobacteraerogenes, Pasteurella* spp,

Corynebacterium spp, *Bacillus anthracis*, *Proteus*, *Escherichia coli*, and *A. aerogenes*. It penetrates most body fluids other than spinal fluid. Also see **AMINOGLYCOSIDE ANTIBIOTICS**.

ADVERSE AND COMMON SIDE EFFECTS: Impairment of vestibular function or irreversible hearing loss may occur if dosage is excessive or use prolonged. Weight loss often precedes ototoxicity. Nephrotoxicity may occur, especially in toxic, poorly hydrated patients. At higher doses, local irritation at the injection site may occur. The drug has also been shown to decrease cardiac output and produce hypotension and bradycardia. Cardiac arrest has been reported in humans overdosed with the drug. Also see **AMINOGLYCOSIDE ANTIBIOTICS**.

DRUG INTERACTIONS: The potential for ototoxicity increases if kanamycin is used with other aminoglycosides. Furosemide and mannitol potentiate ototoxicity. Amphotericin B, vancomycin, cephalosporins, and inhibitors of prostaglandin synthesis (e.g., nonsteroidal anti-inflammatory drugs [NSAIDs]) potentiate nephrotoxicity. Anesthetics and succinylcholine or tubocurare may have an additive neuromuscular blocking effect. Calcium gluconate can be given IV to reverse aminoglycoside-induced neuromuscular blockade or myocardial depression and to restore blood pressure. Penicillins and aminoglycosides should not be mixed in the same syringe because inactivation of the aminoglycoside may result. Extended-spectrum penicillins, especially carbenicillin, inactivate aminoglycosides. NSAIDs can increase serum levels of aminoglycosides, possibly related to decreased urinary output. Also see **AMINOGLYCOSIDE ANTIBIOTICS**.

SUPPLIED AS: VETERINARY PRODUCT
For injection containing 50 and 200 mg/mL

KAOLIN-PECTIN

INDICATIONS: Kaolin-pectin (Kaopectate Suspension♥, K-D-Sol♥★, Kaolin-Pectin★, Kaolin Pectin Suspension★, Kaolin-Pectin Plus Powder★, Kaolin-Pectin Powder★, Kaolin-Pectin Plus★, Kao-Pec★, Kaopectolin★, Kao-Pect +★, Kaopectol★) is a gastrointestinal protectant used in the management of diarrhea. It coats the surface of the gut and exerts a mild demulcent and absorbent effect. It is ineffective in absorbing toxins produced by enteropathogenic bacteria. It appears to act by adding particulate matter to the feces, which serves to improve consistency until the disease spontaneously resolves. Kaolin is a potent coagulation activator and may be of some benefit in treating diarrhea associated with mucosal disruption and hemorrhage, such as coronavirus infection in calves.

ADVERSE AND COMMON SIDE EFFECTS: Kaolin-pectin may cause constipation, especially in poorly hydrated patients.

DRUG INTERACTIONS: None listed for large animals.

SUPPLIED AS: VETERINARY PRODUCTS
Oral suspensions containing 5.8 g kaolin and 268 mg pectin or 130 mg, or 7 g kaolin and 259 mg pectin per fluid ounce (29.6 mL)
Oral suspension containing 197 mg kaolin and 4.33 mg pectin/mL
HUMAN PRODUCT
Oral suspension containing kaolin 197 mg and pectin 4.33 mg/mL

KETAMINE

INDICATIONS: Ketamine (Ketalean♣, Ketaject★, Ketaset♣★, Ketaved★, Rogarsetic♣, Vetaket★, Vetalar♣★, Vetamine★, Vetame★) is a rapid-acting, nonbarbiturate general anesthetic. It is classified as a dissociative anesthetic and is accompanied by marked analgesia in most species. A major safety factor with ketamine is the lack of cardiorespiratory depression. Ketamine may be used in combination with a tranquilizing agent such as xylazine in large animals for induction of general anesthesia for endotracheal intubation. Ketamine combined with xylazine is also an effective anesthetic for short procedures, such as surgical repair of minor wounds or castration of stallions or colts. Muscle relaxation with ketamine alone is poor.

ADVERSE AND COMMON SIDE EFFECTS: Ketamine should not be used as the sole anesthetic agent in large animals. IV injection is followed by extensor rigidity, a "dog-sitting" position, extreme muscle spasm and jerking purposeless movements, an excited facial expression, profuse sweating, and, occasionally, convulsions. If used alone, tremors and tonic spasticity will occur, and laryngeal reflexes remain active. Induction of general anesthesia should only be performed in combination with sedatives and administered only after effects of the sedative are clinically obvious (see **ACEPROMAZINE, DETOMIDINE DIAZEPAM, GUAIFENESIN, XYLAZINE**). Because the eyes remain open and fixed, lubricant should be placed in the eyes during anesthesia. Eye position cannot be used as criteria for anesthetic depth. Other sporadic reports of adverse reaction in horses have included turbulent recovery from anesthesia, or ineffective anesthesia, convulsions, and apparent hallucinations.

DRUG INTERACTIONS: Use of ketamine in humans taking thyroid replacement hormones has been associated with severe hypertension and tachycardia. Ketamine may also potentiate respiratory depression and/or paralysis following use of succinylcholine. Ketamine can be antagonized by administration of a mixture of L-amphetamine and yohimbine.

SUPPLIED AS: VETERINARY PRODUCT
For injection containing 100 mg/mL

KETOCONAZOLE

INDICATIONS: Ketoconazole (Nizoral♣★) is an imidazole derivative used for treating superficial and systemic fungal infections. The
primary effect of imidazoles on fungi is their ability to alter membrane permeability by blocking synthesis of cellular sterols. Ketoconazole has been useful in treating histoplasmosis, coccidioidomycosis, and other systemic fungal infections. The pharmacokinetics of
ketoconazole in normal horses has been studied, but its use for such
diseases as equine sporotrichosis has not, at the time of this writing,
been reported. At the recommended doses in horses, peak serum
concentrations reach 3.76 μg/mL, synovial peak concentrations
reach 0.87 μg/mL, and peak peritoneal concentrations reach 1.62
μg/mL. Penetration into the cerebrospinal fluid appears low.

ADVERSE AND COMMON SIDE EFFECTS: Anorexia, photopho-
bia, gingival bleeding, and paresthesia are untoward effects in people that should be monitored for in animals. Transient elevations in
liver enzymes and jaundice have been reported. Gastrointestinal
side effects may be prevented by administering the drug with food
(which may also serve to increase its absorption) and by dividing the
daily dose and administering the drug two to four times daily. Gynecomastia has also been reported. The drug should not be given to
pregnant animals because its use has been associated with stillbirths
and mummified fetuses. In addition, decreased libido and impotence are reported in humans.

DRUG INTERACTIONS: Rifampin increases metabolic clearance of
ketoconazole. Antacids, cimetidine, ranitidine, and sucralfate decrease the absorption of ketoconazole. It is recommended that these
drugs be administered 2 hours after ketoconazole. Phenytoin may antagonize the actions of ketoconazole. Ketoconazole blunts the cortisol
response to ACTH. Ketoconazole may increase the anticoagulant effects of warfarin. The duration of activity of methylprednisolone or
prednisolone is prolonged with ketoconazole. Ketoconazole may decrease serum concentrations of theophylline in some patients.

SUPPLIED AS: HUMAN PRODUCTS
Tablets containing 200 mg
Suspension containing 20 mg/mL

KETOPROFEN

INDICATIONS: Ketoprofen (Anafen♣, Ketofen★) is a nonsteroidal
anti-inflammatory drug introduced for the treatment of muscu-

loskeletal inflammatory disorders in horses. It is in the class of drugs that include ibuprofen and naproxen, with dose-dependent anti-inflammatory effects in a chronic adjuvant carpitis model in the horse. It also appears equally effective as flunixin meglumine in blocking endotoxin-stimulated cyclo-oxygenase-mediated inflammation. It appears to be less ulcerogenic and less nephrotoxic than flunixin meglumine. Onset of activity occurs within 2 hours with peak response by 12 hours after IV or IM administration.

ADVERSE AND COMMON SIDE EFFECTS: Adverse reactions as reported in horses include injection site swelling, collapse, fever, sweating, and neck swelling. Large overdoses (15- to 25-fold) can result in laminitis, inappetence, depression, icterus, recumbency, and abdominal swelling, but lesser overdoses (to fivefold) appear well tolerated.

DRUG INTERACTIONS: Ketoprofen should not be administered with other drugs because compatibility studies have not been done.

SUPPLIED AS: VETERINARY PRODUCT
For injection containing 100 mg/mL, in 50-mL and 100-mL vials

OTHER USES
Horses
ENDOTOXEMIA
A dose of 0.5 mg/kg; IV every 6 hours appears to be as effective as low dose flunixin meglumine for reduction of endotoxin-mediated circulatory problems.

Cattle
PNEUMONIC PASTEURELLOSIS
Ketoprofen has been shown to modulate inflammation in a model of pneumonic pasteurellosis using 3 mg/kg once daily; IM for 3 days. Its effects blunt the severity of hypoxemia and tachypnea associated with the disease.

LACTULOSE

INDICATIONS: Lactulose (Acilac✚, Cephulac✚★, Cholac★, Chronulac✚★, Comolose-R✚, Constulose★, Constilac★, Duphalac✚★, Enulose★, Gen-Lac✚, Lactulose PSE★ Syrup, Lactulax✚, Lactulose✚, PMS-Lactulose✚) is a synthetic nonabsorbable disaccharide used in the management of hepatic encephalopathy. Enteric bacteria ferment lactulose to acidic by-products, decrease intraluminal pH, and favor the formation of ammonium ions, which are poorly absorbed. Lactulose also acts as a mild osmotic laxative, increases the rate of passage of ingesta, and leads to the reduction of bacterial production of ammonia. Lactulose is unlikely to be effective in the ruminant with hepatic encephalopathy because ruminal degradation of the drug can be expected.

ADVERSE AND COMMON SIDE EFFECTS: No adverse effects have been reported in horses. However, in humans, transient gastric distention, flatulence, and abdominal cramping may occur. With excessive doses, diarrhea may occur.

DRUG INTERACTIONS: Antacids decrease the efficacy of the drug. Neomycin and other oral anti-infectives may inhibit lactulose activity by the reduction or removal of resident colonic bacteria. However, clinical evidence in humans suggests that combined therapy in hepatic encephalopathy may actually be synergistic.

SUPPLIED AS: HUMAN PRODUCT
Syrup containing 10 g/15 mL

LASALOCID

INDICATIONS: Lasalocid (Avatec♣★, Bovatec♣★) is an ionophor antibiotic used for enhancing feed efficiency in cattle. It is also used for the prevention of coccidiosis in cattle and sheep.

ADVERSE AND COMMON SIDE EFFECTS: It may be fatal if ingested by horses or other equines. Lasalocid should not be fed to pigs or dogs. If fed undiluted to cattle it could also be fatal. If fed at five times the recommended levels, a slight, transient diarrhea may occur. A recent report suggests this drug may cause rumenitis if given to newborn calves at a dose of 3 mg/kg; PO.

DRUG INTERACTIONS: None listed.

SUPPLIED AS: VETERINARY PRODUCT
Feed premix containing 150 g/kg

OTHER USES
Cattle
GRAIN BLOAT
1.32 mg/kg daily; PO for the prevention of grain bloat
INTERSTITIAL PNEUMONIA
200 mg/head/day; PO for the prevention of interstitial pneumonia associated with L-tryptophan/3-methyl indole

LEVAMISOLE

INDICATIONS: Levamisole (Levasole♣★, Prohibit★, Ripercol♣, Topasole♣, Totalon★, Tramisol♣★) is a broad-spectrum anthelmintic. It is the only anthelmintic licensed for use in sheep for lungworms. It is not effective against *Mullerius capillarius*. Levamisole may help restore immune function, especially in old or debilitated animals, by increasing the number and function of T lymphocytes and macrophages. Levamisole has been shown to hasten recovery of calves with viral respiratory disease. It has also been reported to stimulate antibody production, increase macrophage phagocytosis, inhibit tumor growth, and stimulate suppressor cell activity, but the clinical applicability of such use in large animals remains poorly established. In cattle and sheep, the efficacy of levamisole is equal, regardless of whether the injectable, bolus, or pour-on formulation is used.

ADVERSE AND COMMON SIDE EFFECTS: Toxic doses produce signs suggestive of organophosphate toxicity, including diarrhea, anorexia, salivation, and muscular tremors. Mild toxicity may cause slight muzzle foam and licking of the lips in cattle. Death from toxicity in sheep and goats is the most commonly reported adverse drug reaction for these species. Such problems have occurred more commonly as a result of using the injectable form rather than oral dosing and use of products formulated for other species. Atropine is only partially effective as an antidote. If toxicity progresses to flaccid paralysis, respiratory assistance should be given until recovery has occurred. The pour-on formulation may cause occasional dermal irritation with scaling and fissures at the site of application. Other reports have included sudden death and injection site pain as adverse reactions to injections; pour-on reactions included frothing at the mouth, paddling, and death, as well as alopecia and exfoliation of the skin.

DRUG INTERACTIONS: The concurrent use of chloramphenicol has led to death in some cases. Pyrantel, diethylcarbamazine, and organophosphate drugs may enhance the toxic effects of levamisole.

SUPPLIED AS: VETERINARY PRODUCTS
For injection containing 136.5 mg/mL
Soluble drench powder containing 11.7 g/packet
Soluble drench containing 13 g/packet
Soluble drench containing 52 g/packet
Soluble drench containing 544.5 g/packet
Soluble drench containing 93.6 g/100g
Oral tablets/boluses containing 184 mg and 2.19 g bolus
Wormer pellets containing 8 g/kg
Pour-on formulation containing 200 mg/mL
Medicated premix containing 500 g/kg

OTHER USES
Horses
RESPIRATORY DISEASE
Levamisole has been used empirically as an immunostimulant for

horses with respiratory disease, based mainly on the drug's immunostimulant effects in laboratory animals.

Sheep
LUNGWORMS
7.5 mg/kg; PO, SC

LEVOTHYROXINE

INDICATIONS: Levothyroxine (Eltroxin✦★, Levo-T✦, Levo-Powder★, Lovoxine★, Levothroid★, Levotabs★, Nutrived T-4 Chewables★, Soloxine✦★, Synthroid✦★, Thyro-Form★, Thyro-Tabs★, Thyroxine-L★, Thyrozine★) is a synthetic form of T_4 used in the treatment of hypothyroid disease. Although hypothyroidism has been incriminated in a number of relatively common diseases in horses, conclusive scientific data to substantiate its occurrence in horses are lacking.

ADVERSE AND COMMON SIDE EFFECTS: Thyroid replacement should be undertaken with caution in animals with hypoadrenocorticism, diabetes mellitus, or congestive heart failure. The increase in metabolism may place undue stress on the heart.

DRUG INTERACTIONS: With the use of thyroid medications, marked hypertension and tachycardia following induction with ketamine has been documented in people.

SUPPLIED AS: VETERINARY PRODUCTS
Tablets containing 0.1, 0.2, 0.3, 0.5, 0.6, and 0.8 mg
Tablets containing 0.4 and 0.7 mg (US only)
Powder (0.22%, US only) containing 1 g T_4 in 454 g powder, 2.3 g T_4 in 1050 g powder, 10 g T_4 in 4.53 kg powder
HUMAN PRODUCTS
Tablets containing 12.5, 25, 50, 75, 88, 100, 112, 125, 150, 175, 200, and 300 mg
Injection containing 200 or 500 µg/vial

LIDOCAINE

INDICATIONS: Lidocaine (Lidocaine Neat✦, Lurocaine✦, Anthracaine★, Lidoject★) is one of the most commonly used local anesthetics in large animals. It is also the drug of choice for the management of ventricular premature contractions or tachycardia.

ADVERSE AND COMMON SIDE EFFECTS: With drug overdose, drowsiness, tremors, nystagmus, seizure, hypotension, and increased atrioventricular conduction with atrial flutter and fibrillation have been reported. The neurologic signs can be controlled with diazepam. Hypokalemia reduces antiarrhythmic effects.

DRUG INTERACTIONS: Cimetidine, propranolol, and quinidine increase activity of lidocaine. Barbiturates decrease lidocaine action via enzyme induction. Phenytoin increases the cardiac depressant effect of lidocaine.

SUPPLIED AS: VETERINARY PRODUCTS
For injection containing 20 mg/mL
To prepare IV infusion using 2% veterinary solution, add 1 g (50 mL) of 2% solution to 1 L D$_5$W, thus providing 1 mg/mL (1,000 mg/mL). With a minidrop (60 drops/mL) IV set, each drop will contain approximately 17 mg.

OTHER USES
Horses
POSTOPERATIVE ILEUS
Horses with ileus after colic surgery can be administered an IV infusion of 1.3 mg/kg in a slow IV bolus, then 0.05 mg/kg/min over a period of 5 to 6 hours. The mechanism of action may be the suppression of afferent neural pathways from the peritoneum, inducing analgesia, some anti-inflammatory properties, and it may also be directly stimulating to smooth muscle. Side effects at this dose are not common but may include trembling, muscle fasciculations, or ataxia, for which decreasing the infusion rate is suggested. Further studies may find that lower doses are equally effective prokinetics and will avoid undesirable side effects.

LINCOMYCIN

See Description of Drugs for Small Animals.

LOPERAMIDE

INDICATIONS: Loperamide (Alti-Loperamide✦, Anti-Diarrheal Formula★, Apo-Loperamide✦, Imodium✦★, Novo-Loperamide✦, PMS-Loperamide Hydrochloride✦) is a narcotic analgesic product that is used as an antidiarrheal agent through its action of prolonging intestinal transit time. It has been used to manage experimental diarrhea in calves in which it merely delays the onset of diarrhea.

ADVERSE AND COMMON SIDE EFFECTS: The drug is relatively safe. Sedation, constipation, and ileus may occur. With chronic use, soft stools, bloody diarrhea, and weight loss have also been reported. The drug should not be used to treat cases of suspected invasive bacterial enteritis, such as salmonellosis, because decreased intestinal transit can delay clearance of the pathogen. Loperamide is also contraindicated in patients with liver disease, obstructive gastrointestinal disease, glaucoma, and obstructive uropathy. The drug should be discontinued if diarrhea has not been controlled within 48 hours.

DRUG INTERACTIONS: None established.

SUPPLIED AS: HUMAN PRODUCTS
Tablets and capsules containing 2 mg
Oral liquid containing 0.2 mg/mL

LUTEINIZING HORMONE

INDICATIONS: Luteinizing hormone (Lutrophin-V❤, L-Tropin❤) is
an anterior pituitary extract that acts to stimulate follicular maturation, estrogen production, and ovulation, provided follicle-stimulating hormone has already acted. Luteinizing hormone is used in cattle to correct ovarian cysts and in mares to treat failure to ovulate.

ADVERSE AND COMMON SIDE EFFECTS: None listed.

DRUG INTERACTIONS: None listed.

SUPPLIED AS: VETERINARY PRODUCTS
For injection containing 25 mg/5-mL vial
For injection containing 25 mg/10-mL vial

MAGNESIUM HYDROXIDE

INDICATIONS: Magnesium hydroxide (Carmilax❤★ Bolets, Carmi-
lax Powder★, Laxade Boluses★, Laxade Powder★, Magnalax Bolus★,
Magne-Lax★, Milk of Magnesia❤★, Polyox II Bolus★, Polyox Pow-
der★, Rumalax★, Rumalax Gel★, Rumen Boluses★) is an oral antacid
and mild laxative. It is used in cattle to treat rumen acidosis and in
horses for treatment of gastric ulceration.

ADVERSE AND COMMON SIDE EFFECTS and **DRUG INTERAC-
TIONS:** See ANTACIDS.

SUPPLIED AS: VETERINARY PRODUCTS
Oral boluses containing 6 and 17 g
Powder containing 361 g★ or 295 g★ per 454 g powder
Powder containing 106 g/340 g
Gel containing 216 g/454 g
Note: Three boluses contain the equivalent magnesium hydroxide to
946 mL of Milk of Magnesia.

HUMAN PRODUCTS
Oral suspension containing 77.5 mg/g
Tablets containing 300 and 600 mg

MAGNESIUM SULFATE

INDICATIONS: Magnesium sulfate❤★ (Epsom salts) is used in
large animals mainly as an oral cathartic.

ADVERSE AND COMMON SIDE EFFECTS: Undiluted magnesium sulfate can cause osmotic damage to intestinal mucosal cells and may induce enteritis.

DRUG INTERACTIONS: None listed.

SUPPLIED AS: CHEMICAL PRODUCT
As salts containing 98% to 100% magnesium sulfate

HUMAN PRODUCTS
For injection containing 40, 80, 100, 125, 200, and 500 mg/mL
For injection containing 1% and 2% in 5% dextrose

OTHER USES
Euthanasia
Magnesium sulfate can be administered IV as a euthanasia solution but should be combined with depressants such as pentobarbital and chloral hydrate to prevent alarm and struggling of the animal.

MANNITOL

INDICATIONS: Mannitol (Mannitol★, Osmitrol♣★) is a potent osmotic diuretic. It is used for the prevention and treatment of oliguria and acute glaucoma and in the management of acute cerebral edema in diseases such as cranial trauma, polioencephalomalacia, or equine neonatal maladjustment. The use of the drug in animals with intracranial injury is controversial. These patients may have a damaged blood–brain barrier, which would allow the drug to leak across into the damaged brain and cause the area to swell further. Mannitol has also been used to enhance the renal elimination of toxins such as aspirin, ethylene glycol, and some barbiturates.

ADVERSE AND COMMON SIDE EFFECTS: Volume overload and pulmonary edema may occur, especially in patients with compromised renal or cardiac disease. Hyponatremia and seizures have been reported with drug overdose. Mannitol is contraindicated in the case of cerebral hemorrhage.

DRUG INTERACTIONS: None established for large animals.

SUPPLIED AS: VETERINARY PRODUCT
For injection containing 180 mg/mL

HUMAN PRODUCT (Osmitrol)
For injection containing 5%, 10%, 15%, 20%, and 25%

OTHER USES
Horses and Ruminants
OLIGURIC RENAL FAILURE
0.25 to 1.0 g/kg; slowly IV

MEBENDAZOLE

INDICATIONS: Mebendazole (Equiverm♣, Vermox♣★) is an anthelmintic useful for the elimination of large roundworms, large and small strongles, and pinworms in horses.

ADVERSE AND COMMON SIDE EFFECTS: None reported for horses.

DRUG INTERACTIONS: None established.

SUPPLIED AS: VETERINARY PRODUCT
Oral paste containing 200 mg/g

HUMAN PRODUCT
Tablets containing 100 mg [Vermox♣★]

OTHER USES
Horses

D. ARNFIELDI
20 mg/kg once daily; PO for 5 days

Sheep
GASTROINTESTINAL NEMATODES, LUNGWORMS, TAPEWORMS
10 mg/kg; PO

MECLOFENAMIC ACID

INDICATIONS: Meclofenamic acid (Arquel♣★) is a nonsteroidal anti-inflammatory drug used in the treatment of acute or chronic osteoarthritic disease in the horse. It has also been used experimentally to prevent respiratory distress in anaphylactic shock in conscious calves. Its onset of action is slow, taking 36 to 96 hours to develop.

ADVERSE AND COMMON SIDE EFFECTS: Toxic signs in the horse (buccal erosions, anorexia, and gastrointestinal disturbances) can result from prolonged, high (12–16 mg/kg) daily doses. Higher than therapeutic doses can lower the packed cell volume. Horses with heavy bot infestation may develop mild colic and diarrhea following meclofenamic acid administration. The drug is contraindicated in animals with gastrointestinal, renal, or hepatic disorders.

DRUG INTERACTIONS: Meclofenamic acid binds to plasma proteins and may displace other drugs, such as warfarin, resulting in adverse reaction to the displaced drug.

SUPPLIED AS: VETERINARY PRODUCTS
Oral granules containing 500 mg in 10-g packet
Oral granules containing 50 mg/g in 100-g jar

MEGESTROL ACETATE

INDICATIONS: Megestrol acetate (Ovaban♣★, Ovarid♣) is a progestational compound marketed for the postponement of estrus and the alleviation of false pregnancy in bitches. The drug is used in horses to treat behavioral problems such as aggression in stallions and nonpregnant mares.

ADVERSE AND COMMON SIDE EFFECTS: The drug should not be given to females with reproductive problems, during pregnancy, or to those with mammary tumors. Information on adverse effects in horses is scant, but in small animals, polyphagia, polydipsia, weight gain, and a change in behavior are common side effects.

DRUG INTERACTIONS: None established.

SUPPLIED AS: VETERINARY PRODUCT (small animal products only)
Tablets containing 5 and 20 mg

MELENGESTROL ACETATE

INDICATIONS: Melengestrol acetate (MGA♣★) is a progestational compound used in feedlot heifers (> 181 kg) to suppress estrus, enhance feed utilization, and to promote growth.

ADVERSE AND COMMON SIDE EFFECTS: Melengestrol should only be used in intact heifers as it is ineffective in steers or spayed heifers. The 3- to 5-day withdrawal of the drug (US recommendation) prior to shipping is thought to predispose to heat at the time of loading for transport.

DRUG INTERACTIONS: Do not use the drug in feed containing pellet binding agents.

SUPPLIED AS: VETERINARY PRODUCT
Premix feed additive containing 200 or 500 mg/kg

OTHER USES
Horses

Melengestrol acetate has also been advocated for treating behavioral problems such as nervousness or sexual aggression in both stallions and mares. Dosage and efficacy was not indicated.

MENADIONE SODIUM BISULFITE (VITAMIN K₃)

INDICATIONS: Menadione sodium bisulfite [menadione, menadione sodium diphosphate, vitamin K_3] (Anti-Blood♣, K-Sol★, K-3

Vite✦) is a synthetic vitamin K compound used for the treatment of prolonged bleeding due to vitamin K deficiency states, as occurs in cattle fed moldy sweet clover containing dicoumarin, or from toxicity due to ingested rodenticides containing dicumarol. Recent literature suggests vitamin K_1 is preferred to treat sweet clover toxicosis because vitamin K_3 may be ineffective in cattle.

ADVERSE AND COMMON SIDE EFFECTS: Menadione sodium bisulfite (vitamin K_3) has resulted in acute renal failure in horses when given at the recommended IV dose of 2.2 to 11 mg/kg.

DRUG INTERACTIONS: None listed.

SUPPLIED AS: VETERINARY PRODUCTS
Soluble powder packet containing 2.5 g menadione sodium bisulfite per 100 g [Anti-Blood✦, K-3 Vite✦]
Feed additive (poultry) containing 12.8 g/lb [K-Sol★]
Injection containing 50 mg/mL [✦]

MEPERIDINE

INDICATIONS: Meperidine/Pethidine (Demerol✦★) is a short-acting narcotic sedative with pharmacologic properties similar to morphine in that it binds to opiate receptors and raises the pain threshold. Unlike morphine, it is no more toxic to the newborn than adult animals. It is used to relieve pain associated with cesarean section in the mare and for its analgesic and sedative properties during calving in cattle. It does not appreciably depress fetal respiration. It is a less potent analgesic than morphine. Meperidine can be used in place of morphine where an analgesic drug is required that does not also depress intestinal motility.

ADVERSE AND COMMON SIDE EFFECTS: The SC route of administration should be avoided because of local irritation and pain at the site of injection. Significant decreases in systemic blood pressure and bronchoconstriction can occur, possibly due to central vagal effects and histamine release.

DRUG INTERACTIONS: Naloxone antagonizes the respiratory depression and toxic effects of meperidine.

SUPPLIED AS: HUMAN PRODUCTS
Tablets containing 50 and 100 mg
Oral solution containing 10 mg/mL
For injection containing 10, 25, 50, 75, and 100 mg/mL

MEPIVACAINE HYDROCHLORIDE

INDICATIONS: Mepivacaine hydrochloride (Carbocaine-V 2%♣★) is a rapid-acting local anesthetic of similar potency to lidocaine, but with a more rapid onset and less toxicity. Its anesthetic effects last several hours and can be prolonged with the addition of epinephrine 1:100,000. It has been used in topical anesthesia of the laryngeal mucosa prior to ventriculectomy in horses.

ADVERSE AND COMMON SIDE EFFECTS: It should not be injected into infected tissues or regions that lack adequate blood circulation such as fibrosed areas. Epidural use should be avoided in hypovolemic animals.

DRUG INTERACTIONS: See LIDOCAINE.

SUPPLIED AS: VETERINARY PRODUCT
For injection containing 2%

METHIONINE

INDICATIONS: Methionine (Ammonil★, D-L-M Tablets★, Equi-Phar DL-Methionine Powder★, Methio-Tabs★, Methigel♣★, D-L-Methionine Powder★, M-200 Tablets♣, M-500 Tablets♣, Methio-Form♣★, Methio Tablets♣, Methio-Vet★) is a urinary acidifying agent used in the treatment and prevention of struvite urolithiasis in small animals. In horses, it is used to promote keratinization and healing of hoof and sole defects, as in chronic laminitis.

ADVERSE AND COMMON SIDE EFFECTS: The drug is contraindicated in patients with renal failure or pancreatic disease. The drug has no place in the treatment of hepatic lipidosis unless caused by choline deficiency, as may occur with pancreatic exocrine insufficiency. It may, in fact, potentiate clinical signs of hepatic encephalopathy by leading to the increased production of mercaptan-like compounds.

DRUG INTERACTIONS: Methionine may increase the renal excretion of quinidine. The antibacterial efficacy of aminoglycosides and erythromycin may be decreased in the presence of an acid urine produced by methionine.

SUPPLIED AS: VETERINARY PRODUCTS
Tablets containing 200 and 500 mg
Gel containing 80 mg/g
Powder as a feed additive containing 100% DL-methionine

METHOCARBAMOL

INDICATIONS: Methocarbamol (Robaxin-V★, Methocarbamol Injection✦) is a centrally acting muscle relaxant that is used as adjunct therapy to rest and physical therapy in the treatment of musculoskeletal injury. It has also been used to reduce muscular spasm associated with tetanus poisoning by strychnine.

ADVERSE AND COMMON SIDE EFFECTS: Excessive salivation, sedation, vomiting, muscular weakness, and ataxia have been reported. Extravascular injection may cause tissue necrosis. The drug should not be given to animals with renal dysfunction or used in pregnant animals.

DRUG INTERACTIONS: Other central nervous system (CNS) depressants may potentiate the CNS depressive effects of methocarbamol.

SUPPLIED AS: VETERINARY PRODUCTS
Tablets containing 500 mg
For injection containing 100 mg/mL

HUMAN PRODUCTS
Tablets containing 500 and 750 mg
For injection containing 100 mg/mL

METHYLCELLULOSE FLAKES

INDICATIONS: Methylcellulose flakes (Citrucel✦★, Entrocel✦, Methylcellulose Tablets★) are hydrophilic, indigestible, nonabsorbable colloid derivatives of cellulose used to soften and bulk the stool. They are also used for treatment of sand impaction in the horse, but psyllium mucilloid may be more effective.

ADVERSE AND COMMON SIDE EFFECTS: Fluid retention can occur with some forms of the flakes.

DRUG INTERACTIONS: None listed.

SUPPLIED AS: HUMAN PRODUCTS
Dry product containing 1 part methylcellulose flakes and 5 parts sugar.
Tablets containing 500 mg
Liquid containing 18 mg/mL

OTHER USES Methylcellulose flakes are also mixed to create a lubricant for obstetric procedures.

METHYLENE BLUE

INDICATIONS: Methylene blue (Methylene Blue Injection♣★, Methylene Blue Tablets♣★, Urolene Blue★★) is used in the treatment of methemoglobinemia, as occurs from the ingestion of nitrate-accumulating plants in ruminants, and chlorate toxicosis in large animals. Although methemoglobinemia is a component of red maple leaf toxicity in horses, methylene blue is reported to be neither necessary nor beneficial for treatment of this specific toxicity.

ADVERSE AND COMMON SIDE EFFECTS: The drug is contraindicated in patients with renal insufficiency. Methylene blue may cause Heinz body hemolytic anemia and, possibly, acute renal failure. In people, additional side effects may include bladder irritation, nausea, vomiting, diarrhea, and abdominal pain. With large IV doses, fever, cardiovascular abnormalities, methemoglobinemia, and profuse sweating may also occur.

DRUG INTERACTIONS: None reported.

SUPPLIED AS: HUMAN PRODUCTS
For injection containing 10 mg/mL
Tablets containing 65 mg
Note: Not approved for use in food-producing animals

METHYLPREDNISOLONE

INDICATIONS: Methylprednisolone (Medrol★, Centramedrin♣, Depo-Medrol♣★, Methysone 40♣, Methylprednisolone Tablets★, Uni-Med♣, Vetacortyl♣) is an intermediate-acting glucocorticoid used for its anti-inflammatory properties. In large animals, it is most often used intra-articularly for nonseptic joint disease, or IM for its anti-inflammatory properties.

ADVERSE AND COMMON SIDE EFFECTS: See GLUCOCORTICOID AGENTS.

DRUG INTERACTIONS: See GLUCOCORTICOID AGENTS.

SUPPLIED AS: VETERINARY PRODUCTS
Tablets containing 1, 2, and 4 mg
For injection containing 20 and 40 mg/mL
HUMAN PRODUCTS
Tablets containing 2, 4, 8, 16, 24, and 32 mg
For injection containing 20, 40, and 80 mg/mL

METHYLSULFONOMETHANE

INDICATIONS: Methylsulfonomethane★ (MSM) is a derivative of dimethyl sulfoxide that has been claimed to promote healing and recovery from disease, athletic injuries, and stress. It is also used in horses to promote hoof keratinization in chronic laminitis. The Food and Drug Administration has questioned its safety and efficacy.

ADVERSE AND COMMON SIDE EFFECTS: None listed.

DRUG INTERACTIONS: None listed.

SUPPLIED AS: VETERINARY PRODUCT
As feed additive powder 9.9 g/10 g★

METOCLOPRAMIDE

INDICATIONS: Metoclopramide (Apo-Metoclop♣, Maxeran♣★, Maxolon★, Metoclopramide Hydrochloride Intensol★, Nu-Metoclopramide♣, Octamide★, Reglan♣★) acts peripherally to enhance the action of acetylcholine at muscarinic synapses and in the central nervous system as a dopamine antagonist. It contributes to lower esophageal sphincter competence and promotes gastric emptying. It is useful in the management of gastric reflux and gastric motility disorders, as in sheep with abomasal emptying defect, and abomasal impaction in cattle. It is also used in the horse to treat intestinal ileus. Pharmacologic studies in ruminants have shown that serum concentrations in goats administered 0.5 mg/kg IM or IV peaked at 15 and 3 minutes, respectively, and declined to nondetectable levels by 120 minutes, with a biologic half-life following IV administration in goats of 36 minutes. Rumen degradation, complexation, or binding reduces the amount of drug available that is administered orally by nearly 50%. Metoclopramide use in ruminants has also been shown to increase serum prolactin, grazing time, and average daily weight gain that had been formerly depressed in cattle grazing toxic fescue. However, because of the short half-life, this would currently need to be formulated as a continuous-release device to be potentially useful in the prevention and treatment of fescue toxicosis.

ADVERSE AND COMMON SIDE EFFECTS: Metoclopramide should not be used in patients with gastric outlet obstruction or those with a history of epilepsy. Side effects in horses may include violent central nervous system (CNS) excitation and severe flatulence. Oral administration in foals has fewer side effects.

DRUG INTERACTIONS: Phenothiazine drugs may potentiate CNS effects. Aspirin, diazepam, and tetracycline absorption may be accelerated. Digoxin absorption may be decreased. Atropine will block the effects of the drug on gastrointestinal motility.

SUPPLIED AS: HUMAN PRODUCTS
Tablets containing 5 and 10 mg
Syrup containing 1 and 2 mg/mL
For injection containing 5 mg/mL

OTHER USES
Sheep

ABOMASAL EMPTYING DEFECT
0.3 mg/kg every 4 to 6 hours; SC

METRONIDAZOLE

INDICATIONS: Metronidazole (Apo-Metronidazole♣, Flagyl♣★, Metric 21★, Metro I.V.★, Novo-Nidazol♣, PMS-Metronidazole♣, Protostat★) is a synthetic antibacterial, antiprotozoal agent that has been used in the treatment of giardiasis, trichomoniasis, amoebiasis, balantidiasis, and trypanosomiasis. It is bactericidal to many anaerobic bacteria including *Bacteroides* spp, *Fusobacterium*, *Clostridium* spp, *Veillonella* spp, *Peptococcus* spp, and *Peptostreptococcus* spp, and has been used for treating anaerobic infections of the respiratory tract, as may occur in aspiration pneumonia and for peritonitis. A recent report suggests that it may be of value for treatment of the anaerobic bacterial component of metritis associated with retained fetal membranes in cattle. The drug may also have immunosuppressive or immunostimulatory properties.

ADVERSE AND COMMON SIDE EFFECTS: Limited information is available regarding adverse effects in large animals. It is potentially hepatotoxic.

DRUG INTERACTIONS: Blood levels may be decreased by concurrent use of phenobarbital or phenytoin and blood levels may be increased by cimetidine use. The effects of oral anticoagulants are potentiated by metronidazole.

SUPPLIED AS: HUMAN PRODUCTS
Tablets containing 250 and 500 mg
Capsules containing 500 mg
For injection containing 500 mg/vial
For injection containing 5 mg/mL

OTHER USES
Cattle

TRICHOMONIASIS
75 mg/kg; IV three times at 12-hour intervals, or as a urethral douche of 1% solution

MICONAZOLE

INDICATIONS: Miconazole (Conofite♣, Micatin♣★, Monistat♣★, Monistat IV★) is an antifungal agent used for the treatment of dermatophytosis in large animals. It has also been described for the treatment of fungal keratitis and fungal pneumonia in horses, but there are no clinical trials available to verify the efficacy and safety of such use.

ADVERSE AND COMMON SIDE EFFECTS: Reactions to topical application are rare but include mild pruritus and pain at the site of application.

DRUG INTERACTIONS: None listed.

SUPPLIED AS: HUMAN PRODUCTS
Cream (2%) for topical use
For injection containing 10 mg/mL★

MINERAL OIL

INDICATIONS: Mineral oil♣★ (or liquid paraffin) is used for the relief of intestinal impaction, particularly in horses. It softens stools by coating the feces and preventing the colonic absorption of water. The agent works at the level of the colon and may take 6 to 12 hours to work effectively. It has also been used to hasten the transit of ingesta, as with grain overload in horses and ruminants, but other products (see **MAGNESIUM SULFATE**) are more appropriate.

ADVERSE AND COMMON SIDE EFFECTS: Mineral oil is contraindicated in patients with intestinal obstruction or dysphagia. A small amount of oil is absorbed, but this is generally of no clinical significance. Because of the lack of taste, accidental aspiration pneumonia may occur.

DRUG INTERACTIONS: Increased absorption may occur if mineral oil is given concurrently with docusate sodium or docusate calcium. Mineral oil may interfere with the action of nonabsorbable sulfonamides.

SUPPLIED AS: VETERINARY PRODUCT
As a liquid for oral use

MONENSIN

INDICATIONS: Monensin (Coban♣★, Rumensin♣★, Rumensin CRC♣) is an ionophor antibiotic used to enhance feed efficiency in cattle. It is also used in cattle and goats to prevent coccidiosis. Recently it has been shown to be effective in reducing subclinical ketosis in dairy cattle, with additional benefits of increased milk production and increased protein content in the milk. As of June 1996 the restriction from use in lactating dairy cattle has been removed from the label in Canada. However, the indications for use remain restricted to treatment of coccidiosis.

ADVERSE AND COMMON SIDE EFFECTS: Monensin can cause fatal cardiomyopathy if ingested by horses or other equines. Monensin also should not be fed to pigs or dogs. If fed undiluted to cattle it could be fatal. If fed at five times the recommended levels to cattle, a slight, transient diarrhea may occur.

DRUG INTERACTIONS: None listed. Monensin can be mixed with melengestrol acetate (MGA♣★) for heifer feeding programs.

SUPPLIED AS: VETERINARY PRODUCTS
Feed additive containing 132.2 or 176 g/kg
Block containing 880 mg/kg
Controlled-release bolus containing 32 g

OTHER USES
Cattle
BLOAT PREVENTION
1.32 mg/kg daily; PO

PNEUMONIA
200 mg/head/day; PO, for prevention of interstitial pneumonia associated with L-tryptophan/3-methyl indole

SUBCLINICAL KETOSIS PREVENTION
200 mg/head/day; PO to dairy cattle for prevention of subclinical ketosis coupled with an increase in milk production

MORANTEL TARTRATE

INDICATIONS: Morantel tartrate (Banminth♣★, Exhelm E♣, Rumatel★) is an anthelmintic used for the removal and control of mature gastrointestinal nematode infections of dairy and beef cattle. Morantel tartrate is not approved for use in lactating cattle in Canada.

ADVERSE AND COMMON SIDE EFFECTS: None listed.

DRUG INTERACTIONS: None listed.

SUPPLIED AS: VETERINARY PRODUCTS
Pellets containing 10 g/kg

Premix containing 10 g/kg, 193.6 g/kg, or 200 mg/g
Bolus containing 2.5 g

OTHER USES
Sheep

OSTERTAGIA and *TRICHURIS* SPP
10 mg/kg; PO. Morantel tartrate is 95% effective in removing gastrointestinal nematodes and 90% effective for *Ostertagia* and *Trichuris* spp.

MORPHINE

INDICATIONS: Morphine (Astramorph★, Duramorph★, Infumorph★, Kadian♣, Morphine HP♣, Morphitec♣, M.O.S-Sulfate♣, MS Contin♣★, MS.IR♣★, Oramorph SR♣★, Rescudose★, RMS★, Roxanol★, Statex♣, and others) is a very effective analgesic narcotic agent. It is used for the management of acute pain and as a preanesthetic agent. In the horse, it has been used for treatment of pain associated with spasmodic colic, but many horses will show undesirable and dangerous central nervous system stimulation and excitement. Morphine can also be used in pleuritis to ease pain associated with respiration.

ADVERSE AND COMMON SIDE EFFECTS: In horses it can cause excitement, restlessness, and loss of coordination.

DRUG INTERACTIONS: Phenothiazines, antihistamines, fentanyl, and parenteral magnesium sulfate may potentiate the depressant effects of morphine.

SUPPLIED AS: HUMAN PRODUCTS
For injection containing 0.5, 1, 2, 3, 4, 5, 8, 10, 15, 25, and 50 mg/mL
Tablets containing 5, 10, 15, 20, 25, 30, 40, 50, 60, and 100 mg
Oral solution containing 1, 2, 4, 5, 10, 20, and 50 mg/mL
Capsules containing 10, 15, 20, 30, 50, 60, 100, and 200 mg
Suppositories containing 5, 10, 20, 30, 60, 100, and 200 mg

OTHER USES
Epidural Analgesia

Morphine can be administered epidurally in small doses (0.05–0.1 mg/kg) to treat acute or chronic pain. Analgesia lasts from 6 to 24 hours. Adverse side effects are usually minimal but may include some central nervous system stimulation.

MOXIDECTIN

INDICATIONS: Moxidectin (Cyadectin♣) is a milbemycin anthelmintic synthesized from the bacterium *Streptomyces cyanogriseus* non *cyanogenus*—from the same family as ivermectin. Whereas ivermectin is found in both fat and liver, moxidectin is sequestered almost exclusively in fat, with a half-life of 12 to 14 days following administration. Moxidectin is highly effective against *Ostertagia* and *Dictyocaulus* (>99.9%) and, slightly less effective against *Cooperia oncophora* (94–96%).

ADVERSE AND COMMON SIDE EFFECTS: None listed.

DRUG INTERACTIONS: None listed.

SUPPLIED AS: VETERINARY PRODUCT
For injection containing 10 mg/mL

NAFCILLIN

INDICATIONS: Nafcillin (Nafoil★, Nallpen★, Unipen✦★) is a β-lactamase-resistant, parenterally administered penicillin effective against gram-positive bacteria, particularly *Staphylococcus aureus* infections resistant to penicillin G. For more information, see **PENICILLIN**.

ADVERSE AND COMMON SIDE EFFECTS: Nausea, vomiting, and diarrhea are reported in people. Rash, pruritus, urticaria, and thrombophlebitis with IV injection are also reported to occur. Experience with the drug in large animals is limited. Also see **PENICILLINS**.

DRUG INTERACTIONS: See PENICILLINS.

SUPPLIED AS: HUMAN PRODUCTS
For injection containing 20 mg/mL, in vials containing 500 mg, 1 g, 2 g, and 10 g
Capsules containing 250 and 500 mg

NALOXONE

INDICATIONS: Naloxone (P/M Naloxone HCl Injection✦★) is a narcotic antagonist. It is the preferred agent for reversal of narcotic-induced depression, including respiratory depression induced by morphine, oxymorphone, meperidine, or fentanyl. Survival times have been shown to increase and mortality rates decrease in animals in endotoxic shock given naloxone. Naloxone increases cardiac output and arterial blood pressure, decreases hemoconcentration and metabolic acidosis, and helps prevent hypoglycemia.

ADVERSE AND COMMON SIDE EFFECTS: At recommended doses, the drug is relatively free of adverse effects. At high doses, seizure activity has been reported. The duration of its action may be less than that of the opioid it is antagonizing; consequently, the animal should be monitored for signs of returning narcosis. The safety of the drug in pregnant animals has not been established although reproductive studies in rats did not reveal any adverse effects.

DRUG INTERACTIONS: Naloxone also reverses the effects of butorphanol and pentazocine.

SUPPLIED AS: VETERINARY PRODUCTS
For injection containing 0.4 mg/mL

NALTREXONE

INDICATIONS: Naltrexone (ReVia♣, Trenonil★) is an opioid antagonist used in horses to prevent cribbing. Naltrexone is a relatively pure antagonist and has higher oral efficacy and longer duration of action than naloxone.

ADVERSE AND COMMON SIDE EFFECTS: High doses in humans may cause mild dysphoria. No information concerning adverse effects is available for horses.

DRUG INTERACTIONS: None listed.

SUPPLIED AS: VETERINARY PRODUCT
For injection containing 20 mg/mL
HUMAN PRODUCT
Tablets containing 50 mg

NAPROXEN

INDICATIONS: Naproxen (Anaprox♣★, Apo-Napro-Na♣, Apo-Naproxen♣, Naprosyn♣★, Naxen♣, Novo-Naprox Sodium♣, Novo-Naprox♣, Nu-Naprox♣, PMS-Naproxen♣, Synflex♣) is an anti-inflammatory compound similar in action to phenylbutazone. It is used for the management of musculoskeletal injuries in horses. Information available for human use suggests the drug is better tolerated than aspirin, indomethacin, or the pyrazolone derivatives, such as phenylbutazone. Naproxen is reported to be superior to phenylbutazone in horses for treatment of inflammatory conditions involving pain and lameness.

ADVERSE AND COMMON SIDE EFFECTS: See **PHENYLBUTAZONE**.

DRUG INTERACTIONS: Naproxen absorption is reduced by the concomitant use of aluminum hydroxide or magnesium hydroxide. See **PHENYLBUTAZONE** for further information.

SUPPLIED AS: HUMAN PRODUCTS
Tablets containing sodium salt 275 and 550 mg
Enteric-coated tablets containing 250, 375, and 500 mg
Tablets containing 125, 250, 275, 375, and 500 mg
Tablets (sustained release) containing 750 mg
Suspension containing 25 mg/mL
Suppositories containing 500 mg

NAQUASONE

INDICATIONS: Naquasone✦★ is a combination of the benzothia-diazide diuretic trichlormethiazide and dexamethasone. This combination of drugs is complementary in the reduction of pre- and postpartum udder edema in cattle. The diuretic action of trichlor-methiazide is to inhibit reabsorption of sodium and chloride in the renal tubules, thereby enhancing excretion of sodium, chloride, and water. Effects on potassium and bicarbonate exchange in the tubules are much less and temporary. In contrast to other benzothiadiazide diuretics, potassium supplementation is not usually necessary. Dex-amethasone may enhance the reduction of udder edema through its anti-inflammatory properties. The injectable form has been used for treatment of inflammatory conditions such as musculoskeletal in-juries in the horse.

ADVERSE AND COMMON SIDE EFFECTS: Electrolyte depletion may occur with prolonged or overzealous therapy. Because of trichlormethiazide, Naquasone is contraindicated in severe renal im-pairment. Naquasone should not be given to animals with bacterial infections unless they are being treated with appropriate antibiotics. The dexamethasone portion of Naquasone may mask signs of infec-tion such as elevation in body temperature. Administration of the injectable product to prepartum cows may cause premature par-turition and retained placenta. Do not administer Naquasone to pregnant mares.

DRUG INTERACTIONS: None listed.

SUPPLIED AS: VETERINARY PRODUCTS
For injection containing 10 mg/mL trichlormethiazide and 0.5 mg/mL dexamethasone acetate
Bolets containing 200 mg trichlormethiazide and 5 mg dexamethasone

NATAMYCIN

INDICATIONS: Natamycin (Natacyn★) is a broad-spectrum anti-fungal agent used in horses for treating ocular fungal infections.

ADVERSE AND COMMON SIDE EFFECTS: Conjunctival chemosis and hyperemia have been reported in humans.

DRUG INTERACTIONS: None listed.

SUPPLIED AS: HUMAN PRODUCT
Ophthalmic 5% suspension

NEOMYCIN

INDICATIONS: Neomycin (Biosol♥★, Neomed 325♥, Neomix♥★, Neo-Ved 200★, Neovet♥★, Neomycin♥★) is an aminoglycoside antibiotic. It is generally less effective than amikacin or gentamicin against many bacteria. It is commonly used as a topical antibiotic and in oral antidiarrheal preparations. Neomycin is used orally in hepatic encephalopathy to reduce nitrogen breakdown by bacterial flora of the gut. Parenteral use of the drug is toxigenic and has been implicated as a major cause of renal failure in cattle. Neomycin is the most common cause of violative tissue residues in young calves in the United States and hence is not used in veal calves.

ADVERSE AND COMMON SIDE EFFECTS: Neomycin is the most nephrotoxic aminoglycoside. The drug is also potentially toxic to the vestibular and auditory nerves. Prolonged oral administration of neomycin to horses can induce diarrhea.

DRUG INTERACTIONS: Orally administered neomycin may decrease the absorption of digitalis, penicillin V and K, and vitamin K.

SUPPLIED AS: VETERINARY PRODUCT
Oral liquid containing 50 and 140 mg/mL
Soluble powder containing 500, 715, and 812 mg/g

OTHER USES
Horses
HEPATIC ENCEPHALOPATHY
50 to 100 mg/kg qid; PO

NEOSTIGMINE

INDICATIONS: Neostigmine methylsulfate (PMS-Neostigmine Methylsulfate♥, Prostigmin♥★, Stimuline♥) is an anticholinesterase used in the diagnosis and treatment of myasthenia gravis. There is marked clinical variability in response to dose. Neostigmine has also been used to stimulate intestinal motility in large animals but is contraindicated in intestinal obstruction. Do not administer the drug to lactating cattle if milk is destined for human consumption.

ADVERSE AND COMMON SIDE EFFECTS: Salivation, urination, and diarrhea may occur if the drug dose is too high. A cholinergic crisis should be treated with atropine (0.4 mg/kg; IM, IV). Neostigmine may precipitate atrial fibrillation in cattle.

DRUG INTERACTIONS: Corticosteroids may decrease the anticholinesterase activity of neostigmine. Neostigmine antagonizes the action of pancuronium and tubocurarine. Atropine antagonizes the muscarinic effects of neostigmine and is often used to treat adverse effects of the drug. Neostigmine may effectively reverse neuromuscular blockade caused by aminoglycosides. Dexpanthenol may have additive effects if given with neostigmine.

SUPPLIED AS: VETERINARY PRODUCT
For injection containing 2 mg/mL

HUMAN PRODUCTS
Tablets containing 15 mg neostigmine bromide
For injection containing 0.5, 1, and 2.5 mg/mL neostigmine methylsulfate

NETILMICIN

INDICATIONS: Netilmicin (Netromycin♥★) is an aminocyclitol antibiotic produced from an analogue of gentamicin. It is used for treatment of serious infections of the respiratory tract, peritonitis, or endometritis caused by *Pseudomonas* or *Serratia* spp.

ADVERSE AND COMMON SIDE EFFECTS AND DRUG INTERACTIONS. See AMINOGLYCOSIDE ANTIBIOTICS.

SUPPLIED AS: HUMAN PRODUCT
For injection containing 25, 50, and 100 mg/mL

NIACIN

INDICATIONS: Niacin (nicotinic acid) and nicotinamide are included in the dry cow ration of dairy cows and early lactating cows to help prevent hepatic lipidosis and ketosis. Niacin (Nu-Keto♥★) alone, or in commercially available compounds (Bovi Plus♥, Lipotinic Boluses★, Ketopro Oral Gel★, Niacin Plus Vitamin Supplement♥) is used as a supplementary nutritive source for animals off feed. Niacin decreases blood ketones and free fatty acids and increases blood glucose. Niacin is proposed to decrease ketosis and increase milk production, but supporting evidence is not strong.

ADVERSE AND COMMON SIDE EFFECTS: None listed.

DRUG INTERACTIONS: Niacin has been used in conjunction with monensin for prevention of ketosis, the latter being recently licensed in Canada for use in lactating dairy cows.

SUPPLIED AS: VETERINARY PRODUCTS
As a feed additive 100%
Boluses containing 6 g niacin/15 g

HUMAN PRODUCTS
Tablets containing 25, 50, 100, 250, 500, 750, and 1,000 mg
Capsules containing 125, 250, 300, 400, and 500 mg
Elixir containing 10 mg/mL

NITROFURANS

INDICATIONS: Nitrofurans are synthetic compounds with antibacterial properties against gram-positive and gram-negative bacteria, although they are used primarily for their gram-negative activity. Nitrofurans have also been used as antifungal and antiprotozoal drugs. Although their exact antibacterial mechanism is not known they may inhibit an enzymatic oxidative process. A number of nitrofurans are available for clinical use, including furazolidone (Furall★, Furazolidone Aerosol Powder★, Norizone♣, Topazone♣), nitrofurantoin (Equifur♣), nitrofurazone (Centrafur♣, Fura-Dressing♣, Fura Ointment♣★, Fura-Sweat♣, Furacin Soluble Dressing♣, Furacin Solution♣, Fura Septin Soluble Dressing★, Furasone Soluble Dressing♣, Fura-Zone Ointment★, Intrafur Solution♣, Niderm Ointment♣, Nitro Ointment♣ NFZ★, Nifulidone 0.2% Ointment♣, Nitro-Fur Solution♣, Nitro-Gel★, Nitrotop★, Nitrozone Ointment★, Nitrofurazone Ointment♣★, Nitrofurazone Soluble Dressing★, Nitrofurazone Soluble Powder★, Nitrofurazone Solution★, Pinkaway Powder♣), and nitrofuraldezone. The antibacterial activities of nitrofurans are reduced in the presence of blood, pus, and milk. The toxic and chemical properties of nitrofurans have limited their widespread use as systemic anti-infective drugs. Nitrofurazone is used locally but is of little value systemically. Nitrofurantoin is rapidly and completely absorbed from the intestinal tract; it is used as a urinary antiseptic. Furazolidone is used for control of various digestive tract infections, including salmonellosis. Nitrofurans are also used in boluses for intrauterine treatment of endometritis and retained placenta.

Because of the carcinogenic activity of nitrofurazone in rats and mice, nitrofuran drugs, including nitrofurantoin, furaltadone, furazolidone, nitrofuraldezone, and nitrofurazone, have been withdrawn from use in food-producing animals by the Food and Drug Administration in the United States and by the Bureau of Veterinary Drugs in Canada. The gravity of this restriction for use in food animals is similar to that of chloramphenicol. However, pinkeye sprays containing nitrofurazones continue to be licensed for use in food-producing animals in the United States.

ADVERSE AND COMMON SIDE EFFECTS: Orally administered nitrofurazone in calves can cause hindlimb paralysis. Higher doses may cause reduction in feed intake or, if administration is prolonged, hyperirritability and convulsions.

DRUG INTERACTIONS: Concurrent use of nitrofurantoin with probenecid may raise plasma levels of nitrofurantoin to undesirable levels and impair its action as a urinary antiseptic.

SUPPLIED AS: VETERINARY PRODUCTS
Nitrofurans are available as oral and parenteral medications and in wound dressing medications. See individual product for detailed information.

NIZATIDINE

INDICATIONS: Nizatidine (Axid♥★) is an H_2-receptor antagonist that has been used in the horse to treat gastric ulceration. Effective doses for use in horses are yet to be established.

ADVERSE AND COMMON SIDE EFFECTS: Side effects are few in humans but may include somnolence and elevated liver enzymes.

DRUG INTERACTIONS: None listed.

SUPPLIED AS: HUMAN PRODUCT
Capsules containing 150 and 300 mg

NOREPINEPHRINE BITARTRATE

INDICATIONS: Norepinephrine (Levophed♥★) is a potent β_1- and α-adrenergic agonist. Its practical use in large animals is limited mainly for the treatment of hypotension due to shock.

ADVERSE AND COMMON SIDE EFFECTS AND DRUG INTERACTIONS: See EPINEPHRINE.

SUPPLIED AS: HUMAN PRODUCT
For injection containing 1 mg/mL

NOVOBIOCIN

INDICATIONS: Novobiocin♥★ is an antibiotic active against gram-positive cocci including staphylococci and some streptococci. Variable effectiveness has been found against *Proteus, Pseudomonas,* and *Pasteurella multocida.* It is marketed in large animals as mastitis preparations as the sole agent (Albadry♣, Biodry★) or in combination with penicillin G (Albacillin Suspension♣★, Albadry Plus★, Novodry Plus Suspension♣) and with penicillin G, polymyxin B, dihydrostreptomycin and hydrocortisone (Special Formula 17900-Forte♣).

ADVERSE AND COMMON SIDE EFFECTS: There are no adverse effects listed for mastitis preparations.

DRUG INTERACTIONS: The elimination of penicillin drugs and the cephalosporins may be decreased.

SUPPLIED AS: VETERINARY PRODUCTS
Mastitis tubes containing 150 mg
Dry treatment tubes containing 400 mg

OMEPRAZOLE

INDICATIONS: Omeprazole (Prilosec★, Losec♣) is a proton pump-inhibitor used for the treatment of esophagitis, erosive gastritis, and gastric ulcers. The drug is 5 to 10 times more potent than cimetidine in inhibiting gastric acid secretion and has a long duration of action (24 hours or more). The drug is more effective than cimetidine in controlling aspirin-induced gastric erosions in dogs. It has cytoprotective (by enhancing mucosal cell prostaglandin production) and acid-reducing properties and may be useful in decreasing gastric hyperacidity. Safety and efficacy in horses have been confirmed in recent studies.

ADVERSE AND COMMON SIDE EFFECTS: In humans nausea, flatulence, vomiting, and diarrhea are reported. Headaches and dizziness have also been reported. Long-term, high-dose administration does not cause clinical, hematologic, or biochemical abnormalities in dogs, but similar studies are as yet unavailable for horses.

DRUG INTERACTIONS: The elimination time of diazepam, phenytoin, and warfarin is increased with chronic administration of omeprazole.

SUPPLIED AS: HUMAN PRODUCTS
Capsules containing 20 mg
Tablets (delayed release) containing 20 mg

ORGOTEIN

INDICATIONS: Orgotein (Palosein♣★) is a superoxide dismutase product of bovine liver origin that scavenges superoxide radicals and has anti-inflammatory effects. Orgotein is used to treat nonseptic joint disease. Orgotein also has anti-inflammatory effects if administered systemically, but this product has not found widespread use in equine medicine. Scientific data supporting its efficacy for use in equine medicine are lacking.

ADVERSE AND COMMON SIDE EFFECTS: Orgotein can induce an intense synovitis, possibly because of the presence of acidic carbohydrate polymer impurities in some products.

DRUG INTERACTIONS: None listed.

SUPPLIED AS: VETERINARY PRODUCT
For injection containing 5 mg as a lyophilized powder

OXFENDAZOLE

INDICATIONS: Oxfendazole (Benzelmin♥★, Equi-Cide★, Synanthic♥★) is a broad-spectrum anthelmintic effective for the removal of ascarids (*Parascaris equorum*), mature and immature pinworms (*Oxyuris equi*), large strongyles including the 4th stage larvae of *Strongylus vulgaris*, and small strongyles of horses. It is effective in cattle for removal and control of lungworms, roundworms (including inhibited forms of *Ostertagia ostertagi*) and adult tapeworms.

ADVERSE AND COMMON SIDE EFFECTS: None listed.

DRUG INTERACTIONS: None listed.

SUPPLIED AS: VETERINARY PRODUCTS
Oral paste containing 4.5 g/dose syringe, 5.4 g/dose syringe, and for cattle 185 mg/g
Suspension containing 90.6 or 225 mg/mL

OTHER USES
Sheep
MONIEZIA
5 mg/kg; PO

OXIBENDAZOLE

INDICATIONS: Oxibendazole (Anthelcide♥, Anthelcide EQ★, Equipar Equine Wormer★) is an equine anthelmintic effective for the removal and control of threadworms (*Strongyloides westeri*), large roundworms (*Parascaris equorum*), mature and L_4 larval stages of pinworms (*Oxyuris equi*), and large and small strongyles.

ADVERSE AND COMMON SIDE EFFECTS: The drug should not be used in debilitated horses or horses suffering from infectious disease, toxemia, or colic. Repeated dosing is not recommended in breeding stallions or pregnant mares. A recent report in horses associated administration with change in fecal consistency, severe diarrhea, abdominal pain, and in one instance, a birth defect.

DRUG INTERACTIONS: None listed.

SUPPLIED AS: VETERINARY PRODUCTS
Oral paste containing 22.7% W/W
Suspension containing 100 mg/mL

OXYMORPHONE

INDICATIONS: Oxymorphone (Numorphan♥★, P/M Oxymorphone HCl★) is a narcotic agent used for sedation, preanesthesia, and the management of pain. It is not commonly used in large animals.

ADVERSE AND COMMON SIDE EFFECTS: Respiratory depression and bradycardia have been reported. The drug should not be used in animals with head trauma because it may increase cerebrospinal fluid pressure.

DRUG INTERACTIONS: Antihistamines, phenothiazines, barbiturates, and anesthetic agents may potentiate central nervous system or respiratory depression.

SUPPLIED AS: VETERINARY PRODUCT
For injection containing 1.5 mg/mL

HUMAN PRODUCTS
For injection containing 1 and 1.5 mg/mL
Suppositories containing 5 mg

OXYTETRACYCLINE

See **TETRACYCLINES**.

OXYTOCIN

INDICATIONS: Oxytocin♥★ is a synthetic pituitary hormone used to stimulate uterine muscle contraction and milk letdown. Because of its action on the uterus, oxytocin is used to speed the normal process of parturition. It is also used to promote postoperative uterine contraction following cesarean section and to control uterine hemorrhage, to aid in the replacement of the prolapsed uterus, and/or evacuation of uterine debris such as retained placenta or pyometra. Oxytocin is also used to treat associated agalactia with acute udder edema in the cow. It is also indicated for evacuation of residual milk and inflammatory secretions in mastitis but is of questionable efficacy. Oxytocin will not stimulate milk formation by the mammary glands. Oxytocin is 10 to 40 times more effective when administered IV as compared to other routes.

ADVERSE AND COMMON SIDE EFFECTS: For prepartum use, the cervix should be fully relaxed. Pretreatment with estrogen before oxytocin may facilitate this. Large doses can produce a marked fall in arterial blood pressure.

DRUG INTERACTIONS: None listed.

SUPPLIED AS: VETERINARY PRODUCT
For injection containing 20 IU/mL

PANCURONIUM

INDICATIONS: Pancuronium (Gen-Pancuronium♣, Pancuronium Bromide Injection★, Pavulon♣★) is a synthetic nondepolarizing neuromuscular blocking agent. It can be used to facilitate mechanical ventilation during the intensive care of large-animal neonates.

ADVERSE AND COMMON SIDE EFFECTS: The drug should be used with caution in patients with compromised renal function and in those in whom tachycardia may be hazardous. Drug toxicity may be treated with mechanical support of ventilation and the use of atropine followed by neostigmine.

DRUG INTERACTIONS: Neuromuscular blockade may be potentiated by aminoglycoside antibiotics (amikacin, gentamicin, kanamycin, neomycin, streptomycin), bacitracin, halothane, isoflurane, lincomycin, magnesium sulfate, polymyxin B, and quinidine. Succinylcholine may hasten the onset of action of pancuronium and potentiate neuromuscular blockade. The action of pancuronium is antagonized by acetylcholine, anticholinesterases, and potassium ion. Theophylline may inhibit or reverse the neuromuscular blocking effect of pancuronium and precipitate arrhythmias.

SUPPLIED AS: HUMAN PRODUCT
For injection containing 1 and 2 mg/mL

PAREGORIC

INDICATIONS: Paregoric (opium tincture★) is a camphorated tincture of opium, used to treat diarrhea in foals and calves. It also has analgesic and sedative properties. It inhibits gastrointestinal motility and intestinal secretion and may enhance intestinal absorption.

ADVERSE AND COMMON SIDE EFFECTS: Opiates should be used with caution in animals with renal insufficiency, adrenocortical insufficiency, hypothyroid disease, and in severely debilitated or geriatric patients. These drugs are contraindicated in cases of diarrhea likely caused by toxins. Cautious use of these drugs is also recommended in cases with trauma to the head or with suspect increased cerebrospinal fluid pressure and in those with significant respiratory disease or hepatic disease. Sedation, constipation, and bloat may occur. Ileus, pancreatitis, and central nervous system (CNS) effects are also reported. Naloxone may be used to reverse adverse effects.

DRUG INTERACTIONS: Antihistamines, phenothiazines, barbiturates, and anesthetic agents may exacerbate CNS or respiratory depression.

SUPPLIED AS: HUMAN PRODUCT
Paregoric (opium tincture; camphorated) containing 2 mg morphine equivalent per 5 mL

PAROMOMYCIN

INDICATIONS: Paromomycin (Humatin♥★) is used for the treatment of *Giardia* and intestinal amoeba. Recent research has shown it to be highly effective and nontoxic when treating calves for cryptosporidiosis. It reduces the duration and severity of diarrhea and eliminates oocyst shedding in experimentally infected neonatal calves.

ADVERSE AND COMMON SIDE EFFECTS: None listed for large animals.

DRUG INTERACTIONS: None known for large animals.

SUPPLIED AS: HUMAN PRODUCT
Capsules containing 250 mg

PENICILLAMINE

INDICATIONS: Penicillamine (Cuprimine♥★, Depen♥★) is a thiol compound that chelates cystine, lead, iron, mercury, and copper and promotes their excretion in the urine. It is principally used in large animals for the management of lead or mercury poisoning and for hepatitis in ruminants associated with progressive copper accumulation. In the case of copper-associated hepatic disease, clinical improvement may take months to years. High cost may restrict its use in large animals.

ADVERSE AND COMMON SIDE EFFECTS: Lethargy, oral lesions, anorexia, proteinuria, and thrombocytopenia have been reported. The drug decreases the strength of skin wound closure by its effect on collagen and should only be used after wound healing is complete. Finally, the drug has been used experimentally in the treatment of renal amyloidosis.

DRUG INTERACTIONS: Phenylbutazone may potentiate hematologic and renal toxicity of the drug. Oral iron may inhibit absorption of the drug.

SUPPLIED AS: HUMAN PRODUCTS
Tablets containing 250 mg penicillamine
Capsules containing 125 and 250 mg penicillamine

PENICILLINS

INDICATIONS: Penicillin is a widely used antibiotic in large animal practice. It is available as the potassium and sodium salts for IV use, the procaine salt for IM or SC administration (Agri-Cillin★, Aquacillin★, Crysticillin★, Co-op Penicillin G Procaine♣, Depocillin♣, Ethacilin♣, Hi-Pencin 300♣, Microcillin★, Pen G Injection★, Pen-Aqueous♣★, Pen-G★, Pen-G Procaine★, Penicillin G Procaine♣★, Penmed♣, Penpro♣, Pfi-Pen★, Procaine Penicillin G♣), the benzathine salt for long-acting use [combined with procaine penicillin] (Ambi-Pen★, Benzapro♣, Crystiben★, Combicillin★, Crysticillin 300 A.S. Veterinary★, Duplocillin LA♣, Duo Pen★, Dura-Pen★, Durapen★, Flo-Cillin★, Longisil♣, PenBP-48★, Pendure Neat♣, Penlong XL♣, Sterile Penicillin G Benzathine-Penicillin G★, Twin-Pen★), or for oral administration as the phenoxymethyl derivative of penicillin, penicillin V (Beepen-VK★, Betapen-VK★, Ledercillin VK★, Pen-Vee K★, V-Cillin K★, Veetids★).

Studies in horses have suggested the site of drug administration may influence blood levels. SC injection may cause irritation and necessitate prolonged withdrawal periods. Long-acting products (benzathine penicillin G with procaine penicillin G) seldom result in therapeutic blood levels.

ADVERSE AND COMMON SIDE EFFECTS: Hypersensitivity reactions to penicillins are the most common untoward reaction and can occur with any penicillin group. Neither procaine nor the long-acting preparations should be administered IV. Untoward reactions to procaine penicillin in horses have been linked to inadvertent IV injection and are likely the effect of the procaine component.

DRUG INTERACTIONS: Various penicillins can inactivate amino-glycosides in vitro. Probenecid markedly decreases the tubular secretion of the penicillins.

SUPPLIED AS: VETERINARY PRODUCTS
For injection as the procaine salt containing 300,000 IU/mL
For injection as the benzathine salt containing 100,000 to 150,000 IU/mL combined with procaine penicillin G containing 100,000 to 150,000 IU/mL.
(Note: For European formulations, 1,000 IU is equivalent to 1 mg penicillin.)
HUMAN PRODUCTS
For injection, potassium or sodium penicillin containing 1, 5, and 10 million units
Tablets of penicillin V containing 125, 250, and 500 mg
Suspension containing 125, 250, and 300 mg/5 mL

OTHER USES
Penicillin is found in numerous combination products with other antibiotics (see **DIHYDROSTREPTOMYCIN/STREPTOMYCIN**) particularly in mastitis preparations and/or corticosteroids or antihistamines for systemic or topical use.

PENTAZOCINE

INDICATIONS: Pentazocine (Talwin♥★) is an opiate-type analgesic. Pentazocine is used in horses as a premedicant and to control pain in minor surgical procedures such as treatment of wounds. IV administration to ponies provides analgesia for 10 to 20 minutes. IM administration prolongs the analgesic effect. Pentazocine has not been as effective as a number of other analgesics (see **FLUNIXIN, XYLAZINE, DETOMIDINE**) when used for controlling colic pain in horses. Pentazocine does not produce profound sedation.

ADVERSE AND COMMON SIDE EFFECTS: A transient fall in systolic blood pressure may occur. High doses can result in muscle tremors, incoordination, hypersensitivity to noise, and muscle hypertonicity in the horse.

DRUG INTERACTIONS: See **MORPHINE**.

SUPPLIED AS: HUMAN PRODUCTS
For injection containing 30 mg/mL
Tablets containing 50 mg

PENTOBARBITAL

INDICATIONS: Pentobarbital (Dolethal♥, Euthansol♥, Euthanyl♥, Euthanyl Forte♥, Pentobarbital Sodium Injection★, Socumb★,

Sodium Pentobarbital Injection★, Somnotol♣) is classified as a short-acting barbiturate that acts to depress the central nervous system. Pentobarbital is used in large animals for the treatment of convulsions, for sedation in most large animals at low doses, and as a humane method of euthanasia. Pentobarbital suppresses sensitivity of the motor endplate of skeletal muscle to acetylcholine, but does not fully relax the abdominal muscles. Ruminants, particularly sheep and goats, metabolize pentobarbital from the plasma at a high rate, which may explain the need for supplemental increments of pentobarbital in anesthesia every 15 to 30 minutes. However, pentobarbital metabolism in sheep cannot be accelerated beyond its already high rate. Barbiturates are potent depressants of cerebral oxygen consumption and depress respiratory centers, particularly when given by IV injection. Most barbiturates can cross the placenta and result in depression of fetal respiration. Caesarean section performed solely with pentobarbital anesthesia results in 100% fetal mortality. Doses of barbiturates four times that producing respiratory arrest may be administered before cardiac arrest occurs. Pentobarbital is not suitable for use alone as a general anesthetic in large animals. Pentobarbital can be used at a low dose for standing sedation in cattle.

ADVERSE AND COMMON SIDE EFFECTS: If used alone for IV anesthesia in the horse or cow, pentobarbital may cause initial excitement. Some horses may rear and fall backward, injuring the poll. Additionally, the animal may injure itself during the prolonged period of recovery while attempting to stand. Barbiturate anesthesia in the horse should not be prolonged for longer than 1 hour, and no more than 5 g of any barbiturate should be given, even to draft breeds. Because pentobarbital is metabolized by the liver, it should not be administered to animals with hepatic disease.

DRUG INTERACTIONS: Pentobarbital may induce a severe cardiodepressant effect if used with streptomycin. Use of chloramphenicol within 25 days of pentobarbital can decrease the rate of pentobarbital metabolism and predispose to overdose of the barbiturate. Duration of sleeping time with pentobarbital is prolonged with concurrent use of sulfonamides, acetylsalicylic acid, or doxycycline. Duration of thiobarbiturate anesthesia appears to be unaffected by prior chloramphenicol administration; caution is still advised if chloramphenicol has been used.

SUPPLIED AS: VETERINARY PRODUCTS
For injection containing 65 mg/mL for general anesthesia
For injection containing 200, 240, 340, 390, and 540 mg/mL for euthanasia

OTHER USES
Cattle
STANDING SEDATION
2 mg/kg IV will give moderate sedation of up to 30 minutes and
mild sedation to 60 minutes after administration.

PENTOXIFYLLINE

INDICATIONS: Pentoxifylline (Trental♥★, Navicon♥) is a xanthine
derivative that improves peripheral blood flow and tissue oxygena-
tion. It also decreases blood viscosity and improves red blood cell
flexibility. A preliminary study in horses demonstrated that the drug
improved selected measures of circulatory flow. Recently, this drug
has been approved for use in Canada for treatment of navicular disease in horses.

ADVERSE AND COMMON SIDE EFFECTS: Information in humans indicates that pentoxifylline should not be used in patients
with marked liver or kidney impairment. It is also contraindicated in
humans with peptic ulcers or intolerance to other xanthines, such as
theophylline. Arrhythmias, edema, hypertension, hypotension, and
abdominal discomfort are reported in humans. Additionally, occasional and transient sweating, behavioral change, conjunctival congestion, edema, pruritus, and epiphora are also reported.

DRUG INTERACTIONS: Erythromycin may decrease hepatic metabolism of pentoxifylline.

SUPPLIED AS: VETERINARY PRODUCT
Oral powder containing 2 g/28.4-g pouch
HUMAN PRODUCT
Tablets containing 400 mg

PENTYLENETETRAZOL

INDICATIONS: Pentylenetetrazol (Metrazol★) is indicated for the
nonspecific treatment of toxic-induced respiratory depression. It is
also used in large animals as an evocative drug challenge for elec-
troencephalographic evaluation of seizure disorders.

ADVERSE AND COMMON SIDE EFFECTS: Overdose of pentylenetetrazol can induce convulsions. Subconvulsive doses of the drug
may activate latent epilepsy.

DRUG INTERACTIONS: None listed.

SUPPLIED AS: HUMAN PRODUCT
For injection containing 100 mg/mL

PHENOBARBITAL

INDICATIONS: Phenobarbital♥★ (Luminal★, Solfoton★) is used in large animals to treat convulsions of cerebrocortical diseases, such as head trauma, neonatal maladjustment of foals, lead poisoning, nervous coccidiosis, polioencephalomalacia, and others.

ADVERSE AND COMMON SIDE EFFECTS: Phenobarbital can cause liver damage, either due to drug allergy or toxic metabolism. See **BARBITURATES**.

DRUG INTERACTIONS: See **BARBITURATES**.

SUPPLIED AS: HUMAN PRODUCTS
For injection containing 30, 60, 65, 120, and 130 mg/mL
Tablets containing 15, 16, 30, 32, 60, 65, and 100 mg
Elixir containing 3 and 4 mg/mL

PHENOXYBENZAMINE

INDICATIONS: Phenoxybenzamine (Dibenzyline★) is a long-acting α-adrenergic blocking agent. The drug may be of use in reducing α-adrenergic-induced arterial spasm in acute laminitis. Its α-adrenergic blocking effects have also been used for treating presumed intestinal hypermotility in horses with diarrhea. However, this can also result in severe hypotension in a volume-depleted animal.

ADVERSE AND COMMON SIDE EFFECTS: In humans hypotension, reflex tachycardia, weakness, miosis, increased intraocular pressure, nausea, and vomiting are reported. In horses mild sedation has been reported.

DRUG INTERACTIONS: Phenoxybenzamine antagonizes the effects of α-adrenergic agonists such as phenylephrine.

SUPPLIED AS: HUMAN PRODUCT
Capsules containing 10 mg phenoxybenzamine

OTHER USES
Horses
DIARRHEA
1 mg/kg IV (diluted in 500 mL saline) over 5 to 10 minutes, followed in 12 hours by 0.5 mg/kg IV (diluted in 500 mL saline). Diarrhea of experimental grain engorgement and some clinical cases of diarrhea in horses have recovered following administration of phenoxybenzamine.

URINARY INCONTINENCE
0.7 mg/kg qid; PO to decrease urethral tone and aid bladder emptying; to be given along with bethanechol at 0.04 to 0.08 mg/kg tid; SC.

PHENYLBUTAZONE

INDICATIONS: Phenylbutazone (Bizolin 200★, Butaject★, Butasone
400♣, Butasone Conc♣, Butazone Injection♣, Butazone Powder♣,
Butequin♣, Butezole♣, Buzone Concentrate♣, Buzone Injectable♣,
Buzone Powder♣, Centrabute Injectable♣, Equipalazone♣, Equi-
Phar★, Equiphen Paste★, Phen-Buta-Vet★, Phenybutazone♣,
Phenybutazone Tablets♣★, Phenylbutazone Injectable♣, Phenylbutazone Injection★★, Phenylbutazone Powder♣, Phenylzone Paste★,
Pro-Bute Injection★, Pro-Bute Tablets★) is a synthetic, nonsteroidal
anti-inflammatory drug (NSAID) used for its antipyretic, anti-inflammatory, and analgesic properties. Phenylbutazone and other NSAIDs
have no direct effect on pain perception; rather they reduce hypersensitivity to pain by reducing the inflammatory response in inflamed tissue. It is particularly useful for alleviating musculoskeletal
lameness in horses. The drug is also used to reduce fever in horses
with viral infection. If the drug is used in febrile disease caused by
bacterial infection, it may mask a failure of response to concurrent antibiotic therapy. Phenylbutazone has not been useful in relieving the
pain of colic. Phenylbutazone has a prolonged half-life in ruminants
(50 hours in cows and 63 hours in bulls) and should be administered
only on alternate days in these animals. Adult goats have a far shorter
half-life of 16 hours. Pharmacokinetic data from goats suggest that
neonatal ruminants within the first 4 weeks of life have dramatic differences in drug distribution, with a half-life of up to 120 hours, necessitating longer dose intervals to avoid drug accumulation.

ADVERSE AND COMMON SIDE EFFECTS: Toxicity can occur in
the horse if administered at a dose greater than the manufacturer's
recommendation, especially if a high dose is maintained for more
than a few days. Signs of toxicity include anorexia, depression, oral
and gastrointestinal ulcers (including the cecum and colon), protein-
losing enteropathy, and death from shock. Neutropenia and severe
depletion of bone marrow neutrophils also occur. Ponies may be
more susceptible to toxicity than horses. Renal papillary necrosis is
also a consequence of toxicity, being more likely to occur in states of
reduced renal blood flow such as dehydration. Although it results in
a high incidence of agranulocytosis in humans, this does not appear
to be a problem in the horse.

DRUG INTERACTIONS: Phenylbutazone is highly bound to
plasma proteins and can displace other drugs that bind to plasma
proteins, such as other anti-inflammatory drugs, sulfonamides, or

anticoagulants such as warfarin, leading to increased pharmacologic effect or toxicity of the displaced drug. Displacement of plasma protein-bound thyroid hormone complicates interpretation of thyroid function tests. Phenylbutazone is contraindicated in animals with cardiac, renal, or hepatic insufficiency.

SUPPLIED AS: VETERINARY PRODUCTS
For injection containing 200 mg/mL
Powder containing 1, 1.5, and 4 g phenylbutazone per 15 g powder
Tablets containing 100 and 200 mg and 1 g
Paste form (apple flavor) containing 1 g/3 mL paste, 6 g/30 g
Granules containing 1 g/pouch
Gel containing 4 g/30 g

OTHER USES
Cattle
MUSCULOSKELETAL PAIN
4.4 to 10 mg/kg; IV, PO for alleviating chronic musculoskeletal pain such as in laminitis, arthritis, or spondylitis. The long elimination half-life of 36 to 65 hours in cattle necessitates dosing at approximately 2-day intervals.

PHENYLEPHRINE

INDICATIONS: Phenylephrine (AK-Dilate♣★, AK-Nefrin★, Dionephrine♣, IsoptoFrin★, Minums Phenylephrine♣, Mydfrin♣★, Neo-Synephrine♣★, Ocu-Nephrin★, Ocu-Phrin★, Phenylephrine♣★, Prefrin♣★, Relief★) is an α-adrenergic agonist used in ophthalmic preparations to enhance pupillary dilation poorly responsive to parasympatholytic drugs. Phenylephrine has been used as a mydriatic in equine recurrent uveitis.

ADVERSE AND COMMON SIDE EFFECTS: Prolonged topical use of phenylephrine has been associated with the development of corneal ulcers.

DRUG INTERACTIONS: Phenylephrine may be ineffective if combined with a parasympatholytic agent. This, however, remains to be clarified.

SUPPLIED AS: HUMAN PRODUCT
Ophthalmic solution containing 0.12%, 2.5%, and 10%

PHENYTOIN

INDICATIONS: Phenytoin or diphenylhydantoin (Dilantin♣★, Diphenylan Sodium★, Novo-Phenytoin♣, Ocusert Pilo★, Phenytoin Sodium Injection♣★, Phenytoin Oral Suspension★) is an anticonvulsant. Phenytoin stops the propagation and spread of neural excitation. The drug may also be used for management of digitalis-induced tachyarrhythmias. The drug has also been suggested as a preventive for the myotonia that occurs with hyperkalemic periodic paralysis of horses and for treatment of Australian Stringhalt. Although phenytoin gives symptomatic relief from myotonia in humans and dogs, it appears to have little if any benefit in horses with myotonia.

ADVERSE AND COMMON SIDE EFFECTS: Vomiting, ataxia, tremors, depression, hypotension, and atrioventricular block are reported in the dog. There is little information on adverse effects in large animals.

DRUG INTERACTIONS: Antacids (aluminum, calcium, and magnesium compounds), antihistamines, barbiturates, calcium gluconate, folic acid, and rifampin decrease serum levels of phenytoin. Serum levels are increased (and the potential for toxicity and loss of seizure control) by chloramphenicol, cimetidine, allopurinol, theophylline, anticoagulants, benzodiazepines, dexamethasone, estrogens, nitrofurantoin, phenothiazines, sulfonamides, salicylates and phenylbutazone. Phenytoin may decrease the activity of corticosteroids, estrogens, quinidine, dopamine, and furosemide.

SUPPLIED AS: HUMAN PRODUCTS
Capsules (extended) containing 30 and 100 mg
Oral suspension containing 6 and 25 mg/mL
Tablets containing 50 mg
For injection containing 50 mg/mL
Capsules containing combinations of 100 mg phenytoin and 15 mg phenobarbital or 100 mg phenytoin and 30 mg phenobarbital♣

OTHER USES
Horses
EXERTIONAL RHABDOMYOLYSIS
Begin with 6 to 8 mg/kg; PO for 3 to 5 days and increase by 1-mg/kg increments until rhabdomyolysis is prevented. Doses should be adjusted to achieve serum levels of 5 to 10 µg/mL. Reduce the dose if the horse appears drowsy.

PILOCARPINE

INDICATIONS: Pilocarpine (Adsorbocarpine★, Akarpine♣★, Diocarpine♣, Isopto Carpine★, Miocarpine♣, Ocu-Carpine★, Pilopine HS♣★, Pilocar★, Piloptic★, Pilostat★) is a cholinergic agent used to treat open-angle glaucoma in humans. Although primary glaucoma in large animals is rare, secondary or acquired glaucoma may occur following periodic ophthalmia of horses or as a sequela to melanoma or squamous cell carcinoma of the eye.

ADVERSE AND COMMON SIDE EFFECTS: Frequent intraconjunctival instillation of pilocarpine can result in sufficient absorption to produce systemic effects. Poisoning from pilocarpine is characterized by exaggeration of parasympathetic effects. See **ORGANOPHOSPHATES** in Description of Drugs for Small Animals.

DRUG INTERACTIONS: None listed.

SUPPLIED AS: HUMAN PRODUCTS
Ophthalmic solution containing 0.25%, 0.5%, 1%, 2%, 3%, 4%, 5%, and 6%
Inserts releasing 20 and 40 μg/hr
Ophthalmic gel containing 4%

PIPERAZINE

INDICATIONS: Piperazine (Alfalfa Pellet Horse Wormer✤, Co-op Wormer 52%✤, Piperazine✤★, Pipfuge★, Polywormerzine 53%✤, Warazine 53%✤, Wonder Wormer for Horses✤) is an anthelmintic used for the eradication of large roundworms, pinworms, and strongyles in horses. Many other more effective anthelmintics, such as parantel pamoate or ivermectin, are presently available.

ADVERSE AND COMMON SIDE EFFECTS: The most common clinical signs of toxicity in decreasing order of frequency are tremors, ataxia, seizures, and weakness. For recent ingestion, activated charcoal and a saline or osmotic cathartic are recommended. The drug should not be given to animals with chronic liver or renal disease. A horse treated with a piperazine/phenothiazine/trichlorfon suffered urticaria and alopecia.

DRUG INTERACTIONS: Piperazine and chlorpromazine may precipitate seizure activity if used at the same time. Piperazine may exaggerate the extrapyramidal effects of phenothiazines. Pyrantel/morantel antagonize the efficacy of piperazine. The concurrent use of laxatives is not recommended because these agents may cause elimination of the drug before it has had an opportunity to work effectively.

SUPPLIED AS: VETERINARY PRODUCTS
Alfalfa pellets containing 50% piperazine
Water additive wormer containing 17, 22, and 34 g/100 mL
Feed or water additive containing 50% and 52.5% piperazine as soluble powder

Tablets containing 50, 80, 110, 125, and 250 mg base piperazine
Capsules containing 120, 125, and 140 mg base piperazine
Paste containing 2.7 g/13 g

PIPERCILLIN

INDICATIONS: Pipercillin (Pipracil♥★) is a third-generation semi-synthetic penicillin.

ADVERSE AND COMMON SIDE EFFECTS AND DRUG INTER-ACTIONS: See PENICILLINS.

SUPPLIED AS: HUMAN PRODUCT
For injection containing 2, 3, 4, and 40 g

POLOXALENE

INDICATIONS: Poloxalene (Bloat Guard♣, Sweet Lix Bloat Guard Block medicated★, Therabloat Drench Concentrate★) is used in the prevention of bloat in ruminants due to legume feeding. It can be top dressed for feed or mixed in the feed. Under severe bloat-producing conditions the dose can be doubled.

ADVERSE AND COMMON SIDE EFFECTS: The expiration date should be strictly observed. If poloxalene is subjected to high environmental temperatures ($>37°C$, or $98.6°F$) for longer than 6 months, spontaneous combustion can occur.

DRUG INTERACTIONS: None listed.

SUPPLIED AS: VETERINARY PRODUCTS
Block containing 6.6% poloxalene
Multiwall bags containing 530 g poloxalene/kg
Oral concentrate containing 25 g/fluid ounce (833 mg/mL)
Liquid containing 99.5% poloxalene

POLYMYXIN B

INDICATIONS: Polymyxin B (Aerosporin♥★) is used in the treatment of gram-negative infections, especially those caused by *Pseudomonas, Pasteurella, Klebsiella, Salmonella, Bordetella*, and *Shigella* organisms. *Proteus* and *Brucella* organisms are frequently resistant. The drug is frequently used as a topical preparation for treating localized infections of the ears or eyes or for instillation in mastitis and intrauterine preparations. Absorption from the gastrointestinal tract is slow. Parenteral use should be restricted to severe urinary tract or systemic infections caused by susceptible coliforms or *Pseudomonas* *aeruginosa.* The drug is often combined with neomycin and bacitracin or tetracycline to broaden its spectrum of activity.

ADVERSE AND COMMON SIDE EFFECTS: Pain at the site of injection, nephrotoxicity, central nervous system signs, and neuromuscular blockade have been reported. Urticaria can occur at the site of contact with polymyxin B, which is nephrotoxic.

DRUG INTERACTIONS: Aminoglycoside antibiotics, bacitracin, and quinidine intensify the nephrotoxic and neurotoxic potential of polymyxin B. Succinylcholine and anesthetics may prolong the neuromuscular blockade and precipitate respiratory paralysis associated with the use of polymyxin B.

SUPPLIED AS: HUMAN PRODUCT
For injection containing 500,000 U/20-mL vial, equivalent to 50 mg polymyxin

POLYSULFATED GLYCOSAMINOGLYCAN (PSGAG)

INDICATIONS: Polysulfated glycosaminoglycan (Adequan Canine♣, Adequan I.A.★, Adequan I.M.★) is a potent proteolytic enzyme inhibitor that diminishes or reverses the processes that result in the loss of cartilaginous mucopolysaccharides. It is recommended for the treatment of noninfectious degenerative and/or traumatic joint dysfunction and associated lameness in the horse. PSGAG improves joint function by stimulating synovial membrane activity, reducing synovial protein levels, and increasing synovial fluid viscosity. Parenteral administration (IM) has been effective for reducing joint inflammation attributable to degenerative joint disease and has the added advantage of minimizing the risk of joint sepsis or postinjection inflammation associated with intra-articular administration.

ADVERSE AND COMMON SIDE EFFECTS: Postinjection joint inflammation may result from hypersensitivity to PSGAG, traumatic injection technique, increased dose or frequency of administration, or combination with other drugs. Joint sepsis is a rare complication of intra-articular injection.

DRUG INTERACTIONS: PSGAG should not be mixed with other drugs. Concomitant use with steroidal or nonsteroidal anti-inflammatory drugs may mask signs of joint sepsis.

SUPPLIED AS: VETERINARY PRODUCT
For injection containing 100 and 250 mg/mL

POTASSIUM CHLORIDE

INDICATIONS: Potassium chloride♣★ (Potassiject★) is used for the treatment of digitalis toxicity and for the treatment of hypokalemia commonly associated with diarrhea, or cattle with metabolic alkalosis as may occur with abomasal disease.

ADVERSE AND COMMON SIDE EFFECTS: If administered IV, potassium chloride should not exceed 0.5 mEq/kg/hr or 2 mEq/kg/day. Oral administration is the preferred route of supplementation. Potassium chloride has an unpleasant taste; gastric intubation for administration may be indicated. Even brief periods of excessively rapid administration can result in fatal cardiac arrhythmias. Electrocardiographic monitoring is advised if IV administration at rates above the guidelines indicated are deemed necessary. Signs of cardiotoxicity include prolongation of the QRS and PR intervals, loss of P waves, peaked T waves, and bradycardia.

DRUG INTERACTIONS: The concurrent use of penicillin G potassium may predispose to severe hyperkalemia.

SUPPLIED AS: VETERINARY PRODUCT
For injection containing 2 mEq/mL

HUMAN PRODUCT
For injection containing 1.5, 2, and 3 mEq/mL
Note: For large-animal use, inexpensive potassium chloride fluids can be mixed using chemical grade sterile potassium chloride and sterile water. Isotonic potassium chloride can be produced by adding 11 g to 1 L distilled water; 1 g of KCl contains 13 mEq potassium.

OTHER USES
Horses
EQUINE PERIODIC PARALYSIS
As a diagnostic test dose at 0.1 g/kg; PO, moving up in 0.025-g/kg increments to 0.2 g/kg; PO for induction of periodic paralysis in susceptible horses. The recent introduction of genetic testing for equine periodic paralysis may make this application obsolete.

PRALIDOXIME

INDICATIONS: Pralidoxime [pyridine-2-aldoxime-methiodide] (Protopam Chloride♣★) or PAM, is part of a group of compounds known as oximes. It is a reactivator of cholinesterase and is used as an antidote for organophosphate poisoning. PAM significantly reverses the combination of organophosphate with cholinesterase. Delay of treatment may be less effective as the phosphorylated enzyme complex of organophosphate to cholinesterase becomes resistant to reactivation by oximes. Atropine should be administered first to block muscarinic receptor sites.

ADVERSE AND COMMON SIDE EFFECTS: High doses of pralidoxime can cause neuromuscular blockade and inhibition of acetylcholinesterase. Rapid IV injection may cause tachycardia and weakness.

DRUG INTERACTIONS: Oximes should not be used in carbamate toxicity because they are ineffective in antagonizing carbamate cholinesterase inhibitors and, because they have weak anticholinesterase properties, may act synergistically with carbamates.

SUPPLIED AS: HUMAN PRODUCT
For injection containing 1 g

PREDNISONE, PREDNISOLONE

INDICATIONS: Prednisone (Deltasone♣, Meticorten Suspension★, Predsone-5♣) and Prednisolone (Cortisate-20★, Predate 50★, Prednisolone Sodium Succinate♣★, Solu-Delta-Cortef♣★, Sterisol-20 Injection★, Uni-Pred 50♣) are intermediate-acting glucocorticoid agents. Prednisone is converted by the liver to prednisolone. Except for cases of liver failure, the drugs can essentially be used interchangeably. Prednisolone is also available in combination with other agents, such as salicylates (Pred-C♣), antibiotics (Chlorasone★, Delta Albaplex♣★, Predbiotic★) or antihistamines (Cortatabs♣, Predniderm♣, Sterolin♣, Temaril-P★, Vanectyl-P♣). Prednisolone is indicated for the treatment of inflammatory conditions of the skin and joints and for supportive care during periods of stress. Prednisolone sodium succinate is also beneficial for the treatment of acute hypersensitivity reactions, atopic and contact dermatitis, summer eczema, and conjunctivitis. This drug is also used in animals with severe overwhelming infections (in combination with appropriate antibiotic therapy) and for the prevention and treatment of adrenal insufficiency and shock (in conjunction with fluid support). Rifampin decreases the half-life of prednisone.

ADVERSE AND COMMON SIDE EFFECTS and **DRUG INTERACTIONS:** See GLUCOCORTICOID AGENTS.

SUPPLIED AS: VETERINARY PRODUCTS
PREDNISOLONE
For injection containing 20 mg/mL prednisolone sodium phosphate
For injection containing 10 and 50 mg/mL prednisolone acetate
Tablets containing 5 mg

For injection containing 10 and 50 mg/mL prednisolone sodium succinate

PREDNISONE
Tablets containing 5 mg prednisone

HUMAN PRODUCTS
Oral solution containing 5 and 15 mg/5 mL prednisolone
Oral solution containing 1 and 5 mg/mL prednisone
Tablets containing 1, 2.5, 5, 10, 20, 25, and 50 mg prednisone
For injection containing 25 and 50 mg/mL prednisolone acetate, 20 mg/mL prednisolone phosphate

PREGNANT MARE'S SERUM GONADOTROPHIN (PMSG)

INDICATIONS: Pregnant mare's serum gonadotrophin [PMSG] (Equinex♣, Folligon♣, PMSG-5000♣) is a complex glycoprotein produced by the endometrial cups of the pregnant mare's uterus. PMSG has high follicle-stimulating hormone (FSH) properties and luteinizing hormone (LH) actions. Due to its FSH activity, it stimulates growth of the interstitial cells of the ovaries as well as growth and maturation of the follicles; hence it is used to induce superovulation for embryo transfer in cows. In the mare, PMSG administration may produce out-of-season estrus (fall and late winter) followed by ovulation if a follicle is palpable on the ovary at the time of injection.

ADVERSE AND COMMON SIDE EFFECTS: Anaphylaxis can occur. Repeated administration may result in decreased efficacy due to the production of antihormone antibodies.

DRUG INTERACTIONS: None listed.

SUPPLIED AS: VETERINARY PRODUCT
For injection containing 5,000 U

OTHER USES
Sheep and Goats
OVULATION INDUCTION
The LH activity of PMSG (400–700 IU; IM) will induce ovulation and thus is used along with intravaginal progestagens for out-of-season breeding or estrus synchronization in sheep and goats.

PRIMIDONE

INDICATIONS: Primidone (Apo-Primidone♣, Myidone★, Mysoline♣, Neurosyn★, Primidone★, Primitabs★, Sertan♣) is an anticonvulsant agent that works by raising the seizure threshold. It can be used to control convulsions due to head trauma or meningitis in horses. The drug is metabolized in the liver to phenobarbital (contributes about 85% of the anticonvulsant activity) and phenylethylmalonamide (which contributes about 15% of the anticonvulsant activity). Primidone is more expensive than phenobarbital and consequently is not commonly used in large animals.

ADVERSE AND COMMON SIDE EFFECTS: Polyuria, polydipsia, and polyphagia are noted during the first few weeks of therapy or when the dose is increased. Sedation and ataxia may occur but tend to resolve with continued treatment. Transient anxiety and agitation at the start of therapy may be observed.

DRUG INTERACTIONS: Acetazolamide may decrease the absorption of primidone. The combination of primidone and phenytoin potentiates hepatotoxicity. The effects of corticosteroids, β-blockers, quinidine, theophylline, and metronidazole may be decreased if used in conjunction with primidone.

SUPPLIED AS: VETERINARY PRODUCT
Tablets containing 50 and 250 mg

HUMAN PRODUCTS
Tablets containing 50, 125, and 250 mg
Oral suspension containing 250 mg/5 mL

PROGESTERONE

INDICATIONS: Progesterone✦★ is a gonadal hormone from the corpus luteum that favors the maintenance of pregnancy. Other actions include induction of mammary tissue growth and secretory changes to the endometrium, which only occur after suitable priming of the target tissue by estrogen. Progesterone inhibits the action of follicle-stimulating hormone (FSH), preventing the development of follicles and blocking ovulation. A number of commercially available drugs have progesterone activity (Centra Progestin✦, Progesterone✦) or similar-acting progestagens [altrenogest] (Regu-Mate✦✦), [medroxyprogesterone acetate] (Veramix Sponges✦), [melengestrol acetate] (MGA Premix✦✦), [megestrol acetate] (Ovaban Tablets✦★, Ovarid Tablets✦). Progesterone is used to treat habitual or threatened abortion and has been used empirically to prevent embryonic death in horses and cattle. Other suggested uses are nymphomania and mammary underdevelopment. As nymphomania is likely due to the presence of cystic ovaries, progesterone is not indicated in such cases. Possibly the most widespread and effective use of progesterone or similar acting compounds has been to control estrus cycles. Progesterone will suppress estrus in large animals and subsequent withdrawal yields a predictable occurrence of estrus.

Specific progestagen products, such as intravaginal sponges for sheep (Veramix Sponges♣) and implants (Synchro-Mate★), assist in timed induction of estrus. Suppression of estrus will also facilitate regular cycles following winter anestrus in mares and facilitate scheduled breeding and help manage mares exhibiting prolonged estrus. Ovulation will occur 5 to 7 days after the onset of estrus. The progestin melengestrol acetate (MGA Premix♣★) has been used as a feed additive to suppress heat in feedlot heifers and for stimulation of growth and improved feed utilization.

ADVERSE AND COMMON SIDE EFFECTS: Progesterones favor closure of the cervix, preventing infections of the uterus draining. Overdosage of progesterone can cause cystic ovaries in cattle. The drug should not be used in lactating dairy cattle.

DRUG INTERACTIONS: None listed.

SUPPLIED AS: VETERINARY PRODUCTS
Medroxyprogesterone-impregnated intravaginal polyurethane sponges containing 60 mg/sponge
Feed additive containing 17.6, 220, 440, and 1,100 mg/kg melengestrol acetate
Tablets containing 5 and 20 mg megestrol acetate
Injection containing 50 mg/mL
Solution containing 2.2 mg/mL altrenenogest
Gel containing 2.15 mg/g altrenogest

OTHER USES
Cattle
GROWTH PROMOTER
Progesterone is a component of growth implants combined with estradiol benzoate (Steer-Oid♣★, Synovex-C♣★, Synovex-S♣★).

INDUCE LACTATION
Progesterone can be administered to open heifers or cows to induce lactation at 0.125 mg/kg bid; SC, in combination with estrogen (17β-estradiol) at 0.05 mg/kg bid; SC, for 7 days.

PROMAZINE

INDICATIONS: Promazine (Primazine★, Promazine Hydrochloride★, Promazine Granules★, Prozine-50★, Sparine★, Tranquazine★) is a phenothiazine tranquilizer that may be used for minor chemical restraint such as floating teeth, loading and transportation of horses, and as a preanesthetic agent in large animals. Acepromazine is a more widely used phenothiazine for large animals.

ADVERSE AND COMMON SIDE EFFECTS AND DRUG INTER-ACTIONS: See **ACEPROMAZINE**.

SUPPLIED AS: VETERINARY PRODUCTS
Soluble granules containing 8 g/10.25 oz
Injection containing 50 mg/mL

HUMAN PRODUCTS
For injection containing 25 and 50 mg/mL
Tablets containing 25, 50, and 100 mg

PROPANTHELINE

INDICATIONS: Propantheline bromide (Pro-Banthine♥★, Propanthel♥) is an anticholinergic agent. It is used in horses to decrease intestinal spasm to facilitate rectal examination. At this time no commercial product is available for parenteral use.

ADVERSE AND COMMON SIDE EFFECTS: Tachycardia, weakness, nausea, constipation, pupillary dilation, and dryness of the mucous membranes may occur. Signs of drug overdose include urinary retention, excitement, hypotension, respiratory failure, paralysis, and coma.

DRUG INTERACTIONS: Antihistamines, procainamide, quinidine, meperidine, benzodiazepines, and the phenothiazines may enhance the activity of propantheline and primidone and long-term corticosteroid use may potentiate the adverse effects of the drug. Propantheline may enhance the activity of nitrofurantoin, thiazide diuretics, and sympathomimetic drugs. Propantheline delays the absorption of, but increases serum levels of, ranitidine and it may decrease the absorption of cimetidine.

SUPPLIED AS: HUMAN PRODUCT
Tablets containing 7.5 and 15 mg

PROPARACAINE

INDICATIONS: Proparacaine (AK-Taine★, Alcaine♥★, Diocaine♥, Kainair★, Ocu-Caine★, Ophthetic♥★, Ophthaine★, Spectro-Caine★) is a local anesthetic used for desensitization of the cornea and conjunctiva. Unlike some topical anesthetics, proparacaine produces little or no initial irritation.

ADVERSE AND COMMON SIDE EFFECTS: Proparacaine is generally safe for patients with hypersensitivities to other local anesthetics. However, in humans there are rare occurrences of immediate hyperallergic corneal reactions with development of diffuse epithelial keratitis.

DRUG INTERACTIONS: None listed.

SUPPLIED AS: HUMAN PRODUCT
Ophthalmic solution containing 0.5%

PROPOFOL

INDICATIONS: Propofol (Diprivan♥★, Rapinovet ♥★) is a hypnotic agent given IV to induce and maintain anesthesia. The drug is rapidly metabolized by the liver, which results in rapid recovery from anesthesia. It has been used satisfactorily in foals premedicated with xylazine to induce anesthesia for restraint during magnetic resonance imaging. Some respiratory depression does occur during the anesthesia.

ADVERSE AND COMMON SIDE EFFECTS: None listed. It is very susceptible to bacterial growth and should be discarded within 6 hours of opening.

DRUG INTERACTIONS: None listed.

SUPPLIED AS: VETERINARY PRODUCT
For injection containing 10 mg/mL
HUMAN PRODUCT
For injection containing 10 mg/mL

PROPRANOLOL

INDICATIONS: Propranolol (Apo-Propranolol♥, Detensol♥, Dom-Propranolol♥, Inderal♥★, Novo-Propranolol♥, Nu-Propranolol♥, PMS-Propranolol♥) is a nonselective β_1- and β_2-blocking agent. Its use in large animals is restricted to the management of tachycardia in the horse.

ADVERSE AND COMMON SIDE EFFECTS: Propranolol is contraindicated in patients with congestive heart failure unless it is secondary to a tachyarrhythmia responsive to β-blockade. The drug is also contraindicated in those with second- or third-degree heart block and sinus bradycardia and with bronchoconstrictive lung disease, for example, horses with chronic obstructive pulmonary disease (COPD). Adverse effects including bradycardia, central nervous system effects, gastrointestinal effects, and dermatologic and hematologic effects are common in humans.

DRUG INTERACTIONS: Antacids delay gastrointestinal absorption of propranolol. Antiarrhythmic effects of quinidine, procainamide, and lidocaine are enhanced by propranolol, but toxic effects may be additive. Serum levels of propranolol are increased by cimetidine. The hypotensive effects of propranolol are reduced by nonsteroidal anti-inflammatory drugs and enhanced by phenothiazines, cimetidine, furosemide, and other diuretics. Propranolol may potentiate the effects of neuromuscular blocking agents and theophylline.

SUPPLIED AS: HUMAN PRODUCTS
Tablets containing 10, 20, 40, 60, 80, 90, and 120 mg
Tablets (extended release) containing 60, 80, 120, and 160 mg
For injection containing 1 mg/mL
Solution containing 4, 8, and 80 mg/mL

PROPYLENE GLYCOL

INDICATIONS: Propylene glycol is used alone (Propylene Glycol♣★) or combined with other medications (Domcol Solution♣, Ketoban Oral Solution and Gel★, Keto Plus Gel★, PCE Glycol♣, Co-op Ketox♣, Co-op Ketox Liquid Plus♣, Glycol-P♣, Ketopar♣ Ketoroid♣) for the treatment and prevention of ketosis (acetonemia) in cows and sheep (pregnancy toxemia). Given orally, propylene glycol is a glucose precursor in ruminants. The drug is also administered to ruminants in combination with other medications (Bloat-Pac7★, Veterinary Surfactant★) for the management of pasture bloat.

ADVERSE AND COMMON SIDE EFFECTS: Overuse may have a deleterious effect on rumen flora, decrease rumen motility, and cause diarrhea.

DRUG INTERACTIONS: None listed.

SUPPLIED AS: VETERINARY PRODUCTS
Liquid as propylene glycol 100%
Propylene glycol in combination with other products such as cobalt, choline chloride ethylenediamine dihydroiodide, and potassium iodide for ketosis therapy♣, or with dioctyl sodium succinate for treatment of bloat★

OTHER USES
Horses
MUCOLYTIC
Propylene glycol can be used in horses as a mucolytic for disrupting respiratory mucus. This requires use of a nebulizer and can cause airway irritation and bronchoconstriction. Propylene glycol is also used as a base for many products. See **DIOCTYL SODIUM SULFOSUCCINATE** in propylene glycol.

PROSTAGLANDIN F₂α

INDICATIONS: Prostaglandin $F_{2\alpha}$ ($PGF_{2\alpha}$) is available as a number of natural (dinoprost tromethamine; Lutalyse♥★) or synthetic compounds such as cloprostenol (Estrumate♥★, Planate♥), fluprostenol (Equimate★), and fenprostalene (Synchrocept B♥, Bovilene★). Prostaglandin $F_{2\alpha}$ administration causes functional and morphologic regression of the corpus luteum if it is at least 4 or 5 days old. Estrus usually follows 2 to 5 days after treatment, followed by ovulation and normal fertility. $PGF_{2\alpha}$ is used to manipulate the estrus cycle for planned breeding, to aid in evacuation of pyometra, and in cattle to induce abortion. It is also used in goats to treat hydrometra (pseudo-pregnancy). Due to the seasonal polyestrus nature of the mare, the efficacy of $PGF_{2\alpha}$ in the mare may vary with the time of year it is administered.

ADVERSE AND COMMON SIDE EFFECTS: Specific products are available for horses and for cattle. $PGF_{2\alpha}$ should not be given to cows that may be pregnant unless to induce abortion; 95% of cows up to 4½ months into pregnancy will abort, as will some cattle in later gestation. Because $PGF_{2\alpha}$ can be absorbed through the skin, care should be taken in handling the product, particularly for women of child-bearing age and asthmatics. Some products used in mares may cause sweating, increased heart rate, and abdominal discomfort. These signs abate within 30 minutes to 1 hour. A low incidence of clostridial infection at the site of injection has been reported following prostaglandin administration. Only cattle with functional corpus luteum can be expected to respond to cloprostenol.

DRUG INTERACTIONS: None listed.

SUPPLIED AS: VETERINARY PRODUCTS
For injection containing 5 mg/mL prostaglandin $F_{2\alpha}$ (dinoprost tromethamine) [Lutalyse♥★]
For injection containing 88 mg cloprostenol/mL [Planate♥, for swine] and 250 mg/mL cloprostenol [Estrumate♥★]
For injection containing 50 mg/mL fluprostenol [Equimate★]
For injection containing 0.5 mg/mL fenprostalene [Synchrocept B♥, Bovilene★]

PROTAMINE SULFATE

INDICATIONS: Protamine sulfate♥★ is a low molecular weight protein that antagonizes the anticoagulant effects of heparin; the effect of heparin on platelet aggregation may persist. It is used to reverse severe bleeding associated with excessive anticoagulation caused by heparin. Protamine sulfate given in the absence of heparin has its own anticoagulant activity.

ADVERSE AND COMMON SIDE EFFECTS: It must be given only by the IV route and administered slowly. Rapid administration may cause dyspnea, bradycardia, and hypotension, possibly from the release of endogenous histamine. Hypersensitivity reactions may also occur. These effects are minimized if the drug is injected slowly over a 3- to 10-minute period. A rebound effect leading to prolonged bleeding may occur several hours after heparin has apparently been neutralized. The cause may be due to release of heparin from the heparin-protamine complex or release of additional heparin from extravascular spaces.

DRUG INTERACTIONS: None reported.

SUPPLIED AS: HUMAN PRODUCT
For injection containing 10 mg/mL

PSYLLIUM MUCILLOID

INDICATIONS: Psyllium mucilloid (Equine Psyllium★, Equi-Phar Sweet Psyllium★, Sandex Crumbles★, Vetasyl★★, Metamucil★★, Novo-Mucilax♣, and others) is a hydrophilic substance that forms a gelatinous mass when mixed with water. It is used for the treatment of sand impaction colic in horses. The gel lubricates and binds the sand, moving it distally, clearing the impaction. After initial doses are mixed with water, the mucilloid can be mixed with sweet feed.

ADVERSE AND COMMON SIDE EFFECTS: Once in contact with water, the mucilloid quickly forms a gel and becomes difficult to pump through a nasogastric tube. Side effects are minimal. Temporary cramping, flatulence, and bloating may occur. It should, however, not be used in patients with abdominal pain, vomiting, nausea, or fecal impaction.

DRUG INTERACTIONS: None established.

SUPPLIED AS: VETERINARY PRODUCTS
Capsules containing 250, 400, and 495 mg
Powder containing 2 or 3.75 oz/scoop (100%)

HUMAN PRODUCT
Powder containing 3, 3.4, or 6 g/rounded teaspoonful

PYRANTEL

INDICATIONS: Pyrantel [pyrantel pamoate] (Equi-Phar Horse and Colt Wormer★, Nemex Tabs★, Nemex-2★, Pyran♣, Pyr-A-Pam♣, Strongid-P Paste♣★, Strongid-T♣★, Sure Shot Liquid Wormer★), [pyrantel tartrate] (Banminth Premix♣, Banminth For Horses &

Colts★, Purina Colt and Horse Wormer★, Strongid-C♣★) is an anthelmintic effective against the adult forms of the large and small strongyles and ascarids of horses. It is also an effective broad-spectrum anthelmintic for ruminants, including the adult forms of *Haemonchus contortus* in sheep and goats. Pyrantel is a cholinesterase inhibitor and has a wide margin of safety. The tartrate salt is generally administered dry in the feed rather than in solution to minimize absorption of this highly soluble form.

ADVERSE AND COMMON SIDE EFFECTS: Cautious use of the drug is advised in patients with liver dysfunction, malnutrition, dehydration, or anemia. There is one report of a horse exhibiting abdominal pain after administration.

DRUG INTERACTIONS: Because of its cholinergic properties, it has been suggested that pyrantel should not be used concurrently with levamisole, organophosphates, or diethylcarbamazine. However, there appears to be no clinical evidence to substantiate this and labeling for pyrantel products indicates safety for simultaneous use with insecticides, tranquilizers, muscle relaxants, and central nervous system depressants. Piperazine and pyrantel have antagonistic actions and should not be used together.

SUPPLIED AS: VETERINARY PRODUCTS
Paste containing 3.58 g/premeasured syringe
Liquid containing 2.27, 4.54, and 50 mg/mL
Tablets containing 22.7, 35, 113.5, and 125 mg
Granules containing 10.6 g/kg
Premix containing 10.8% (swine) and 1.25% (equine)

OTHER USES
Horses
TAPEWORMS
13.3 mg/kg; PO
Pyrantel is also available in combination with trichlorfon [Strongid Plus] to remove bots as well as intestinal worms.

PYRIMETHAMINE

INDICATIONS: Pyrimethamine (Daraprim♣★, Quinnoxine-S♣) is used in combination with the sulfonamides, such as sulfadiazine, in the treatment of equine protozoal myelitis. Pyrimethamine inhibits folic acid metabolism in the parasite and appears to increase the activity of the sulfonamide against the sporozoan parasite.

ADVERSE AND COMMON SIDE EFFECTS: Problems are rare at the recommended dose, but depression, anorexia, vomiting, and re-

versible bone marrow suppression (anemia, leukopenia, and thrombocytopenia) may occur within 4 to 6 days of initiation of therapy
with the pyrimethamine-sulfonamide combination. The anemia that
develops over long-term administration is seldom of clinical significance. Bone marrow suppression may be mitigated by the concurrent administration of folic acid (75 mg; IM per horse every 3 days),
or by supplementing the diet with brewer's yeast.

DRUG INTERACTIONS: Pyrimethamine is synergistic with sulfonamides. Pyrimethamine is highly bound to plasma protein and may
displace other drugs, such as phenylbutazone or warfarin, thereby
interfering with their action.

SUPPLIED AS: VETERINARY PRODUCT
Water additive for poultry containing 9.8 g/L, combined with sulfaquinoxaline 32.5 g/L [Quinnoxine-S♣]

HUMAN PRODUCT
Tablets containing 25 mg

QUINIDINE

INDICATIONS: Quinidine bisulfate (Biquin♣★), quinidine gluconate (Quinaglute★, Quinate♣), quinidine polygalacturonate (Car-
dioquin♣★) and quinidine sulfate (Apo-Quinidine♣, Quinidex♣★,
Quinora★) is used in the management of atrial fibrillation in horses
and cattle. The IV route has recently been advocated as a more rapid
mode of treatment in horses, using the gluconate form, but is considerably more expensive and less likely to be effective in long-
standing atrial fibrillation. Although quinidine is also useful in treating atrial fibrillation in cattle, they will usually convert to normal
sinus rhythm without treatment once the initiating disease (e.g., gastrointestinal problems) is resolved.

ADVERSE AND COMMON SIDE EFFECTS: The drug is contraindicated in patients with myasthenia gravis, digitalis intoxication, heart block, and escape beats. Anorexia, diarrhea, vagolytic response, urine retention, weakness, hypotension, and decreased
cardiac contractility are reported. Sinus node suppression, ventricular tachycardia, atrioventricular block, prolongation of the PR, QRS,
and QT intervals are also reported. A paradoxical acceleration in
ventricular rate may occur, especially when the drug is used to treat
patients with atrial flutter or fibrillation. In these cases it is often
used after patients have first been given a digitalis glycoside. Quinidine intoxication can be antagonized by rapid alkalinization of the
blood with sodium bicarbonate. Drug dose should be decreased in
cases with liver disease, congestive heart failure, hyperkalemia, or
hypoalbuminemia.

DRUG INTERACTIONS: Quinidine increases serum digoxin levels. Cimetidine increases serum quinidine levels. Phenothiazines potentiate the cardiac depressive effects of quinidine. Quinidine potentiates the neuromuscular blocking effects of curariform and depolarizing blocking agents as well as those induced by neomycin and kanamycin. Anticholinergic drugs have additive vagolytic effects. Phenobarbital and phenytoin decrease the half-life of quinidine, necessitating readjustment of drug dose. Sodium bicarbonate, antacids, and thiazide diuretics prolong the half-life of quinidine, predisposing to toxicity. Quinidine may enhance the hypotensive effects of β-blocking agents and vasodilators.

SUPPLIED AS: HUMAN PRODUCTS
Tablets containing 200 and 300 mg quinidine sulfate
Tablets containing 275 mg quinidine polygalacturonate (200 mg quinidine sulfate)
Tablets (sustained release) containing 300 mg quinidine sulfate
Tablets containing 250 mg quinidine bisulfate (200 mg quinidine sulfate)
For injection containing 190 mg/mL quinidine sulfate
Tablets containing 325 mg quinidine gluconate
Tablets (sustained release) containing 324 mg quinidine gluconate
For injection containing 80 mg/mL quinidine gluconate

RANITIDINE

INDICATIONS: Ranitidine (Alti-Ranitidine HCl♣, Apo-Ranitidine♣, Novo-Ranitidine♣, Nu-Ranit♣, Zantac-C♣, Zantac♣★) is an H_2-receptor antagonist that reduces gastric acid secretion in a dose-dependent competitive manner by blocking histamine-induced gastric acid secretion. The H_2 blockers (see also **CIMETIDINE**) are highly selective in action and virtually without effect on H_1 receptors. Although the H_2 receptors are widely distributed throughout the body, the extragastric receptors appear to be of only minor physiologic importance. The H_2 blockers also inhibit, at least partially, gastric secretion elicited by muscarinic agonists and gastrin. Ranitidine is used in horses to treat gastric ulcers and as a preventive measure for animals considered at risk for the development of gastric ulcers, such as sick neonatal foals. Its effects are longer lasting than cimetidine, but ranitidine is considerably more expensive. Ranitidine lacks the antiandrogenic activity that may occur with cimetidine and can be substituted for cimetidine. Treatment should continue for 10 to 20 days.

Ranitidine has been shown experimentally to increase abomasal pH in sheep. The IV route caused a greater increase and for a longer period of time than oral dosing. Peak increase in abomasal pH with IV dosing occurred at 4 to 6 hours, with pH remaining above baseline for 24 to 36 hours. From this information it may be possible to use this drug in the treatment of abomasal ulceration in ruminants on a once-daily dosage regimen.

ADVERSE AND COMMON SIDE EFFECTS: Adverse reactions are low in incidence and relatively minor, and include skin rash, diarrhea, constipation, and loss of libido. Rapid IV injection may cause profound bradycardia. Lower than recommended doses will alleviate clinical signs of gastric ulceration, but significant ulceration may continue unabated.

DRUG INTERACTIONS: Concurrent use of H_2 blockers with warfarin, phenytoin, theophylline, phenobarbital, diazepam, propranolol, and imipramine may result in the accumulation of the latter drugs through impairment of the hepatic metabolism. Ranitidine has fewer effects on hepatic drug metabolism by the cytochrome P-450 system than does cimetidine.

SUPPLIED AS: HUMAN PRODUCTS
Tablets containing 150 and 300 mg
Capsules containing 150 and 300 mg
Oral syrup containing 15 mg/mL
For injection containing 25 mg/mL

RESERPINE

INDICATIONS: Reserpine (Novo-Reserpine✚, Reserpine Tablets★, Serpalan★, Serpasil✚) has been used in horses for its taming effect of highly spirited horses, producing a state of indifference to environmental stimuli. Its mode of action is as a catecholamine-depleting agent that causes a severe reduction of the neuronal stores of norepinephrine. It has fallen out of favor in veterinary medicine. It is currently used in humans for treating hypertension and psychiatric disorders. The onset of action of reserpine is long: 24 to 48 hours after oral administration and 1 to 2 hours after IV injection. However, only the tablets are commercially available in North America; the injectable product for veterinary use is found in New Zealand.

Its use is prohibited for competitions, but may be of value in some situations on the farm where prolonged continuous sedative and calming effects are desired.

ADVERSE AND COMMON SIDE EFFECTS: None listed.

DRUG INTERACTIONS: None listed.

SUPPLIED AS: HUMAN PRODUCT
Tablets containing 0.1 and 0.25 mg

RIFAMPIN

INDICATIONS: Rifampin (Rifadin✦★, Rofact✦, Rimactane✦★) is an antibiotic that is very lipid soluble and attains good intracellular concentrations. It can be used alone for treatment of bacterial endocarditis or osteomyelitis in large animals or in combination with other agents such as erythromycin to reduce the frequency of acquired resistance. It is used in the treatment of internal abscesses, such as those caused by *Rhodococcus equi* or *Corynebacterium pseudotuberculosis* infections. Adult ruminants have prolonged oral absorption similar to adult horses, possibly relating to the time required for the drug to pass through the rumen. Recent studies in foals have shown that they have up to a threefold longer elimination time than adult horses, which suggests lower than currently recommended doses may still be clinically effective.

ADVERSE AND COMMON SIDE EFFECTS: If given IV to horses, even slowly over 10 minutes, adverse reactions such as weakness, slight to profuse sweating, defecation, and apprehension may occur. In humans, hepatopathy and discoloration of the urine, feces, saliva, tears, and sweat are reported. Although rare, anorexia, vomiting, diarrhea, thrombocytopenia, hemolytic anemia, interstitial nephritis, and bloody/cloudy urine, as well as death have also been reported.

DRUG INTERACTIONS: Rifampin decreases the half-life of prednisone, digoxin, barbiturates, quinidine, ketoconazole, oral anticoagulants, and other drugs subject to metabolism by hepatic microsomal enzymes. Combination with halothane or isoniazid may cause hepatotoxicity.

SUPPLIED AS: HUMAN PRODUCTS
Capsules containing 150 and 300 mg
Injection containing 600 mg

ROMIFIDINE

INDICATIONS: Romifidine (Sedivet✦) is a potent, semisynthetic α_2-agonist with sedative effects like xylazine and detomidine, but is longer lasting and produces less ataxia. Its use in horses is indicated to facilitate handling, examination, and minor treatments. It provides dose-dependent sedation and tolerance to pain. Lowering of the head is the first sign of sedation, followed by lethargy, reduced sensitivity to environmental stimuli, and immobility. The onset of sedation occurs within 1 to 2 minutes and lasts 40 to 80 minutes. When used as a premedicant agent, it is given 8 to 10 minutes prior to general anesthesia. Clinically useful sedation of 60 minutes occurs with the concurrent administration of butorphanol.

ADVERSE AND COMMON SIDE EFFECTS: A prolonged reduction in blood pressure and heart rate with partial atrioventricular (AV) block occur following administration. This can be prevented by the IV administration of atropine at 0.01 mg/kg 3 to 5 minutes before romifidine administration. Following administration, occasional sweating and diuresis may occur. As with the other α_2-sympathomimetics, sedated horses may show increased skin sensitivity to the hind legs. Its use is contraindicated in horses with preexisting AV block, respiratory disease, advanced liver or kidney disease, or endotoxic or traumatic shock. Its safety has not been established for use in breeding horses.

DRUG INTERACTIONS: None listed.

SUPPLIED AS: VETERINARY PRODUCT
For injection containing 10 mg/mL in 20-mL multidose vials.

SODIUM BICARBONATE

INDICATIONS: Sodium bicarbonate✦★ (Bicarboject★, Neutralyzer★) is indicated for the treatment of metabolic acidosis as occurs commonly in neonatal diarrhea of large animals. It is also indicated for the management of hyperkalemia and hypercalcemia.

ADVERSE AND COMMON SIDE EFFECTS: The agent is contraindicated in cases with alkalosis, significant chloride loss associated with gastric or abomasal reflux, or with hypocalcemia where infusion of this agent will predispose to hypocalcemic tetany. Sodium bicarbonate should be used with caution in those with potential volume overload, for example, congestive heart failure and renal disease. Hypercapnia predisposing to ventricular fibrillation may occur in patients during cardiopulmonary resuscitation if adequate ventilatory support is not given. The use of this drug may cause metabolic alkalosis, hypokalemia, hypocalcemia, hypernatremia, volume overload and paradoxical cerebrospinal fluid (CSF) acidosis leading to respiratory arrest. Myocardial depression and peripheral vasodilation leading to hypotension, hyperosmolality, CSF acidosis, increased intracranial pressure, and intracranial hemorrhage have been reported.

DRUG INTERACTIONS: If sodium bicarbonate is mixed with calcium-containing fluids, insoluble complexes may form. The action of epinephrine is impaired if it is mixed with sodium bicarbonate. Oral sodium bicarbonate may reduce the absorption of anticholinergic agents, cimetidine, ranitidine, iron products, ketoconazole, and tetracycline antibiotics and reduce the efficacy of sucralfate. Orally administered drugs are best given 2 hours before or after sodium bicarbonate.

SUPPLIED AS: VETERINARY PRODUCTS
For injection containing 8.4% (1 mEq/mL)
For injection containing 7.5% (0.89 mEq/mL)
Paste containing 2.27 g/454-g tube
For "home mixed" solutions, a 1.3% (13 g/L) solution of sodium bicarbonate is approximately isotonic. One gram of sodium bicarbonate contains 12 mEq of sodium and 12 mEq of bicarbonate.

HUMAN PRODUCTS
Tablets containing 325 mg (5 grain) and 650 mg (10 grain)
Tablets containing 500 mg
For injection containing 4% (0.48 mEq/mL), 4.2% (0.5 mEq/mL), 5% (0.595 mEq/mL), 7.5% (0.9 mEq/mL), and 8.4% (1 mEq/mL)

OTHER USES
Horses
PRERACE
Sodium bicarbonate is used as an oral prerace medication ("milkshake") to enhance performance. Doses of 0.4 g/kg PO (and reportedly considerably higher) have been given within 3.5 hours of race time. Studies of its effect as a performance enhancer have led to inconsistent results. High doses or excessive dietary supplementation of sodium bicarbonate can produce metabolic alkalosis and reduce clinical and cardiovascular effects of carbohydrate overloading in horses. Further, it is considered unethical and illegal to administer this medication prerace, and administration by nonmedical personnel has occasionally resulted in lethal aspiration pneumonia.

SODIUM CHLORIDE

INDICATIONS: Sodium chloride (Hypersaline E★, Hyper Saline Solution 8X★, Hypertonic Saline★, Physiologic Saline♣, Physiological Saline Solution♣, Physiologic Saline Solution★, Saline 0.9%★, Saline Solution★, Sterile Saline Solution★) is recommended for the treatment of hyponatremia, hypochloremic metabolic alkalosis, and the restoration of normovolemia and the promotion of urinary calcium excretion. Isotonic sodium chloride (0.9%) remains in the extracelluar space (two-thirds in the interstitial space, one-third in the intravascular space) after IV injection. Half-strength saline (0.45%) is directed into the intracellular space (one-third) and extracellular space (two-thirds) after IV administration and is a suggested treatment for animals with hypernatremia. Hypertonic saline (7.5%) has been successfully used to reverse the pathologic effects of hemorrhagic/hypovolemic shock in ruminants and the horse. It is a suggested treatment for abomasal metabolic alkalosis associated with abomasal problems in ruminants. It has also been advocated as adjunctive treatment for corneal ulceration in horses.

ADVERSE AND COMMON SIDE EFFECTS: Excessive volumes of 0.9% saline may cause hyperchloremic metabolic acidosis and hypokalemia, especially in patients with diarrhea in which sodium loss is greater than chloride and in those patients in whom the kidney can not excrete the excess chloride load. Volume overload and pulmonary edema is a potential concern in animals with cardiac or renal insufficiency. Hypernatremia may also occur and lead to irritability, lethargy, weakness, ataxia, stupor, coma, and seizure.

DRUG INTERACTIONS: Glucocorticoids and corticotropin may predispose to sodium retention and volume overload especially in patients with congestive heart failure.

SUPPLIED AS: VETERINARY PRODUCTS
For injection containing 7, 7.2, and 7.5 g /100mL★
For injection containing 0.9 g/100 mL

HUMAN PRODUCTS
For injection containing 0.45% (77 mEq/L)
For injection containing 0.9% (154 mEq/L) (isotonic)
For injection containing 3% (513 mEq/L)
For injection containing 5% (855 mEq/L)
Oral tablets containing 650 mg

OTHER USES
Horses and Ruminants
HYPOVOLEMIC SHOCK
7.5% saline: 4 to 5 mL/kg slowly over 8 to 10 minutes or longer; IV (Note: Hypertonic saline is available commercially as 7%, 7.2%, and 7.5 % in the United States, or can be prepared as 7.5% saline by withdrawing 882 mL from a 3-L bag of 0.9% saline and adding 882 mL of 23.4% saline back to the original 3-L bag.)

SODIUM CROMOGLYCATE

INDICATIONS: Sodium cromoglycate (Intal♣★) is reported to inhibit degranulation of mast cells and release of proinflammatory mediators. It is used as an aerosol to inhibit both the immediate and nonimmediate bronchoconstriction reactions to inhaled allergens. It has no intrinsic bronchodilator or anti-inflammatory activity. Inhalation of sodium cromoglycate 20 to 30 minutes before antigen inhalation challenge prevents the induction of airway obstruction in horses with recurrent airway obstruction (heaves, chronic obstructive pulmonary disease). Four consecutive daily treatments ameliorated clinical signs of heaves in horses for over 3 weeks. Thus, it is advocated for prevention of occurrence of clinical signs of airway obstruction in horses, by administration in advance of a predictable antigen exposure. However, clinical experience suggests that only selected horses will respond to the treatment, possibly because of variations in type and stage of immune hyperreactivity between horses.

ADVERSE AND COMMON SIDE EFFECTS: The most frequently reported adverse effects in humans were irritation to the throat, cough, wheeze, and nausea. Bronchospasm, nasal congestion, and laryngeal and pharyngeal irritation have been reported. Other adverse reactions that occur infrequently include anaphylaxis, angioedema, dizziness, dysuria, joint swelling, lacrimation, urticaria, and myopathy. Adverse effects in horses have not been described.

DRUG INTERACTIONS: None reported.

SUPPLIED AS: HUMAN PRODUCTS
As aerosol in spincaps, containing 20 mg/dose
As solution for nebulization containing 10 mg/mL

SODIUM IODIDE

INDICATIONS: Sodium iodide (Iodoject★, Sodide♣, Sodium Iodide 20% Injection♣★, Sodium Iodide Solution 20%♣★, Sodium Iodine 20%♣, Sodium Iodide Sterile Solution★) is used in large animals as an aid in the treatment of actinomycosis or actinobacillosis, as an expectorant, and in treatment of ringworm and necrotic stomatitis.

ADVERSE AND COMMON SIDE EFFECTS: Adverse effects include anorexia, lacrimation, depression, cardiomegaly, and cutaneous reactions that are generally reversible when the drug dose is decreased. The drug is contraindicated in hyperthyroidism, advanced pregnancy, and acute metal poisoning. Avoid SC or IM injection. This drug is not to be used in lactating dairy cattle (U.S.).

DRUG INTERACTIONS: None reported.

SUPPLIED AS: VETERINARY PRODUCT
For injection containing 200 mg/mL [20%]

SODIUM SULFATE

INDICATIONS: Sodium sulfate♣★ [Glauber's salt] is used in ruminants as a preventive for urolithiasis. It is also administered as a cathartic for large animals. When administered it should be mixed as a 6% solution and given by stomach tube. Sodium sulfate is also indicated to help mobilize excessive hepatic copper in sheep.

ADVERSE AND COMMON SIDE EFFECTS: Excessive doses can result in profuse diarrhea and abdominal discomfort.

DRUG INTERACTIONS: None listed.

SUPPLIED AS: Commercially available as Glauber's salt.

SODIUM THIOSULFATE

INDICATIONS: Sodium thiosulfate♣ is used as an antidote for heavy metal poisoning and has been used to treat cattle in field outbreaks of copper poisoning.

ADVERSE AND COMMON SIDE EFFECTS: None listed.

DRUG INTERACTIONS: None listed.

SUPPLIED AS: HUMAN PRODUCT
For injection containing 25%

SPECTINOMYCIN

INDICATIONS: Spectinomycin (Spectam♣, Spectam Injectable♣, Spectam Oral Solution♣, Spectam Scour-Halt♣★, Spectam Soluble Powder♣, Spectam Water Soluble★, Spectinomycin Oral♣★, Trobicin♣★) is an aminocyclitol antibiotic similar in action to aminoglycosides and is used in poultry to treat fowl cholera and chronic respiratory disease due to *Mycoplasma gallisepticum* and in swine to treat diarrhea due to *Escherichia coli*. Spectinomycin has been used by clinicians to treat granular vulvitis in cattle caused by ureaplasma infections, and by equine practitioners to treat pneumonia. Little scientific data are available concerning its use in horses, cattle, sheep, or goats.

ADVERSE AND COMMON SIDE EFFECTS: Neuromuscular blockade is a rare side effect that can be reversed by parenteral calcium administration. Local myositis may occur at the injection site. Recent reports of its use in cattle have described adverse reactions of respiratory distress, weakness, and death following administration of water soluble spectinomycin by the IV route. Recent veterinarian reports from the Food and Drug Administration have indicated sudden death, epistaxis, dyspnea, and shock in cattle treated orally or parenterally.

DRUG INTERACTIONS: Antagonism may occur if the drug is used concurrently with chloramphenicol or tetracycline. Spectinomycin combined with lincomycin acts synergistically against mycoplasma organisms.

SUPPLIED AS: VETERINARY PRODUCTS
For injection containing 100 mg/mL
Oral solution containing 50 mg/mL
Soluble powder containing 500 mg/g

HUMAN PRODUCT
For injection containing 2 g

OTHER USES Spectinomycin can also be found in combination with lincomycin (Linco-Spectin, L-S20, L-S100♣), but lincomycin has been associated with lethal complications in horses and sheep and thus this formulation should be strictly avoided.

STANOZOLOL

INDICATIONS: Stanozolol (Winstrol-V♥★) is an anabolic steroid with strong anabolic and weak androgenic activity. It is potentially useful as an adjunct to the management of catabolic disease states. The drug has been recommended to stimulate erythropoiesis, arouse appetite, promote weight gain, and increase strength and vitality. The efficacy of promoting these positive changes is questionable and prolonged treatment (3–6 months) may be required before a response in the erythron is seen. The drug is most commonly used in horses to enhance athletic performance. Also see **ANABOLIC STEROIDS**, under Description of Drugs for Small Animals.

ADVERSE AND COMMON SIDE EFFECTS: The drug should be used with caution in animals with cardiac or renal insufficiency and those with hypercalcemia. It may promote sodium and water retention and exacerbate azotemia; it may also promote hypercalcemia, hyperphosphatemia, and hyperkalemia. The drug is potentially hepatotoxic. Stanozolol should not be used in pregnant animals because of possible masculinization of fetuses.

DRUG INTERACTIONS: Anabolic agents may potentiate the effect of anticoagulants.

SUPPLIED AS: VETERINARY PRODUCTS
Tablets containing 2 mg
For injection containing 50 mg/mL

SUCRALFATE

INDICATIONS: Sucralfate (Apo-Sucralfate♣, Carafate★, Novo-Sucralfate♣, Nu-Sucralfate♣, Sulcrate♣, Sucrate Suspension Plus♣) accelerates the healing of oral, esophageal, gastric, and duodenal ulcers. It forms a complex with proteinaceous exudates that adheres to the ulcer, providing a protective barrier to the penetration of gastric acid. Sucralfate stimulates prostaglandin production, increases mucous production and mucosal turnover, inactivates pepsin, and absorbs bile acids. Sucralfate may be useful for the prevention of nonsteroidal anti-inflammatory-induced ulceration. Sucralfate is used in large animals, mainly in foals to treat or prevent gastric ulceration.

ADVERSE AND COMMON SIDE EFFECTS: Side effects are rare. Constipation is the only significant problem reported in small animals.

DRUG INTERACTIONS: Antacids and H_2-blocking agents decrease gastric pH and reduce the efficacy of sucralfate and should be given at least one-half hour after giving sucralfate. Sucralfate decreases the bioavailability of digoxin, cimetidine, ranitidine, ketoconazole, phenytoin, theophylline, and tetracycline antibiotics. Concurrent oral drug administration should be separated by 2 hours. Sucralfate decreases gastrointestinal absorption of ciproflaxacin and norfloxacin.

SUPPLIED AS: HUMAN PRODUCTS
Tablets containing 1 g sucralfate
Suspension containing 1 g/5 mL

SULFADIMETHOXINE

INDICATIONS: Sulfadimethoxine (Albon★, Albon SR★, Bactrovet★, Di-Methox★, S-125 Tablets♣, S-250 Tablets♣, Sulfadimethoxine Injection-40%★) is a sulfonamide drug used for the treatment of respiratory, genitourinary, enteric, and soft tissue infections caused by susceptible organisms including *Streptococcus*, *Staphylococcus*, *Escherichia*, *Salmonella*, *Klebsiella*, *Proteus*, and *Shigella*.

ADVERSE AND COMMON SIDE EFFECTS: See SULFONAMIDES.

DRUG INTERACTIONS: IM injection is associated with pain and poor blood drug levels and is not recommended. See SULFONAMIDES.

SUPPLIED AS: VETERINARY PRODUCTS
Tablets containing 125, 250, and 500 mg
Oral suspension containing 50 and 125 mg/mL
Injection containing 400 mg/mL
Boluses containing 5 and 15 g
Slow-release boluses containing 12.5 g
Premix containing 6.6%

SULFAMETHAZINE

INDICATIONS: Sulfamethazine (Bovazine SR Bolus★, Calfspan♣, Hava-Span♣, Sodium Sulfamethazine Antibacterial Soluble Powder★, Sodium Sulfamethazine 25%♣, Sodium Sulfamethazine Solution 12.5% and 25%♣, Sulfa-Max III Cattle Bolus★, Sulfa-Max III Calf Bolus★, SulfaSure SR★, SulfaSure SR Calf Bolus★, SulfaTech SR★, SulfaTech SR Calf Bolus★, Sulfamethazine Bolus♣, Sulfa 25♣, Sulmet★, SustainIII♣★, SustainIII Cattle Bolus★, SustainIII Calf Bolus★) is a sulfonamide antimicrobial used for treatment of a wide variety of bacterial infections in large animals. Various formulations can be used for addition to water for mass medication (e.g., Sodium Sulfamethazine 25%♣, Sulmet★) and others for individual treatment with sustained-release products (e.g., SustainIII♣★).

ADVERSE AND COMMON SIDE EFFECTS: See SULFONAMIDES.

DRUG INTERACTIONS: See SULFONAMIDES.

SUPPLIED AS: VETERINARY PRODUCTS
Water additive containing 12.5 and 25 g/100 mL
Bolus containing 2.5, 5, 15, and 15.6 g
Sustained-release bolus form containing 8, 8.25, 22.5, 27, 30, and 32.1 g
Powder in 1-lb (454-g) packets

OTHER USES Sulfamethazine is also found in combination with a number of medications, either with other sulfa drugs (Sulfalean♣, Bi-Sulfas♣, Triple Sulfa♣), or other antibacterials (AureoS-700♣★), or vitamins and minerals (Super Chlor 250♣).

SULFONAMIDES

INDICATIONS: The sulfonamides are bacteriostatic drugs that are effective against streptococci, *Bacillus*, *Corynebacterium*, *Nocardia*, *Brucella*, *Campylobacter*, *Pasteurella*, and *Chlamydia*. *Pseudomonas*, *Serratia*, and *Klebsiella* are generally resistant. The sulfonamides readily enter the cerebrospinal fluid (CSF) and are effective in treating meningeal infections. These drugs are ineffective in the presence of pus and necrotic tissue.
Sulfonamides are classified according to their duration of effect. Short-acting sulfonamides require dosing at 8-hour intervals and include sulfadiazine, sulfamerazine, sulfamethazine, and sulfamethoxazole; they are generally indicated in the treatment of systemic and urinary tract infections. Intermediate-acting sulfonamides require dosing every 12 to 24 hours and include sulfisoxazole and sulfadimethoxine, which are primarily indicated in the treatment of urinary tract infections. The long-acting sulfonamides require dosing every few days and include sulfadoxine; they have been primarily used in people for the treatment of chronic bronchitis and urinary tract infections.

ADVERSE AND COMMON SIDE EFFECTS: Precipitation and crystalluria are not generally a problem in veterinary patients, but sulfonamides should be used with caution in patients with preexisting renal disease, especially if complicated by dehydration or metabolic acidosis. Pruritus and photosensitization have been reported and alopecia may occur with long-term use. Other reported conditions associated with the use of these drugs include polyarthritis, urticaria, facial swelling, fever, hemolytic anemia, polydipsia, polyuria, hepatitis, diarrhea, anorexia, and seizure activity. Hypersensitivity, including anaphylaxis, although rare, has also been documented.

DRUG INTERACTIONS: Antacids decrease the absorption of sulfonamides. Methenamine and other acidifying agents increase the risk of sulfonamide crystallization in the urine. Paraminobenzoic acid and local anesthetics may antagonize sulfonamide action. Phenothiazines may increase the toxic effects of sulfonamide.

SUPPLIED AS: VETERINARY PRODUCTS
See individual product.

SULFONAMIDES: POTENTIATED

INDICATIONS: The combinations of a sulfonamide with trimethoprim or pyrimethamine are referred to as "potentiated sulfonamides," such as trimethoprim-sulfadiazine (Di-Trim★, Tribrissen♣★, Uniprim★) or trimethoprim-sulfadoxine (Trivetrin♣, Borgal♣, Biotrim♣, Trimadox♣); they greatly enhance antimicrobial activity. Another example of a potentiated sulfa is the sulfadimethoxine-ormetoprim combination (Primor★, Rofenaid 40★, Romet♣★). This agent is indicated in the treatment of skin and soft tissue infections caused by *Staphylococcus aureus* and *Escherichia coli*. A large-animal formulation is not available. Potentiated sulfonamides are bactericidal antibacterial combinations recommended for the treatment of alimentary tract, respiratory, and urinary tract infections and skin and soft tissue infections caused by susceptible organisms including *E. coli*, *Enterobacter*, *Klebsiella*, *Streptococcus*, *Staphylococcus*, *Pasteurella*, *Proteus*, *Clostridia*, *Salmonella*, *Shigella*, *Brucella*, *Actinomyces*, *Corynebacterium*, *Bordetella*, *Neisseria*, and *Vibrio* organisms. A combination product is available for treating food animals in Canada, but is not approved in the United States. Although the dose interval for ruminants is once daily, the half-life of trimethoprim has been reported to be extremely short in the ruminating animal, which suggests more frequent treatment may be indicated. Absorption of oral products from the gastrointestinal tract in horses is good; however, peak serum concentration can vary significantly between individual horses.

ADVERSE AND COMMON SIDE EFFECTS: The drug should not be used in animals with marked liver disease or blood dyscrasias or in those with sulfonamide sensitivity. Anemia, leukopenia, thrombocytopenia, anorexia, and ataxia have been noted at higher doses. Supplementation of folic acid (75 mg; IM every 3 days to an adult horse) may protect the patient against the anemia and leukopenia that accompany the interference of folic acid metabolism.

Trimethoprim may cause increases in serum creatinine, via competition for sites of excretion. There have been several reports of death after IV administration to horses, presumably due to vagal stimulation and subsequent bradycardia and vasodilation. However, this may also be related to the acute deaths in association with concurrent administration of detomidine, which has been reported in the Nordic countries.

DRUG INTERACTIONS: Antacids may decrease the bioavailability of trimethoprim-sulfa if administered concurrently. Trimethoprim-sulfadiazine may prolong clotting times in patients receiving warfarin. Sulfonamides may increase the effects of phenylbutazone, phenytoin, salicylates, thiazide diuretics, and probenicid.

SUPPLIED AS: VETERINARY PRODUCTS
For injection containing 40 mg/mL trimethoprim and 200 mg/mL sulfadiazine or sulfadoxine
For injection containing 80 mg/mL trimethoprim and 400 mg/mL sulfadiazine
Bolus containing 200 mg trimethoprim and 1 g sulfadiazine
Oral paste containing 67 mg/g trimethoprim and 333 mg/g sulfadiazine
Oral suspension containing 9.1 mg trimethoprim and 45.5 mg sulfadiazine
Oral powder containing 67 mg/g trimethoprim and 333 mg/g sulfadiazine

SYNERGISTIN

INDICATIONS: Synergistin♣ is a combination of ampicillin trihydrate and sulbactam benzathine, a β-lactamase inhibitor. Sulbactam has poor intrinsic antimicrobial activity, but binds to β-lactamases, preventing the destruction of ampicillin. It is approved for use in cattle for the treatment of bacterial pneumonia and pneumonic pasteurellosis and is indicated in the treatment of bacterial infections resistant to ampicillin alone because of production of β-lactamase.

ADVERSE AND COMMON SIDE EFFECTS: Anaphylaxis can occur.

DRUG INTERACTIONS: None listed.

SUPPLIED AS: VETERINARY PRODUCT
For injection containing 120 mg ampicillin trihydrate with 60 mg sulbactam benzathine/mL

OTHER USES
Horses

Synergistin is also used in horses for the treatment of bacterial infections such as pneumonia, although it is not approved for use in this species. The drug combination has been effective in treating experimentally induced gram-negative pneumonia in foals.

TERBUTALINE

INDICATIONS: Terbutaline (Bricanyl♣★, Brethane★, Brethine★) is a synthetic adrenergic stimulant with selective β_2- and negligible β_1-agonist activity. It is useful as a bronchodilator and has been used for testing for anhidrosis in horses by assessing sweat response to intradermal injections of gradually reducing concentrations.

ADVERSE AND COMMON SIDE EFFECTS: The drug should not be given to patients with tachycardia associated with digitalis intoxication. The drug should be used with caution in patients with hypertension, cardiac arrhythmias, or renal or hepatic dysfunction. Side effects may include tachycardia, hypotension or hypertension, tremor, fatigue, or seizure activity.

DRUG INTERACTIONS: Propranolol antagonizes the bronchodilating effect of terbutaline. Use with other sympathetic agents may potentiate the risk of arrhythmias.

SUPPLIED AS: HUMAN PRODUCTS
Tablets containing 2.5 and 5 mg
For injection containing 1 mg/mL
Aerosol containing 0.20 mg/actuation
Turbuhaler containing 0.5 mg/inhalation

TESTOSTERONE AND ESTRADIOL

INDICATIONS: Testosterone and estradiol (Anadiol★, Implus-H♣★, Implus-H Heifer Implant★, Synovex-H♣, Uni-Bol♣) are used in large animals to improve weight gain and muscle mass. Products designed for the horse (Anadiol♣) are used as anabolic agents where the potential adverse masculinizing effects of testosterone alone are undesirable. Implant pellets are used in heifers to stimulate weight gain and feed efficiency. Use is recommended for heifers weighing 185 to 365 kg. Maximal growth will be attained with good quality stock free of parasitism and disease.

ADVERSE AND COMMON SIDE EFFECTS: Anadiol is not recommended for use in stallions. Treatment in mares should not occur within 6 months prior to the breeding season. Implants are not intended for use in dairy heifers or breeding animals. The drug is not recommended for use in ovariectomized heifers. Bulling, vaginal and rectal prolapse, udder development, ventral edema, and elevated tail heads are occasional reported side effects. Implants should only be placed in the ear. Implantation at other sites may result in condemnation of the carcass.

DRUG INTERACTIONS: None listed.

SUPPLIED AS: VETERINARY PRODUCTS
For injection containing 100 mg/mL testosterone, 7.5 mg/mL estradiol enanthate, and 1 mg/mL estradiol benzoate
Implant pellets containing 200 mg testosterone propionate and 20 mg estradiol benzoate

TESTOSTERONE

INDICATIONS: Testosterone (Anatest♣, Ini-Test♣, Uni-Test Suspension♣, Veto-Test♣) is a potent anabolic hormone used in horses to improve weight gain, strength, and performance. It is used in other animals to treat impotence and cryptorchidism and to suppress lactation.

ADVERSE AND COMMON SIDE EFFECTS: Testosterone is not recommended for use in stallions. Stop treatment in mares at least 6 months prior to the breeding season.

DRUG INTERACTIONS: None listed.

SUPPLIED AS: VETERINARY PRODUCT
For injection containing 100 mg/mL in proprionate or aqueous suspension

OTHER USES
Sheep
ULCERATIVE POSTHITIS
Testosterone propionate is useful for reducing the incidence and severity of ulcerative posthitis in sheep at an implant dose of 100 mg every 3 months.

TETANUS ANTITOXIN

INDICATIONS: Tetanus antitoxin♣★ is prepared from the blood of horses hyperimmunized with the toxin of *Clostridium tetani*. It is used for the prevention of tetanus in animals that have suffered a penetrating wound and are of unknown immune status. Preventive doses confer immediate passive immunity that lasts 7 to 14 days. The antitoxin will not affect toxin already bound in the nervous system but may bind to circulating toxin. Concurrent treatment of the site of infection is necessary. Animals that survive tetanus remain susceptible to the disease as the dose of toxin required for clinical disease is less than that necessary to prime the immune system.

ADVERSE AND COMMON SIDE EFFECTS: Biologics of equine origin have been associated with the development of hepatitis (Theiler's disease) in horses.

DRUG INTERACTIONS: None listed.

SUPPLIED AS: VETERINARY PRODUCT
For injection containing 1,500 U

OTHER USES
Horses

Intrathecal tetanus antitoxin has been advocated for treatment of tetanus in horses, but the efficacy has not been established.

TETRACYCLINE

INDICATIONS: Tetracyclines (Action 200★, Agrimycin★, Alamycin LA♥, Aureomycin♥★, Biocyl★, Bio-Mycin♥★, Chlorosol-50♥, Chlora-cycline★, CLTC 100MR★, CTC★, Duramycin★, Fermycin Soluble★, Intracin♥, Kelamycin Intrauterine Suspension♥, Liquamast♥, Liquamycin LA200♥★, Liquamycin/LP♥, Liquamast Aerosol♥, Maxim-200★, Medamycin★, Onycin♥, Oxy 1000♥, Oxysol♥, Oxy LA♥, Oxy LP♥, Oxy-Mycin★, OT200★, Oxytet♥★, Oxy-Tet★, Oxytetracycline♥★, Oxymycine LP♥, Oxymycine LA♥, Oxytetracycline♥★, Oxyvet♥, Oxyject 100★, Oxy Tetra Forte♥, Oxyshot LA★, Panamycin 500 Bolus★, Promycin★, Procure 200★, Solu-Tet★, Terramycin♥★, Terra-Vet★, Tetracycline Hydrochloride♥★, Tetra♥, Tetrachel 250♥, Tetralean♥, Tetramed♥, Tetrabol♥, Tetraject♥, and many others) are broad-spectrum antibiotics that inhibit most gram-positive bacteria, some gram-negative bacteria, rickettsiae, mycoplasmas, spirochetes, and actinomycetes. At high doses, some antiprotozoal activity has also been observed. Tetracyclines are used for the treatment of a number of bacterial infections in large animals, including pneumonia, metritis, mastitis, tetanus, and foot rot, as well as systemic diseases such as anaplasmosis, leptospirosis, and brucellosis. Long-acting products have been effective in treating infectious bovine keratoconjunctivitis caused by *Moraxella bovis* and for prophylaxis in the reduction of incidence and severity of pneumonic pasteurellosis (shipping fever) in feedlot cattle. Tetracyclines (e.g., rolitetracycline) have been used for postbreeding infusions in cattle. Tetracyclines are found in highest concentration in the kidney, liver, spleen, and lung and are deposited at sites of ossification. Tetracyclines are most effective against rapidly growing organisms. Bacteri-al resistance to tetracyclines develops readily and persists for longer periods than most other antibiotics. Tetracycline is the generic name for these compounds and also the name of the specific semisynthetic compound. Naturally occurring tetracyclines are oxytetracycline and chlortetracycline. Chlortetracycline is mainly an oral product. Newer tetracyclines include doxycycline and rolitetracycline.

High doses of oxytetracycline have been used with some success to treat flexural limb deformities in foals. Objective evaluation of this treatment has recently shown its value in obtaining short-term moderate decrease in metacarpophalangeal joint angle in newborns within 36 hours of birth. The possible mechanism of action is unknown; however, chelation of calcium, or alternatively, a neuromuscular blocking effect has been suggested.

ADVERSE AND COMMON SIDE EFFECTS: Tetracycline is irritating if administered IM. Chlortetracycline causes severe tissue irritation if injected IM. Oral administration of tetracyclines to cattle may cause bloat or digestive upset. Oral administration in horses upsets gastrointestinal flora and may result in colitis. Parenteral administration to horses under periods of stress, as with the postoperative period, may also predispose to colitis, but occurs less frequently than with oral administration. High doses of tetracyclines have been incriminated in causing renal failure in feedlot cattle. Infusion of chlortetracycline into the udder of cows during the dry period may cause udder damage. Occasional hypersensitivity reactions may occur.

DRUG INTERACTIONS: Absorption of oral tetracycline products is impaired by milk products, aluminum hydroxide gels, sodium bicarbonate, calcium and magnesium salts, and iron preparations.

SUPPLIED AS: VETERINARY PRODUCTS
Chlortetracycline
Powders for administering in feed or water containing 25, 50, and 100 g/lb; 55, 110, and 220 g/kg
Boluses containing 500 mg
Tablets containing 25 mg
Oxytetracycline
For injection containing 50 mg/mL, 100 mg/mL
For injection in long-acting formulation containing 200 mg/mL
Aerosol containing 426 mg/6.4 g
Premix containing 110, 220, 250, and 440 g/kg
Powder for water additive containing 10, 22, 25, 25.6, 88, 100, 102.4,

204.8, and 500 g/packet
Tablets containing 250 mg
Mastitis infusions containing 426 mg/5mL and 30 mg/g
Intrauterine infusions containing 50 mg/mL
Tetracycline
Water additive containing 25, 102.4, and 324 g/lb; 55, 62.5, 250, and 1,000 mg/g
Liquid containing 100 mg/mL
Bolus containing 500 mg

HUMAN PRODUCT
Rolitetracycline
For injection containing 275 mg/vial

OTHER USES
Horses
FLEXURAL LIMB DEFORMITIES
3 g (44 mg/kg) oxytetracycline to foals younger than 1 week; IV once, or repeated in 24 hours

Sheep
LEPTOSPIROSIS
200 to 400 mg/head/day in the feed for 2 to 3 weeks for leptospirosis outbreaks

THIABENDAZOLE

INDICATIONS: Thiabendazole (Mintezol♥★) is extensively used for gastrointestinal parasitism in a wide range of hosts. Despite development of newer benzimidazoles and other anthelmintics, thiabendazole is still widely used as a ruminant anthelmintic. Thiabendazole has excellent efficacy against all major gastrointestinal nematodes of sheep, cattle, and goats, with the exception of whipworms. Thiabendazole is also effective against most mature gastrointestinal parasites of horses but is generally ineffective against filarial parasites such as *Onchocerca* or *Setaria*.

ADVERSE AND COMMON SIDE EFFECTS: None listed for large animal use.

DRUG INTERACTIONS: Thiabendazole may compete with theophylline and aminophylline for metabolism in the liver, resulting in increased serum levels of the latter two drugs.

SUPPLIED AS: VETERINARY PRODUCTS
At the time of writing, these have been discontinued.

HUMAN PRODUCTS
Tablets containing 500 mg
Suspension containing 500 mg/5 mL

OTHER USES
Horses
CHRONIC DIARRHEA
500 mg/kg thiabendazole; PO, repeated on successive days
This is suggested in some literature as a reliable cure for chronic diarrhea, but clinical experience suggests that it has little effect.

STRONGYLUS VULGARIS
440 mg/kg; PO on 2 successive days has been advocated for treatment of the somatic forms of *Strongylus vulgaris*.

THIAMINE

INDICATIONS: Thiamine or vitamin B$_1$ (B-1★, T-Dex♣, Thiamine Hydrochloride Injection♣★, Thiamine HCl Injection♣★, T Sol♣, Ultra-B$_1$♣) is used for the treatment of vitamin B$_1$ deficiencies in animals. In ruminants the most common manifestation of vitamin B$_1$ deficiency is polioencephalomalacia. Response to treatment of ruminants is rapid. There is usually insufficient thiamine in multiple vitamin injectables for treatment of polioencephalomalacia.

ADVERSE AND COMMON SIDE EFFECTS: Rapid IV administration can result in anaphylaxis. Dilution in D$_5$W or 0.9% saline is advised.

DRUG INTERACTIONS: None listed.

SUPPLIED AS: VETERINARY PRODUCTS
For injection containing 100, 200, and 500 mg/mL
Powder containing 16,677 mg/kg, 17,600 mg/kg, or 1,000 mg/30g
Liquid containing 1 g/30 mL

OTHER USES
Ruminants
LEAD TOXICITY
20 mg/kg daily; SC for 15 days

THIOBARBITURATES

INDICATIONS: Thiobarbiturates [thiopental] (Induthol♣, Pentothal♣★, Pentothal Sodium♣) are ultrashort-acting barbiturate anesthetics used for induction of anesthesia in large animals and for short surgical procedures, such as castration. Duration of anesthesia is 10 to 25 minutes, with recovery in 30 to 90 minutes. During the period of induction, a brief period of excitement may occur. The brief period of anesthetic action is due to rapid distribution of the drug from the plasma into various tissues. Large or repeated doses will prolong anesthesia as plasma levels remain near that of fat and tissues. Metabolism of thiobarbiturates is slow, and repeated doses will prolong the time to recovery. Barbiturate anesthesia in the horse should not be prolonged for longer than 1 hour, and no more than 5 g of any barbiturate should be given, even to draft breeds. Thiobarbiturates are reconstituted with water to form a solution for IV use. Once reconstituted the solution quality deteriorates within 1 week or less, depending on a number of storage factors. Ponies may require higher doses than horses. In goats, thiobarbiturates are useful for short procedures, such as castration or tattooing.

ADVERSE AND COMMON SIDE EFFECTS: Respiratory centers are depressed, but approximately 16 times as much drug is required to stop the myocardium as to paralyze respiration. SC or perivascular injection with thiobarbiturates, particularly at 5% or 10% concentration, is irritating and may result in severe tissue reaction, including abscess formation and tissue slough. Areas of perivascular injection should be treated with saline for dilution and hyaluronidase to promote dispersion. Thiobarbiturates can trigger cardiac arrhythmias such as ventricular fibrillation. Pretreatment with acepromazine or chlorpromazine will considerably lessen this risk. Intracarotid injection can result in cerebrovascular endothelial injury and subsequent brain necrosis. Recovery from anesthesia in horses is often accompanied by violent excitement, which can be prevented with premedication with a phenothiazine.

DRUG INTERACTIONS: Reinduction of thiobarbiturate anesthesia can occur with administration of high doses of phenylbutazone or aspirin through displacement of thiobarbiturates from plasma proteins. These products are physically unstable with acids, acidic salts, and oxidizing agents.

SUPPLIED AS: VETERINARY PRODUCT
For injection containing 5 g thiopental

HUMAN PRODUCTS
For injection containing 1, 2.5, and 5 g
Vials for injection containing 0.5 and 1 g

TICARCILLIN

INDICATIONS: Ticarcillin (Ticar♣, Ticillin★) is an extended-spectrum parenteral penicillin antibiotic with activity similar to, but more potent than, carbenicillin. In humans, the drug is active against gram-negative bacteria including *Klebsiella pneumoniae*, *Proteus mirabilis* and *vulgaris*, *Escherichia coli*, *Enterobacter aerogenes*, *Serratia marcescens*, *Pseudomonas aeruginosa*, and *Bacteroides fragilis*, and gram-positive organisms including *Staphylococcus aureus*, coagulase-positive staphylococci, enterococci, and streptococcal organisms. Bacterial susceptibility is similar in veterinary medicine. The antibiotic is available in combination with clavulanic acid (Timentin★) that is effective against many penicillinase-producing strains of bacteria. Ticarcillin is available for intrauterine infusion in the horse.

ADVERSE AND COMMON SIDE EFFECTS: Use of the drug is contraindicated in animals with hypersensitivity to penicillins or the cephalosporins. IM injection may cause pain. Also see **PENICILLINS**. One horse developed laminitis after parenteral treatment.

DRUG INTERACTIONS: Ticarcillin is physically and/or chemically incompatible with aminoglycosides and can inactivate the drug in vitro. Also see **PENICILLINS**.

SUPPLIED AS: VETERINARY PRODUCT
For intrauterine infusion containing 6 g/50-mL vial

HUMAN PRODUCT
For injection containing 1, 3, 6, 20, and 30 g

TILMICOSIN

INDICATIONS: Tilmicosin (Micotil✦) is a long-acting macrolide antibiotic used for the treatment of and mortality reduction in bovine respiratory disease caused by *Pasteurella hemolytica* and *Pasteurella multocida*. It is also approved for treatment of pneumonic pasteurellosis in lambs associated with *P. hemolytica*. Its spectrum of activity is predominantly gram-positive organisms, with some gram-negative organisms and several mycoplasmas.

ADVERSE AND COMMON SIDE EFFECTS: Avoid contact with eyes. IV injection in cattle and administration to swine has been fatal. The dosage in calves less than 70 kg has not been established. Do not inject more than 25 mL per site. Swelling at the site of injection may occur under normal conditions but is mild and transient. Reports of sudden death, injection site swelling, collapse, anaphylaxis, and lameness have been associated reactions to parenteral injections in cattle. Human injection may result in severe adverse reaction, particularly if doses are large.

DRUG INTERACTIONS: None listed.

SUPPLIED AS: VETERINARY PRODUCT
For injection containing 300 mg/mL

TOBRAMYCIN

INDICATIONS: Tobramycin (Nebcin♥★) is an aminoglycoside antibiotic. It is closely related to gentamicin in spectrum, activity, and pharmacologic properties, but it is more active against some strains of *Pseudomonas* that are resistant to gentamicin, and it is less nephrotoxic. Also see **AMINOGLYCOSIDE ANTIBIOTICS**.

ADVERSE AND COMMON SIDE EFFECTS: See AMINOGLYCOSIDE ANTIBIOTICS.

DRUG INTERACTIONS: Tobramycin should not be mixed with other drugs. Also see **AMINOGLYCOSIDE ANTIBIOTICS**.

SUPPLIED AS: HUMAN PRODUCTS
For injection containing 10 and 40 mg/mL
For injection in premeasured syringes containing 60 and 80 mg
Bulk vials containing 1.2 g

TOLAZOLINE

INDICATIONS: Tolazoline (Priscoline★, Tolazine♥) is an α_2-adrenoceptor antagonist that has been used to reverse xylazine-induced (via caudal epidural administration) rumen hypomotility, and partially antagonize xylazine-induced cardiopulmonary depression without affecting sedation or local (S3–coccyx) analgesic effects. It has also been used in horses (7.5 mg/kg; IV) to antagonize ventricular bradycardia and atrioventricular conduction disturbances and central nervous system depression associated with xylazine administration. Tolazoline in this instance may cause a persistent, mild systemic hypertension.

ADVERSE AND COMMON SIDE EFFECTS: Tachycardia, peripheral vasodilation, and hyperalgesia of the lips may occur. Piloerection may be noted in the rump and neck. Clear lacrimal and nasal discharges may be noted, as well as signs of apprehension.

DRUG INTERACTIONS: Blood pressure may fall followed by an exaggerated rebound if combined with epinephrine or norepinephrine.

SUPPLIED AS: VETERINARY PRODUCT
For injection containing 100 mg/mL

HUMAN PRODUCTS
For injection containing 25 mg/mL
Tablets containing 25 mg

TRIAMCINOLONE

INDICATIONS: Triamcinolone (Aristocort♣★, Aristospan★, Amcort★, Articulose★, Centracort★, Cortalone★, Kenaject★, Kenalog♣★, Scheinpharm Triamcine-A♣, Tac-3★, Tac-40★, Triam-A★, Triamonide 40★, Tri-Kort★, Trilog★, Triam-Forte★, Triamolone★, Trilone★, Tristoject★, Vetalog★) is a potent glucocorticoid. The drug is indicated for the treatment of arthritic and related disorders and for the treatment of allergic and dermatologic conditions responsive to corticosteroids. It is used predominantly for horses with noninfectious soft tissue injuries and arthritis and for allergic respiratory disease. Also see **GLUCOCORTICOIDS**.

ADVERSE AND COMMON SIDE EFFECTS: Subconjunctival injection may be associated with granuloma formation requiring surgical excision. Also see **GLUCOCORTICOIDS**.

DRUG INTERACTIONS: See **GLUCOCORTICOIDS**.

SUPPLIED AS: HUMAN PRODUCTS
Tablets containing 1, 2, 4, and 8 mg
Syrup containing 2 mg/5 mL and 4 mg/mL
For injection containing 3, 10, and 40 mg/mL
For intralesional injection containing 25 mg/mL

OTHER USES
Horses
CHRONIC OBSTRUCTIVE PULMONARY DISEASE
Triamcinolone is used by some clinicians for reducing the clinical signs of small airway disease. However, as for other glucocorticoids, iatrogenic induction of laminitis can occur.

TRICHLORFON

INDICATIONS: Trichlorfon (Neguvon♣) is a organophosphate insecticide. It is used topically for the control of lice and grubs (*Hypoderma bovis, Hypoderma lineatum*) in cattle. Trichlorfon is also used alone or in combination with anthelmintics such as febantel (Negabot-Plus Paste♣) and pyrantel pamoate (Strongid Plus♣) in oral wormers for inclusion of stomach bots in the antiparasitic spectrum in horses. For further information, see **ORGANOPHOSPHATES**.

SUPPLIED AS: VETERINARY PRODUCTS
Pour-on liquid containing 8% trichlorfon
Oral combination products. See individual products.

TRIFLURIDINE

INDICATION: Trifluridine (Viroptic Ophthalmic Solution♣★) is a halogenated pyrimidine used in humans for the treatment of ocular herpes viral infections. Although this may have theoretical use for treatment of bovine herpes virus-I or equine herpes virus ocular manifestations, resolution generally occurs without treatment.

ADVERSE AND COMMON SIDE EFFECTS: Burning or stinging on instillation or palpebral edema are reported. Rarely, superficial punctate keratopathy, epithelial keratopathy, stromal edema, keratitis sicca, hyperemia, or increased intraocular pressure has been reported in humans.

DRUG INTERACTIONS: None listed.

SUPPLIED AS: HUMAN PRODUCT
Ophthalmic solution containing 1%

TROPICAMIDE

INDICATIONS: Tropicamide (Diotrope♣, L-Picamide★, Mydriacyl♣★, Ocu-Tropic★, PMS-Tropicamide♣, Tropicacyl♣★) is a synthetic tertiary amine antimuscarinic compound with properties similar to atropine. Tropicamide is a short-acting ophthalmic preparation used to dilate the pupil for short-acting relief of pain of ciliary spasm associated with uveitis and for fundoscopic examination.

ADVERSE AND COMMON SIDE EFFECTS AND DRUG INTERACTIONS: See ATROPINE.

SUPPLIED AS: HUMAN PRODUCT
Ophthalmic solution containing 0.5% and 1.0%

TYLOSIN

INDICATIONS: Tylosin (Tylan♣★, Tylocine♣, Tylosin♣★) is a macrolide antibiotic with activity against gram-negative and gram-positive bacteria, spirochetes, chlamydiae, and mycoplasma organisms. This drug is frequently used in large animals for the treatment of swine dysentery. However, tylosin is also effective in the treatment of bovine respiratory disease complex, foot rot, diphtheria and metritis in cattle, pneumonia, arthritis, chlamydial abortion in sheep, and other infectious problems caused by tylosin-susceptible organisms.

ADVERSE AND COMMON SIDE EFFECTS: Anorexia, diarrhea, and local pain with IM injection are reported. Do not inject more than 10 mL per site. Injection of tylosin in horses has been fatal.

DRUG INTERACTIONS: Tylosin may increase serum digitalis levels.

SUPPLIED AS: VETERINARY PRODUCTS
Tablets containing 200 mg
For injection containing 50 and 200 mg/mL
Soluble powder water additive containing 1 g/g (100%) as tylosin tartrate
Soluble powder for feed additive containing 22, 88, and 220 g/kg as tylosin phosphate

VANCOMYCIN

INDICATIONS: Vancomycin (Lyphocin★, Vancocin♥★, Vancoled★) is an antibiotic primarily effective against gram-positive organisms, including methicillin-resistant strains. It acts at the bacterial cell wall and is unrelated chemically to any other available antibiotics. Oral absorption is poor. Although a dosage has been published for use in horses, little information is available on its efficacy or safety.

ADVERSE AND COMMON SIDE EFFECTS: Hypersensitivity, flushing, neutropenia, and thrombocytopenia have been reported, as have phlebitis and pain at the site of injection. Vancomycin is ototoxic and nephrotoxic.

DRUG INTERACTIONS: Avoid concurrent administration of other nephrotoxic drugs.

SUPPLIED AS: HUMAN PRODUCTS
For injection containing 500 mg and 1, 5, and 10 g
Capsules containing 125 and 250 mg

VASOPRESSIN

INDICATIONS: Vasopressin (Pitressin★, Pressyn♥) is a synthetic form of vasopressin or antidiuretic hormone. It is used in the management of diabetes insipidus. In one report of idiopathic diabetes insipidus in a horse, it was found to be effective in decreasing water consumption and increasing urinary concentration for 24 hours. Otherwise its use in large animals is limited. It has been effective in inducing closure of the esophageal groove, which may have clinical implications to administer oral medication directly into the abomasum of ruminants.

ADVERSE AND COMMON SIDE EFFECTS: Abdominal pain, bronchial constriction, fluid retention, hyponatremia, pain at the site of injection, and the formation of sterile abscesses have been reported.

DRUG INTERACTIONS: Large doses of epinephrine or heparin may antagonize the effects of pitressin.

SUPPLIED AS: HUMAN PRODUCT
For injection containing 20 pressor U/mL

VITAMIN A

INDICATIONS: Vitamin A (A-500♣) is a generic term for compounds possessing the biologic activity of retinol. It is present in considerable amounts in green forage plants. Vitamin A functions mainly to maintain normal structure and function of epithelial cells and ocular structures such as the retina and cornea that are important for normal vision. Deficiency in large animals on forage diets is uncommon, but signs may manifest as increased keratinization of epithelial surfaces, keratinization of mucous-secreting surfaces such as the respiratory or gastrointestinal tract. Night blindness, excessive lacrimation, and corneal keratinization may also occur with deficiency. A single injection may last several months, and the liver can store approximately a 3- to 6-month supply of vitamin A. For parenteral use the drug is combined with vitamin D (Co-op A-D Injectable♣, Poten A.D.♣, Vitamin A-D-500★, Vita-Ject A-D 500★, Vitamin A-D♣, Vitamin A-D Injectable★★, Vitamin AD Injection★, Vitamin AD-500♣, Vitamin AD Injectable♣).

ADVERSE AND COMMON SIDE EFFECTS: Toxicity can occur with excess dietary or parenteral supplementation, with clinical signs resembling deficiency states. Administration of combination products of vitamin A and D have been as associated with collapse or abortion in cattle.

DRUG INTERACTIONS: None listed.

SUPPLIED AS: VETERINARY PRODUCT
For injection containing 500,000 IU/mL combined with 75,000 IU/mL vitamin D_3

VITAMIN D_3

INDICATIONS: Vitamin D_3 (High-D Dispersible★, Hydro-Vit D_3♣, Soln-Vit D_3♣, Vita-D♣, Poten-D♣, Downer-D♣) increases intestinal and renal calcium absorption and mobilizes calcium from the bone. It is used in pregnant cows to prevent milk fever. Knowledge of the exact date of expected calving is essential because vitamin D must be administered between 2 and 8 days prepartum for optimal effect. Maximal effect occurs between 48 to 96 hours and wanes during the following 96 hours. The drug is also contained in combination with vitamin A (Vitamin A-D-500★, Vitamin AD 500♣, Vitamin A-D In-jectable★, Vitamin AD Injection★, and others), but the concentration of vitamin D is insufficient for use as a preventive for parturient paresis. Vitamin D is also available in combination with calcium chloride (Cal Oral Plus★) for oral calcium supplementation.

ADVERSE AND COMMON SIDE EFFECTS: Administration to cows not in the immediate prepartum state and at high dosages can result in vascular calcification and/or renal calcium deposition.

DRUG INTERACTIONS: None listed.

SUPPLIED AS: VETERINARY PRODUCTS
Water additive containing 66,667, 80,000, or 160,000 IU/kg
For injection containing 500,000 and 1,000,000 IU/mL
For injection containing 75,000 IU/mL combined with 500,000 IU/mL vitamin A
Oral suspension containing 2,400 U combined with 400 mg/mL calcium chloride

VITAMIN E-SELENIUM

INDICATIONS: Vitamin E-selenium (Alphasel Powder♣, Bo Se★ In-jectable, Dystosel♣, Dystosel DS♣, Equ-SeE★, E-Se Injectable★★, E-Sel♣, Mu-Se Injectable★★, Selenium-E♣, Selepherol♣, Selon-E♣, Super SeE★, Ultra-Sel♣, Vetre-Sel-E♣) is a combination product used in the treatment and prevention of white muscle disease (nutritional myopathy) in calves and sheep and for myositis due to selenium-tocopherol deficiency in horses.

ADVERSE AND COMMON SIDE EFFECTS: Selenium is toxic if given in excess. Vitamin E has low toxicity. Administer only to animals known to be ingesting subnormal levels of selenium. Anaphylactic reactions have occurred occasionally, particularly if the drug is given by IV injection in horses. Treat the animal immediately with epinephrine. Some products will cause transitory local muscle soreness. Injection site abscess has also been reported in cattle and horses. Additionally, abortion, diarrhea, and bloat have been noted in cattle; dyspnea, abdominal pain, polypnea, head shaking or swelling, and tachycardia have been described in horses.

DRUG INTERACTIONS: None indicated.

SUPPLIED AS: VETERINARY PRODUCTS
For injection containing 2.5 mg selenium and 68 IU vitamin E/mL
For injection containing 3 mg selenium and 136 IU vitamin E/mL
For injection containing 5 mg selenium and 68 IU vitamin E/mL

For injection containing 6 mg selenium and 136 IU vitamin E/mL
Feed additive containing 90.7 mg selenium and 20,000 IU vitamin E/lb
Feed additive containing 40 mg selenium and 35,000 IU vitamin E/kg
Powder containing 85 µg sodium selenite and 35 IU vitamin E/g

OTHER USES
Horses

Vitamin E-selenium has been used for prevention of exertional rhabdomyolysis in horses and the empirical treatment of ionophor toxicity, but there is little evidence to support its use in these diseases.
Vitamin E is also advocated for treatment and prevention of equine degenerative myelopathy. The optimal success of this treatment has been with recognition and treatment at early stages of the disease, with the horse less than 12 months of age.
Treatment: 6,000 IU/250 to 500 kg; PO daily
Prophylaxis: 1,500 to 2,000 IU; PO daily per foal
For the equine athlete, vitamin E has been advocated in feed supplementation at 80 to 100 IU/kg dry matter feed.

Cattle

Vitamin E-selenium given 1 month prior to calving (2.5–3.75 mg selenium content of the combination; SC or IM) has reduced the incidence of retained placentas in selenium-deficient herds.

VITAMIN K₁

INDICATIONS: Vitamin K_1 [phytonadione] (Veta-K1✚, Vita-Ject Vitamin K_1 Injectable★, Vitamin K_1★) is a naturally occurring vitamin K compound used for the treatment of prolonged bleeding due to vitamin K deficiency states, as occur in cattle fed moldy sweet clover containing anti-vitamin K compounds such as bishydroxycoumarin, or from toxicity from ingested rodenticides containing dicoumarol. The drug is also indicated in horses receiving excess warfarin and in animals with hepatocellular disease. The primary function of vitamin K is to promote hepatic biosynthesis of prothrombin (factor II), as well as factors VII, IX, and X. Vitamin K_1 is more effective than menadione (vitamin K_3) in countering bleeding problems associated with vitamin K deficiency. The prothrombin time should be shortened within 1 to 2 hours of administration and can be monitored for response to therapy. Bleeding should be controlled in 3 to 6 hours and the prothrombin time may be normal in 12 to 24 hours. The smallest effective dose should be used to minimize the risk of allergic reaction. In severe bleeding, whole blood transfusion or plasma transfusion may also be warranted.

ADVERSE AND COMMON SIDE EFFECTS: Severe, sometimes fatal, reactions can occur if given IV, even if precautions such as dilution of vitamin K and slow infusions have been observed. Hypersensitivity can also occur from other ingredients of this product. Pain or swelling at the site of injection may occur. Keep the drug out of sunlight at all times.

DRUG INTERACTIONS: Vitamin K_1 will not counteract the anticoagulant effects of heparin.

SUPPLIED AS: VETERINARY PRODUCTS
For injection containing 10 mg/mL phytonadione
Oral capsule containing 25 mg

WARFARIN

INDICATIONS: Warfarin (Coumadin♥★, Panwarfin★, Soferin★, Warfilone♥) is an anticoagulant. It interferes with clotting by depressing hepatic synthesis of vitamin K-dependent coagulation factors II, VII, IX, and X. It is suggested as a maintenance therapy for navicular disease in horses. Monitoring of the one-stage prothrombin time is necessary because hemorrhage is a potential serious side effect. Efficacy in treating navicular disease is said to be 40% to 80%. However, problems inherent with such treatment have kept it from wide acceptance.

ADVERSE AND COMMON SIDE EFFECTS: The drug is contraindicated in patients with preexisting bleeding tendencies, gastrointestinal ulceration, or those undergoing surgery. Vitamin K_1 should always be readily available when this drug is used.

DRUG INTERACTIONS: Drugs that may enhance the anticoagulant effect of warfarin include allopurinol, aminoglycosides, anabolic steroids, oral antibiotics, chloramphenicol, cimetidine, diuretics, erythromycin, metronidazole, mineral oil, miconazole, neomycin, nonsteroidal anti-inflammatory drugs, potassium products, quinidine, sulfonamides, tetracyclines, and vitamin E.
Drugs that may decrease anticoagulant response include barbiturates, corticosteroids, diuretics, griseofulvin, laxatives, rifampin, vitamin C, and dietary vitamin K.

SUPPLIED AS: HUMAN PRODUCT
Tablets containing 1, 2, 2.5, 4, 5, 7.5, and 10 mg

XYLAZINE

INDICATIONS: Xylazine (Anased♥★, Cervizine★, Rompun♥★, Gemini★, Gemini SA★, Solvazine Injection★, Tranquived★, Xylaject★, Xylamax♥, Xylazine Injection★, Xylazine HCL★) is a tranquilizing agent characterized in the horse by a rapid onset, good to excellent sedation, excellent analgesia of 15 to 30 minutes duration, and a smooth recovery. Xylazine is particularly potent as a short-acting analgesic in horses with colic. The duration of sedation in ruminants is longer than in horses.

ADVERSE AND COMMON SIDE EFFECTS: Ruminants are particularly sensitive to the sedative effects of xylazine. Temporary salivation, diuresis, ruminal stasis, and diarrhea have been observed in cattle. Use of the drug is contraindicated in animals receiving epinephrine or those with ventricular arrhythmias. It should be used with caution in animals with heart disease, hypotension, shock, respiratory dysfunction, severe hepatic or renal disease, a history of seizure activity, or those severely debilitated. Bradycardia may be prevented by the administration of atropine or glycopyrrolate. Xylazine induces a modest catecholamine release and may result in patchy sweating and elevated blood glucose in the horse. The drug may precipitate early parturition and retained placenta if used in the last trimester of pregnancy. Repeated doses of xylazine in tympanic colic should be avoided because it can have detrimental effects by decreasing intestinal motility. Draft breeds of horses may be more sensitive to the effects of xylazine. Movement in response to sharp auditory stimuli may be observed. Occasionally, parenteral administration to equines may not induce effective sedation.

DRUG INTERACTIONS: Xylazine sensitizes the heart to epinephrine-induced arrhythmias, especially in the face of halothane anesthesia. Other central nervous system (CNS) depressants, including barbiturates, narcotics, and phenothiazines may potentiate CNS and respiratory depression. Yohimbine (Yobine♥★ at 0.12 mg/kg; slowly IV) can be used in horses to antagonize the effects of xylazine, shorten recovery times, and reduce anesthetic-related complications. Avoid perivascular or intracarotid injection.

SUPPLIED AS: VETERINARY PRODUCT
For injection containing 20 and 100 mg/mL

OTHER USES
Horses
EPIDURAL ANALGESIA
0.17 to 0. 22 mg/kg diluted to a 10-mL volume using 0.9% saline, given epidurally into the first or second coccygeal space. Analgesia duration is approximately 3.5 hours and at the lower dose hind end ataxia is not reported to occur.

Cattle
EPIDURAL ANALGESIA
0.05 mg/kg diluted to a 5-mL volume using 0.9% saline, given epidurally into the first caudal intervertebral space. Trials in our hospital have had less than favorable response to this mode of analgesia.

YOHIMBINE

INDICATIONS: Yohimbine (Antagonil♣★, Yobine♣★) is a competitive α_2-adrenergic blocking agent used for reversal of the effects of xylazine and detomidine. It is also used empirically in horses in combination with parasympathomimetics such as bethanechol to treat ileus presumed to be caused by adrenergic stimulation.

ADVERSE AND COMMON SIDE EFFECTS: Signs of sympathomimetic stimulation, including sweating, increased heart rate and blood pressure, muscle tremors, and irritability have been noted in humans and laboratory animals. Adverse effects are yet to be described in large animals.

DRUG INTERACTIONS: None listed.

SUPPLIED AS: VETERINARY PRODUCT
For injection containing 2 and 5 mg/mL

OTHER USES
Horses
GASTROINTESTINAL ILEUS
Slow IV administration (75 µg/kg) of yohimbine has been used to counteract negative propulsive effects of endotoxin on the gastrointestinal tract, presumed mediated through α_2-adrenoreceptors. This regimen has restored intestinal electromechanical activity after induced ileus in Shetland ponies.

ZERANOL

INDICATIONS: Zeranol (Ralgro♣★) is a hormone implant used in cattle for growth promotion and improving feed efficiency. Zeranol acts by stimulating increased secretion of endogenous somatotropin.

ADVERSE AND COMMON SIDE EFFECTS: None listed. Zeranol may not be as effective if used in animals with poor husbandry or parasite control.

DRUG INTERACTIONS: None listed.

SUPPLIED AS: VETERINARY PRODUCT
Implants containing 36 mg zeranol

OTHER USES
Sheep
Zeranol can be used in rams to reduce the incidence of ulcerative posthitis, but it is not as effective as testosterone.

Part III

Exotics

Part II

Exotics

Handbook of Veterinary Drugs, Second Edition, edited by Dana Allen,
Lippincott–Raven Publishers, Philadelphia. © 1998

Section 7

Introduction: Chemotherapeutics in Avian and Exotic Pet Practice

Provision of optimum medical care to avian and the less traditional, or exotic, pet species requires both the art and the science of veterinary medicine. Very few drugs are licensed or specifically formulated for use in birds, small mammals, or reptiles. Despite increasing research on the pharmacokinetics and efficacy of medications in these species, the majority of dosage regimes are still empirical and derived, sometimes very roughly, from other species. It is essential that the veterinarian be knowledgeable about the mode of action and reported side effects of a given drug to assess its appropriateness for a novel patient or treatment situation. Owners must be aware that the vast majority of medications are off-label and that a guarantee of either safety or efficacy is impossible in all situations. Veterinarians must remain abreast of the current literature pertaining to the treatment of exotic pets and adjust or discard recommendations that are shown to be inappropriate. Contributions to the literature by practitioners, particularly on observed efficacy, adverse effects, or applications of new drugs to exotic animal practice, assist in promoting rational, effective, and safe treatment regimens.

The dosages in this book are derived from information in the published literature, including texts, refereed journal articles, and less formal communications such as letters to the editor or "In My Experience" style comments. Nonrefereed material often provides the first information on the application of new drugs and on adverse or unexpected side effects.

The Drug Description section summarizes information on the use of a particular drug in a given group of animals. Summarized pharmacokinetic details are provided to help the reader judge the applicability of research results to a particular clinical situation. Drug dosages derived from pharmacokinetic work or efficacy trials in exotic species are marked with an asterisk in the dosage tables. Because of the format of this book, specific references are not included, but are available from the author on request. Readers are referred to the Small Animal or Large Animal sections for general information on the characteristics and use of particular drugs in the more common domestic species and for the commercial availability of drugs used in standard veterinary practice.

ALLOMETRIC SCALING

Allometric scaling is a mathematical technique used to adapt drug dosage and frequency of administration from one species of animal to another. Metabolic rates and many other physiologic processes that affect pharmacokinetic parameters are exponentially rather than linearly associated with body weight or mass. Hence, the direct application of a mg/kg dose from a small animal, or species with a high metabolic rate, to a large animal, or species with a slower metabolic rate, may result in a considerable overdosage. Underdosage could occur if the calculation is reversed, that is, from a large to a small species of animal. Allometric scaling formulas multiply an exponential function of lean body weight by a constant (K). Vertebrates are placed in five very broad K groups, the value of K reflecting mean core body temperature and basal energy requirements, as follows:

Reptiles (at 37°C): 10
Marsupials: 49
Placental mammals: 70
Nonpasserine birds: 78
Passerine birds: 129

Although metabolic scaling has been used extensively to determine treatment protocols, it is important to recognize the underlying assumptions. It is assumed that all animals absorb, distribute, and metabolize a given drug in the same manner. This is untrue in many instances; for example, the absorption of an orally administered compound is likely to be very different among a herbivorous reptile, a carnivorous mammal, and a granivorous bird. Quantitative differences in excretory pathways make allometric scaling of aminoglycoside and penicillin doses from mammals to birds inappropriate. Physiologic mechanisms vary even within a vertebrate class, for example, between aquatic and terrestrial reptiles, or temperate and highly xerophilic birds. The half-life of gentamicin correlates with body size for some, but not all, avian species. It is well recognized that pharmacokinetic parameters in reptiles are significantly affected by changes in ambient, and hence body, temperature. The K value used to scale allometric doses for reptiles was determined for an ambient temperature of 37°C and may be inappropriate for other environmental situations. It is, therefore, likely that the most valid allometric extrapolations will be between species with similar basic physiologic mechanisms and for drugs metabolized and excreted by processes that are closely related to basal metabolic rate.

The following calculations incorporate the K value of 70 (appropriate for placental mammals) and illustrate how to use allometric scaling to extrapolate drug dosage rate and frequency of administration from a control species in which this information is known, to one in which it is not.

1. The specific minimum energy cost (SMEC) is calculated for both the animal in which drug dosage is known (control) and the patient to be treated.

$$SMEC = 70 \, (W_{kg}^{-0.25})$$

2. The SMEC dose rate (dose per metabolic energy unit) for the control animal is calculated by dividing the drug's dose rate (mg/kg) for that species by its SMEC ($SMEC_{control}$).

$$SMEC \text{ dose rate (mg/kg)} = Dose_{control}(mg/kg)/SMEC_{control}$$

3. The dose rate for the patient is calculated by multiplying the $SMEC_{patient}$ by the SMEC dose rate.

$$Dose_{patient}(mg/kg) = SMEC_{patient} \times SMEC \text{ dose rate}(mg/kg)$$

4. Treatment frequency is allometrically scaled in a similar fashion to determine the frequency of administration within a 24-hour period, or the number of times the dose should be administered.

$$SMEC \text{ frequency} = \text{treatment frequency}_{control}/SMEC_{control}$$

5. The frequency of administration for a 24-hour period for the patient is calculated by multiplying the SMEC frequency by the $SMEC_{patient}$.

$$Frequency_{patient} = SMEC \text{ frequency} \times SMEC_{patient}$$

Handbook of Veterinary Drugs, Second Edition, edited by Dana Allen,
Lippincott–Raven Publishers, Philadelphia. © 1998

Section 8

The Use of Chemotherapeutic Agents in Rodents and Rabbits

Few drugs are licensed for use in rabbits and rodents; therefore, most of the drugs listed are off-label applications and should be recognized as such. The susceptibility of rabbits and rodents, particularly guinea pigs and hamsters, to antimicrobial toxicity is particularly important. Disturbances in the intestinal microflora caused by narrow-spectrum antimicrobial agents can lead to overgrowth of gram-negative or gram-positive anaerobic bacteria, causing enterotoxemia and death.

Drugs can be administered orally, parenterally, or topically to rabbits and rodents. Medication of the drinking water has been traditionally advocated for use in laboratory animals due to the ease of administration to large groups and the relative unimportance of any particular individual. In pet practice this approach is seldom justified. Direct individual dosing for each patient is preferred because the amount to be administered can be accurately determined based on the weight, age, sex, disease status, hydration status, and metabolic rate of the individual patient. Because of the small size of most rodents, it is essential that drugs be diluted sufficiently to enable accurate dosage. Consultation with a pharmacy may be necessary to determine the appropriate diluent.

Direct administration of oral suspensions is readily feasible. Some animals will lick flavored medications from a syringe. Alternatively, the liquid can be administered directly into the side of the mouth. Owners must be shown appropriate technique so that all medication is received by the patient and to ensure their own and the patient's safety. Medication can also be mixed with preferred foods or treats; however, it may be difficult to ensure complete consumption if the size of the offering is too great. The effectiveness of this route also depends on the palatability of a given medication to the individual being treated. Rabbits and rodents are difficult to medicate with intact tablets or capsules.

Subcutaneous injection is the preferred route of administration for parenteral medications. Larger volumes of drug can be administered as compared to the intramuscular route, and irritating compounds can be diluted to reduce tissue damage. The preferred site for subcutaneous injection is the loose skin over the back and shoulders and the dorsal flank area in rabbits. Sites for intramuscular injection include the large lumbar muscles cranial to the pelvis in rabbits and the biceps and quadriceps muscles of the cranial thigh in all species. Injection into the caudal thigh is not recommended because damage to the sciatic nerve can occur, with subsequent lameness and self-mutilation. Intravenous injections in all species but the rabbit are difficult.

Topical drugs are used to treat rabbits and rodents, but caution is necessary. Because of the fastidious grooming habits of most individuals, it is essential that compounds used be nontoxic if ingested. Because of their small size, and hence greater ratio of surface area to volume, rodents are more susceptible to the toxic side effects of any drug administered topically, particularly those containing steroids or organophosphates.

Handbook of Veterinary Drugs, Second Edition, edited by Dana Allen,
Lippincott–Raven Publishers, Philadelphia. © 1998

Section 9

Common Dosages for Rodents and Rabbits

The following table lists drugs and doses as recommended for use in rodents and rabbits in clinical practice. This information is derived from the published literature pertaining to pet and laboratory animals. A few pharmacokinetic trials have been carried out, primarily in rabbits; however, almost all doses are empirical and off-label. Small rodent species other than those specifically listed are also seen in veterinary practice. The veterinarian should attempt to match these animals with a species listed in this table in order to most safely extrapolate drug dosage regimens. Matching should be particularly based on similar gastrointestinal form and function in order to minimize the possibility of antimicrobial toxicity.

Drug	Rabbits	Guinea Pigs	Chinchillas
Acepromazine	1 to 5 mg/kg; IM	0.5 to 5 mg/kg; SC, IM	0.5 to 1 mg/kg; IM
Acetaminophen	200 to 500 mg/kg; PO		
Amikacin	8 to 16 mg/kg total dose; once daily to divided tid; SC, IM, IV	10 to 15 mg/kg total per day, once daily to divided tid; SC, IM, IV	10 to 15 mg/kg total per day, once daily to divided tid; SC, IM, IV
Amitraz (Mitaban) make up as per package directions		Apply topically 3 to 6 treatments 14 days apart	
Ampicillin		Do not use	
Amprolium 9.6% solution	1 mL/7 kg once daily for 5 days; PO 0.5 mL/500 mL drinking water for 10 days		
Aspirin	100 mg/kg q 4 to 6 hr; PO	80 mg/kg q 4 hr; PO	

Hamsters	Gerbils	Rats	Mice
0.5 to 5 mg/kg; SC, IM	Do not use	0.5 to 2.5 mg/kg; SC, IM	0.5 to 2.5 mg/kg; SC, IM
		100 to 300 mg/kg q 4 hr; PO	300 mg/kg q 4 hr; PO
10 to 20 mg/kg total daily dose; once daily to divided tid; IM, SC	10 to 20 mg/kg total daily dose; once daily to divided tid; IM, SC	10 to 20 mg/kg total daily dose; once daily to divided tid; IM, SC	10 to 20 mg/kg total daily dose; once daily to divided tid; IM, SC
Apply topically 3 to 6 treatments 14 days apart			
Do not use.	20 to 100 mg/kg divided tid; PO, SC	20 to 100 mg/kg divided tid; PO, SC	20 to 100 mg/kg divided tid; PO, SC
240 mg/kg; PO	240 mg/kg; PO	100 mg/kg q 4 hr; PO	120 to 300 mg/kg q 4 hr; PO

Drug	Rabbits	Guinea Pigs	Chinchillas
Atropine	0.1 to 2 mg/kg; IM, SC (see also glyco-pyrrolate)	0.05 to 0.2 mg/kg; SC	
	1% atropine plus 10% phenyl-ephrine ophthalmic drops to dilate pig-mented eyes	1% atropine ophthalmic drops to dilate pig-mented eyes	1% atropine (±10% phenyl-ephrine) ophthalmic drops to dilate pig-mented eyes
	2 to 10 mg/kg q 20 min as necessary for organo-phosphate toxicity; IM, SC		
Buprenorphine	0.01 to 0.1 mg/kg bid–tid; SC, IM, IV	0.05 to 0.1 mg/kg bid–tid; SC, IM	
Butorphanol	0.1 to 0.5 mg/kg q 2 to 4 hr; SC, IM, IV	2 mg/kg q 2 to 4 hr; SC, IM	
Calcium EDTA	27.5 mg/kg qid for 5 days; SC; dilute to 10 mg/mL with saline. Repeat if necessary.		25 to 30 mg/kg bid–qid for 5 days; SC
Carbaryl 5% powder	Dust lightly once weekly.	Dust lightly once weekly.	Dust lightly once weekly.
Chloramphenicol palmitate	50 mg/kg bid; PO	50 mg/kg bid; PO	50 mg/kg bid; PO
Chloramphenicol succinate	30 to 50 mg/kg bid; IM, SC	30 to 50 mg/kg bid; IM, SC	30 to 50 mg/kg bid; IM, SC
Chlorpromazine		25 mg/kg; SC	

Hamsters	Gerbils	Rats	Mice
0.04 to 0.05 mg/kg; SC, IM	0.04 to 0.05 mg/kg; SC, IM	0.04 to 0.05 mg/kg; SC, IM (see also glyco-pyrrolate)	0.02 to 0.05 mg/kg; SC, IM
1% atropine (±10% phenyl-ephrine) ophthalmic drops to dilate pigmented eyes	1% atropine (±10% phenyl-ephrine) ophthalmic drops to dilate pig-mented eyes	1% atropine (±10% phenyl-ephrine) ophthalmic drops to dilate pig-mented eyes	1% atropine (±10% phenyl-ephrine) ophthalmic drops to dilate pig-mented eyes
0.05 to 1.0 mg/kg bid–tid; SC, IM	0.05 to 1.0 mg/kg bid–tid; SC, IM	0.05 to 1.0 mg/kg bid–tid; SC, IM	0.05 to 2.5 mg/kg bid–tid; SC, IM
2 mg/kg q 2 to 4 hr; SC, IM	2 mg/kg q 2 to 4 hr; SC, IM	0.5 to 5 mg/kg q 2 to 6 hr; SC, IM	1 to 5 mg/kg q 2 to 6 hr; SC, IM
Dust lightly once weekly	Dust lightly once weekly	Dust lightly once weekly	Dust lightly once weekly
50 to 200 mg/kg tid; PO	50 to 200 mg/kg tid; PO	50 to 200 mg/kg tid; PO	50 to 200 mg/kg tid; PO
30 to 50 mg/kg bid; IM, SC	30 to 50 mg/kg bid; IM, SC	30 to 50 mg/kg bid; IM, SC	30 to 50 mg/kg bid; IM, SC
		20 to 30 mg/kg; SC	

Drug	Rabbits	Guinea Pigs	Chinchillas
Chlortetracycline	50 mg/kg bid; PO		50 mg/kg bid; PO
Cholestyramine	2 g in 20 mL water once daily by gavage (2.5–3.8-kg animal)		
Chorionic gonado-trophin		100 IU once, re-peat in 10 to 14 days; IM	
Cimetidine	5 to 10 mg/kg bid–tid; PO, SC, IM, IV	5 to 10 mg/kg bid–tid; PO, SC, IM, IV	5 to 10 mg/kg bid–qid; PO, SC, IM, IV
Ciprofloxacin	5 to 15 mg/kg bid; PO	5 to 15 mg/kg bid; PO	5 to 15 mg/kg bid; PO
Cisapride	0.5 mg/kg once daily to tid; PO, SC		0.5 mg/kg tid; PO
Clotrimazole	Topical applica-tion to shaved skin as needed		
Codeine			
Copper sulfate	1% topically applied as a dip		
Dexamethasone	0.5 to 2.0 mg/kg bid; PO, SC, IM. Wean off dosage at end of treatment.	0.1 to 0.6 mg/kg; IM	
Diazepam	1 to 5 mg/kg; IM, IV	1 to 5 mg/kg; IM	1 to 3 mg/kg; IM
Dichlorvos impregnated resin strip	Follow package directions for room size, hang in room for 24 hr once weekly for 6 wk.		

Hamsters	Gerbils	Rats	Mice
20 mg/kg bid; IM, SC		6 to 10 mg/kg bid; SC, IM	25 mg/kg bid; SC, IM
5 to 10 mg/kg bid–qid; PO, SC, IM	5 to 10 mg/kg bid–qid; PO, SC, IM	5 to 10 mg/kg bid–qid; PO, SC, IM	5 to 10 mg/kg bid–qid; PO, SC, IM
10 mg/kg bid; PO	10 mg/kg bid; PO	10 mg/kg bid; PO	10 mg/kg bid; PO
		60 mg/kg qid; SC	10 to 20 mg/kg qid; SC
0.1 to 0.6 mg/kg; IM	0.1 to 0.6 mg/kg; IM	0.1 to 0.6 mg/kg; IM	0.1 to 0.6 mg/kg; IM
3 to 5 mg/kg; IM	3 to 5 mg/kg; IM	3 to 5 mg/kg; IM	3 to 5 mg/kg; IM
1-in. square laid on cage for 24 hr once weekly for 6 wk	1-in. square laid on cage for 24 hr once weekly for 6 wk	1-in. square laid on cage for 24 hr once weekly for 6 wk	1-in. square laid on cage for 24 hr once weekly for 6 wk

Drug	Rabbits	Guinea Pigs	Chinchillas
Diethylstilbestrol	0.5 mg/kg PO once to twice per week as needed		
Dimetridazole	0.2 mg/mL drinking water		0.8 mg/mL drinking water
Diovol Plus	1 to 2 mL as needed; PO	0.5 to 1 mL as needed; PO	1 mL as needed; PO
Dipyrone	6 to 12 mg/kg bid–tid; PO, SC, IM		
Doxapram	2 to 5 mg/kg as needed; IV		5 to 10 mg/kg; IV
Doxycycline	2.5 mg/kg bid; PO 4 mg/kg once daily; PO 100 to 200 mg/L drinking water for 14 days	2.5 mg/kg bid; PO	2.5 mg/kg bid; PO
Enilconazole	Apply topically as required		
Enrofloxacin	5 to 15 mg/kg bid; PO, SC, IM	2.5 to 10 mg/kg bid; PO, SC, IM	2.5 to 10 mg/kg bid; PO, SC, IM
Erythromycin	Do not use.	Do not use.	Do not use.
Fenbendazole	20 mg/kg once daily for 5 days; PO 10 to 20 mg/kg; PO once, repeat in 10 to 14 days	20 mg/kg once daily for 5 days; PO	20 mg/kg once daily for 5 days; PO 50 to 100 mg/kg once; PO
Flunixin	0.3 to 2.0 mg/kg once daily to bid for no more than 3 days; deep IM, PO	2.5 mg/kg once daily to bid; IM	

Hamsters	Gerbils	Rats	Mice
0.5 mg/mL drinking water	0.5 mg/mL drinking water	1 mg/mL drinking water	1 mg/mL drinking water
0.1 to 0.3 mL as needed; PO	0.1 to 0.3 mL as needed; PO	0.1 to 0.3 mL as needed; PO	0.1 to 0.3 mL as needed; PO
5 to 10 mg/kg; IV	5 to 10 mg/kg; IV	5 to 10 mg/kg; IV	5 to 10 mg/kg; IV
2.5 mg/kg bid; PO	2.5 mg/kg bid; PO	2.5 to 5 mg/kg bid for 7 to 21 days; PO	2.5 to 5 mg/kg bid; PO
10 mg/kg bid for 5 to 7 days; PO, IM		2.5 to 10 mg/kg bid; PO, SC, IM	2.5 to 10 mg/kg bid; PO, SC, IM
500 mg/gal drinking water continuously			
20 mg/kg once daily for 5 days; PO	20 mg/kg once daily for 5 days; PO	20 mg/kg once daily for 5 days; PO	20 mg/kg once daily for 5 days; PO
2.5 mg/kg once daily to bid; IM	2.5 mg/kg once daily to bid; IM	2.5 mg/kg once daily to bid; IM	2.5 mg/kg once daily to bid; IM

Drug	Rabbits	Guinea Pigs	Chinchillas
Furosemide	2 to 5 mg/kg bid; PO, SC, IM, IV	2 to 5 mg/kg bid; PO, SC	2 to 5 mg/kg bid; PO, SC
Gentamicin	5 to 8 mg/kg total dose; once daily to divided tid; SC, IM, IV	5 to 8 mg/kg total dose; once daily to divided tid; SC, IM, IV	5 to 8 mg/kg total dose; once daily to divided tid; SC, IM, IV
Glycopyrrolate	0.01 to 0.05 mg/kg; SC, IM	0.01 to 0.05 mg/kg; SC, IM	
Griseofulvin	25 mg/kg once daily or divided bid for 28 to 40 days; PO	25 mg/kg once daily for 14 to 28 days; PO	25 mg/kg once daily for 28 to 40 days; PO
Halothane	Anesthetic	Anesthetic	Anesthetic
Ibuprofen	7.5 to 20 mg/kg q 4 hr; PO	10 mg/kg q 4 hr; IM	
Innovar-Vet 10% solution	0.1 to 0.3 mL/kg; SC, IM	0.4 to 0.8 mL/kg; SC, IM	
Innovar-Vet 10% solution and xylazine		0.2 to 0.4 mL/kg + 20 mg/kg IM	
Isoflurane	Anesthetic of choice	Anesthetic of choice	Anesthetic of choice
Ivermectin	200 to 400 µg/kg once, repeat in 10 to 14 days; PO, SC. For ear mites, divide dose in two and apply topically into each ear. At least two doses up to 18 days apart.	300 to 500 µg/kg once, repeat in 8 to 10 days; PO, SC	200 to 400 µg/kg once, repeat in 8 to 10 days; PO, SC

Hamsters	Gerbils	Rats	Mice
2 to 5 mg/kg bid; PO, SC	2 to 5 mg/kg bid; PO, SC	2 to 5 mg/kg bid; PO, SC	2 to 5 mg/kg bid; PO, SC
5 to 8 mg/kg total dose; once daily to divided tid; SC, IM	5 to 8 mg/kg total dose; once daily to divided tid; SC, IM	5 to 8 mg/kg total dose; once daily to divided tid; SC, IM, IV	5 to 8 mg/kg total dose; once daily to divided tid; SC, IM, IV
0.01 to 0.05 mg/kg; SC, IM	0.01 to 0.05 mg/kg; SC, IM	0.01 to 0.05 mg/kg; SC, IM	0.01 to 0.05 mg/kg; SC, IM
25 mg/kg once daily for 14 to 28 days; PO	25 mg/kg once daily for 14 to 28 days; PO	25 mg/kg once daily for 14 to 28 days; PO	25 mg/kg once daily for 14 to 28 days; PO
Anesthetic	Anesthetic	Anesthetic	Anesthetic
		10 to 30 mg/kg q 4 hr; PO	7 to 15 mg/kg q 4 hr; PO
Do not use.	Do not use.	0.1 to 0.5 mL/kg; SC, IM	0.1 to 0.5 mL/kg; SC, IM
		0.1 to 0.15 mL/kg + 20 mg/kg IM	
Anesthetic of choice	Anesthetic of choice	Anesthetic of choice	Anesthetic of choice
200 to 400 µg/kg, repeat in 8 to 10 days; PO, SC	200 to 400 µg/kg, repeat in 8 to 10 days; PO, SC	200 to 400 µg/kg, repeat in 8 to 10 days; PO, SC	200 to 400 µg/kg, repeat in 8 to 10 days; PO, SC
			2 mg/kg once, repeat in 10 days; PO, SC (for pinworms)

Drug	Rabbits	Guinea Pigs	Chinchillas
Ketamine	20 to 50 mg/kg; IM	20 to 60 mg/kg; IM, IP	20 to 60 mg/kg; IM, IP
Ketamine and acepromazine	25 to 40 mg/kg + 0.25 to 1.0 mg/kg; IM	20 to 50 mg/kg + 0.5 to 1.0 mg/kg; IM	20 to 40 mg/kg + 0.5 mg/kg; IM
Ketamine and diazepam	20 to 40 mg/kg + 5 to 10 mg/kg; IM	20 to 50 mg/kg + 3 to 5 mg/kg; IM	20 to 40 mg/kg + 3 to 5 mg/kg; IM
Ketamine and xylazine	20 to 40 mg/kg + 3 to 5 mg/kg; IM 10 mg/kg + 3 mg/kg; IV	20 to 44 mg/kg + 3 to 5 mg/kg; IM	35 mg/kg + 5 mg/kg; IM
Lime sulfur 2.5% solution	Apply once weekly for 4 to 6 wk.	Apply once weekly for 4 to 6 wk.	
Lindane (0.03% solution)	Dip once weekly for 3 wk.	Dip once weekly for 3 wk.	
Malathion (2% solution)	Dip q 10 days for 3 wk.	Dip q 10 days for 3 wk.	
MECA	1 part MECA : 1 part activator : 10 parts water; applied topically as a dip or spray		
Meperidine	5 to 20 mg/kg q 2 to 6 hr as needed; SC, IM, IV	10 to 20 mg/kg q 2 to 6 hr as needed; SC, IM	10 to 20 mg/kg q 2 to 6 hr as needed; SC, IM
Metoclopramide	0.5 mg/kg tid–qid; PO, SC		
Metronidazole	20 to 60 mg/kg bid for 3 to 5 days; PO	20 to 60 mg/kg bid–tid; PO	20 to 60 mg/kg bid–tid; PO

Hamsters	Gerbils	Rats	Mice
40 to 200 mg/kg; IP	40 to 100 mg/kg; IP	40 to 100 mg/kg; IM, IP	40 to 80 mg/kg; IP
50 to 150 mg/kg + 2.5 to 5.0 mg/kg; IM	Do not use	50 to 150 mg/kg + 2.5 to 5.0 mg/kg; IM	50 to 150 mg/kg + 2.5 to 5.0 mg/kg; IM
40 to 150 mg/kg + 5 mg/kg; IM	40 to 150 mg/kg + 3 to 5 mg/kg; IM	40 to 100 mg/kg + 3 to 5 mg/kg; IM	40 to 150 mg/kg + 3 to 5 mg/kg; IM
50 to 150 mg/kg + 5 to 10 mg/kg; IM	50 to 70 mg/kg + 2 to 3 mg/kg; IM	90 mg/kg +5 mg/kg; IM	50 to 150 mg/kg + 5 to 10 mg/kg; IM
		Dip once weekly for 3 wk.	Dip once weekly for 3 wk.
		Dip q 10 days for 3 wk.	Dip q 10 days for 3 wk.
10 to 20 mg/kg q 2 to 6 hr as needed; SC, IM	10 to 20 mg/kg q 2 to 6 hr as needed; SC, IM	10 to 50 mg/kg q 2 to 3 hr as needed; SC, IM	10 to 20 mg/kg q 2 to 3 hr as needed; SC, IM
20 to 60 mg/kg bid–tid; PO 7.5 mg/70 to 90 g hamster tid; PO	20 to 60 mg/kg bid–tid; PO	10 to 60 mg/kg bid–tid; PO 10 to 40 mg/rat once daily; PO	10 to 60 mg/kg bid–tid; PO 2.5 mg/mL drinking water for 5 days

Drug	Rabbits	Guinea Pigs	Chinchillas
Miconazole	Apply topically as required.		
Midazolam	1 to 2 mg/kg; SC, IM	1 to 5 mg/kg; SC, IM	
Nalbuphine	1 to 2 mg/kg q 4 hr as required; SC, IM	1 to 4 mg/kg q 3 hr as required; SC, IM	
Naloxone	0.2 mg/kg; IM, IV	0.2 mg/kg; IM, IV	
Neomycin	30 mg/kg bid; PO	30 mg/kg once daily; PO	15 mg/kg bid; PO
Oxymorphone	0.05 to 0.2 mg/kg bid–tid; SC, IM	0.2 to 0.5 mg/kg tid–qid; SC, IM	
Oxytetracycline	15 mg/kg tid; SC, IM		50 mg/kg bid; PO
Oxytocin	1 to 2 U/rabbit; SC, IM	1 U/guinea pig; SC, IM	1 U/chinchilla; SC, IM
Penicillin G, procaine	20,000 to 60,000 U/kg once daily; SC, IM		
Penicillin G, benzathine, and procaine	47,000 to 84,000 U/kg once per week for 3 treatments; SC, IM		
Pentazocine	5 to 10 mg/kg q 4 hr; SC, IM, IV	10 mg/kg q 2 to 4 hr; SC, IM, IV	
Piperazine adipate	500 mg/kg once daily for 2 days; PO	4 to 7 mg/mL drinking water for 3 to 10 days	500 mg/kg once daily for 2 days; PO

Hamsters	Gerbils	Rats	Mice
1 to 5 mg/kg; SC, IM	1 to 5 mg/kg; SC, IM	1 to 5 mg/kg; SC, IM	1 to 5 mg/kg; SC, IM
4 to 8 mg/kg q 3 hr as required; SC, IM	4 to 8 mg/kg q 3 hr as required; SC, IM	1 to 4 mg/kg q 3 hr as required; SC, IM	4 to 8 mg/kg q 3 hr as required; SC, IM
0.2 mg/kg; IM, IP, IV	0.2 mg/kg; IM, IP, IV	0.2 mg/kg; IM, IP, IV	0.2 mg/kg; IM, IP, IV
100 mg/kg once daily; PO	100 mg/kg once daily; PO	50 mg/kg once daily; PO	50 mg/kg once daily; PO
0.2 to 0.5 mg/kg tid–qid; SC, IM	0.2 to 0.5 mg/kg tid–qid; SC, IM	0.2 to 0.5 mg/kg tid–qid; SC, IM	0.2 to 0.5 mg/kg tid–qid; SC, IM
16 mg/kg once daily; SC	20 mg/kg once daily, SC 10 mg/kg tid; PO	6 to 10 mg/kg bid, IM 10 to 20 mg/kg tid; PO	10 to 20 mg/kg tid; PO
0.2 to 0.3 U/kg; SC, IM	0.2 to 0.3 U/kg; SC, IM	1 U/kg; SC, IM	
		22,000 U once daily; IM	
10 mg/kg q 2 to 4 hr; SC, IM	10 mg/kg q 2 to 4 hr; SC, IM	10 mg/kg q 2 to 4 hr; SC, IM, IV	10 mg/kg q 2 to 4 hr; SC, IM, IV
3 to 5 mg/mL drinking water for 7 days, off 7 days, on 7 days	3 to 5 mg/mL drinking water for 7 days, off 7 days, on 7 days	4 to 7 mg/mL drinking water for 3 to 10 days	4 to 7 mg/mL drinking water for 3 to 10 days

Drug	Rabbits	Guinea Pigs	Chinchillas
Piperazine citrate	100 mg/100 mL drinking water for 1 day, repeat in 10 to 14 days	10 mg/mL drinking water for 7 days, off 7 days, on 7 days	
	100 to 200 mg/kg once daily for 2 days, or once and repeat in 10 to 14 days; PO		100 mg/kg once daily for 7 days; PO
Praziquantel	5 to 10 mg/kg once, repeat in 10 days; PO, SC, IM	5 to 10 mg/kg once, repeat in 10 days; PO, SC, IM	5 to 10 mg/kg once, repeat in 10 days; PO, SC, IM
Prednisone	0.5 to 2 mg/kg; PO	0.5 to 2 mg/kg; PO, SC	0.5 to 2 mg/kg; PO, SC
Pyrethrin products (0.05% shampoo)	Once weekly for 4 wk.	Once weekly for 4 wk.	Once weekly for 4 wk.
Stanozolol	1 to 2 mg/rabbit once; PO		
Sulfadimethoxine	25 to 50 mg/kg once daily, or 50 mg/kg loading dose followed by 25 mg/kg once daily for 9 days; PO	25 to 50 mg/kg once daily for 10 to 14 days; PO	25 to 50 mg/kg once daily for 10 to 14 days; PO
Sulfamethazine	1 to 5 mg/mL drinking water	1 to 5 mg/mL drinking water	1 to 5 mg/mL drinking water
Sulfaquinoxaline	1 mg/mL drinking water	1 mg/mL drinking water	
T-61	0.3 mL/kg; IV, IC	0.3 mL/kg; IV, IC	0.3 mL/kg; IV, IC

Hamsters	Gerbils	Rats	Mice
10 mg/mL drinking water for 7 days, off 7 days, on 7 days	4 to 5 mg/mL drinking water for 7 days, off 7 days, on 7 days	4 to 5 mg/mL drinking water for 7 days, off 7 days, on 7 days	4 to 5 mg/mL drinking water for 7 days, off 7 days, on 7 days
5.1 to 11.4 mg/kg once, repeat in 10 days; PO, SC, IM	5.1 to 11.4 mg/kg once, repeat in 10 days; PO, SC, IM	5.1 to 11.4 mg/kg once, repeat in 10 days; PO, SC, IM	25 mg/kg once, repeat in 10 days; PO, SC, IM
0.5 to 2 mg/kg; PO	0.5 to 2 mg/kg; PO	0.5 to 2 mg/kg; PO	0.5 to 2 mg/kg; PO
Once weekly for 4 wk.	Once weekly for 4 wk.	Once weekly for 4 wk.	Once weekly for 4 wk.
25 to 50 mg/kg once daily for 10 to 14 days; PO			
1 to 5 mg/mL drinking water	1 to 5 mg/mL drinking water	1 to 5 mg/mL drinking water	1 to 5 mg/mL drinking water
1 mg/mL drinking water	1 mg/mL drinking water	1 mg/mL drinking water	
0.3 mL/kg; IV, IC	0.3 mL/kg; IV, IC	0.3 mL/kg; IV, IC	0.3 mL/kg; IV, IC

Drug	Rabbits	Guinea Pigs	Chinchillas
Tetracycline	50 mg/kg bid–tid; PO	10 to 20 mg/kg tid; PO	50 mg/kg bid–tid; PO
Thiabendazole	50 to 100 g/kg once daily for 5 days; PO	100 mg/kg once daily for 5 days; PO	50 to 100 mg/kg once daily for 5 days; PO
Thiamylal	30 to 40 mg/kg; IV		
Thiopental	15 to 20 mg/kg; IV	20 to 55 mg/kg; IP	40 mg/kg; IP
Tiletamine-zolazepam	Do not use	20 to 60 mg/kg; IM	20 to 40 mg/kg; IM
Tresaderm (dexamethasone, neomycin, thiabendazole)	Instill 3 drops in ear bid for 7 days, for ear mites; in combination with ivermectin		
Trimethoprim sulfadiazine	30 mg/kg once daily–bid; SC	30 mg/kg once daily–bid; SC	30 mg/kg once daily–bid; SC
Trimethoprim sulfamethoxazole	15 to 30 mg/kg; bid; PO	15 mg/kg bid; PO	15 to 30 mg/kg bid; PO
Tropicamide 1%	Topically to dilate albinotic eyes		
Tylosin	10 mg/kg bid; SC, PO, IM		
Verapamil	200 µg/kg at surgery and q 8 hr for 9 doses total; IV, IP		
Viokase (amylase, lipase, protease)	1 tsp viokase + 3 tbsp yogurt; let stand 15 min, then give 2 to 3 mL bid; PO		

Hamsters	Gerbils	Rats	Mice
10 to 20 mg/kg tid; PO	10 to 20 mg/kg tid; PO	10 to 20 mg/kg tid; PO	10 to 20 mg/kg tid; PO
100 mg/kg once daily for 5 days; PO	100 mg/kg once daily for 5 days; PO	100 mg/kg once daily for 5 days; PO	100 mg/kg once daily for 5 days; PO
			20 to 50 mg/kg; IP
40 mg/kg; IP		40 mg/kg; IP	25 to 50 mg/kg; IP
50 to 80 mg/kg; IM	50 to 80 mg/kg; IM	10 to 30 mg/kg; IM	50 to 80 mg/kg; IM
30 mg/kg once daily; SC	30 mg/kg once daily; SC	30 mg/kg once daily; SC	30 mg/kg once daily; SC
15 to 30 mg/kg bid; PO	15 to 30 mg/kg bid; PO	15 to 30 mg/kg bid; PO	15 to 30 mg/kg bid; PO
Topically to dilate albinotic eyes	Topically to dilate albinotic eyes	Topically to dilate albinotic eyes	Topically to dilate albinotic eyes
2 to 8 mg/kg bid; PO, SC, IM	10 mg/kg bid; PO, SC, IM	10 mg/kg bid; PO, SC, IM	10 mg/kg bid; PO, SC, IM

Drug	Rabbits	Guinea Pigs	Chinchillas
Vitamin C		10 to 30 mg/kg daily for maintenance; up to 50 mg/kg for treatment of deficiency; PO, SC, IM 200 to 1,000 mg/mL drinking water	
Vitamin K₁	1 to 10 mg/kg as needed; IM	1 to 10 mg/kg as needed; IM	1 to 10 mg/kg as needed; IM
Xenodyne	Apply topically as needed	Apply topically as needed	Apply topically as needed
Xylazine (see Ketamine)			
Yohimbine	0.2 mg/kg; IV 0.5 mg/kg; IM	0.2 mg/kg; IV 0.5 mg/kg; IM	

Hamsters	Gerbils	Rats	Mice
1 to 10 mg/kg as needed; IM	1 to 10 mg/kg as needed; IM	1 to 10 mg/kg as needed; IM	1 to 10 mg/kg as needed; IM
Apply topically as needed	Apply topically as needed	Apply topically as needed	Apply topically as needed
0.2 mg/kg; IV	0.2 mg/kg; IV	0.2 mg/kg; IV	0.2 mg/kg; IV
0.5 mg/kg; IM	0.5 mg/kg; IM	0.5 mg/kg; IM	0.5 mg/kg; IM

Handbook of Veterinary Drugs, Second Edition, edited by Dana Allen,
Lippincott–Raven Publishers, Philadelphia. © 1998

Section 10

Description of Drugs for Rodents and Rabbits

ACEPROMAZINE

INDICATIONS: Acepromazine [formerly Acetylpromazine] (AC
Promazine ✦, Atravet ✦ ★, PromAce ★) is a phenothiazine drug used
as a sedative and preanesthetic agent. For more information, see
ACEPROMAZINE in the Small Animal section.

ADVERSE AND COMMON SIDE EFFECTS: The use of acepromazine may precipitate seizures in gerbils. Hypotension may occur
at the higher dosages.

ACETAMINOPHEN

INDICATIONS: Acetaminophen (Atasol ★, Tempra ✦ ★, Tylenol ✦ ★)
is an antipyretic, analgesic agent with weak anti-inflammatory properties. See **ACETAMINOPHEN** in the Small Animal section.

ADVERSE AND COMMON SIDE EFFECTS: Acetaminophen has
not been used extensively in rabbits and rodents; therefore, little information is available regarding toxicity. Published dosages are very
high as compared to those for the dog and the cat. See **ACETA-
MINOPHEN** in the Small Animal section for details on toxicity in
these species.

ACETYLSALICYLIC ACID

See **ASPIRIN**.

AMIKACIN

INDICATIONS: Amikacin (Amiglyde-V ✚ ★, Amikin ✚ ★) is an aminoglycoside antibiotic indicated in the treatment of infections caused by many gram-negative bacteria including susceptible strains of *Escherichia coli, Klebsiella* spp, *Proteus* spp, and *Pseudomonas* spp. For more information, see **AMIKACIN** and **AMINOGLYCO-SIDE ANTIBIOTICS** in the Small Animal section.

ADVERSE AND COMMON SIDE EFFECTS: Nephrotoxicity may occur, especially in animals that are dehydrated, have electrolyte imbalances, or have preexisting renal disease. Concurrent administration of fluids is recommended, especially in gerbils.

AMITRAZ

INDICATIONS: Amitraz (Mitaban ✚ ★) is indicated for the eradication of demodicosis in hamsters and sarcoptic mange in guinea pigs. The drug is used topically. For more information, see **AMITRAZ** in the Small Animal section.

ADVERSE AND COMMON SIDE EFFECTS: Use with caution because application has resulted in death, perhaps due to overdosage.

AMPICILLIN

INDICATIONS: Ampicillin (Omnipen★, Penbriton ✚, Polyflex ✚ ★) is indicated in the treatment of bacterial diseases, including some Pasteurella infections. For more information, see **AMPICILLIN** and **PENICILLIN ANTIBIOTICS** in the Small Animal section.

ADVERSE AND COMMON SIDE EFFECTS: This drug is used rarely for rodents because its administration can cause fatal enterotoxemia secondary to reduction of intestinal flora (anaerobes, lactobacilli, and streptococci) and clostridial and coliform overgrowth. This is seen most commonly in hamsters, guinea pigs, and rabbits; mice, rats, and gerbils may also be affected. Oral therapy is more toxic than parenteral administration.

AMPROLIUM

INDICATIONS: Amprolium (Amprol ✚, Corid ★) is an antiprotozoal agent placed in the drinking water as a coccidiostat and for the treatment of hepatic and intestinal coccidiosis in rabbits. For more information, see **AMPROLIUM** in the Small Animal section.

ADVERSE AND COMMON SIDE EFFECTS: Amprolium is a thiamine inhibitor and may rarely cause thiamine deficiency.

ASCORBIC ACID

INDICATIONS: Vitamin C, or ascorbic acid (Apo-C ♣, Redoxon ♣), is used to treat vitamin C deficiency in guinea pigs and as a supportive measure in anorectic or ill guinea pigs. Guinea pigs must receive adequate amounts of vitamin C on a daily basis. For more information, see **ASCORBIC ACID** in the Small Animal section.

ADVERSE AND COMMON SIDE EFFECTS: Overdosage with vitamin C may cause diarrhea. Precipitation of urate, oxalate, or cysteine crystals in urine has been reported.

DRUG INTERACTIONS: The urinary acidification that results from vitamin C administration may decrease the excretion of other drugs, such as sulfonamides. The potency of vitamin C in both feed and water declines over time. Medicated drinking water should be made fresh daily. Contact with metal watering systems accelerates deterioration; glass or plastic containers are suggested.

SUPPLIED AS: VETERINARY PRODUCT
For injection 250 mg/mL [Vitamin C ♣ ★]

HUMAN PRODUCT
Tablets containing 100, 250, 500, or 1,000 mg ♣ ★

OTHER USES: Vitamin C has also been used at a dosage of 30 mg/kg/day to induce urinary acidification in the treatment of struvite urolithiasis. It is not indicated for the treatment of other forms of urolithiasis.

ASPIRIN

INDICATIONS: Aspirin (ASA) or acetylsalicylic acid (Ecotrin ♣, Entrophen ♣, and many others) is an effective analgesic, antipyretic, and nonsteroidal anti-inflammatory agent. Aspirin has a wide volume of tissue distribution in rabbits and a half-life of 9.7 hours when administered orally. For more information, see **ASPIRIN** in the Small Animal section.

ADVERSE AND COMMON SIDE EFFECTS: Gastric upset may occur after several treatments.

ATROPINE

INDICATIONS: Atropine ♣ ★ is an anticholinergic, antispasmodic, and mydriatic drug used as a preanesthetic to reduce salivation and to treat organophosphate toxicity. For more information, see **ATROPINE** in the Small Animal section.

ADVERSE AND COMMON SIDE EFFECTS: Because many rabbits and rats possess serum atropinesterase, atropine may be ineffective or effective only at very high doses in these species. Glycopyrrolate metabolism is not affected and may therefore be a more effective choice. In guinea pigs atropine may cause hypertension, thereby increasing the tendency for hemorrhage during surgery.

OTHER USES: Atropine is used to treat organophosphate toxicity. One fourth of the dose is given IV if possible, the remainder IM or SC. Atropine ophthalmic drops, alone or in combination with phenylephrine, are used to induce mydriasis in animals with pigmented eyes.

BUPRENORPHINE HYDROCHLORIDE

INDICATIONS: Buprenorphine hydrochloride (Buprenex ★) is a partial opiate agonist used for its analgesic properties. Buprenorphine can also be used to reverse the effects of μ-opioids such as fentanyl, yet still provide postprocedural analgesia. For further information, see **BUPRENORPHINE** in the Small Animal section.

ADVERSE AND COMMON SIDE EFFECTS: Respiratory depression may occur. The drug is resistant to antagonism by naloxone. For further information, see **BUPRENORPHINE** in the Small Animal section.

DRUG INTERACTIONS: For further information, see **BUPRENORPHINE** in the Small Animal section.

BUTORPHANOL

INDICATIONS: Butorphanol (Torbugesic ✦ ★, Torbutrol ✦ ★) is a narcotic agonist/antagonist analgesic with potent antitussive activity in some species. In rabbits, the elimination half-life was 3.16 hours after SC administration and 1.64 hours after IV use. Butorphanol can also be used to reverse the effects of μ-opioids such as fentanyl, yet still provide postprocedural analgesia. For more information, see **BUTORPHANOL** in the Small Animal section.

ADVERSE AND COMMON SIDE EFFECTS: Butorphanol is contraindicated in pregnant and lactating rats because it increases nervousness and decreases newborn caretaking behavior.

CALCIUM EDTA

INDICATIONS: Calcium disodium EDTA (Calcium Disodium Versenate ✦ ★), is a chelating agent used for the treatment of lead toxicity in rabbits and chinchillas. Prior to administration, calcium EDTA is diluted to a 1% solution using 5% dextrose in water or saline. Two 5-day courses of treatment 1 week apart may be necessary.

ADVERSE AND COMMON SIDE EFFECTS and **DRUG INTER-ACTIONS:** See **CALCIUM EDTA** in the Small Animal section.

CARBARYL

INDICATIONS: Carbaryl (Sevin ♣, Zodiac Flea and Tick Power ♣, and others), a carbamate insecticide and cholinesterase inhibitor, is used in the eradication of arthropod ectoparasites including *Cheyletiella, Chirodiscoides, Myobia, Myocoptes, Radfordia, Psorergates,* and *Liponyssus* spp. For more information, see **CARBAMATE INSECTICIDES** in the Small Animal section.

ADVERSE AND COMMON SIDE EFFECTS: Carbaryl is the least toxic of the carbamate insecticides; however, caution against over-dosage should be taken, especially in young rodents. Even low doses of this drug may inhibit breeding. Atropine will counter toxic effects. Diazepam may also help reduce the severity of clinical signs.

SUPPLIED AS: VETERINARY PRODUCTS
Numerous dusting powders containing 5% carbaryl ♣ ★
Spray containing 2.5% carbaryl [D-F-T Spray ★]
Shampoo containing 0.5% carbaryl [Mycodex Pet Shampoo ★]

CHLORAMPHENICOL

INDICATIONS: Chloramphenicol (Azramycine ♣, Chlor Palm ♣, Chlor Tablets ♣, Chloromycetin ♣ ★, Karomycin Palmitate ♣, Viceton ★, and many others) is a bacteriostatic antibiotic with activity against a number of pathogens. It is one of the common first-line drugs for the treatment of bacterial infections in rabbits and rodents. Chloramphenicol has also been used in rabbits for the treatment of *Treponema* sp. infections. Disruption of intestinal microflora has not been associated with the use of this drug. For more information, see **CHLORAMPHENICOL** in the Small Animal section.

ADVERSE AND COMMON SIDE EFFECTS: Treatment in the drinking water has been recommended for colony situations, but this may cause reduced water intake, especially in chinchillas, rabbits, and guinea pigs, due to the bitter taste. Owners should be warned to take precautions to avoid human contact with the drug.

CHLORPROMAZINE

INDICATIONS: Chlorpromazine (Largactil ♣, Thorazine ★) is a phenothiazine derivative used as a preanesthetic, sedative, and antiemetic agent. For more information, see **CHLORPROMAZINE** in the Small Animal section.

ADVERSE AND COMMON SIDE EFFECTS: Chlorpromazine may precipitate seizures in gerbils. It is hypotensive and may cause hypothermia and hyperglycemia.

DRUG INTERACTIONS: Do not use epinephrine with chlorpromazine.

CHLORTETRACYCLINE

INDICATIONS: Chlortetracycline (Aureomycin ♣ ★, Fermycin ★, and others) is a broad-spectrum bacteriostatic antibiotic with activity against gram-positive and gram-negative organisms, chlamydiae, rickettsiae, mycoplasmas, and many anaerobes. For more information, see **TETRACYCLINE ANTIBIOTICS** in the Small Animal section.

DRUG INTERACTIONS: Oral absorption is inhibited by calcium-, magnesium-, and iron-containing substances.

SUPPLIED AS: VETERINARY PRODUCTS
Water-soluble powder containing
55 mg/g [Aureomycin ♣]
25.6 g/6.4 oz, 102.4 g/25.6 oz [Fermycin Soluble ★]
Tablets containing 25 mg [Aureomycin Tablets ★]
Many agricultural feed additives

CHOLESTYRAMINE

INDICATIONS: Cholestyramine (Alti-Cholestyramine ♣, Novo-Cholamine ♣, PMS-Cholestyramine ♣, Questran ★) is a quaternary amine ion resin capable of binding bacterial toxins. It has been used experimentally in rabbits and hamsters to prevent mortality after administration of clindamycin, an antibiotic known to result in disturbance of the normal enteric bacterial flora and fatal enterotoxemia. Rabbits treated with cholestyramine for 21 days after a dose of clindamycin did not show any evidence of gastrointestinal disease, in contrast with control animals. With a similar experimental protocol, hamsters remained healthy while receiving cholestyramine, but died after discontinuation of treatment. This suggests that their enteric flora had not regained a normal balance. The use of cholestyramine in clinical practice has not been well documented as yet.

SUPPLIED AS: HUMAN PRODUCT
Powder for oral suspension containing 4 g/packet [Alti-Cholestyramine ♣, Novo-Cholamine ♣, PMS-Cholestyramine ♣, Questran ★]

CHORIONIC GONADOTROPHIN

INDICATIONS: Chorionic gonadotrophin [human chorionic gonadotrophin, HCG] (A.P.L. ♣, Chorionad ♣, Chorionic Gonadotropin ★, Chorulon ♣ ★, Follutein ★) is a gonadal-stimulating hormone obtained from the urine of pregnant women. It has been used to stimulate ovulation in rabbits and to reduce the size of ovarian cysts in guinea pigs prior to surgical removal. For more information, see **CHORIONIC GONADOTROPHIN** in the Large Animal section.

ADVERSE AND COMMON SIDE EFFECTS: Chorionic gonadotrophin is a foreign protein and can cause anaphylaxis when administered parenterally. Continued administration may result in antihormone antibody production and loss of effectiveness.

SUPPLIED AS: VETERINARY PRODUCTS
For injection containing 5,000 [Chorulon ♣ ★, Chorionic Gonadotropin ★] and 10,000 [A.P.L. ♣, Chorionad ♣, Progron 10,000 ♣, Follutein ★, Chorionic Gonadotropin ★] USP units per vial.

CIMETIDINE

INDICATIONS: Cimetidine (Tagamet ♣ ★), a histamine (H_2) blocking agent, reduces gastric acid secretion and is used in the treatment of gastric ulceration. For more information, see **CIMETIDINE** in the Small Animal section.

CIPROFLOXACIN

INDICATIONS: Ciprofloxacin (Cipro ♣ ★) is a fluoroquinolone antibiotic with activity against *Escherichia coli, Klebsiella, Proteus, Pseudomonas, Staphylococcus, Salmonella, Shigella, Yersinia, Campylobacter,* and *Vibrio* species. It has little activity against anaerobic cocci or *Clostridia* or *Bacteroides* organisms. Ciprofloxacin has not been associated with disruption of the normal enteric flora. Ciprofloxacin ophthalmic drops can be used in rabbits in combination with systemic antibiotic therapy for the treatment of ocular and upper respiratory infections by *Pasteurella multocida*. See also **CIPROFLOXACIN** and **FLUOROQUINOLONE ANTIBIOTICS** in the Small Animal section.

ADVERSE AND COMMON SIDE EFFECTS: See **FLUOROQUINOLONE ANTIBIOTICS** in the Small Animal section. Ciprofloxacin tablets are commonly used as the basis of an oral suspension; however, the stability of the resulting product has not been thoroughly investigated.

DRUG INTERACTIONS: Absorption is hindered by antacid preparations. See **CIPROFLOXACIN** and **FLUOROQUINOLONE ANTIBIOTICS** in the Small Animal section.

CISAPRIDE

INDICATIONS: Cisapride (Prepulsid ✤, Propulsid ★) is chemically related to metoclopramide and is used in rabbits to stimulate gastrointestinal motility in animals with gastric impaction, gastric stasis, or gastric trichobezoars. It stimulates gastrointestinal motility by increasing acetylcholine release. The drug is generally given 15 to 30 minutes before a meal. Cisapride has also been used in the treatment of constipation in chinchillas. See **CISAPRIDE** in the Small Animal section.

ADVERSE AND COMMON SIDE EFFECTS: Use of the drug is contraindicated in animals with gastrointestinal hemorrhage, complete gastric or intestinal obstruction, or perforation. See **CISAPRIDE** in the Small Animal section.

DRUG INTERACTIONS: Because cisapride increases gastric emptying, absorption of drugs from the stomach may be decreased, whereas absorption from the small bowel may be increased. See **CISAPRIDE** in the Small Animal section.

CLOTRIMAZOLE

INDICATIONS: Clotrimazole (Canesten ✤, Lotrimin ★, Mycelex ★) is a topical imidazole useful in the treatment of localized dermatophytosis in rabbits. See **CLOTRIMAZOLE** in the Small Animal section.

ADVERSE AND COMMON SIDE EFFECTS: See **CLOTRIMAZOLE** in the Small Animal section.

CODEINE

INDICATIONS: Codeine (Methylmorphine ★, Paveral ✤, Tylenol No. 1 ✤) is an analgesic with antitussive properties. For more information, see **CODEINE** in the Small Animal section.

ADVERSE AND COMMON SIDE EFFECTS: Codeine depresses the respiratory drive, increases airway resistance, and dries respiratory secretions. Treatment with this drug may precipitate respiratory insufficiency.

COPPER SULFATE

INDICATIONS: Copper sulfate (commercial product) has been used topically to control dermatophytosis caused by *Trichophyton mentagrophytes* in a commercial rabbitry where treatment of individual animals with griseofulvin was not feasible. Animals were dipped in a 1% solution six times over a 26-day period. The number of carriers and extent of clinical signs were greatly reduced, but the infection was not completely eliminated. Also see **COPPER SULFATE** in the Large Animal section.

ADVERSE AND COMMON SIDE EFFECTS: The animal's eyes should be protected by a compound such as petroleum jelly during the dipping procedure.

DEXAMETHASONE

INDICATIONS: Dexamethasone (Azium ♣ ★, Azium SP ♣ ★, Dex-5 ♣) is a glucocorticoid anti-inflammatory agent. For more information, see **DEXAMETHASONE** in the Small Animal section.

ADVERSE AND COMMON SIDE EFFECTS: Dexamethasone may cause gastrointestinal irritation and ulceration. The drug must be used with extreme caution in small rodents to avoid overdosage; begin treatment with a low dose and increase if necessary.

DIAZEPAM

INDICATIONS: Diazepam (Valium ♣ ★, Valrelease ★) is an effective sedative, preanesthetic, and anticonvulsant. For more information, see **DIAZEPAM** in the Small Animal section.

DRUG INTERACTIONS: Diazepam is commonly used in combination with ketamine for sedation and anesthesia.

DICHLORVOS IMPREGNATED RESIN STRIPS

INDICATIONS: Dichlorvos (Vapona No Pest Strip and many others) is a cholinesterase inhibitor anthelmintic and insecticide. It is used as an impregnated resin strip that is hung in the animal's environment to eliminate arthropod ectoparasites including *Myobia, Myocoptes, Radfordia, Liponyssus, Cheyletiella,* and *Chirodiscoides* spp. For more information, see **DICHLORVOS** in the Small Animal section.

ADVERSE AND COMMON SIDE EFFECTS: It is essential to follow manufacturer's instructions in order to prevent excessive air concentrations and overdosage.

SUPPLIED AS: COMMERCIAL PRODUCTS
Impregnated resin strips containing 20% dichlorvos [Vapona No Pest Strip, Black Flag Insect Strip, and many others]

DIETHYLSTILBESTROL

INDICATIONS: Diethylstilbestrol (Stilboestrol ♣) has been used to treat urinary incontinence in spayed rabbits. See **DIETHYLSTIL-BESTROL** in the Small Animal section.

DIMETRIDAZOLE

INDICATIONS: Dimetridazole (Emtryl ♣) is an antimicrobial agent used for the prevention of clostridial enterotoxemia in rabbits.

SUPPLIED AS: VETERINARY PRODUCTS
Water-soluble powder with 40% W/W [Emtryl Soluble ♣]
Feed additives [Dimetridazole 30% Premix ♣, Emtryl Premix ♣]

DIOVOL PLUS

INDICATIONS: Diovol Plus ♣ is an antacid, antiflatulent compound containing aluminum and magnesium hydroxide, and simethicone, which is used to reduce excess gas production in gastrointestinal disturbances in rabbits and rodents. For more information, see **ANTACIDS** and **ALUMINUM HYDROXIDE** in the Small Animal section.

ADVERSE AND COMMON SIDE EFFECTS: Diovol Plus should not be used in animals with impaired renal function or with alkalosis or hypermagnesemia. For further information, see **ANTACIDS** in the Small Animal section.

DRUG INTERACTIONS: Diovol Plus should not be administered concurrently with tetracycline antibiotics or compounds containing iron.

SUPPLIED AS: HUMAN PRODUCTS
Suspension containing, per 5 mL, 200 mg aluminum hydroxide, 200 mg magnesium hydroxide, and 25 mg simethicone [Diovol Plus ♣]
Tablets containing 100 mg magnesium hydroxide, 300 mg aluminum hydroxide and magnesium carbonate co-dried, and 25 mg simethicone [Diovol Plus ♣]
Numerous other nonprescription medications containing the same ingredients

DIPYRONE

INDICATIONS: Dipyrone (Novolate ♣ and generic products ★) is an anti-inflammatory, antipyretic drug and an antispasmodic and analgesic agent. For more information, see **DIPYRONE** in the Small Animal section.

DOXAPRAM

INDICATIONS: Doxapram (Dopram-V ♣ ★) is used to stimulate respiration during anesthesia, to reduce anesthetic recovery time in patients with postanesthetic respiratory depression, and to stimulate respiration in neonates. For more information, see **DOXAPRAM** in the Small Animal section.

DOXYCYCLINE

INDICATIONS: Doxycycline (Vibramycin ♣ ★, Vibravet ♣) is a long-acting, lipid-soluble tetracycline antibiotic used in the treatment of bacterial, rickettsial, chlamydial, and mycoplasmal infections. Doxycycline has greater activity against anaerobes and facultative intracellular bacteria than other tetracyclines. It is useful in patients with renal failure because it is excreted by the intestine. For more information, see **TETRACYCLINE ANTIBIOTICS** in the Small Animal section.

DRUG INTERACTIONS: Combined oral therapy with doxycycline (5 mg/kg) and enrofloxacin (10 mg/kg) has been recommended for the treatment of *Mycoplasma pulmonis* pneumonia in mice and rats.

ENILCONAZOLE

INDICATIONS: Enilconazole (Imaverol ♣) is a topical imidazole antifungal agent that has been used in the treatment of dermatophytosis. See **ENILCONAZOLE** in the Small Animal section.

ADVERSE AND COMMON SIDE EFFECTS: See ENILCONAZOLE in the Small Animal section.

ENROFLOXACIN

INDICATIONS: Enrofloxacin (Baytril ♣ ★) is a fluoroquinolone antibiotic with activity against *Escherichia coli*, *Klebsiella pneumoniae*, *Staphylococcus aureus* and *epidermidis*, *Pasteurella multocida*, and *Proteus mirabilis* as well as *Mycoplasma* spp. Pharmacokinetic trials in rabbits suggest that a dose of 5 mg/kg orally or SC every 12 hours should result in effective tissue concentrations against *P. multocida*. A 14-day course of SC injections at this dosage resulted in resolution of clinical signs and elimination of *Pasteurella* organisms from the respiratory tract. *P. multocida* was still isolated from the tympanic bulla of one animal, suggesting a higher dose may be necessary for the treatment of infections in this site. Oral treatment with 200 mg enrofloxacin/L of drinking water for 14 days also resolved clinical signs of respiratory infection, but organisms could still be cultured from the respiratory tract at necropsy. Enrofloxacin at the above dosages did not eliminate *Bordetella bronchiseptica* from the nasal passages. In another study enrofloxacin in the water at 100 mg/L significantly reduced mortality resulting from inoculation with a septicemic form of *P. multocida*, without adversely affecting water consumption. The oral route of administration results in slower absorption and lower peak blood levels than the SC route, but a longer interdosing interval. Long-term treatment (i.e., months) may be necessary to treat chronic severe pasteurellosis. Enrofloxacin has not been associated with disruption of enteric microflora in rabbits.

Enrofloxacin has been recommended for the treatment of hamsters with proliferative enteritis caused by *Lawsonia intracellularis*. For more information, see **ENROFLOXACIN** in the Small Animal section.

ADVERSE AND COMMON SIDE EFFECTS: Parenteral enrofloxacin injection may result in tissue necrosis and sloughing, especially via the SC route. Oral administration is preferred for long-term therapy. Enrofloxacin has been reported to cause cartilage damage and arthropathy in young guinea pigs and rabbits.

DRUG INTERACTIONS: Combined oral therapy with doxycycline (5 mg/kg) and enrofloxacin (10 mg/kg) has been recommended for the treatment of *Mycoplasma pulmonis* pneumonia in mice and rats.

ERYTHROMYCIN

INDICATIONS: Erythromycin (Gallimycin ✤ ★) has been used in drinking water to prevent enteritis in hamster colonies. For information on the injectable use of erythromycin, see **ERYTHROMYCIN** in the Small Animal section.

ADVERSE AND COMMON SIDE EFFECTS: Dosages greater than 500 mg/gallon can cause enteropathy. Erythromycin is not safe for administration to rabbits, guinea pigs, and chinchillas because disruption of enteric microflora may result.

SUPPLIED AS: VETERINARY PRODUCT
Several formulations of water-soluble powder for use in drinking water [Gallimycin ✤ ★]

FENBENDAZOLE

INDICATIONS: Fenbendazole (Panacur ✤ ★) is an anthelmintic recommended for the elimination of nematodes. It is well tolerated in rabbits and rodents. For more information, see **FENBENDAZOLE** in the Small Animal section.

FENTANYL-DROPERIDOL

See **INNOVAR-VET**

FLUNIXIN MEGLUMINE

INDICATIONS: Flunixin meglumine (Banamine ♣ ★) is a potent antiprostaglandin with anti-inflammatory and antipyretic properties that make it useful in the treatment of inflammation and pain associated with musculoskeletal disease. Its analgesic properties are considered superior to those of aspirin, meperidine, pentazocine, codeine phosphate, and phenylbutazone. See **FLUNIXIN** in the Small Animal section.

ADVERSE AND COMMON SIDE EFFECTS: Parenteral injection can be irritating; injections should be made deep into the largest muscle mass available. This can be a significant problem in small rodents with minimal muscle mass. The efficacy of flunixin in rabbits and rodents has been questioned.

DRUG INTERACTIONS: Also see **FLUNIXIN** in the Small Animal section.

FUROSEMIDE

INDICATIONS: Furosemide (Lasix ♣ ★) is a potent loop diuretic that is effective in reducing pulmonary edema of cardiac origin and promoting diuresis. For more information, see **FUROSEMIDE** in the Small Animal section.

GENTAMICIN

INDICATIONS: Gentamicin (Gentocin ♣ ★) is an aminoglycoside antibiotic used in the treatment of bacterial infections, especially with gram-negative organisms. For more information, see **GENTAMICIN** in the Small Animal section. The half-life of gentamicin administered IV to rabbits was found to be approximately 1 hour, suggesting that therapeutic blood levels are not maintained with commonly recommended dosage schedules. Suppression of bacterial growth continues after blood levels drop below the minimum inhibitory concentration, thus extending the effect of the drug.

ADVERSE AND COMMON SIDE EFFECTS: Concurrent administration of fluids is recommended to prevent renal toxicity, especially in gerbils. A dose of 40 mg/kg of gentamicin, administered IM once daily to rabbits for 5 days, resulted in mild to moderate acute renal tubular necrosis. This damage was prevented by concurrent dosage with 10 or 100 mg of vitamin B_6 (pyridoxine HCl), which also reduced gentamicin serum levels although not below therapeutic levels. Gentamicin is also ototoxic, especially in albino guinea pigs.

OTHER USES: Gentamicin has been used to prevent or treat enterotoxemia caused by the administration of inappropriate antibiotics.

GLYCOPYRROLATE

INDICATIONS: Glycopyrrolate (Robinul-V ★, Robinul ✚ ★) is an anticholinergic agent used in preanesthetic regimens to reduce salivary, tracheobronchial, and pharyngeal secretions; to reduce the volume and acidity of gastric secretion; and to inhibit cardiac vagal inhibitory reflexes during anesthetic induction and intubation. Experimental work using a relatively high dose (0.1 mg/kg IM) has shown glycopyrrolate to be an effective anticholinergic agent in rabbits. In rats, glycopyrrolate was also shown to be a more potent vagolytic agent and to have a more prolonged effect than atropine.

ADVERSE AND COMMON SIDE EFFECTS and **DRUG INTERACTIONS:** See **GLYCOPYRROLATE** and **ATROPINE** in the Small Animal section.

GRISEOFULVIN

INDICATIONS: Griseofulvin (Fulvicin U/F ✚ ★) is used for the treatment of dermatophyte infections, including *Trichophyton* and *Microsporum* spp. For more information, see **GRISEOFULVIN** in the Small Animal section.

ADVERSE AND COMMON SIDE EFFECTS: The drug is teratogenic and should not be used in pregnant animals. Diarrhea, leukopenia, and anorexia have also been reported.

HALOTHANE

INDICATIONS: Halothane (Fluothane ✚ ★, Halothane ✚ ★) is an inhalant drug used for the induction of general anesthesia. For more information, see **HALOTHANE** in the Small Animal section.

IBUPROFEN

INDICATIONS: Ibuprofen (Advil ✚ ★, Motrin ✚ ★) is a nonsteroidal anti-inflammatory agent with antipyretic and analgesic properties. Its use has been described in rabbits and, to a limited extent, in small rodents. Use of the drug may prevent adhesion formation after abdominal surgery. See **IBUPROFEN** in the Small Animal section.

ADVERSE AND COMMON SIDE EFFECTS: The drug causes gastric irritation and ulceration, whose severity varies among species. See **IBUPROFEN** in the Small Animal section.

DRUG INTERACTIONS: See **IBUPROFEN** in the Small Animal section.

INNOVAR-VET

INDICATIONS: Innovar-Vet ♣ ★ is a combination of droperidol and fentanyl citrate. The drug has tranquilizing and analgesic properties and is used as a preanesthetic sedative or as an anesthetic induction agent. For more information, see **INNOVAR-VET** in the Small Animal section.

ADVERSE AND COMMON SIDE EFFECTS: The drug is very irritating to tissues and may induce self-mutilation when given IM. Innovar-vet is not recommended for use in hamsters or gerbils. Deaths, lameness, and self-mutilation have been reported in guinea pigs at doses of 0.88 mL/kg.

DRUG INTERACTIONS: Innovar-vet is commonly used in combination with xylazine.

ISOFLURANE

INDICATIONS: Isoflurane (Forane ♣ ★, Isoflo ♣ ★) is the inhalant anesthetic agent of choice for rabbits and rodents because of its rapid induction and recovery times and cardiovascular stability. For more information, see **ISOFLURANE** in the Small Animal section.

IVERMECTIN

INDICATIONS: Ivermectin (Heartgard ♣ ★, Ivomec ♣ ★, Eqvalan ♣ ★) is used for the eradication of endo- and ectoparasites including *Myobia musculi*, *Myocoptes musculinus*, *Radfordia* spp, *Trixacarus caviae*, *Psoroptes cuniculi*, and others. Several research reports have detailed the effectiveness of ivermectin against ear mites (*Psoroptes cuniculi*) in rabbits and *M. musculinus* and *Mycoptes musculi* in mice. Ivermectin has been also been used successfully in rabbits to treat *Cheyletiella parasitovorax* and *Obeliscoides cuniculi*, but was found to be relatively ineffective against pinworms (*Passaluris ambiguus*). A very high dose, 2.0 mg/kg (2,000 µg/kg) orally twice at a 10-day interval, was necessary to eliminate pinworms in mice. For more information, see **IVERMECTIN** in the Small Animal section.

ADVERSE AND COMMON SIDE EFFECTS: Toxicity has not been seen after oral administration of the recommended dose. Parenteral administration may result in discomfort at the site of injection.

KETAMINE

INDICATIONS: Ketamine (Ketaset ✤ ★, Vetalar ✤ ★) is a nonbarbiturate dissociative anesthetic best used in combination with other agents. For more information, see **KETAMINE** in the Small Animal section.

ADVERSE AND COMMON SIDE EFFECTS: Ketamine is a tissue irritant when given IM. Its use has been associated with nerve damage and self-mutilation in guinea pigs. In rabbits, ketamine should be diluted and injected with caution to avoid the sciatic nerve. In small rodents, the drug is best diluted and administered intraperitoneally into the left lower abdominal quadrant. The animal's forequarters should be tilted down during injection to move the abdominal organs forward and avoid injection into a loop of bowel.

DRUG INTERACTIONS: Ketamine is commonly used in combination with xylazine, diazepam, and acepromazine. Bedding animals on softwood shavings may induce hepatic microsomal enzymes that can alter metabolism of the drug and reduce the duration of anesthesia.

LIME SULFUR

INDICATIONS: Lime sulfur, or calcium polysulfide, is a topical insecticide used in the treatment of ectoparasites including *Trixacarus caviae* and sarcoptic and *Notoedres* sp. mites in rabbits.

ADVERSE AND COMMON SIDE EFFECTS: Lime sulfur is a very safe preparation, especially in young or very small animals, but has a strong odor. Posttreatment, transient pruritus may result from a hypersensitivity reaction to the dead mites and their antigens. Short-acting corticosteroids may help relieve pruritus.

DRUG INTERACTIONS: None reported.

SUPPLIED AS: COMMERCIAL PRODUCT
Lime sulfur (calcium polysulfide) liquid or powder

LINDANE

INDICATIONS: Lindane (Kwellada ✤, Lindane ✤, Happy Jack Kennel Dip ★) is a chlorinated hydrocarbon insecticide used topically for the treatment of ectoparasites including *Trixacarus caviae*, *Notoedres* spp, and *Sarcoptes* in rabbits. For more information, see **CHLORINATED HYDROCARBONS** in the Small Animal section.

SUPPLIED AS: VETERINARY PRODUCTS
Topical insecticidal compounds containing 12.89% lindane [Happy Jack Kennel Dip ★]

HUMAN PRODUCTS
Topical lotions and shampoos containing 1% lindane [Kwellada ✤,
PMS Lindane ✤, Lindane ★]

MALATHION

INDICATIONS: Malathion (Adams Flea and Tick Dip ★, Flea and
Tick Dip ★, Malathion 50 ✤) is an organophosphate insecticide used
for the treatment of ectoparasites including *Cheyletiella, Chirodis-
coides, Myobia, Myocoptes, Radfordia, Psorergates,* and *Liponyssus* spp.
For more information, see **ORGANOPHOSPHATE INSECTI-
CIDES** in the Small Animal section.

ADVERSE AND COMMON SIDE EFFECTS: Caution must be
taken against overdose in young rodents. Toxicity has been reported
in rabbits after treatment with a 2% dip. Breeding may be inhibited
after treatment with this chemical.

SUPPLIED AS: VETERINARY PRODUCTS
Topical insecticidal compounds containing 53% malathion [Adams
Flea and Tick Dip ★, Flea and Tick Dip ★]; 53.4% malathion
[Malathion 50 ✤]

MECA (METASTABILIZED CHLOROUS
ACID/CHLORIDE DIOXIDE)

INDICATIONS: MECA is a commercial disinfectant that has been
used topically to control dermatophytosis caused by *Trichophyton
mentagrophytes* in a commercial rabbitry where treatment of individual animals with griseofulvin was not feasible. Animals were dipped
in or sprayed with a solution of 1 part base compound, 1 part activator, and 10 parts water six times over a 26-day period. The number of
carriers and extent of clinical signs were greatly reduced, but the infection was not completely eliminated. Spraying was more effective
than dipping, perhaps because the compound was massaged into
the fur after the spray was applied.

ADVERSE AND COMMON SIDE EFFECTS: The animal's eyes
should be protected by a compound such as petroleum jelly during
the dipping procedure.

SUPPLIED AS: COMMERCIAL PRODUCT
MECA ★

MEPERIDINE

INDICATIONS: Meperidine (Demerol ✤ ★) is a short-acting narcotic
analgesic used for the relief of moderate to severe pain and as a pre-

anesthetic. For more information, see **MEPERIDINE** in the Small Animal section.

METHOXYFLURANE

INDICATIONS: Methoxyflurane (Metafane ✦ ★) is used for induction and maintenance of general anesthesia. For more information, see **METHOXYFLURANE** in the Small Animal section.

ADVERSE AND COMMON SIDE EFFECTS: "Squirming" is seen in guinea pigs in stage 3, or deep anesthesia, giving a false impression of insufficient anesthetic depth. Other clinical indicators of anesthetic level, such as jaw tone and toe pinch reflex, should also be monitored in this species. Isoflurane is now considered the anesthetic of choice for rabbits and small rodents.

METOCLOPRAMIDE

INDICATIONS: Metoclopramide (Maxeran ✦, Reglan ✦ ★) is an antiemetic agent that contributes to lower esophageal sphincter competence and promotes gastric emptying. It is useful in the management of gastric impaction, gastric stasis, and gastric trichobezoars in rabbits. For more information, see **METOCLOPRAMIDE** in the Small Animal section.

ADVERSE AND COMMON SIDE EFFECTS: Metoclopramide should not be used in animals with gastrointestinal hemorrhage, obstruction, or perforation.

DRUG INTERACTIONS: Metoclopramide may decrease gastric and increase small intestinal absorption of drugs.

METRONIDAZOLE

INDICATIONS: Metronidazole (Flagyl ✦ ★) is a synthetic antibacterial, antiprotozoal agent with activity against anaerobic bacteria. It has been used to treat giardiasis and enteric infections in rabbits and rodents. For more information, see **METRONIDAZOLE** in the Small Animal section.

ADVERSE AND COMMON SIDE EFFECTS: An anecdotal report links the use of metronidazole in chinchillas to subsequent liver failure.

MICONAZOLE

INDICATIONS: Miconazole (Micatin ✦, Monistat ✦, numerous others ★) is a topical imidazole antifungal agent useful in the treatment of localized dermatophytosis. Its use in rabbits has been described.

ADVERSE AND COMMON SIDE EFFECTS and **DRUG INTER-ACTIONS:** None reported in rabbits.

SUPPLIED AS: HUMAN PRODUCTS
Cream, powder, and aerosol formulations for topical use [Micatin ✤, Monistat ✤, numerous others ★]

MIDAZOLAM

INDICATIONS: Midazolam (Versed ✤ ★) is a short-acting parenteral benzodiazepine, central nervous system depressant with sedative-hypnotic, anxiolytic, muscle-relaxing, and anticonvulsant properties. It is used as a preanesthetic, in combination with ketamine for anesthesia, and alone as an anticonvulsant agent. The drug is two to three times more potent than diazepam and has a shorter half-life. Midazolam is administered intramuscularly, in contrast to diazepam, and is preferred in rodents and rabbits for this reason.

ADVERSE AND COMMON SIDE EFFECTS: No significant cardiovascular effects are noted. Respiratory depression and dose-dependent sedation occur.

DRUG INTERACTIONS: See **MIDAZOLAM** in the Small Animal section.

NALBUPHINE

INDICATIONS: Nalbuphine (Nubain ✤ ★, Nalbuphine HCl ★) is a mixed opioid agonist/antagonist used as an analgesic agent. Nalbuphine can also be used to reverse the effects of μ-opioids such as fentanyl, yet still provide postprocedural analgesia.

SUPPLIED AS: HUMAN PRODUCTS
For injection containing 10 and 20 mg/mL [Nubain ✤ ★, Nalbuphine HCl ★]

NALOXONE

INDICATIONS: Naloxone (P/M Naloxone ✤ ★) is a narcotic antagonist used for reversal of narcotic-induced depression, including respiratory depression induced by morphine, oxymorphone, meperidine, or fentanyl (Innovar-Vet). Any analgesic effect of the narcotic agent is also reversed. For more information, see **NALOXONE** in the Small Animal section.

NEOMYCIN

INDICATIONS: Neomycin (Biosol-M ✤, Mycifradin ✤ ★) is an aminoglycoside antibiotic generally used as a topical antibiotic and orally for its local antibiotic effects. Systemic use of the drug is toxic. For more information, see **NEOMYCIN** in the Small Animal section.

DRUG INTERACTIONS: Neomycin has a neuromuscular blocking action that enhances the activity of skeletal muscle relaxants and general anesthetics.

OXYMORPHONE

INDICATIONS: Oxymorphone (Numorphan ♣ ★, P/M Oxymorphone ★) is a narcotic agent used for sedation, preanesthesia, and the management of pain. Pain relief lasts 2 to 4 hours following IM or IV injection. It is about 10 times more potent an analgesic than morphine, causes less sedation, and does not suppress the cough reflex.

ADVERSE AND COMMON SIDE EFFECTS: Respiratory depression and bradycardia are reported. See **OXYMORPHONE** in the Small Animal section. Overdosage and adverse effects of the drug can be reversed with naloxone.

DRUG INTERACTIONS: See **OXYMORPHONE** in the Small Animal section.

OXYTETRACYCLINE

INDICATIONS: Oxytetracycline (Liquamycin ♣ ★, Terramycin ♣ ★) is a short-acting, water-soluble tetracycline with activity against a broad range of gram-positive and gram-negative organisms as well as chlamydia, rickettsia, and mycoplasma. For more information, see **OXYTETRACYCLINE** and **TETRACYCLINE ANTIBIOTICS** in the Small Animal section.

ADVERSE AND COMMON SIDE EFFECTS: In a pharmacokinetic study of oxytetracycline in healthy rabbits, depression, diarrhea, and anorexia resulted within 1 day of the administration of 30 mg/kg, IM, given every 8 hours. No toxic effects were seen in animals given 15 mg/kg in the same manner. This suggests a very narrow safety margin in this species.

OXYTOCIN

INDICATIONS: Oxytocin (Pitocin ★, Syntocinon ♣ ★) is used for the induction of parturition and to stimulate milk letdown. For more information, see **OXYTOCIN** in the Small Animal section.

DRUG INTERACTIONS: The activity of oxytocin on the uterus is strongly influenced by circulating levels of estrogen and progesterone. The response of the uterus to oxytocin is greatest when estrogen levels are high. Epinephrine reduces the effect of oxytocin. If uterine inertia is suspected, the animal should be pretreated with calcium gluconate 30 minutes before administration of oxytocin. See also **OXYTOCIN** in the Small Animal section.

PENICILLIN G; PROCAINE, BENZATHINE

INDICATIONS: Procaine penicillin G and the combination of benzathine and procaine penicillin G are the repository forms of penicillin G. For more information, see **PENICILLIN ANTIBIOTICS** in the Small Animal section. The drugs are used to treat treponematosis in rabbits.

ADVERSE AND COMMON SIDE EFFECTS: The use of penicillin antibiotics can result in a reduction in intestinal anaerobes, lactobacilli, and streptococci allowing overgrowth of clostridial or coliform agents and the development of enteritis and enterotoxemia. Hamsters and guinea pigs are the most susceptible to this condition; mice, rats, gerbils, and rabbits are somewhat more resistant.

PENTAZOCINE

INDICATIONS: Pentazocine (Talwin-V ★, Talwin ✦ ★) is a narcotic agonist used in the management of moderate to severe pain. Pentazocine can also be used to reverse the effects of μ-opioids such as fentanyl, yet still provide postprocedural analgesia. For more information, see **PENTAZOCINE** in the Small Animal section.

PIPERAZINE

INDICATIONS: Piperazine (Hartz Once a Month ★, Once a Month Roundworm Treatment ✦, Pipa-Tabs , Purina Liquid Wormer ★) is an anthelmintic used for the eradication of ascarids and some nodular worms. It is moderately effective against pinworms. It can be used in the drinking water to treat large groups of animals. For more information, see **PIPERAZINE** in the Small Animal section.

SUPPLIED AS: VETERINARY PRODUCTS
See Small Animal section
Numerous powder and liquid formulations for use in drinking water

PRAZIQUANTEL

INDICATIONS: Praziquantel (Droncit ✦ ★) is an anthelmintic used for the elimination of cestodes and trematodes. For more information, see **PRAZIQUANTEL** in the Small Animal section.

PREDNISONE

INDICATIONS: Prednisone (Deltasone ✚ ★) is an intermediate-acting glucocorticoid used as an anti-inflammatory agent. For more information, see **PREDNISONE** and **GLUCOCORTICOID AGENTS** in the Small Animal section.

ADVERSE AND COMMON SIDE EFFECTS: Prednisone must be used with extreme caution in small rodents to prevent overdosage. Overdosage may result in gastrointestinal irritation and ulceration, depression of the immune system, polyuria, polydipsia, polyphagia, and hepatic lipidosis.

PYRETHRIN-CONTAINING PRODUCTS

INDICATIONS: Pyrethrin-containing products (Sectrol ✚ ★, Ovitrol ✚ ★, Vetatix ✚, and many others) are naturally occurring insecticides derived from the plant *Chrysanthemum cinerariae-folium*, and are commonly used for control of ectoparasites including fleas and, in rabbits, *Cheyletiella parasitovorax*. These drugs are γ-aminobutyric acid agonists that stimulate the insect's central nervous system causing muscular excitation, convulsions, and paralysis. Insect mortality is enhanced when these products are combined with piperonyl butoxide (e.g., Sectrol and Ovitrol). Piperonyl butoxide inhibits pyrethrin metabolism. Shampoo and flea powder containing 0.05 to 0.15% pyrethrin are the products most frequently used to treat rabbits and rodents.

Insecticidal shampoos such as Vetatix are effective against various ectoparasites in rabbits and rodents including fur mice and lice. For more information, see **PYRETHRIN-CONTAINING PRODUCTS** in the Small Animal section.

ADVERSE AND COMMON SIDE EFFECTS: These products are relatively nontoxic to mammals. Vetatix may be irritating to eyes; instill ointment in eyes before bathing.

SUPPLIED AS: VETERINARY PRODUCTS
Shampoo containing 0.05% pyrethrins, 0.12% piperonyl butoxide, and 0.20% N-octyl bicycloheptene dicarboximide [Vetatix shampoo ✚]
Numerous veterinary products in powder, spray, and shampoo formulations containing varying percentages of pyrethrin and piperonyl butoxide. Some products also contain carbaryl and other insecticidal compounds.

STANOZOLOL

INDICATIONS: Stanozolol (Winstrol-V ✤ ★) is an anabolic steroid with strong anabolic and weak androgenic activity. It is potentially useful as an adjunct to the management of catabolic disease states. See **STANOZOLOL** and **ANABOLIC STEROIDS** in the Small Animal section.

ADVERSE AND COMMON SIDE EFFECTS and **DRUG INTERACTIONS:** See **STANOZOLOL** and **ANABOLIC STEROIDS** in the Small Animal section.

SULFADIMETHOXINE
SULFAMETHAZINE
SULFAQUINOXALINE

INDICATIONS: The sulfonamides are oral bacteriostatic antibiotics and coccidiostats. They are used for the prevention and treatment of intestinal coccidiosis and, in rabbits, hepatic coccidiosis due to *Eimeria stiedae*. For more information, see **SULFADIMETHOXINE** and **SULFONAMIDE ANTIBIOTICS** in the Small Animal section.

ADVERSE AND COMMON SIDE EFFECTS: Sulfamerazine depresses thyroid activity in rats. Crystalluria may occur in acid urine. Chronic treatment with sulfamerazine may result in alterations in intestinal flora leading to malnutrition and vitamin deficiency, especially vitamin K.

SUPPLIED AS: VETERINARY PRODUCTS
Sulfamethazine: Various formulations for oral use in drinking water [Sulmet ✤ ★, Sulfamethazine ★, and others]
Sulfaquinoxaline: Various liquid and powder formulations for oral use in drinking water [Sulfaquinoxaline 19.2% concentrate ✤, Purina Sulfa-Nox Liquid ★, and others]

T-61

INDICATIONS: T-61 Euthanasia Solution ✤ is a nonnarcotic euthanasia agent that has a narcotic-like action while paralyzing the respiratory center and striated skeletal and respiratory muscles.

ADVERSE AND COMMON SIDE EFFECTS: Vocalization and muscular activity are seen in some species.

SUPPLIED AS: VETERINARY PRODUCT
Solution for IV and intrapulmonary injection containing 200 mg/L
[T-61 Euthanasia Solution ✦]

TETRACYCLINE

INDICATIONS: Tetracycline (Panmycin Aquadrops Liquid ✦ ★) is a
bacteriostatic antibiotic effective against many aerobic and anaerobic
gram-positive and gram-negative bacteria, spirochetes, mycoplasmas, and rickettsial organisms. Tetracycline has been recommended
for the treatment of treponemiasis and listeriosis in rabbits. For more
information, see **TETRACYCLINE ANTIBIOTICS** in the Small Animal section.

ADVERSE AND COMMON SIDE EFFECTS: Tetracycline should
be used with caution in hamsters, although it has been recommended for the treatment of young hamsters with proliferative
ileitis caused by *Lawsonia intracellularis*. Tetracycline has been added
to the drinking water for many purposes; however, antibiotic blood
levels are often below minimum inhibitory concentration levels for
relevant bacteria. Even a dose of 1,600 mg/L did not result in significant blood levels in rabbits.

SUPPLIED AS: VETERINARY PRODUCTS
For oral administration containing 100 mg/mL [Panmycin Aquadrops
Liquid ✦ ★]
For injection containing 100 [Tetroxy ✦] and 200 mg/mL [Tetraject ✦]
Numerous liquid and powder formulations for use in drinking
water

THIABENDAZOLE

INDICATIONS: Thiabendazole (Equizole ★, Mintezol ★, Thibenzole ★)
is a broad-spectrum anthelmintic drug with antipyretic and anti-inflammatory effects and fungicidal activity. It is well tolerated by rabbits and rodents and has been highly effective for the treatment
of *Obeliscoides cuniculi* in rabbits. For more information, see **THI-
ABENDAZOLE** in the Small Animal section and **TRESADERM** in
this section.

THIAMYLAL SODIUM

INDICATIONS: Thiamylal sodium (Anestatal ★) is an ultrashort-
acting thiobarbiturate general anesthetic agent, which has been used
intraperitoneally in rodents. For more information, see **THIAMY-
LAL SODIUM** and **BARBITURATES** in the Small Animal section.

THIOPENTAL SODIUM

INDICATIONS: Thiopental sodium (Veterinary Pentothal kit ★, Pentothal ✦ ★) is an ultrashort-acting thiobarbiturate used for procedures requiring general anesthesia of short duration. For more information, see **THIOPENTAL SODIUM** and **BARBITURATES** in the Small Animal section.

TILETAMINE + ZOLAZEPAM

INDICATIONS: Tiletamine zolazepam (Telazol ★) is an injectable dissociative anesthetic/tranquilizer combination useful for sedation and restraint, and anesthetic induction or anesthesia of short duration (30 minutes) requiring mild to moderate analgesia. It has been used primarily in rats and mice, although central nervous system (CNS) excitation may occur.

ADVERSE AND COMMON SIDE EFFECTS: This combination is contraindicated in rabbits because the tiletamine fraction is nephrotoxic. CNS depression and poor anesthesia occur in guinea pigs.

TRESADERM

INDICATIONS: Tresaderm ✦ ★ is a dermatologic solution containing thiabendazole, dexamethasone, and neomycin sulfate that is indicated for the treatment of chronic dermatoses and otitis externa of bacterial, mycotic, and parasitic origin. In rabbits the drug is used to treat otitis externa caused by *Psoroptes cuniculi* infestation, often in combination with topical or systemic ivermectin.

ADVERSE AND COMMON SIDE EFFECTS: In dogs, transient discomfort has been reported when the drug is applied to denuded areas. Hypersensitivity to neomycin has also been described. Tresaderm should be used with caution in small rodents to avoid overdosage with dexamethasone.

SUPPLIED AS: VETERINARY PRODUCT
Topical solution [Tresaderm ✦ ★]

TRIMETHOPRIM SULFADIAZINE
TRIMETHOPRIM SULFADOXINE
TRIMETHOPRIM SULFAMETHOXAZOLE

INDICATIONS: Trimethoprim plus sulfadiazine (or sulfadiazine), sulfadoxine, and sulfamethoxazole (Tribrissen ✦ ★, Trivetrin ✦,

Septra ✦ ★, Bactrim ✦ ★, and others) are bactericidal antibiotic combinations used commonly as first-line drugs for the treatment of rabbits and small rodents. They are also effective in the treatment of hepatic coccidiosis in rabbits. For more information, see **TRIMETHOPRIM SULFADIAZINE** in the Small Animal section.

ADVERSE AND COMMON SIDE EFFECTS: The use of trimethoprim-sulfonamide combinations may depress thyroid activity in rats.

SUPPLIED AS: VETERINARY PRODUCTS
For injection containing 40 mg/mL trimethoprim and 200 mg/mL sulfadiazine [Tribrissen 24% ✦]
For injection containing 40 mg/mL trimethoprim and 200 mg/mL sulfadoxine [Bimotrin ✦, Borgal ✦, Trimidox ✦, Trivetrin ✦]
For injection containing 80 mg/mL trimethoprim and 400 mg/mL sulfadiazine [Tribrissen 48% ✦]
Tablets containing trimethoprim plus sulfadiazine in the following combinations: 5 + 25, 20 + 100, 80 + 400 [DiTrim ★, Tribrissen ✦ ★]
Oral suspension containing 9.1 mg trimethoprim and 45.5 mg sulfadiazine/ml [Tribrissen ✦]

HUMAN PRODUCTS
Oral suspensions containing 40 mg trimethoprim and 200 mg sulfamethoxazole/5 mL [Bactrim ✦ ★, Septra ✦ ★, and many others]
Oral suspensions containing 45 mg trimethoprim and 205 mg sulfadiazine/5 mL [Coptin ✦]

TROPICAMIDE

INDICATIONS: Tropicamide is used to induce mydriasis in animals that lack ocular pigmentation.

SUPPLIED AS: HUMAN PRODUCTS
For topical ophthalmic use containing 0.5% [Diotrope ✦, Tropicamide ✦, Mydriacyl ✦ ★, OcuTropic ★, and others] and 1.0% [Diotrope ✦, Tropicamide ✦, Mydriacyl ✦]

TYLOSIN

INDICATIONS: Tylosin (Tylan ✦ ★, Tylocine ✦, Tylosin ★) is a macrolide antibiotic. It has activity against some gram-negative and gram-positive bacteria, spirochetes, chlamydiae, and mycoplasma organisms. The drug has been used in drinking water to treat *Mycoplasma pulmonis* pneumonia in rats. For more information, see **TYLOSIN** in the Small Animal section.

ADVERSE AND COMMON SIDE EFFECTS: The use of tylosin may result in colonic overgrowth of nonsusceptible bacteria causing diarrhea.

VERAPAMIL

Verapamil (Isoptin ♣ ★) is a calcium channel-blocking agent used in the management of atrial flutter, atrial fibrillation, and atrial tachycardia. The drug has been used experimentally and, to a limited extent, clinically to decrease adhesion formation after abdominal surgery in rabbits. No adverse effects on cardiopulmonary function or wound healing were noted.

SUPPLIED AS: HUMAN PRODUCT
For injection containing 2.5 mg/mL [Isoptin ♣ ★]

VIOKASE-V

INDICATIONS: Viokase ♣ ★ is a mixture containing standardized activities of the pancreatic enzymes lipase, amylase, and protease that is used for the management of pancreatic exocrine insufficiency. Viokase is used in rabbits to help dissolve gastric trichobezoars. It appears most effective early in the clinical course.

ADVERSE AND COMMON SIDE EFFECTS: Viokase may cause mucosal irritation or dermatitis if allowed to remain on the skin around the mouth after oral administration.

SUPPLIED AS: VETERINARY PRODUCT
Powder or tablets containing lipase, protease, and amylase [Viokase-V ★]

HUMAN PRODUCT
Powder or tablets containing lipase, protease, and amylase [Viokase ♣ ★]

VITAMIN C

See **ASCORBIC ACID**

VITAMIN K

INDICATIONS: Vitamin K_1 or phytonadione (Aqua-Mephyton ★, Mephyton ★, Konakion ★, Veta-K1 ♣ ★) is used to treat coagulopathies due to fat-soluble vitamin malabsorption such as occurs with long-term use of antibacterial agents, and vitamin K antagonism caused by salicylates, coumarins, and indanediones, including warfarin and brodifacoum poisoning. For more information, see **VITAMIN K** in the Small Animal section.

XENODYNE

INDICATIONS: Xenodyne ♣ is a topical antibacterial solution containing iodine. It is used in the management of cutaneous wounds and infections. Xenodyne has greater epidermal penetration than other iodine-containing preparations.

ADVERSE AND COMMON SIDE EFFECTS: Because of the degree of epidermal penetration, hyperiodinism is possible.

SUPPLIED AS: VETERINARY PRODUCT
Xenodyne 1% (0.5% titratable) iodine ♣ solution and spray

XYLAZINE

INDICATIONS: Xylazine (Anased ♣ ★, Rompun ♣ ★) is an injectable anesthetic agent commonly used in conjunction with ketamine for anesthesia of rodents and rabbits. For more information, see **XYLAZINE** in the Small Animal section.

YOHIMBINE

INDICATIONS: Yohimbine (Yobine ♣ ★, Antagonil ♣ ★) can be used to antagonize the effects of xylazine to shorten anesthetic recovery times and reduce anesthetic-related complications. For more information, see **XYLAZINE** in the Small Animal section.

SUPPLIED AS: VETERINARY PRODUCTS
For injection containing 2 [Yobine ♣ ★] and 5 [Antagonil ♣ ★] mg/mL

Handbook of Veterinary Drugs, Second Edition, edited by Dana Allen,
Lippincott–Raven Publishers, Philadelphia. © 1998

Section 11

The Use of Chemotherapeutic Agents in Ferrets

Medical therapy for ferrets has generally been derived from recommendations for domestic cats. Similarities in body size and gastrointestinal form and function make feline dosages reasonable starting points for extrapolation. Administration of oral liquids is generally simpler than pilling. The ferret should be firmly scruffed to ensure that the owner is not bitten and that the full dose of medication is administered. Small volumes of liquid preparations and some ground tablets or capsule contents can be mixed with food; however, palatability and taste preferences vary significantly among products and individuals, respectively. Strong-tasting malt products, such as feline nutritional supplement pastes, can be good vehicles for disguising medications.

Ferrets have relatively little muscle mass for their size; subcutaneous injections are preferred over the intramuscular route. This is especially the case when large volumes or repeated injections are required. Intravenous injections can be made into the cephalic, lateral saphenous, and sometimes jugular veins; however, excellent restraint or even general anesthesia will be required.

Although all the drugs and dosages listed in this section have been used in ferrets, the majority of the general indications and adverse and common side effects listed are based on what is known in dogs and cats. Information pertaining specifically to use in ferrets is described in the appropriate section, as available.

Handbook of Veterinary Drugs, Second Edition, edited by Dana Allen,
Lippincott–Raven Publishers, Philadelphia. © 1998

Section 12

Common Dosages for Ferrets

Drug	Dosage	Indications
Amikacin	8 to 16 mg/kg total per day, once daily or divided bid–tid; SC, IM, IV	General antibiotic therapy. See precautions for aminoglycosides.
Aminophylline	4 mg/kg bid; PO, IM	Bronchodilation
Amitraz	Apply to affected skin 3 to 6 times, at 14-day intervals	Ectoparasite control, especially mites
Amoxicillin	10 to 20 mg/kg once daily or bid; PO, SC	General antibiotic therapy; also used in combination with metronidazole and gastric protectants and/or H_2 blockers for *Helicobacter pylori* gastritis
Amphotericin B	0.4 to 0.8 mg/kg once weekly; IV; to a total dose of 7 to 25 mg **OR** Follow published canine protocols	Systemic antifungal therapy

Drug	Dosage	Indications
Ampicillin	5 to 10 mg/kg bid; SC, IM, IV	General antibiotic therapy
Ascorbic acid	50 to 100 mg/kg bid; PO	Supportive therapy, antioxidant
Aspirin	10 to 20 mg/kg bid; PO	Analgesia, anti-inflammatory, anticoagulant
Atropine	0.05 mg/kg; IM	Preanesthetic, parasympatholytic
	2 to 10 mg/kg as needed; SC	Organophosphate toxicity
Bismuth subsalicylate	0.25 to 1 mL/kg tid–qid; PO	Gastric protectant
Buprenorphine	0.01 to 0.05 mg/kg bid–tid as needed; SC, IM, IV	Analgesic
Butorphanol tartrate	0.05 to 0.5 mg/kg bid–tid as needed; SC, IM	Analgesic
Carbaryl (0.5% shampoo, 5.0% powder)	Treat once weekly for 3 to 6 wk	Ectoparasite control
Cefadroxil	10 to 20 mg/kg bid; PO	General antibiotic therapy
Cephalexin	15 to 25 mg/kg bid–tid; PO	General antibiotic therapy
Chloramphenicol	50 mg/kg bid; PO (palmitate), SC, IM (succinate)	General antibiotic therapy; treatment of choice for proliferative bowel disease with minimum 14-day course
Chlorpheniramine	1 to 2 mg/kg bid–tid; PO	Antihistamine
Chorionic gonadatrophin	100 IU once after 2nd wk of estrus, repeat in 2 wk if needed; IM	To terminate estrus
Cimetidine	10 mg/kg tid; PO, SC, IM, slow IV	Histamine (H_2)-blocking agent for gastric ulcer therapy

Drug	Dosage	Indications
Ciprofloxacin	5 to 15 mg/kg bid; PO	General antibiotic therapy
Cisapride	0.5 mg/kg tid; PO	Gastrointestinal motility stimulant
Clavulanic acid and amoxicillin	10 to 20 mg/kg bid–tid; PO	General antibiotic therapy
Clindamycin	5.5 to 10 mg/kg bid; PO	General antibiotic therapy
Cloxacillin	10 mg/kg qid; PO, IM, IV	General antibiotic therapy
Dexamethasone sodium phosphate	4 to 8 mg/kg once; IM, IV	Shock therapy
Dextrose	0.5 to 2 mL of 50% in slow IV bolus to effect. Continuous IV infusion of 5% dextrose in crystalloid fluids.	Hypoglycemia caused by insulinoma
Diazepam	1 to 2 mg/kg as needed; IM, IV	For seizure control and sedation
Diazoxide	5 mg per ferret bid initially, up to 30 mg/kg bid as necessary; PO	For treatment of insulinoma, in combination with prednisone
Diethylcarbamazine	5 to 11 mg/kg once daily; PO	Daily heartworm preventive
Digoxin elixir	0.005 to 0.01 mg/kg once daily to bid; PO. Adjust dose as necessary.	Management of congestive heart failure and cardiomyopathy
Diltiazem	1.5 to 7.5 mg/kg once daily to qod; PO. Adjust dose as necessary.	Management of congestive heart failure due to cardiomyopathy
Diphenhydramine	0.5 to 2 mg/kg bid–tid; PO; bid; IM	Antihistamine
Doxapram	5 to 11 mg/kg; IV	Respiratory stimulant
Enalapril	0.25 to 0.5 mg/kg once daily to qod; PO	Management of congestive heart failure and cardiomyopathy

Drug	Dosage	Indications
Enrofloxacin	5 to 15 mg/kg bid; PO, SC, IM	General antibiotic therapy
Erythromycin	10 mg/kg qid; PO	General antibiotic therapy
Flunixin meglumine	0.5 to 2 mg/kg once daily; PO, deep IM, IV; maximum 3 days	Nonsteroidal anti-inflammatory
Furosemide	1 to 4 mg/kg bid–tid; PO, SC, IM, IV	Diuretic, management of congestive heart failure
Gentamicin	4 to 8 mg/kg total per day, once daily or divided bid–tid; SC, IM, IV	General antibiotic therapy. See precautions for aminoglycosides.
GnRH	20 µg once after 2nd wk of estrus, repeat in 2 wk if needed; IM	To terminate estrus
Griseofulvin	25 mg/kg once daily for 3 to 6 wk; PO	Systemic antifungal therapy
Hydroxyzine hydrochloride	2 mg/kg tid; PO	Antihistamine
Insulin, NPH	0.1 to 0.5 U/kg bid initially, increase dose as necessary; SC, IM	For treatment of diabetes mellitus. Monitor blood/urine glucose.
Iron dextran	10 mg/kg once weekly as needed; IM	For iron deficiency anemia
Ivermectin	200 to 400 µg/kg twice at 14-day intervals; PO, SC	General parasite control
	500 to 1,000 µg/kg divided into 2 doses; massage into each ear	Control of ear mites
	6 µg/kg once monthly; PO	Heartworm prevention
Kaolin-pectin	1 to 2 mL/kg q 2 to 6 hr as needed; PO	Gastrointestinal protectant

Drug	Dosage	Indications
Ketoconazole	10 to 30 mg/kg once daily to bid; PO	Systemic antifungal therapy; management of adrenal neoplasia when surgical removal not possible
Lactulose (syrup)	1.5 to 3 mL/kg bid; PO	In hepatic disease to decrease blood ammonia levels; laxative
Lime sulfur	Dilute 1:40 in water, wash once weekly for 6 wk	Ectoparasite control, especially mites
Lincomycin	10 to 15 mg/kg tid; PO 10 mg/kg bid; IM	General antibiotic therapy
Meperidine	5 to 10 mg/kg as needed q 2 to 4 hr; SC, IM, IV	Analgesic
Metoclopramide	0.2 to 1 mg/kg tid–qid; PO, SC	Gastric motility disorders
Metronidazole	10 to 20 mg/kg bid; PO	Antibacterial agent with good anaerobic spectrum
	20 mg/kg bid; PO for 10 days	Giardiasis
Milbemycin oxime	1.15 to 2.33 mg/kg once monthly; PO	Heartworm prevention
Mitotane	50 mg once daily; PO, for 7 days, then q 72 hr as needed	Management of adrenal neoplasia when surgical removal not possible
Neomycin	10 to 20 mg/kg bid–qid; PO	Local antibiotic therapy in the gastrointestinal tract
Nitroglycerine	1/8-in. length of 2% ointment applied topically; once daily–bid	Management of congestive heart failure
Oxymorphone	0.05 to 0.2 mg/kg bid–tid; SC, IM, IV	Analgesia

Drug	Dosage	Indications
Oxytetracycline	20 mg/kg tid; PO	General antibiotic therapy
Oxytocin	0.2 to 3 U/kg once; SC, IM	Stimulate uterine motility or milk letdown
Penicillin G, Procaine	40,000 U/kg once daily or divided bid; IM	General antibiotic therapy
Penicillin G, Na or K	20,000 U/kg q 4 hr; SC, IM, IV 40,000 U/kg tid; PO	General antibiotic therapy
Pentazocine	5 to 10 mg/kg q 4 hr; IM	Analgesia
Phenobarbital elixir	1 to 2 mg/kg bid–tid for seizure control, titrate dose for maintenance; PO	Control and prevention of seizures
Piperazine	50 to 100 mg/kg once, repeat in 2 wk; PO	Gastrointestinal parasitism, especially nematodes
Praziquantel	12.5 mg (½ of 23-mg tablet) once, repeat in 2 wk; PO 5 to 10 mg/kg once, repeat in 2 wk; SC	Gastrointestinal cestodes
Prednisone, prednisolone	0.5 to 1.0 mg/kg once daily–bid, reduce dosage and frequency for long-term therapy; PO, IM	Anti-inflammatory
	0.5 to 2.5 mg/kg bid; PO, IM. Start at low dose, increase as necessary.	Treatment of hypoglycemia due to insulinoma. Reduce dosage if combined with diazoxide therapy.
Propranolol	0.5 to 2 mg/kg once daily to bid; PO, SC	Medical management of cardiomyopathy
Prostaglandin $F_{2\alpha}$	0.5 mg as needed; IM	Treatment of metritis
Pyrantel pamoate	4.4 mg/kg once, repeat in 2 wk; PO	Treatment of gastrointestinal nematodes

Drug	Dosage	Indications
Pyrethrin products	Use topically as directed once weekly as needed	Treatment of ecto-parasites, especially fleas
Stanozolol	10 mg/kg once weekly as required; IM	Anabolic steroid
Sucralfate	25 mg/kg to 125 mg/ferret tid–qid; PO	Treatment of gastric ulceration
Sulfadimethoxine	25 mg/kg once daily; PO, SC, IM 50 mg/kg once, then 25 mg/kg daily for 9 days; PO	General antibiotic therapy Treatment of gastro-intestinal coccidiosis
Sulfasalazine	10 to 20 mg/kg bid; PO	Inflammatory bowel disease
Tetracycline	25 mg/kg bid–tid; PO	General antibiotic therapy
Theophylline (elixir)	4.25 mg/kg bid–tid; PO	Bronchodilation
Thiacetarsamide	2.2 mg/kg bid for 2 days; IV	Adulticide for heart-worm treatment (see precautions)
Trimethoprim-sulfonamide combinations	15 to 30 mg/kg bid; PO, SC 30 mg/kg once daily for 2 wk; PO	General antibiotic therapy Treatment of gastro-intestinal coccidiosis
Tylosin	10 mg/kg once daily–bid; PO	General antibiotic therapy
Vitamin B complex	Dose to thiamine content at 1 to 2 mg/kg as needed; IM	Vitamin B supplementation
Vitamin C		See Ascorbic Acid

Handbook of Veterinary Drugs, Second Edition, edited by Dana Allen,
Lippincott–Raven Publishers, Philadelphia. © 1998

Section 13

Description of Drugs for Ferrets

AMIKACIN

INDICATIONS: Amikacin (Amiglyde-V ♣ ★, Amikin ♣ ★) is an
amino-glycoside antibiotic indicated for the treatment of various soft
tissue infections. Measurement of serum amikacin levels is helpful in
dogs and cats to ensure appropriate dosage; recommended peak and
trough levels for these species are likely adequate approximations of
those for ferrets. See also **AMIKACIN** and **AMINOGLYCOSIDE
ANTIBIOTICS** in the Small Animal section.

ADVERSE AND COMMON SIDE EFFECTS: Like other aminoglycosides, amikacin has nephrotoxic, neurotoxic, and ototoxic potential. An increase in the efficacy and a decrease in toxicity may occur
when the total dose is given once daily. Neuromuscular blockade
and acute renal failure can occur after IV injection. Aminoglycosides
administered IV should be diluted with saline or sterile water and
administered over 20 minutes.

AMINOPHYLLINE

INDICATIONS: Aminophylline (Phylloconton ♣ ★ and generics) is
a bronchodilator principally used for the management of cough
caused by bronchospasm. It has mild inotropic properties and mild,
transient diuretic activity.

ADVERSE AND COMMON SIDE EFFECTS: See **AMINO-PHYLLINE** and **THEOPHYLLINE** in the Small Animal section for information on effects and usage in dogs and cats. The drug should be used with caution in ferrets with cardiac disease, systemic hypertension, cardiac arrhythmias, gastrointestinal tract ulcers, impaired renal or hepatic function, diabetes mellitus, hyperthyroid disease, and glaucoma.

DRUG INTERACTIONS: See **AMINOPHYLLINE** and **THEOPHYLLINE** in the Small Animal section. Aminophylline should not be mixed in a syringe with other drugs.

AMITRAZ

INDICATIONS: Amitraz (Mitaban ♣ ★) is indicated for the eradication of demodicosis and sarcoptic mange. The drug is classified as a monoamine oxidase (MAO) inhibitor (causes a buildup of norepinephrine in the central nervous system) although the exact mechanism of its action is unknown. It also inhibits prostaglandin synthesis and is an α-adrenergic agonist.

ADVERSE AND COMMON SIDE EFFECTS: The most common side effects of mild toxicosis are ataxia and depression. Other side effects may include transient sedation, mydriasis, hypersalivation, transient pruritus (due to effect of dead mites), hypothermia or hyperthermia, vomiting, diarrhea, and occasionally bradycardia. Clinical signs of severe toxicosis may include hypotension, hyperglycemia, mydriasis, and hypothermia. Puppies are especially sensitive and cats may become toxic even when treated aurally. Safe use of the drug in pregnant bitches and puppies less than 4 months of age has not been established and is not recommended.

DRUG INTERACTIONS: In small animals, atropine potentiates the pressor effects of amitraz and may cause hypertension and cardiac arrhythmias, and potentiate ileus and gastric distention. Yohimbine (0.1 mg/kg; IV) is a safe and effective antidote. See **AMITRAZ** in the Small Animal section.

AMOXICILLIN

INDICATIONS: Amoxicillin (Amoxi-Tabs ★, Amoxi-Drop ★, Amoxi-Inject ★, Amoxil ♣ ★, Moxilean ♣, Robamox-V ★) is a penicillin antibiotic indicated for the treatment of genitourinary, gastrointestinal, respiratory, and skin/soft tissue infections. Amoxicillin is specifically indicated in ferrets, in combination with metronidazole, gastric protectants (e.g., bismuth subsalicylate), and H_2-receptor blockers (e.g., cimetidine), for the treatment of gastritis and gastric ulcers caused by *Helicobacter mustelae*.

Amoxicillin has the same antibacterial spectrum as ampicillin but is better absorbed from the gastrointestinal tract and has a more rapid bactericidal activity and a longer duration of action. For more information, see **PENICILLIN ANTIBIOTICS** in the Small Animal section.

ADVERSE AND COMMON SIDE EFFECTS: None specifically described in the ferret; see **PENICILLIN ANTIBIOTICS** in the Small Animal section for general information.

DRUG INTERACTIONS: See PENICILLIN ANTIBIOTICS in the Small Animal section for general information.

AMPHOTERICIN B

INDICATIONS: Amphotericin B (Fungizone ♣ ★) is an effective systemically administered antifungal agent whose use has been described for the treatment of blastomycosis and cryptococcosis in ferrets.

ADVERSE AND COMMON SIDE EFFECTS: The most important side effect is renal dysfunction. Serum urea and creatinine levels and urinalyses should be monitored frequently throughout the treatment regimen. See **AMPHOTERICIN B** in the Small Animal section for details on regimens designed to reduce nephrotoxicity. In the ferret it may be difficult to obtain IV access over a prolonged treatment period.

DRUG INTERACTIONS: A number of significant drug interactions exist; see **AMPHOTERICIN B** in the Small Animal section. Ketoconazole appears to potentiate the efficacy of amphotericin B against blastomycosis and histoplasmosis; combined therapy has been recommended for the treatment of blastomycosis in ferrets.

AMPICILLIN

INDICATIONS: Ampicillin (Omnipen ★, Penbriton ♣, Polyflex ♣ ★) is a penicillin antibiotic indicated in the treatment of urinary tract, gastrointestinal tract, and respiratory tract infections susceptible to the antibiotic. Ampicillin has increased antibacterial activity against many gram-negative bacteria not affected by the natural penicillins or penicillinase-resistant penicillins, including some strains of Escherichia coli and Klebsiella. Ampicillin also has activity against anaerobic bacteria, including clostridial organisms. Ampicillin is susceptible to β-lactamase–producing bacteria (e.g., Staphylococcus aureus). For information concerning adverse and common side effects, see **PENICILLIN ANTIBIOTICS** in the Small Animal section.

DRUG INTERACTIONS: In patients with impaired renal function, the administration of ampicillin concurrently with an aminoglycoside may reduce the efficacy of the aminoglycoside. Do not administer ampicillin with bacteriostatic drugs (e.g., chloramphenicol, erythromycin, or tetracyclines) because the combination may reduce the bactericidal activity of the ampicillin.

ASCORBIC ACID

INDICATIONS: Ascorbic acid or vitamin C (Apo-C ✦, Redoxon ✦) is essential for the synthesis and maintenance of collagen and intercellular ground substance of body tissue cells, blood vessels, bone, cartilage, tendons, and teeth. It is also important in wound healing and resistance to infection. It may influence the immune response. In ferrets, administration of ascorbic acid has been recommended for general support in immunosuppressive diseases and during chemotherapy for lymphoma.

ADVERSE AND COMMON SIDE EFFECTS: See ASCORBIC ACID in the Small Animal section. Chelated, buffered, or ester forms may cause less gastrointestinal irritation. Vitamin C is bitter and must be mixed with strongly flavored food treats to disguise the taste.

DRUG INTERACTIONS: See ASCORBIC ACID in the Small Animal section.

ASPIRIN

INDICATIONS: Aspirin (ASA) or acetylsalicylic acid (Ecotrin ✦, Entrophen ✦, and many others) is an effective analgesic for the management of mild to moderate nonvisceral pain, and an antipyretic and anti-inflammatory agent. It has been used in conjunction with thiacetarsamide in the treatment of heartworm disease for its antiplatelet activity.

ADVERSE AND COMMON SIDE EFFECTS: Specific toxic effects have not been described in the ferret. See ASPIRIN in the Small Animal section for general information.

DRUG INTERACTIONS: See ASPIRIN in the Small Animal section for general information, with particular reference to treatment of cardiac disease, control of blood insulin levels, and concurrent glucocorticoid administration.

ATROPINE

INDICATIONS: Atropine ✦ ★ is an anticholinergic, antispasmodic, and mydriatic drug. It is indicated in the treatment of sinus bradycardia, sinus block or arrest, and incomplete atrioventricular block.

It is a parasympatholytic agent that causes relaxation of the gastrointestinal, biliary, and genitourinary tracts and suppresses salivary, gastric, and respiratory tract secretions (given preoperatively). Atropine is a mydriatic and cycloplegic agent, making it useful in the management of ocular inflammation. It is also used in the treatment of organophosphate and carbamate poisoning.

BISMUTH SUBSALICYLATE

INDICATIONS: Bismuth subsalicylate (Pepto-Bismol ♣ ★) is used in the treatment of diarrhea and, in combination with amoxicillin and metronidazole, for the treatment of gastritis and gastric ulcers associated with infection by *Helicobacter mustelae*. It inhibits the synthesis of prostaglandins responsible for gastrointestinal tract hypermotility and inflammation. The drug may also have antibacterial and antisecretory properties. Bismuth subsalicylate relieves indigestion by forming insoluble complexes with offending noxious agents and by forming a protective coating.

ADVERSE AND COMMON SIDE EFFECTS: See **BISMUTH SUBSALICYLATE** and **ASPIRIN** in the Small Animal section.

DRUG INTERACTIONS: The antimicrobial action of tetracyclines may be reduced if these drugs are used concurrently. It is advised that tetracycline be given at least 2 hours before or after bismuth administration.

BUPRENORPHINE HYDROCHLORIDE

INDICATIONS: Buprenorphine hydrochloride (Buprenex★) is a partial opiate agonist with analgesic properties. Analgesia lasts 4 to 8 hours in dogs and cats.

ADVERSE AND COMMON SIDE EFFECTS: Respiratory depression may occur. Opiates should be used with caution in animals with severe renal insufficiency, head trauma, central nervous system (CNS) dysfunction, and in debilitated or geriatric patients. The drug is resistant to antagonism by naloxone.

DRUG INTERACTIONS: The concurrent use of other CNS depressants (anesthetics, antihistamines, tranquilizers) may potentiate CNS and respiratory depression. This drug may inhibit the analgesic effects of opiate agonists (e.g., morphine).

BUTORPHANOL

INDICATIONS: Butorphanol (Torbugesic ♣ ★, Torbutrol ♣ ★) is a narcotic agonist/antagonist analgesic that is also used as a preanesthetic. Butorphanol has potent antitussive activity in dogs. See **BUTORPHANOL** in the Small Animal section for further information.

ADVERSE AND COMMON SIDE EFFECTS: Butorphanol has minimal cardiovascular effects and causes only slight respiratory depression. Alone it causes little sedation. All opiates should be used with caution in debilitated animals and those with head trauma, increased cerebrospinal fluid pressure, hypothyroidism, severe renal disease, or adrenocortical insufficiency.

DRUG INTERACTIONS: See **BUTORPHANOL** in the Small Animal section.

CARBARYL

INDICATIONS: Carbaryl (Sevin ♣, Zodiac Flea and Tick Power ♣, and others) is a carbamate insecticide and cholinesterase inhibitor used in the eradication of arthropod ectoparasites, including mites, lice, fleas, and ticks.

ADVERSE AND COMMON SIDE EFFECTS: Toxicity results from cholinesterase inhibition and is treated by administration of atropine. Clinical signs include miosis, salivation, frequent urination and defecation, vomiting, bronchoconstriction, ataxia, incoordination, muscle tremors, convulsions, respiratory depression, paralysis, and possibly death. Carbamate products should not be used on immature ferrets or in pregnant or nursing animals. See **CARBAMATE INSECTICIDES** in the Small Animal section.

DRUG INTERACTIONS: SEE **CARBAMATE INSECTICIDES** in the Small Animal section.

SUPPLIED AS: VETERINARY PRODUCTS
Numerous dusting powders containing 5% carbaryl ♣ ★
Spray containing 2.5% carbaryl [D-F-T Spray ★]
Shampoo containing 0.5% carbaryl [Mycodex Pet Shampoo★]

CEFADROXIL

INDICATIONS: Cefadroxil (Cefa-Tabs ♣ ★, Cefa-Drops ♣ ★) is a broad-spectrum, first-generation cephalosporin antibiotic. For more information see **CEFADROXIL** and **CEPHALOSPORIN ANTIBIOTICS** in the Small Animal section.

ADVERSE AND COMMON SIDE EFFECTS: See **CEFADROXIL** and **CEPHALOSPORIN ANTIBIOTICS** in the Small Animal section.

DRUG INTERACTIONS: See **CEPHALOSPORIN ANTIBIOTICS** in the Small Animal section.

CEPHALEXIN

INDICATIONS: Cephalexin (Keflex ♣ ★) is a broad-spectrum, first-generation cephalosporin antibiotic. For more information see **CEPHALOSPORIN ANTIBIOTICS** in the Small Animal section.

ADVERSE AND COMMON SIDE EFFECTS: In addition to the side effects noted for the **CEPHALOSPORIN ANTIBIOTICS**, cephalexin has been reported to cause salivation, tachypnea, and excitability in dogs and vomiting and fever in cats. See **CEPHALOSPORIN ANTIBIOTICS** in the Small Animal section.

DRUG INTERACTIONS: See **CEPHALOSPORIN ANTIBIOTICS** in the Small Animal section.

CHLORAMPHENICOL

INDICATIONS: Chloramphenicol (Azramycine ♣, Chlor Palm ♣, Chlor Tablets ♣, Chloromycetin ♣ ★, Karomycin Palmitate ♣, Viceton★, and many others) is a bacteriostatic antibiotic with activity against a wide range of pathogens. It is well absorbed following oral administration and widely distributed throughout the body. See **CHLORAMPHENICOL** in the Small Animal section for further details.

  Chloramphenicol is the treatment of choice for proliferative bowel disease in ferrets, which is currently believed to be caused by *Lawsonia intracellularis*, a *Campylobacter*-like organism. Treatment may be curative, but some animals remain carriers and may relapse.

ADVERSE AND COMMON SIDE EFFECTS: The most common side effect in dogs and cats following oral administration is gastrointestinal upset manifested by transient depression, anorexia, nausea, vomiting, or diarrhea. Adverse reactions may also include a reversible bone marrow suppression and nonregenerative anemia, thrombocytopenia, and leukopenia; however, these have not been specifically described in the ferret.

  Owners must be cautioned as to the potential for adverse reactions by humans exposed to chloramphenicol.

DRUG INTERACTIONS: A number of significant drug interactions exist. See **CHLORAMPHENICOL** in the Small Animal section.

CHLORPHENIRAMINE MALEATE

INDICATIONS: Chlorpheniramine (Chlor-Trimeton ★, Chlor-Tripolon ♣) is an antihistamine used in the ferret to control sneezing and coughing resulting from influenza-viral infection. For additional information see **CHLORPHENIRAMINE MALEATE** and **ANTIHISTAMINES** in the Small Animal section.

ADVERSE AND COMMON SIDE EFFECTS: The most common adverse effects in dogs and cats are lethargy and somnolence. Anorexia, vomiting, and diarrhea may also occur. For additional information see **CHLORPHENIRAMINE MALEATE** and **ANTIHISTAMINES** in the Small Animal section.

DRUG INTERACTIONS: See **CHLORPHENIRAMINE MALEATE** and **ANTIHISTAMINES** in the Small Animal section.

CHORIONIC GONADOTROPHIN

INDICATIONS: Chorionic gonadotrophin [human chorionic gonadotrophin, HCG] (A.P.L. ♣, Chorionad ♣, Chorionic Gonadotropin ★, Chorulon ♣ ★, Follutein ★) is a gonadal-stimulating hormone obtained from the urine of pregnant women. It is used in ferrets to terminate estrus. A single dose of 100 IU most closely simulated copulation-induced ovulation in experimental trials. Treatment is most effective if administered after the second week of estrus. Ovulation should occur within 35 hours, and signs of estrus such as vulvar swelling should disappear within 21 to 30 days. Restoration of bone marrow activity after persistent estrus may require several weeks. For more information, see **CHORIONIC GONADOTROPHIN** in the Large Animal section.

ADVERSE AND COMMON SIDE EFFECTS: The drug may not be effective if the ferret has been in heat for a prolonged period (i.e., longer than 1 month). Chorionic gonadotrophin is a foreign protein and can cause anaphylaxis when administered parenterally. Continued administration may result in antihormone antibody production and loss of effectiveness.

SUPPLIED AS: VETERINARY PRODUCTS
For injection containing 5,000 [Chorulon ♣ ★, Chorionic Gonadotropin ★] and 10,000 [A.P.L. ♣, Chorionad ♣ Progron 10,000 ♣, Follutein ★, Chorionic Gonadotropin ★] USP units per vial

CIMETIDINE

INDICATIONS: Cimetidine (Tagamet ♣ ★) is a histamine (H_2)-blocking agent that reduces gastric acid secretion and is useful in the management of gastric and duodenal ulceration. In ferrets cimetidine is most often used in combination with antibiotics (i.e., amoxicillin and metronidazole) and gastric protectants in the treatment of gastritis and gastric ulceration associated with infection by *Helicobacter mustelae*. See **CIMETIDINE** in the Small Animal section for further details on indications.

ADVERSE AND COMMON SIDE EFFECTS: Adverse effects in small animals appear rare. Ferrets dislike the taste of the oral elixir. See **CIMETIDINE** in the Small Animal section.

DRUG INTERACTIONS: When using combined therapy in ferrets, it is important to note that antacids may reduce gastrointestinal absorption of cimetidine and if used should be given no less than 1 hour before or after cimetidine. Because sucralfate can absorb drugs, it is recommended that cimetidine be given parenterally or that dosage times be staggered by about 2 hours. Cimetidine also decreases the metabolism and/or absorption of many drugs by interfering with hepatic microenzyme systems and altering gastric pH. See **CIMETIDINE** in the Small Animal section.

CIPROFLOXACIN

INDICATIONS: Ciprofloxacin (Cipro ♣ ★) is a fluoroquinolone antibiotic with activity against a range of gram-negative bacteria and some spirochetes. See **CIPROFLOXACIN** and **FLUOROQUINO-LONE ANTIBIOTICS** in the Small Animal section.

ADVERSE AND COMMON SIDE EFFECTS: See **FLUORO-QUINOLONE ANTIBIOTICS** in the Small Animal section. Some reports describe the use of ciprofloxacin tablets to formulate an oral suspension; however, the stability and potency of this suspension over time have not been described.

DRUG INTERACTIONS: Absorption is hindered by antacid preparations. See **FLUOROQUINOLONE ANTIBIOTICS** in the Small Animal section.

CISAPRIDE

INDICATIONS: Cisapride (Prepulsid ♣, Propulsid ★) is chemically related to metoclopramide and may be useful in cases of gastroesophageal reflux and to stimulate gastrointestinal motility in cases of primary motility disorders. See **CISAPRIDE** in the Small Animal section.

ADVERSE AND COMMON SIDE EFFECTS: See **CISAPRIDE** in the Small Animal section.

DRUG INTERACTIONS: Because cisapride increases gastric emptying, absorption of drugs from the stomach may be decreased, whereas absorption from the small bowel may be increased. See **CISAPRIDE** in the Small Animal section.

CLAVULANIC ACID + AMOXICILLIN

INDICATIONS: Clavamox ♣ ★ (amoxicillin/clavulanate) is an amoxicillin and clavulanic acid combination. See **CLAVAMOX** and see **PENICILLIN ANTIBIOTICS** in the Small Animal section for information on antibacterial spectrum and tissue distribution.

ADVERSE AND COMMON SIDE EFFECTS: The drug combination is contraindicated in animals with sensitivity to the penicillins or the cephalosporin antibiotics. See also **PENICILLIN ANTIBIOTICS** in the Small Animal section.

DRUG INTERACTIONS: See PENICILLIN ANTIBIOTICS in the Small Animal section.

CLINDAMYCIN

INDICATIONS: Clindamycin (Antirobe ♣ ★, Cleocin ★) is a lincosamide antibiotic with activity against a wide variety of pathogenic agents. See **CLINDAMYCIN** in the Small Animal section for information on antibacterial spectrum and tissue distribution. Clindamycin has been recommended for the treatment of bone and dental disease in ferrets.

ADVERSE AND COMMON SIDE EFFECTS: Adverse effects may include vomiting and diarrhea (sometimes hemorrhagic) following oral use of the drug and local pain after IM injection. See **CLINDAMYCIN** in the Small Animal section for further details.

DRUG INTERACTIONS: See CLINDAMYCIN in the Small Animal section.

CLOXACILLIN

INDICATIONS: Cloxacillin (Cloxapen ★, Orbenin ♣, Tegopen ♣ ★) is a penicillin antibiotic used primarily against gram-positive, β-lactamase–producing bacteria, especially *Staphylococcus* spp. For further information, see **PENICILLIN ANTIBIOTICS** in the Small Animal section.

ADVERSE AND COMMON SIDE EFFECTS: See PENICILLIN ANTIBIOTICS in the Small Animal section.

DRUG INTERACTIONS: See PENICILLIN ANTIBIOTICS in the Small Animal section.

DEXAMETHASONE

INDICATIONS: Dexamethasone (Azium ♣ ★, Azium SP ♣ ★, Dex-5 ♣) is a glucocorticoid used in small animal medicine for the treatment of a variety of conditions. The most frequently published indications for its use in ferrets include prior to blood transfusion, immediate use after adrenalectomy, and shock. For further information, see **DEXAMETHASONE** and **GLUCOCORTICOID AGENTS** in the Small Animal section.

ADVERSE AND COMMON SIDE EFFECTS and **DRUG INTERACTIONS:** See **DEXAMETHASONE** and **GLUCOCORTICOID AGENTS** in the Small Animal section.

DEXTROSE

INDICATIONS: Dextrose ✚ ★ is used to treat hypoglycemia in ferrets with insulinomas. Dextrose is administered IV during hypoglycemic episodes that are not responsive to oral therapy, and during and for several days after surgical removal of an insulinoma. Blood glucose levels should be monitored postoperatively to determine when therapy should be discontinued.

ADVERSE AND COMMON SIDE EFFECTS: When 50% dextrose is used as an IV bolus, it is important to cease administration once clinical signs resolve because rapid elevations in blood glucose can result in rebound hyperinsulinemia.

DRUG INTERACTIONS: None described.

SUPPLIED AS: VETERINARY PRODUCT
For IV injection containing 50% dextrose

DIAZEPAM

INDICATIONS: Diazepam (Valium ✚ ★, Valrelease ★) is an effective anticonvulsant for the control of seizure in status epilepticus. The drug is also used as a preanesthetic and to stimulate appetite. See **DIAZEPAM** in the Small Animal section for further information.

ADVERSE AND COMMON SIDE EFFECTS: The benzodiazepines are generally safe drugs. They have minimal cardiopulmonary effects and are short-acting agents. Dose-related sedation, ataxia, excitement, and sometimes paradoxical aggression may occur. The benzodiazepines should not be used for more than 2 days to stimulate appetite. See **DIAZEPAM** in the Small Animal section for further information.

DRUG INTERACTIONS: See **DIAZEPAM** in the Small Animal section.

DIAZOXIDE

INDICATIONS: Diazoxide (Proglycem ✦ ★) is an antihypertensive agent used in ferrets in conjunction with prednisone for the management of hypoglycemia resulting from islet cell tumors (insulinomas). It inhibits pancreatic insulin secretion, enhances epinephrine-induced glycogenolysis, and inhibits peripheral glucose utilization.

ADVERSE AND COMMON SIDE EFFECTS: Side effects are primarily anorexia, vomiting, and diarrhea. Other possible side effects include diabetes mellitus, anemia, agranulocytosis, thrombocytopenia, sodium and fluid retention, and cardiac arrhythmias.

DRUG INTERACTIONS: Prednisone is used initially to prevent hypoglycemic episodes. Diazoxide is added to the regimen when prednisone is no longer efficacious. Medical treatment should be used in conjunction with dietary manipulation (i.e., frequent high protein/ low carbohydrate meals). For more information, see **DIAZOXIDE** in the Small Animal section.

DIETHYLCARBAMAZINE

INDICATIONS: Diethylcarbamazine [DEC] (Carbam ★, Filaribits ✦ ★) has been recommended for the prevention of heartworm disease in ferrets.

ADVERSE AND COMMON SIDE EFFECTS: Vomiting and diarrhea are occasionally noted in dogs. Administration with food reduces this problem. Do not use in microfilaremic animals because hypersensitivity or anaphylaxis and death may occur.

DRUG INTERACTIONS: Levamisole and pyrantel may enhance the toxic effects of DEC and vice versa.

DIGOXIN

INDICATIONS: Digoxin (Lanoxin ★, Cardoxin ✦ ★) decreases sympathetic nerve activity and is a positive inotropic and negative chronotropic agent. Digoxin is used in ferrets to improve cardiac output in conditions of congestive heart failure and cardiomyopathy. Therapeutic blood digoxin levels for ferrets have not been specifically defined; however, those for dogs and cats provide approximate guidelines. See **DIGOXIN** in the Small Animal section for further information.

ADVERSE AND COMMON SIDE EFFECTS: A variety of toxic effects have been described in dogs and cats. Serum levels should be monitored to evaluate dosage. See **DIGOXIN** in the Small Animal section for further information.

DRUG INTERACTIONS: Interactions exist with a number of drugs which, for example, affect potassium levels and hepatic and gastric function. See **DIGOXIN** in the Small Animal section for further information.

DILTIAZEM

INDICATIONS: Diltiazem (Cardizem ♣ ★) is a calcium channel-blocking agent whose use has been described in ferrets for the treatment of hypertrophic cardiomyopathy. See **DILTIAZEM** in the Small Animal section for further information.

ADVERSE AND COMMON SIDE EFFECTS: See **DILTIAZEM** in the Small Animal section.

DRUG INTERACTIONS: Diltiazem is reported to increase serum digoxin levels in humans. See **DILTIAZEM** in the Small Animal section for further information.

DIPHENHYDRAMINE

INDICATIONS: Diphenhydramine (Benadryl ♣ ★) is an antihistamine that has been used in ferrets to reduce coughing and sneezing associated with influenza-viral infection and to guard against the effects of histamine release from mast cell tumors. For further information, refer to **DIPHENHYDRAMINE** and **ANTIHISTAMINES** in the Small Animal section.

DOXAPRAM

INDICATIONS: Doxapram (Dopram-V ♣ ★) is used to stimulate respiration in patients with postanesthetic respiratory depression or apnea and to encourage the return of laryngopharyngeal reflexes in patients with mild to moderate respiratory and central nervous system depression due to anesthetic overdose. In the neonate, doxapram may be used to stimulate respiration following dystocia or Cesarean section.

ADVERSE AND COMMON SIDE EFFECTS: See **DOXAPRAM** in the Small Animal section.

DRUG INTERACTIONS: Halothane and enflurane may precipitate arrhythmias. It is recommended that doxapram use be delayed about 10 minutes after discontinuation of these anesthetic agents. See **DOXAPRAM** in the Small Animal section.

ENALAPRIL

INDICATIONS: Enalapril (Enacard ♣ ★, Vasotec ♣ ★) is an angiotensin-converting enzyme (ACE) inhibitor used for its vasodilatory properties in the treatment of congestive heart failure. For more information, see **ENALAPRIL** in the Small Animal section.

ADVERSE AND COMMON SIDE EFFECTS: Lethargy, anorexia, and weakness resulting from hypotension have been reported in the ferret. Treatment should be initiated with a low dose, which can be increased if no adverse effects are noted. A range of other effects have been described in small animals. For more information, see **ENALAPRIL** in the Small Animal section.

DRUG INTERACTIONS: See **ENALAPRIL** in the Small Animal section for further information, especially with respect to concurrent use of diuretic agents.

ENROFLOXACIN

INDICATIONS: Enrofloxacin (Baytril ♣ ★) is a fluoroquinolone antibiotic with activity against a wide range of pathogenic agents. The injectable product can be compounded into an oral formulation using a palatable liquid syrup base. See **ENROFLOXACIN** in the Small Animal section for further details on antibacterial spectrum.

ADVERSE AND COMMON SIDE EFFECTS: Induction of cartilage damage in growing ferrets has not been specifically described; however, caution should be applied when prescribing this drug for young growing kits or pregnant females. Enrofloxacin administered by injection can cause marked myonecrosis; oral treatment is preferred whenever possible. For more information on adverse effects in dogs and cats, see **ENROFLOXACIN** and **FLUOROQUINOLONE ANTIBIOTICS** in the Small Animal section.

DRUG INTERACTIONS: Absorption is hindered by antacid preparations as well as sucralfate. See **ENROFLOXACIN** and **FLUOROQUINOLONE ANTIBIOTICS** in the Small Animal section for details on other interactions.

ERYTHROMYCIN

INDICATIONS: Erythromycin (Erythro-100 ★) is a macrolide antibiotic with primary activity against gram-positive bacteria. It is effective against streptococci, staphylococci, *Erysipelothrix*, *Clostridium*, *Bacteroides*, *Borrelia*, and *Fusobacterium*, as well as *Pasteurella* and *Bordetella* organisms. The drug also has activity against *Campylobacter fetus*, mycoplasmas, chlamydiae, rickettsiae, spirochetes, some atypical mycobacteria, *Leptospira*, and amoebae.

ADVERSE AND COMMON SIDE EFFECTS: Adverse effects are rare but have been reported; see **ERYTHROMYCIN** in the Small Animal section. All parenteral preparations are irritating at the site of injection.

DRUG INTERACTIONS: Kaolin, pectin, and bismuth decrease gastrointestinal tract absorption of the drug. A number of significant drug interactions exist; see **ERYTHROMYCIN** in the Small Animal section.

FLUNIXIN MEGLUMINE

INDICATIONS: Flunixin meglumine (Banamine ✦ ★) is a potent antiprostaglandin with anti-inflammatory and antipyretic properties that make it useful in the treatment of inflammation and pain associated with musculoskeletal disease. For further information, see **FLUNIXIN MEGLUMINE** in the Small Animal section.

ADVERSE AND COMMON SIDE EFFECTS: Flunixin should be administered for no more than 3 consecutive days. Gastric ulceration may be exacerbated by the concurrent use of prednisone. As IM injection can be irritating; injections should be made deep into large muscle bundles. For further information, see **FLUNIXIN MEGLUMINE** in the Small Animal section.

DRUG INTERACTIONS: None established. Concurrent use of methoxyflurane may predispose to acute renal tubular necrosis.

FUROSEMIDE

INDICATIONS: Furosemide (Lasix ✦ ★) is a potent loop diuretic used in ferrets to reduce preload and pulmonary edema in patients with congestive heart failure and cardiomyopathy. For further information, see **FUROSEMIDE** in the Small Animal section.

ADVERSE AND COMMON SIDE EFFECTS: A number of adverse effects have been described in dogs and cats. See **FUROSEMIDE** in the Small Animal section for further information.

DRUG INTERACTIONS: A number of drug interactions exist. See **FUROSEMIDE** in the Small Animal section for further information.

GENTAMICIN

INDICATIONS: Gentamicin (Gentocin ✦ ★) is an aminoglycoside antibiotic. See **GENTAMICIN** in the Small Animal section for details on drug pharmacokinetics in the dog and cat.

ADVERSE AND COMMON SIDE EFFECTS and **DRUG INTER-ACTIONS:** See **GENTAMICIN** and **AMINOGLYCOSIDE AN-TIBIOTICS** in the Small Animal section.

GNRH/GONADORELIN

INDICATIONS: Gonadorelin (Cystorelin ✦ ★, Factrel ✦ ★) is used in ferrets to terminate estrus. It is most effective if administered after the second week of estrus. Vulvar swelling should reduce in 2 to 3 weeks; restoration of bone marrow activity after persistent estrus may require several weeks. See **GONADORELIN** in the Small Animal section for information on use in dogs and cats.

ADVERSE AND COMMON SIDE EFFECTS: None reported.

DRUG INTERACTIONS: None reported.

GRISEOFULVIN

INDICATIONS: Griseofulvin (Fulvicin U/F ✦ ★) is used for the treatment of dermatophyte infections. The drug is detectable in the skin within 4 to 8 hours of oral administration. High dietary fat facilitates absorption.

ADVERSE AND COMMON SIDE EFFECTS: Nausea, vomiting, and diarrhea are the most common side effects. Hepatotoxicity and photosensitization also have been reported but are rare. The drug may inhibit spermatogenesis and is potentially teratogenic and mutagenic in a number of species.

HYDROXYZINE

INDICATIONS: Hydroxyzine (Atarax ✦ ★) is an anxiolytic, antihistaminic agent. The drug also has anticholinergic, antiemetic, and bronchodilator effects. It has been used in small animals primarily for its antihistaminic properties. For more information concerning **ADVERSE AND COMMON SIDE EFFECTS** and **DRUG INTERACTIONS**, see **ANTIHISTAMINES** in the Small Animal section.

ADVERSE AND COMMON SIDE EFFECTS: Transitory drowsiness is the most common side effect. Other adverse effects may include fine rapid tremors, seizures, xerostomia, hypotension, diarrhea, and decreased appetite.

DRUG INTERACTIONS: Barbiturates and other sedatives may potentiate central nervous system depression.

INSULIN

INDICATIONS: Insulin preparations ♣ ★ are used in the management of diabetes mellitus. The various types of beef-pork insulin and their properties are described under **INSULIN** in the Small Animal section. NPH insulin is the form most commonly prescribed for use in ferrets.

ADVERSE AND COMMON SIDE EFFECTS and **DRUG INTERACTIONS:** See INSULIN in the Small Animal section.

IRON DEXTRAN

INDICATIONS: Iron dextran is indicated for the treatment of iron deficiency anemia.

ADVERSE AND COMMON SIDE EFFECTS: An IM injection can be irritating. Allergic reactions and anaphylaxis have occasionally been reported in humans.

DRUG INTERACTIONS: Clinical response may be delayed in patients concurrently receiving chloramphenicol.

SUPPLIED AS: VETERINARY PRODUCTS
For injection containing 100 and 200 mg elemental iron/mL [Ferrodex★, Ironol-100♣, and generic products]

IVERMECTIN

INDICATIONS: Ivermectin (Heartgard ♣ ★, Ivomec ♣ ★, Eqvalan ♣ ★) is used for the eradication of parasites including enteric nematodes and ectoparasites, especially sarcoptic mange and, by topical installation, ear mites.

Ivermectin is also used for the prevention of infection by *Dirofilaria immitis* [Heartgard] and as a microfilaricide. The American Heartworm Association recommends a monthly oral dose of 6 μg/kg beginning 1 month before the onset of the transmission season and continuing throughout the period of exposure. Experimental work suggested that the minimum effective dose to prevent maturation of *D. immitis* larvae is between 12.5 and 50 μg/kg. Ivermectin liquid can be diluted in propylene glycol to make an oral solution of convenient volume. The diluted solution must also be protected from light.

One report in the literature describes the successful treatment of eosinophilic gastroenteritis with two doses of ivermectin (400 μg/kg) administered SC at a 2-week interval.

ADVERSE AND COMMON SIDE EFFECTS: Ivermectin has a wide margin of safety.

DRUG INTERACTIONS: None.

KAOLIN-PECTIN

INDICATIONS: Kaolin-pectin (Kaopectate ✚ ★, others) is a gastro-intestinal protectant used in the management of diarrhea. It coats the surface of the gut and exerts a mild demulcent and absorbent effect. It is actually relatively ineffective in absorbing toxins produced by enteropathogenic bacteria. It appears to act by adding particulate matter to the feces, which improves consistency until the disease spontaneously resolves. Kaolin is a potent coagulation activator and may be of some benefit in treating diarrhea associated with mucosal disruption and hemorrhage.

ADVERSE AND COMMON SIDE EFFECTS: Kaolin-pectin may cause constipation, especially in poorly hydrated patients.

DRUG INTERACTIONS: The absorption of lincomycin is decreased if given concurrently with kaolin-pectin. Administer kaolin-pectin 2 hours before or 3 to 4 hours after. Absorption of digoxin may also be hindered by kaolin-pectin.

KETOCONAZOLE

INDICATIONS: Ketoconazole (Nizoral ✚ ★) is used in the treatment of a variety of topical and systemic mycotic infections, sometimes in combination with amphotericin B. The drug has also been used in ferrets, with varying success, for the treatment of hyperadrenocor-ticism when surgical removal of the affected gland is not possible. Ketoconazole effectively blocks cortisol synthesis in dogs with pituitary-dependent hyperadrenocorticism as well as those with adrenocortical tumors.

ADVERSE AND COMMON SIDE EFFECTS: Gastrointestinal side effects in dogs may be prevented by administering the drug with food (which may also serve to increase its absorption) and by dividing the daily dose and administering the drug two to four times daily.

DRUG INTERACTIONS: See **KETOCONAZOLE** in the Small Animal section.

LACTULOSE

INDICATIONS: Lactulose (Cephulac ✚ ★, Chronulac ✚ ★) is a syn-thetic nonabsorbable disaccharide. It acts as a mild osmotic laxative, increases the rate of passage of ingesta, and reduces bacterial production of ammonia, making it useful in the management of hepatic encephalopathy. Enteric bacteria ferment lactulose to acidic byproducts, which decrease intraluminal pH, and favor the formation of ammonium ions, which are poorly absorbed.

ADVERSE AND COMMON SIDE EFFECTS and **DRUG INTERACTIONS:** See **LACTULOSE** in the Small Animal section.

LIME SULFUR

INDICATIONS: Lime sulfur, or calcium polysulfide, is a topical insecticide used in the treatment of sarcoptic mange. It may be safer than ivermectin for the treatment of young kits.

ADVERSE AND COMMON SIDE EFFECTS: Lime sulfur is a very safe preparation, but it has a strong odor.

DRUG INTERACTIONS: None reported.

SUPPLIED AS: COMMERCIAL PRODUCT
Lime sulfur (calcium polysulfide) liquid or powder

LINCOMYCIN

INDICATIONS: Lincomycin (Lincocin ✦ ★) is a lincosamide antibiotic. For information on antibacterial spectrum and indications for use in dogs, see **LINCOMYCIN** in the Small Animal section.

ADVERSE AND COMMON SIDE EFFECTS: Vomiting and loose stools may occur. Hemorrhagic diarrhea is infrequent in dogs. Pain at the injection site is reported.

DRUG INTERACTIONS: Kaolin, pectin, and bismuth subsalicylate decrease gastrointestinal absorption. For further information, see **LINCOMYCIN** in the Small Animal section.

MEGESTROL ACETATE

INDICATIONS: Megestrol acetate or MGA (Ovaban ✦ ★, Ovarid ✦) is a progestational compound that is contraindicated in ferrets because it predisposes to pyometra. See also **MEGESTROL ACETATE** in the Small Animal section.

MEPERIDINE

INDICATIONS: Meperidine (Demerol ✦ ★) is a short-acting narcotic analgesic used for the relief of moderate to severe pain or as a preanesthetic. See **MEPERIDINE** in the Small Animal section for further details.

ADVERSE AND COMMON SIDE EFFECTS: A number of adverse effects have been described. See **MEPERIDINE** in the Small Animal section for further details. The drug is quite irritating given SC.

DRUG INTERACTIONS: Central nervous system depression or stimulation induced by meperidine may be potentiated by amphetamines, barbiturates, or cimetidine. See **MEPERIDINE** in the Small Animal section for further details.

METOCLOPRAMIDE

INDICATIONS: Metoclopramide (Maxeran ✿, Reglan ✿ ★) is an antiemetic agent with central (chemoreceptor trigger zone) and peripheral activity. It contributes to lower esophageal sphincter competence and promotes gastric emptying. It is useful in the management of vomiting, gastroesophageal reflux, and gastric motility disorders.

ADVERSE AND COMMON SIDE EFFECTS: Metoclopramide should not be used in patients with gastric outlet obstruction or those with a history of epilepsy. Renal disease may increase blood levels of the drug. Central nervous system (CNS) reactions include increased frequency of seizure activity, vertigo, hyperactivity, depression, and disorientation.

DRUG INTERACTIONS: Phenothiazine drugs may potentiate CNS effects. Digoxin, cimetidine, tetracycline, narcotic agents, and sedatives enhance CNS effects. Digoxin absorption may also be decreased, whereas acetaminophen, aspirin, diazepam, and tetracycline absorption may be accelerated. Atropine will block the effects of the drug on gastrointestinal tract motility.

METRONIDAZOLE

INDICATIONS: Metronidazole (Flagyl ✿ ★) is a synthetic antibacterial and antiprotozoal agent that is used for the treatment of giardiasis in ferrets. It is also bactericidal to many anaerobic bacteria.

Metronidazole is specifically indicated, in combination with amoxicillin, gastric protectants (e.g., bismuth subsalicylate), and H_2 receptor blockers (e.g., cimetidine), for the treatment of gastritis and gastric ulcers caused by *Helicobacter mustelae*. It has also been recommended for the treatment of hepatitis, in combination with a broad-spectrum antibiotic, and as an adjunct to chloramphenicol therapy for proliferative bowel disease. It has been described that the addition of sucrose to oral preparations reduces the aftertaste. For further information, see **METRONIDAZOLE** in the Small Animal section.

ADVERSE AND COMMON SIDE EFFECTS: See METRONIDAZOLE in the Small Animal section for details on adverse effects reported in dogs. The tablets have a bitter taste and should not be crushed before use. The drug may also be mutagenic and should not be given to pregnant animals.

DRUG INTERACTIONS: See **METRONIDAZOLE** in the Small Animal section.

MILBEMYCIN

INDICATIONS: Milbemycin oxime (Interceptor ✦ ★) is an anthelmintic used in the prevention of heartworm caused by *Dirofilaria immitis*, as a microfilaricide, and for the control of gastrointestinal parasites. For more information, see **MILBEMYCIN** in the Small Animal section.

ADVERSE AND COMMON SIDE EFFECTS: None described in ferrets. See **MILBEMYCIN** in the Small Animal section.

DRUG INTERACTIONS: None reported.

MITOTANE

INDICATIONS: Mitotane or o,p'-DDD (Lysodren ✦ ★) is indicated in the treatment of pituitary-dependent hyperadrenocorticism in dogs and has been used with variable success to treat ferrets with adrenal neoplasia. Surgical removal of the tumor is preferable to medical management in most cases. See **MITOTANE** in the Small Animal section.

ADVERSE AND COMMON SIDE EFFECTS: The most significant side effect described in ferrets is the development of severe hypoglycemia, presumably due to a reduction in negative feedback on a previously subclinical insulinoma. The possible emergence of this problem should be addressed when mitotane is dispensed. See also **MITOTANE** in the Small Animal section.

DRUG INTERACTIONS: See **MITOTANE** in the Small Animal section.

SUPPLIED AS: HUMAN PRODUCT
Tablets containing 500 mg (a pharmacist can reformulate capsules to the required dosage)

NEOMYCIN

INDICATIONS: Neomycin (Biosol-M ✤, Mycifradin ✤ ★), an aminoglycoside antibiotic, is most often used topically and orally for its local antibiotic effects in the gastrointestinal tract. It is generally less effective against many bacteria than amikacin or gentamicin. The drug is very toxic when used systemically.

ADVERSE AND COMMON SIDE EFFECTS: Neomycin is the most nephrotoxic aminoglycoside. The drug is also potentially toxic to the vestibular and auditory nerves. Ototoxicity is especially a concern if the drug is instilled into external ear canals with ruptured tympanic membranes. It may also cause a contact hypersensitivity and otitis externa. Neomycin may decrease cardiac output and produce hypotension.

DRUG INTERACTIONS: Orally administered neomycin may decrease the absorption of digitalis, methotrexate, penicillin V and K, and vitamin K.

NITROGLYCERIN

INDICATIONS: Nitroglycerin (Nitro-Bid ✤ ★, Nitrol ✤ ★) is a venous vasodilator used in the medical management of congestive heart failure and cardiomyopathy in ferrets, especially when pulmonary edema is present. Apply the ointment to a relatively hairless or shaved area of skin.

ADVERSE AND COMMON SIDE EFFECTS: Rash and hypotension are reported.

DRUG INTERACTIONS: Use of calcium channel-blocking agents (e.g., verapamil and diltiazem), β-blocking agents (e.g., propranolol, atenolol, or metoprolol), and phenothiazine drugs may potentiate hypotension.

OXYMORPHONE

INDICATIONS: Oxymorphone (Numorphan ✤ ★, P/M Oxymorphone★) is a narcotic agent used for sedation, preanesthesia, and the management of pain. See **OXYMORPHONE** in the Small Animal section for further details.

ADVERSE AND COMMON SIDE EFFECTS and **DRUG INTERACTIONS:** See OXYMORPHONE in the Small Animal section for further details on adverse effects. Adverse effects of the drug can be reversed with naloxone.

OXYTETRACYCLINE

INDICATIONS: Oxytetracycline (Liquamycin ✤ ★, Terramycin ✤ ★) is a short-acting, water-soluble tetracycline. For more information, see **OXYTETRACYCLINE** and **TETRACYCLINE ANTIBIOTICS** in the Small Animal section.

ADVERSE AND COMMON SIDE EFFECTS: Oxytetracycline may cause discoloration of the teeth in young animals. High doses or prolonged use may cause delayed bone growth and healing. Tetracyclines cause nausea, anorexia, vomiting, and diarrhea in small animals.

DRUG INTERACTIONS: A number of oral preparations interfere with the absorption of tetracyclines. See **OXYTETRACYCLINE** and **TETRACYCLINE ANTIBIOTICS** in the Small Animal section for further details.

OXYTOCIN

INDICATIONS: Oxytocin (Pitocin ★, Syntocinon ✤ ★) is a hormone of the posterior pituitary gland used in ferrets to stimulate milk letdown and help expel retained fetuses.

ADVERSE AND COMMON SIDE EFFECTS: The drug is contraindicated in animals with dystocia due to abnormal presentation of the fetus or in those with a closed cervix. See **OXYTOCIN** in the Small Animal section.

DRUG INTERACTIONS: See **OXYTOCIN** in the Small Animal section.

PENICILLIN G AND V

INDICATIONS: Penicillin antibiotics, including penicillin G and V, are effective bactericidal antibiotics used for the treatment of gram-positive and gram-negative infections. Penicillin drugs are widely distributed throughout the body to most body fluids and bone except the brain and cerebrospinal fluid unless inflamed. Penicillin G is effective against most gram-positive organisms. Penicillin V has the same spectrum but is more reliably absorbed from the gastrointestinal tract.

ADVERSE AND COMMON SIDE EFFECTS: Toxicity is rare in dogs and cats. See **PENICILLIN ANTIBIOTICS** in the Small Animal section. Sensitivity to one penicillin implies sensitivity to all penicillins.

DRUG INTERACTIONS: See **PENICILLIN ANTIBIOTICS** in the Small Animal section. Food and antacids decrease the absorption of orally administered penicillins. The drug should be given 1 hour before or 2 hours after feeding.

PENTAZOCINE

INDICATIONS: Pentazocine (Talwin-V ★, Talwin ♣ ★) is a narcotic agonist used in the management of moderate to severe pain. The drug does not depress respiration and produces little or no sedation at therapeutic doses. See **PENTAZOCINE** in the Small Animal section for further details.

ADVERSE AND COMMON SIDE EFFECTS: See PENTAZOCINE in the Small Animal section for further details. Side effects can be reversed with naloxone.

DRUG INTERACTIONS: Do not mix pentazocine with soluble barbiturates because precipitation will occur.

PHENOBARBITAL

INDICATIONS: Phenobarbital is the drug of choice for the control of seizure activity in small animals. Therapeutic blood phenobarbital levels for ferrets have not been specifically defined; however, those for dogs and cats provide approximate guidelines. See **PHENOBARBITAL** and **BARBITURATES** in the Small Animal section for further indications and information on pharmacokinetics.

ADVERSE AND COMMON SIDE EFFECTS: Initially, sedation and ataxia may be noted, especially at higher doses. These effects tend to resolve with continued treatment. For further information on treatment of drug overdose, see **PHENOBARBITAL** in the Small Animal section.

DRUG INTERACTIONS: Interactions exist with a number of compounds. See **PHENOBARBITAL** in the Small Animal section.

PIPERAZINE

INDICATIONS: Piperazine (Hartz Once a Month ★, Once a Month Roundworm Treatment ♣, Pipa-Tabs ★, Purina Liquid Wormer ★) is an anthelmintic used for the eradication of roundworms.

ADVERSE AND COMMON SIDE EFFECTS: See PIPERAZINE in the Small Animal section.

DRUG INTERACTIONS: See **PIPERAZINE** in the Small Animal section. The concurrent use of laxatives is not recommended because these agents may cause elimination of the drug before it has had an opportunity to work effectively.

PRAZIQUANTEL

INDICATIONS: Praziquantel (Droncit ✦ ★) is an anthelmintic used to eliminate tapeworms. After use of the drug, the parasite loses its ability to resist digestion by the host and because of this, it is common to see only disintegrated and partially digested pieces of tapeworm in the stool.

ADVERSE AND COMMON SIDE EFFECTS: The drug is very safe but is not recommended for use in puppies or kittens younger than 4 weeks of age. Drug overdose may be associated with anorexia, vomiting, salivation, diarrhea, and depression.

DRUG INTERACTIONS: None reported.

PREDNISOLONE
PREDNISOLONE SODIUM SUCCINATE
PREDNISONE

INDICATIONS: Prednisolone (Delta-Cortef ★) and prednisone (Deltasone ✦ ★) are intermediate-acting glucocorticoid agents. Prednisone is converted by the liver to prednisolone. Except for cases of liver failure, the drugs can essentially be used interchangeably. These drugs are indicated for the treatment of a number of medical problems including inflammatory and allergic conditions, acute hypersensitivity reactions, severe overwhelming infections with toxicity (in combination with appropriate antibiotic therapy), for supportive care during periods of stress, and for the prevention and treatment of adrenal insufficiency and shock (in conjunction with fluid support). For further information, see **PREDNISOLONE/PREDNISOLONE SODIUM SUCCINATE/PREDNISONE** in the Small Animal section.

OTHER USES
Postadrenalectomy

Glucocorticoid administration has been described during and immediately after adrenalectomy in the ferret; however, it has also been stated that routine treatment is likely unnecessary. Published regimens include dosage with 0.25 to 0.5 mg/kg bid orally for 5 to 10 days, after which the dose is gradually tapered over a period of several weeks to several months. Steroid administration should be based on evidence of clinical need.

Insulinoma

In ferrets, prednisone is used for the initial management of hypoglycemia associated with islet cell neoplasia (insulinoma). Diazoxide is added to the regimen when prednisone alone is no longer efficacious. Medical treatment should be in conjunction with dietary manipulation, that is, frequent high protein/low carbohydrate meals.

Eosinophilic Gastroenteritis

Prednisone is one of the recommended treatments for eosinophilic gastroenteritis in ferrets. Treatment is initiated with doses ranging from 1.5 to 2.5 mg/kg orally once daily until clinical signs abate, usually in approximately 7 days, and then the ferret is gradually weaned off therapy. Some animals may require long-term or even permanent therapy.

Lymphosarcoma

Prednisone can be used palliatively in ferrets with lymphoma to reduce the size of tumor masses and reduce clinical signs such as diarrhea. An oral dose of 2 mg/kg once daily is most commonly recommended. Detailed regimens that also incorporate viscristine and cyclophosphamide are published elsewhere.

ADVERSE AND COMMON SIDE EFFECTS and **DRUG INTERACTIONS:** See GLUCOCORTICOID AGENTS in the Small Animal section.

PROPRANOLOL

INDICATIONS: Propranolol (Inderal ✤ ★) is a nonselective β_1- and β_2-blocking agent. It has been used in ferrets primarily for the medical management of hypertrophic cardiomyopathy. Diltiazem may be a more effective choice. See **PROPRANOLOL** in the Small Animal section.

ADVERSE AND COMMON SIDE EFFECTS and **DRUG INTERACTIONS:** See PROPRANOLOL in the Small Animal section.

PROSTAGLANDIN F$_{2\alpha}$

INDICATIONS: Prostaglandin F$_{2\alpha}$ (Lutalyse ✤ ★) has been used in the treatment of metritis in the ferret. The drug causes contraction of the myometrium and relaxation of the cervix. Reduction in uterine size and improvement in clinical signs are not evident for at least 48 hours after the start of therapy. It also has been used as an abortifacient in small animals.

ADVERSE AND COMMON SIDE EFFECTS: See PROSTAGLAN-DIN $F_{2\alpha}$ in the Small Animal section.

DRUG INTERACTIONS: The concurrent use of estrogens is not recommended because estrogens enhance the effects of the drug on the uterus.

PYRANTEL PAMOATE

INDICATIONS: Pyrantel pamoate (Pyr-A-Pam ♣, Pyran ♣, Nemex ★) is an anthelmintic used to eradicate enteric nematodes. Pyrantel is a cholinesterase inhibitor.

ADVERSE AND COMMON SIDE EFFECTS: Cautious use of the drug is advised in patients with liver dysfunction, malnutrition, dehydration, and anemia. Although the drug is considered safe, vomiting may occur.

DRUG INTERACTIONS: The drug should not be used concurrently with levamisole because of similar mechanisms of action and potential toxicity. Adverse effects may be potentiated by the concurrent use of organophosphates or diethylcarbamazine. Piperazine and pyrantel have antagonistic actions and should not be used together.

PYRETHRIN-CONTAINING PRODUCTS

INDICATIONS: Pyrethrin-containing products (Sectrol ♣ ★, Ovitrol ♣ ★, and many others) are naturally occurring insecticides derived from the plant *Chrysanthemum cinerariae-folium*, and are commonly used for flea control. These drugs are γ-aminobutyric acid (GABA) agonists that stimulate the insect's central nervous system, causing muscular excitation, convulsions, and paralysis. Insect mortality is enhanced when these products are combined with piperonyl butoxide (e.g., Sectrol and Ovitrol). Piperonyl butoxide inhibits pyrethrin metabolism.

ADVERSE AND COMMON SIDE EFFECTS: These products are relatively nontoxic to mammals. See **PYRETHRIN-CONTAINING PRODUCTS** in the Small Animal section.

DRUG INTERACTIONS: See PYRETHRIN-CONTAINING PRODUCTS in the Small Animal section.

SUPPLIED AS: VETERINARY PRODUCTS
Powder, spray, and shampoo formulations containing varying percentages of pyrethrin and piperonyl butoxide. Some products also contain carbaryl and other insecticidal compounds.

STANOZOLOL

INDICATIONS: Stanozolol (Winstrol-V ♣ ★) is an anabolic steroid with strong anabolic and weak androgenic activity. It is potentially useful as an adjunct to the management of catabolic disease states. The drug has been recommended to stimulate erythropoiesis, arouse appetite, promote weight gain, and increase strength and vitality. The efficacy of promoting these positive changes is variable and prolonged treatment (3–6 months) may be required before a response in the erythron is seen. Also see **ANABOLIC STEROIDS and STANOZOLOL** in the Small Animal section.

ADVERSE AND COMMON SIDE EFFECTS and **DRUG INTER-ACTIONS:** See **STANOZOLOL** in the Small Animal section.

SUCRALFATE

INDICATIONS: Sucralfate (Carafate ★, Sulcrate ♣) accelerates the healing of oral, esophageal, gastric, and duodenal ulcers and has been used in ferrets for the treatment of gastritis and gastric ulcers. See **SUCRALFATE** in the Small Animal section.

ADVERSE AND COMMON SIDE EFFECTS: Side effects are rare. Constipation is the only significant problem reported in small animals.

DRUG INTERACTIONS: Antacids and H_2-blocking agents decrease gastric pH and reduce the efficacy of sucralfate and should be spaced apart by at least 30 minutes. See **SUCRALFATE** in the Small Animal section.

SULFADIMETHOXINE

INDICATIONS: Sulfadimethoxine (Albon ★, SULFA 125 and 250 ♣) is a sulfonamide antibiotic used most commonly in ferrets for the eradication of coccidiosis. See **SULFADIMETHOXINE** in the Small Animal section for further information.

ADVERSE AND COMMON SIDE EFFECTS: See SULFONAMIDE ANTIBIOTICS in the Small Animal section.

DRUG INTERACTIONS: Although injectable formats are available, IM injection is associated with pain and poor blood drug levels and is not recommended. See **SULFONAMIDE ANTIBIOTICS** in the Small Animal section.

SUPPLIED AS: VETERINARY PRODUCTS
Oral tablets: see Small Animal section.
Numerous powder and liquid large animal and poultry formulations for use in the drinking water ★.

SULFASALAZINE

INDICATIONS: Sulfasalazine (Azulfidine ★, Salazopyrin ✦) has been used in the treatment of inflammatory bowel disease in the ferret. In the colon, bacteria degrade the drug to release aminosalicylic acid, which has an anti-inflammatory effect, and sulfapyridine. See **SULFASALAZINE** in the Small Animal section for further details on mode of action.

ADVERSE AND COMMON SIDE EFFECTS: See SULFASALAZINE in the Small Animal section.

DRUG INTERACTIONS: Antibiotics may alter metabolism of sulfasalazine by altering intestinal flora, and antacids may decrease absorption. See **SULFASALAZINE** in the Small Animal section for specific drug interactions.

TETRACYCLINE

INDICATIONS: The tetracycline antibiotics exert a bacteriostatic effect against many aerobic and anaerobic gram-positive and gram-negative bacteria, spirochetes, mycoplasmas, and rickettsial organisms. Tetracycline itself is short-acting and water soluble. Tetracycline antibiotics are especially useful against *Leptospira, Chlamydia, Brucella, Mycoplasma, Pseudomonas, Rickettsia,* and *Actinomyces* organisms. They are also used in the treatment of protozoan infections.

Tetracycline has been suggested for the treatment of proliferative bowel disease in ferrets; however, chloramphenicol is thought to be more effective.

ADVERSE AND COMMON SIDE EFFECTS and **DRUG INTERACTIONS:** See **TETRACYCLINE ANTIBIOTICS** in the Small Animal section.

SUPPLIED AS: VETERINARY PRODUCT
For oral administration containing 100 mg/mL [Panmycin Aquadrops Liquid✦★]

THEOPHYLLINE

INDICATIONS: Theophylline (Theo-Dur ✦ ★, Theolair ✦ ★, Quibron-T/SR ✦ ★, Slo-Bid ✦ ★) is a bronchodilator indicated for the management of cough due to bronchospasm. See **THEOPHYLLINE** in the Small Animal section.

ADVERSE AND COMMON SIDE EFFECTS: A number of contraindications to treatment and side effects have been noted in small animals. See **THEOPHYLLINE** in the Small Animal section.

DRUG INTERACTIONS: A number of interactions exist. See **THEO-PHYLLINE** in the Small Animal section.

THIACETARSAMIDE

INDICATIONS: Thiacetarsamide (Caparsolate ♣ ★) has been used to a limited extent in ferrets for the eradication of adult heartworms (*Dirofilaria immitis*).

ADVERSE AND COMMON SIDE EFFECTS: A number of adverse effects have been described in dogs and cats; see **THIACETARS-AMIDE** in the Small Animal section. Thromboembolism is a significant posttreatment complication in ferrets. Heparin therapy is recommended to reduce the occurrence of this: 100 U per ferret once daily; SC for up to 5 days before and for 14 to 21 days after administration of thiacetarsamide. After 3 weeks of heparin therapy, aspirin (22 mg/kg once daily; SC) can be administered for an additional 3 months.

DRUG INTERACTIONS: Glucocorticoids may have a protective effect on adult heartworms, decreasing the efficacy of thiacetarsamide. In addition, glucocorticoids may cause increased pulmonary vascular intimal proliferation, predisposing to obstruction. Despite this, prednisolone (1 mg/kg once daily; PO for 7 to 14 days) or prednisolone (2.2 mg/kg once daily; PO for 3 months) have been suggested as alternatives to posttreatment heparin therapy.

TRIMETHOPRIM-SULFONAMIDE COMBINATIONS

INDICATIONS: Trimethoprim-sulfonamide combinations, i.e., sulfadiazine (Tribrissen ♣ ★, Trivetrin ♣, Septra ♣ ★, Bactrim ♣ ★, and others) and sulfamethoxazole, are bactericidal antibiotics recommended for the treatment of infections by susceptible organisms in a variety of soft tissues, especially the respiratory and urinary tracts, and for the treatment of intestinal coccidiosis.

ADVERSE AND COMMON SIDE EFFECTS: None are specifically described in the ferret. Excessive salivation may occur in animals given uncoated tablets.

DRUG INTERACTIONS: Antacids may decrease the bioavailability of oral trimethoprim-sulfa if administered concurrently.

SUPPLIED AS: VETERINARY PRODUCTS
For injection containing 40 mg/mL trimethoprim and 200 mg/mL sulfadiazine [Tribrissen 24% ♣]

For injection containing 40 mg/mL trimethoprim and 200 mg/mL sulfadoxine [Bimotrin ♣, Borgal ♣, Trimidox ♣, Trivetrin ♣]
For injection containing 80 mg/mL trimethoprim and 400 mg/mL sulfadiazine [Tribrissen 48% ♣]
Tablets containing trimethoprim plus sulfadiazine in the following combinations: 5 + 25, 20 + 100, 80 + 400 [DiTrim★, Tribrissen ♣ ★]
Oral suspension containing 9.1 mg trimethoprim and 45.5 mg sulfa-diazine/mL [Tribrissen ♣]

HUMAN PRODUCTS
Oral suspensions containing 40 mg trimethoprim and 200 mg sul-famethoxazole/5 mL [Bactrim ♣ ★, Septra ♣ ★, and many others]
Oral suspensions containing 45 mg trimethoprim and 205 mg sulfa-diazine/5 mL [Coptin ♣]

TYLOSIN

INDICATIONS: Tylosin (Tylan ♣ ★, Tylocine ♣, Tylosin ★) is a macrolide antibiotic with activity against gram-negative and gram-positive bacteria, spirochetes, chlamydiae, and mycoplasma organisms. The drug has been used to manage canine and feline colitis and has been recommended for the treatment of proliferative bowel disease in the ferret.

ADVERSE AND COMMON SIDE EFFECTS: Anorexia, diarrhea, and local pain with IM injection are reported in dogs and cats.

DRUG INTERACTIONS: Tylosin may increase serum digitalis levels.

VITAMIN B COMPLEX

INDICATIONS: Vitamin B complex ♣ ★ is used as a component of supportive therapy.

ADVERSE AND COMMON SIDE EFFECTS AND DRUG INTER-ACTIONS: See **THIAMINE** in the Small Animal section.

SUPPLIED AS: VETERINARY PRODUCT
For injection containing various vitamin level combinations [Vita-min B Complex ♣ ★, Vita-Jec B Complex Fortified ★, Vita-Jec B Com-plex ★, Compound 150 ♣, Hi-Po B Complex ★, Vitamin B Complex Forte ★, Vitamin B Complex Fortified ★, Vitamin B Complex Forti-fied injection ★, Vitamin B Complex injection ★]
Oral syrup [V.A.L. Syrup ★]

VITAMIN C

See **ASCORBIC ACID**

Handbook of Veterinary Drugs, Second Edition, edited by Dana Allen,
Lippincott–Raven Publishers, Philadelphia. © 1998

Section 14

The Use of Chemotherapeutic Agents in Reptilian Medicine

CHOICE OF MEDICATION

Recommendations for the use of chemotherapeutic agents in reptiles are primarily based on clinical experience rather than on controlled or pharmacokinetic studies. Many are derived from mammalian doses and have not been adapted for the variations in body size and metabolic rate that occur in reptiles. Information on safety and efficacy is likewise derived. For a given drug, suggested dosage and frequency and routes of administration often vary widely from one report to another. Generalizations across the classes of reptiles are made; however, the appropriateness of this has seldom been investigated. Because reptiles are ectothermic, ambient or body temperature has a significant effect on absorption, distribution, excretion, and toxicity of administered medications. These factors have rarely been considered by investigators. No medications are specifically designed or registered for use in reptiles; therefore, all treatments are "extralabel" and require the discretion and experience of the veterinarian. Despite these problems, chemotherapeutic agents are widely and effectively used for the treatment of disease in reptiles. The compounds listed in this text are those recommended in the literature and currently marketed in Canada or the United States. Unfortunately, for most species/drug combinations, there is no single "right" dose. Where a particular drug has been recommended for use in a particular species, or for a particular medical condition, this has been noted. Dosages based on pharmacokinetic or controlled efficacy trials are noted with an asterisk in the table. General information and drug availability are provided in the Small Animal section, as noted, or in the reptile section itself.

ROUTES OF ADMINISTRATION

Medications are administered to reptiles primarily via the oral, subcutaneous, and intramuscular routes. Venous access in many species is difficult or impossible to obtain. Oral medications can be administered in the food (e.g., by injection into a prey species), by mixing with a prepared diet, directly into the oral cavity, especially in some lizards, or by direct gastric or esophageal intubation. Opening the mouth to pass a stomach tube may not be possible in some turtles or tortoises. It is advised that parenteral injections be administered to the cranial half of the body. Reptiles have a renal portal system: the blood from the posterior portions of the body passes through renal peritubular venous plexii before entering the general circulation. This circulatory pattern could result in the immediate excretion of a drug filtered or secreted through the kidney or, because of high local drug concentrations, in increased nephrotoxicity. These concerns have not been substantiated by the very few studies that have touched on renal physiology in relation to drug therapy, but until there is more documented information, the veterinarian is advised to continue the practice of using the anterior half of the body whenever feasible. In snakes, intramuscular injections are made into the epaxial muscles on either side of the dorsal spinous processes. In lizards and chelonians, the muscles of the forelegs are generally used. Small specimens may not have adequate muscle mass for repeated injections and other routes must be considered. Subcutaneous administration is a common alternative. Some injectable compounds (e.g., calcium) can be diluted in saline or other isotonic fluids and administered intracoelomically. Caution must be taken to avoid injuring the coelomic viscera with the needle or catheter.

ENVIRONMENTAL TEMPERATURE

As ectotherms, reptiles rely on external means to maintain body temperature. It has been shown that metabolism, the immune system, healing, and resistance to infection are all highly influenced by temperature. It is, therefore, essential that animals are held at appropriate ambient temperatures during treatment. The upper end of the preferred optimum temperature (POT) range is generally recommended; the specific temperature zone will vary considerably among species. Between 25° and 30°C is commonly selected for many temperate and tropical reptiles. Ambient temperature also affects drug pharmacokinetics and the blood concentration of the antibiotic necessary for successful bacterial elimination. The in vitro minimum inhibitory concentration values for some reptile pathogens have been shown to decrease with increasing environmental temperature. Unfortunately, there has been insufficient research to allow these factors to be adjusted on a routine clinical basis.

Handbook of Veterinary Drugs, Second Edition, edited by Dana Allen,
Lippincott–Raven Publishers, Philadelphia. © 1998

Section 15

Common Dosages for Reptiles

Drug	Dosage	Indication/Species
Albendazole	50 to 75 mg/kg; PO	nematodiasis
Amikacin	*5 mg/kg loading dose, then 2.5 mg/kg q 72 hr; IM	gopher snakes at 25° and 37°C
	*3.5 mg/kg once; IM	ball pythons at 25° and 37°C
	*5 mg/kg q 48 hr; IM	gopher tortoises at 30°C
	*2.25 mg/kg frequency not specified; IM	juvenile American alligators at 22°C
	2.5 or 5 mg/kg initial dose, then 2.5 mg/kg q 72 hr; IM	common recommendation for snakes and lizards
	2 mg/10 mL saline	for nebulization
Amitraz	2 mL/L water as pour on	ticks on mountain tortoises
Amoxicillin	22 mg/kg once to twice daily; PO	

Drug	Dosage	Indication/Species
Amphotericin B	5 mg nebulized in 150 mL saline twice daily for 1 hr for 7 days 1 mg/kg diluted with water or saline once daily for 14 to 28 days; intratracheally	for mycotic pneumonia
Ampicillin	*50 mg/kg bid–tid; IM 3 to 10 mg/kg once to twice daily; PO, SC, IM	spur-tailed tortoises at 27°C
Ascorbic acid	10 to 25 mg/kg; SC, IM 100 to 250 mg/kg; IM	
Atropine sulfate	0.01 to 0.04 mg/kg; SC, IM 0.02 to 0.04 mg/kg bid for at least 10 days; SC 0.04 to 0.1 mg/kg as needed	preanesthetic excess oral/respiratory mucus in boid snakes organophosphate toxicity
Calcitonin	50 U/kg once weekly for 2 treatments; IM	metabolic bone disease
Calcium products—oral	230 to 500 mg/kg q 12 to 24 hr; PO	calcium deficiency, metabolic bone disease
Calcium products—parenteral	500 mg/kg (diluted to 10%) once or at 12- to 48-hr intervals as necessary; intracoelomic 10 to 100 mg/kg (diluted from 1% to 10%) once to twice daily or as needed; SC, IM, IV	calcium deficiency, metabolic bone disease, before oxytocin or vasotocin to treat hypocalcemic egg binding
Calcium EDTA	2 mg/kg; IM	lead poisoning in a snapping turtle
Carbaryl	2.5% solution in alcohol; apply topically 5% dusting powder; rinse after 30 minutes	ectoparasites

Drug	Dosage	Indication/Species
Carbenicillin	*400 mg/kg once daily; IM *400 mg/kg 48 hr; IM 100 to 400 mg/kg once daily; IM	snakes at 30°C tortoises at 30°C commonly reported range of dosage
Cefotaxime	20 to 40 mg/kg once daily to q 72 hr; IM	commonly reported range of dosage
Ceftazidime	*20 mg/kg q 72 hr; IM	snakes at 30°C
Cefuroxime	50 mg/kg q 48 hr; IM 100 mg/kg once daily; IM	snakes at 30°C
Cephalothin	20 to 40 mg/kg bid; IM	
Chloramphenicol palmitate	100 mg/kg once daily; PO	
Chloramphenicol succinate	*40 mg/kg once daily; SC *50 mg/kg; SC 20 to 50 mg/kg once daily or 7 to 20 mg/kg bid; SC, IM	gopher snakes at 24°C snakes at 26°C. Dosing frequency from 14 to 99 hr depending on species of snake. See description of drug for details. commonly reported range of dosage
Chlorhexidine (2% solution)	1:20 or 1:30 dilution in water, swab on affected area bid for at least 10 to 14 days 20 mL/US gallon water (5.5 mL/L)	mouth rot in snakes topically for bacterial shell disease in chelonians or mycotic dermatitis in iguanas
Chlortetracycline	200 mg/kg once daily; PO	
Ciprofloxacin	5 mg/kg once daily; PO	common kingsnakes
Clindamycin	5 mg/kg once daily; PO	common kingsnakes
Dexamethasone	0.0625 to 0.25 mg/kg; IM, IV	septic shock, trauma

Drug	Dosage	Indication/Species
Dichlorvos	12.5 mg/kg once daily for 2 days; PO	ascarids
Dichlorvos impregnated resin strip	0.5 to 6.0 mm/10 ft³ of cage space. Treat for 2 to 5 days, repeat in 14 days if required.	ectoparasites
Diethylcarbamazine citrate	50 mg/kg once, repeat at 2- to 3-wk intervals; PO	ascarids
	3 mg/kg once daily for 1 to 2 mo; PO	microfilaria
Diloxanide	0.5 g/kg single dose; PO	amebiasis
Dimetridazole	100 mg/kg single dose, repeat in 2 wk; PO	amebae and flagellates
	40 mg/kg single dose, repeat in 2 wk; PO	sensitive snake species (e.g., tricolor king, indigo, milk, Uracoan rattler)
	20 to 40 mg/kg once daily for 5 days; repeat in 2 wk; PO	amebiasis, trichomoniasis in snakes
	20 mg/kg once daily for 10 days; PO	
	60 to 100 mg/kg once daily for 5 days, repeat in 2 wk; PO	
Doxapram	0.25 mL/kg; IV	to stimulate respiration during anesthesia and anesthetic recovery
Doxycycline	5 to 10 mg/kg once daily for 10 to 45 days; PO	respiratory syndrome of desert tortoises
	*50 mg/kg once, then 25 mg/kg in 8 days if necessary; IM	spur-tailed tortoises at 27°C
Emetine HCl	0.5 mg/kg once daily for 10 days; SC, IM	tissue amebiasis
	2.5 or 5.5 mg/kg once daily for 5 to 7 days; SC, IM	
Enrofloxacin	*10 mg/kg loading dose, then 5 mg/kg q 48 hr; IM	for sensitive gram-negative bacteria, juvenile Burmese pythons at 26°C

Drug	Dosage	Indication/Species
Enrofloxacin (continued)	*10 mg/kg q 48 hr; IM	for *Pseudomonas* spp, juvenile Burmese pythons at 26°C
	*5 mg/kg q 24 to 48 hr	for respiratory pasteurellosis and other infections in gopher tortoises at 30°C
	*5 mg/kg q 24 hr; IM	for susceptible gram-negative organisms, Indian star tortoises at 26° to 30°C
	*5 mg/kg q 12 hr; IM	for *Pseudomonas* and *Citrobacter* spp, Indian star tortoises at 26° to 30°C
	5 or 10 mg/kg once daily or q 48 hr; PO, SC, IM	commonly reported range of dosage
	5 mg/kg q 48 hr; IM + 50 mg enrofloxacin/250 mL sterile water or saline, flush each nostril with 1 to 3 mL q 24 to 48 hr until no nasal discharge is visible	upper respiratory disease in desert tortoises (combined parenteral and topical administration)
Febantel + praziquantel (Vercom)	0.5 to 1 mL/kg once, repeat in 14 days; PO	nematodes in prehensile-tailed skinks
Fenbendazole	*10 to 100 mg/kg q 14 days for a maximum of 4 treatments; PO	nematodiasis in ball pythons
	50 to 100 mg/kg, repeat in 2 wk; PO	commonly reported range of dosage
	100 mg/kg once daily for 3 days, repeat the 3 treatments in 3 wk; PO	ascarids in box turtles
	100 mg/kg once; per cloaca	oxyurid infestations in tortoises
Gentamicin sulfate	*2.5 mg/kg at a minimum of 72-hr intervals; SC	gopher snakes at 24°C

Drug	Dosage	Indication/Species
Gentamicin sulfate (continued)	*2.5 to 3 mg/kg loading dose, then 1.5 mg/kg q 96 hr	blood pythons
	*10 mg/kg q 48 to 72 hr for no more than 2 wks; IM	red-eared slider and western painted turtles at 26°C
	*6 mg/kg q 3 to 5 days; IM	red-eared slider turtles at 24°C
	*3 mg/kg q 72 hr	box turtles at 21° to 29°C
	*1.75 mg/kg q 96 hr; IM	juvenile American alligators at 22°C
	2.5 to 4 mg/kg q 72 to 96 hr; IM	commonly reported range of dosage
	10 to 20 mg/15 mL saline; nebulize for 30 min twice daily	respiratory disease in tortoises
	2 mg/10 mL saline for nebulization	respiratory disease
Glucose	3 g/kg; PO	hypoglycemia in crocodilians
Glycopyrrolate	0.01 mg/kg once; SC	preanesthetic
	0.01 mg/kg once daily; SC	to reduce oral and respiratory mucus in boid snakes
Itraconazole	23.5 mg/kg; PO with food	spiny lizards
Ivermectin	*200 μg/kg, repeat in 2 wk, maximum of 4 treatments; PO	ball pythons
	200 to 400 μg/kg, repeat in 2 wk; IM, SC, PO	commonly reported range of dosage
	200 μg/kg weekly for 3 wk; SC	skin mites in snakes
	5 mg/L water sprayed on the skin as one treatment	skin mites in snakes
	1,000 μg/kg once, or repeat in 14 to 16 days; PO	to eliminate shedding of pentastome eggs in Tokay and Standings day geckos

Drug	Dosage	Indication/Species
Ivermectin (continued)		Ivermectin can be toxic to chelonians even at low dosage—use with extreme care and with knowledge of species sensitivity.
Kanamycin sulfate	10 to 15 mg/kg once daily; IM, IV, wound flush	
Ketoconazole	*15 mg/kg once daily; PO	gopher tortoises at 27°C
	15 to 50 mg/kg once daily to bid for 14 to 28 days; PO	commonly reported range of dosage
	25 mg/kg once daily for 2 wk; PO	mycotic dermatitis and pneumonia in chelonians
	50 mg/kg once daily for 2 wk; PO	mycotic dermatitis in crocodilians
	50 mg/kg + 50 mg/kg thiabendazole once daily for 2 wk; PO	mycotic pneumonia in juvenile green sea turtles
Levamisole	5 to 20 mg/kg, repeat in 2 to 3 wk; SC, IM, intracoelomically	ascarids, acanthocephalans, pentastomes, rhabdias
Lincomycin	6 mg/kg once to twice daily; IM	commonly reported range of dosage
	10 mg/kg bid; PO	snakes
Mebendazole	20 to 25 mg/kg, repeat in 2 wk; PO	nematodiasis; commonly reported range of dosage
	50 to 100 mg/kg, repeat in 2 wk; PO	nematodiasis; skinks, snakes, and other species
Meperidine	*2 to 4 mg/kg; intracoelomically	pain reduction in Nile crocodiles
Metronidazole	40 to 100 mg/kg, repeat in 2 wk; PO	amebiasis, trichomonas and other flagellates; commonly reported range of dosage

Drug	Dosage	Indication/Species
Metronidazole (continued)	40 mg/kg, repeat in 2 wk; PO	sensitive snake species (e.g., tricolor king, indigo, milk, whipsnakes, racers, Uracoan rattlers)
	50 to 100 mg/kg once; PO	to stimulate appetite in snakes
	75 to 275 mg/kg once daily for 3 days, or weekly; PO	commonly reported range of dosage
	60 to 80 mg/kg once daily for 3 treatments; SC	chelonians less than 1 kg
Midazolam	*1.5 to 2.5 mg/kg; IM	sedation in red-eared slider turtles at 24° to 27°C
	*2 mg/kg combined with 20 to 40 mg/kg of ketamine; IM	sedation and anesthesia in snapping turtles at 21°C
Milbemycin	0.25 to 0.5 mg/kg; PO, SC	nematodiasis in red-eared slider, Gulf coast box, and ornate box turtles
Neomycin	2.5 mg/kg once to twice daily; PO	with methscopalamine (Biosol-M)
Nystatin	100,000 U/kg once daily for 10 days; PO	oral candidiasis, gastrointestinal yeast infections
Oxytetracycline HCl	6 to 12 mg/kg once daily; PO, IM	
Oxytocin	1 to 20 U/kg; IM; repeat in 2 to 4 hr as necessary	commonly reported range of dosage
Paromomycin	25 to 110 mg/kg once daily for up to 4 wk; PO 25 or 55 mg/kg once, repeat in 7 or 14 days, respectively; PO	amebiasis in snakes
Penicillin G	10,000 to 20,000 U/kg tid–qid; SC, IM 20,000 to 80,000 U/kg, IM, as a wound flush	

Drug	Dosage	Indication/Species
Penicillin, benzathine	10,000 U/kg q 48 to 96 hr; IM	
Penicillin, benzathine/ procaine	10,000 U/kg q 24 to 72 hr; IM	
Piperacillin	*100 mg/kg q 48 hr; IM	blood pythons at 28° to 30°C
	100 to 200 mg/kg once daily or q 48 hr; IM	commonly reported range of dosage
Piperazine	40 to 60 mg/kg once daily, repeat in 10 to 14 days; PO	nematodes
Polymyxin B	1 to 2 mg/kg once daily; IM	
Praziquantel	3.5 to 8 mg/kg, repeat in 14 days; PO, IM, SC	cestodes, trematodes
Praziquantel plus febantel (Vercom)	0.5 to 1 mL/kg, repeat in 2 wk; PO	nematodes in prehensile-tailed skinks
Prednisolone sodium succinate	5 to 10 mg/kg as required; IM, IV	septic shock
Propranolol	1 mg/kg; intracoelomically	to stimulate egg laying, in conjunction with vasotocin and prostaglandin, in plateus lizards
Prostaglandin $F_2\alpha$	25 μg/kg; intracoelomically	to stimulate nesting behavior and egg laying, in conjunction with vasotocin and propranolol, in plateus lizards
Prostaglandin E_2	0.09 mg/kg intracloacally, near cervix	to stimulate oviposition in a spotted python, in conjunction with prostaglandin $F_2\alpha$
Pyrethrin	0.09% spray; saturate animal for 5 min, then soak in water for 30 min	mites on chuckwallas

Drug	Dosage	Indication/Species
Pyrethrin (continued)	1% permethrin; spray lightly then blot off excess. Wash animals and repeat in 10 days if required.	mites on snakes
Selenium	0.028 mg/kg (route not stated)	presumptive myopathy in a green iguana
Silver sulfadiazine	topically (oral and cutaneous)	mouth rot in snakes, burns
Streptomycin sulfate	5 to 10 mg/kg bid; IM, topically	cutaneous wounds and infections
Sulfadiazine	75 mg/kg once on day 1, then 45 mg/kg on days 2 to 6; PO 25 mg/kg once daily for 7 to 21 days; PO	intestinal and biliary coccidia
Sulfadimethoxine	90 mg/kg once on day 1, then 45 mg/kg once daily for an additional 4 to 6 days; PO, IM 90 mg/kg q second day for 3 treatments; PO 30 mg/kg once on day 1, then 15 mg/kg once daily for an additional 3 days; IM 75 mg/kg once on day 1, then 40 mg/kg once daily for an additional 5 days; PO, IM	intestinal and biliary coccidia
Sulfadimidine (33%)	0.3 to 0.6 mL/kg once on day 1, then the same or one-half the dose once daily for an additional 9 days; PO	intestinal and biliary coccidia
Sulfamethazine	75 or 90 mg/kg once on day 1, then 40 or 45 mg/kg once daily for an additional 4 to 5 treatments; PO 25 mg/kg once daily for 7 to 21 days; PO	intestinal and biliary coccidia

Drug	Dosage	Indication/Species
Sulfame-thoxydiazine	80 mg/kg once, then 40 mg/kg once daily for an additional 4 treatments; SC, IM	intestinal and biliary coccidia
Sulfamerazine	25 mg/kg once daily for 21 days; PO	intestinal and biliary coccidia
Sulfaquinoxyline	75 mg/kg once on day 1, then 40 mg/kg once daily for an additional 6 treatments; PO, IM	intestinal and biliary coccidia
Tetracycline	10 mg/kg once daily; PO 25 to 50 mg/kg once to twice daily; PO, SC, IM	snakes, crocodilians
Thiabendazole	50 to 100 mg/kg, repeat in 2 wk; PO	nematodiasis
Tiletamine-zolazepam	*15 mg/kg; IM	for minor chemical restraint in American alligators
	4 to 9 mg/kg; IM	tranquilizer, light anesthetic, preanesthetic in reptiles, especially Eastern box turtles
	5 to 40 mg/kg; IM	chemical restraint and immobilization in chameleons
	10 to 30 mg/kg; IM	chemical restraint and induction agent in iguanas
Tobramycin	2.5 mg/kg q 72 hr; IM 2.5 mg/kg bid; IM	chameleons
Tolnaftate	1% cream bid; topically	mycotic dermatitis
Trimethoprim-sulfadiazine, sulfadoxine, sulfamethoxazole	15 to 30 mg/kg once to twice daily; PO, SC, IM	antibacterial therapy
	15 to 30 mg/kg once daily for 2 days, then q 2nd day for 3 wk; SC, IM	middle ear infections in box turtles
	30 mg/kg once daily for 7 days; PO, SC, IM	enteric coccidia

Drug	Dosage	Indication/Species
Trimethoprim-sulfadiazine, sulfadoxine, sulfamethoxazole (continued)	30 mg/kg; PO or IM once on day 1, then 15 mg/kg; IM or 30 mg/kg; PO q 48 hr for up to an additional 14 treatments	enteric coccidia
	30 to 60 mg/kg once daily for 2 mo; PO	may reduce infection by cryptosporidia in snakes
Tylosin	5 mg/kg once daily for up to 60 days; IM	
	25 mg/kg once daily; PO, IM	
Vasotocin	0.01 to 1 µg/kg; intracoelomically	to stimulate egg laying
Vitamin A	10,000 to 11,000 IU/kg once; SC, IM	vitamin A deficiency in chelonians
	2,000 IU/kg once weekly for 4 to 6 wk; SC	box turtles
	5 IU/10 g; SC, IM	
	2,000 IU/kg once daily each third day for 2 wk, then once weekly for 2 treatments; SC, IM	
	10,000 IU/300 g loading dose, then 2,000 IU/300 g weekly for 2 to 3 treatments; PO	box turtles
Vitamin B complex	0.5 mL/kg; PO	nutritional supplement, appetite stimulant
	0.25 to 0.5 mL/kg; SC, IM	
Vitamin B_1 (Thiamine)	1.5 mg/kg once daily for 2 wk	
Vitamin B_{12} (Cyanocobalamin)	50 µg/kg; SC, IM	
	10 to 2,500 mg depending on body weight; IM	
Vitamin C—see Ascorbic Acid		
Vitamin D_3	100 to 200 IU/kg once weekly; IM	metabolic bone disease in iguanas
	1500 to 1650 IU/kg single dose; IM	hypovitaminosis D
	7500 IU q 2 wk as needed; IM	tortoises

Drug	Dosage	Indication/Species
Vitamin E	50 to 100 mg/kg as needed; IM 50 to 800 IU/kg 1 to 3 times per wk	nutritional muscular dystrophy steatitis in aquatic chelonians and crocodilians
Vitamin K	0.25 to 0.5 mg/kg; IM	vitamin K deficiency in crocodilians, aid in coagulation factor production

Handbook of Veterinary Drugs, Second Edition, edited by Dana Allen,
Lippincott–Raven Publishers, Philadelphia. © 1998

Section 16

Description of Drugs for Reptiles

ALBENDAZOLE

INDICATIONS: Albendazole (Valbazen ♣ ★) is an anthelmintic used in the oral treatment of nematodiasis. For more information, see **ALBENDAZOLE** in the Small Animal section.

AMIKACIN

INDICATIONS: Amikacin (Amiglyde-V ♣ ★, Amikin ♣ ★) is an amino-glycoside antibiotic indicated in the treatment of superficial and systemic bacterial infections, especially those caused by gram-negative organisms such as *Pseudomonas* and *Aeromonas* spp. The drug can also be nebulized in saline for treatment of pneumonia. For more information, see **AMIKACIN** in the Small Animal section.

Experimental pharmacokinetic studies have been carried out in several species of reptiles. In gopher snakes at 25° and 37°C the rate of absorption and the elimination half-life (71.9 and 75.4 hours, respectively) of amikacin were similar. At the higher temperature, greater volume of distribution and renal clearance resulted in lower serum concentrations of the drug.

Studies in ball pythons held at 25° or 37°C did not show an effect of temperature on amikacin clearance. A dose of 3.48 mg/kg was recommended to achieve serum minimal inhibitory concentration values effective against most gram-negative bacteria, but it was felt that a much higher dosage, i.e., 12 mg/kg, would be required for

Pseudomonas aeruginosa. Amikacin serum levels remained above recommended interdosing trough concentrations for more than 6 days, resulting in the authors' suggestion that treatment consist of a single dose.

In gopher tortoises held at 30°C, a pharmacokinetic study suggested a dosage of 5 mg/kg IM every 48 hours. Tortoises acclimated to 20°C had a similar volume of distribution; however, slower elimination of the drug resulted in amikacin accumulation.

The pharmacokinetics of amikacin were also studied in juvenile American alligators held at a water temperature of 22°C. The half-life of amikacin administered at 1.75 and 2.25 mg/kg IM was shorter than that reported in gopher snakes, suggesting that more frequent dosing is necessary in alligators. The higher dose was recommended to achieve serum levels effective against *Pseudomonas* spp.

ADVERSE AND COMMON SIDE EFFECTS: Nephrotoxicity is reputed to be of concern; however, no reports of this were found. Snakes necropsied 6 days after being administered a single dose of 5 mg/kg did not show histologic evidence of renal disease. During treatment, it is essential to maintain hydration through ensuring the availability of fresh water or by administration of oral, intracoelomic, or SC isotonic fluids. For prolonged therapy, monitoring of plasma or serum uric acid levels may be appropriate. Determination of blood amikacin levels would be helpful. Neurotoxicity has been reported. It has been suggested that a single high dose may give therapeutic levels for several weeks and be less toxic than multiple small doses. Most recent pharmacokinetic studies suggest that the majority of currently published dosage regimes may result in the accumulation of amikacin over time.

DRUG INTERACTIONS: Amikacin is often used in combination with penicillins and cephalosporins such as ampicillin, carbenicillin, piperacillin, and cefotaxime. In vitro exposure to carbenicillin is less inactivating to amikacin than to gentamicin; therefore, amikacin may be a better choice for combination therapy.

AMITRAZ

INDICATIONS: Amitraz (Mitaban ✤ ★) has been used for the removal of *Amblyomma* ticks from mountain tortoises (*Geochelone pardalis*). The emulsion was poured over the tortoises' front and rear carapace openings while they were on their backs, left for a few minutes, then allowed to drain off. The ticks detached and died over 3 to 4 days, after which the tortoises were washed. For more information, see **AMITRAZ** in the Small Animal section.

AMOXICILLIN

INDICATIONS: Amoxicillin (Amoxi-Tabs ★, Amoxi-Drop ★, Amoxi-Inject ★, Amoxil ✦ ★, Moxilean ✦, Robamox-V ★) is indicated for the treatment of superficial and systemic bacterial infections. For more information, see **AMOXICILLIN** in the Small Animal section.

AMPHOTERICIN B

INDICATIONS: Amphotericin B (Fungizone ✦ ★) is an effective antifungal agent that has been used for the treatment of mycotic pneumonia via nebulization or intratracheal infusion. When used parenterally, the drug is highly nephrotoxic in most species. For more information, see **AMPHOTERICIN B** in the Small Animal section.

AMPICILLIN

INDICATIONS: Ampicillin (Omnipen ★, Penbriton ✦, Polyflex ✦ ★) has been recommended for the treatment of bacterial infections including *Pasteurella testudinis* pneumonia in tortoises and ulcerative shell disease in chelonians. For more information, see **AMPICILLIN** in the Small Animal section.

One experimental study looked at the pharmacokinetics of 50 and 100 mg/kg of ampicillin administered IM to spur-tailed tortoises held at 27°C, and compared blood levels with minimal inhibitory concentrations for a range of bacteria isolated from reptiles. Blood levels and drug elimination were similar with both dosage levels; "therapeutic serum levels" of 3 µg/mL were maintained for approximately 8 hours. These dosages were considered appropriate for the treatment of infections by *Staphylococcus* spp, but not *Salmonella* or *Klebsiella* spp. In two animals secondary peaks of blood antibiotic levels were noted; these were attributed to reabsorption of water and ampicillin from the bladder. A range of doses for ampicillin in reptiles has been published in formularies and case reports; most are substantially lower than this.

DRUG INTERACTIONS: Ampicillin is frequently used in combination with aminoglycosides to increase antibacterial spectrum and effectiveness. Lizards and tortoises have been reported cleared of enteric *Salmonella* spp by oral treatment with a combination of 250 mg chloramphenicol and 75 mg ampicillin daily for 10 days.

ASCORBIC ACID

INDICATIONS: Vitamin C (✦ ★) is used as a general supplement for sick reptiles. Vitamin C is sometimes recommended in addition to antibiotic therapy for the treatment of mouth rot in snakes; however, the efficacy is unknown. Vitamin C has also been used in the treatment of splitting skin syndrome in some large constrictors. Because snakes can manufacture vitamin C in their kidneys and intestines, a true deficiency may not occur and treatment is somewhat controversial.

SUPPLIED AS: VETERINARY PRODUCT
For injection 250 mg/mL [Vitamin C✦ ★]

ATROPINE

INDICATIONS: Atropine ✦ ★ is an anticholinergic, antispasmodic, and mydriatic drug used as a preanesthetic and in the treatment of bradycardia and organophosphate toxicity. Its use has also been recommended, in combination with antibiotic therapy, to reduce oral and respiratory mucus in boid snakes with infectious stomatitis or respiratory disease. For more information, see **ATROPINE** in the Small Animal section.

CALCITONIN SALMON

INDICATIONS: Calcitonin (Calcimar ✦ ★) inhibits bone resorption and antagonizes parathormone. In reptiles it is used in the treatment of metabolic bone disease, in conjunction with calcium and vitamin D_3 supplementation and husbandry changes. Most case reports refer to use in the green iguana. For more information, see **CALCITONIN SALMON** in the Small Animal section.

ADVERSE AND COMMON SIDE EFFECTS: Calcitonin should only be used in animals whose blood calcium levels are within normal reference range. Use may otherwise precipitate acute hypocalcemia.

CALCIUM BOROGLUCONATE
CALCIUM GLUBIONATE
CALCIUM GLUCONATE
CALCIUM GLYCEROPHOSPHATE
CALCIUM LACTATE

INDICATIONS: Calcium products are used for the treatment of hypocalcemia and metabolic bone disease, and for the pretreatment of uterine inertia and egg binding prior to the administration of oxytocin or vasotocin. The management of animals with metabolic bone disease should also include vitamin D_3 supplementation and diet and husbandry correction. Calcium glubionate (Neo-Calglucon ★), gluconate (Calcet ✚ ★), and lactate ✚ ★ can be administered orally. Calcium glubionate should be given before feeding to enhance calcium absorption. Calcium gluconate and a glycerophosphate/lactate combination are administered IV, or, if venous access is unavailable, IM, SC, or intracoelomically in a diluted form. For more information, see **CALCIUM GLUCONATE** or **CALCIUM LACTATE** in the Small Animal section.

ADVERSE AND COMMON SIDE EFFECTS: Parenteral calcium can rarely be administered IV; IM and SC injection can result in inflammation, necrosis, and sloughing. This is especially true with large volumes and high concentrations of solution. Intracoelomic administration may result in mild peritonitis and precipitation of calcium on the peritoneal surfaces.

SUPPLIED AS: HUMAN PRODUCTS
Calcium glubionate: oral solution containing 115 mg elemental calcium/5 mL [Neo-Calglucon Syrup ★], 110 mg elemental calcium/5 mL [Calcium Sandoz ✚]
Calcium glycerophosphate powder
Calcium glycerophosphate/lactate: parenteral solution containing 5 mg of each element/mL [Calphosan ★]
VETERINARY PRODUCTS
Calcium glycerophosphate/lactate: solution containing 50 mg/10 mL of each element for IM and SC use [Calphosan Solution★], and IM, SC, and IV use [Cal-pho-sol solution SA ★]
Calcium gluconate or borogluconate: numerous solutions for IV, SC, intraperitoneal use (see individual product information for recommended route of administration) containing 230 mg/mL [23% solution ✚ ★] and 257.5 mg/mL [25.7% solution ✚ ★]

CALCIUM EDTA

INDICATIONS: Calcium disodium EDTA (Calcium Disodium Versenate ✚ ★) is a favored chelating agent for the treatment of lead toxicity in a variety of species. This medication was successfully used in a snapping turtle with elevated blood lead levels and clinical signs consistent with lead poisoning. A dosage of approximately 2 mg/kg was administered every 6 to 13 days for four treatments. For more information, see **CALCIUM EDTA** in the Small Animal section.

CARBARYL

INDICATIONS: Carbaryl (Sevin ✚, Zodiac Flea and Tick Power ✚, and others) is a carbamate insecticide and cholinesterase inhibitor used in the eradication of arthropod ectoparasites, including mites and ticks. A 2.5% solution in alcohol can be used as a topical wipe. Care should be taken to avoid the eyes and mouth. The 5% powder can be applied to environmental surfaces with which the animal has no direct contact, and has been used topically with caution. The powder should be thoroughly rinsed off after approximately 30 minutes of skin contact. For more information, see **CARBAMATE INSECTICIDES** in the Small Animal section.

CARBENICILLIN

INDICATIONS: Carbenicillin (Geopen ✤ ★, Pyopen ✤ ★) is an extended spectrum, penicillinase-sensitive, semisynthetic penicillin used for the treatment of a variety of bacterial infections. It is effective against *Pseudomonas* and *Aeromonas* spp. For more information, see **CARBENICILLIN** in the Small Animal section.

In an experimental study in snakes held at 30°C, carbenicillin administered IM at 400 mg/kg reached peak blood levels in 1 hour; therapeutic levels (defined as > 50 to 60 µg/mL) persisted for at least 12 hours. The authors suggested that previously recommended dosages of approximately 100 mg/kg would not provide effective blood levels and suggested treatment with 400 mg/kg once daily. In a similar study performed in two species of tortoises, also held at 30°C, carbenicillin was rapidly absorbed from the injection site. Thirty-seven hours after injection blood antibiotic levels began to rise again. This was attributed to reabsorption of unchanged drug from the bladder, where urine can be held for long periods of time. Although maintenance of blood levels could be erratic, the authors recommended carbenicillin as a clinically effective drug in tortoises and suggested a dose of 400 mg/kg every 48 hours.

ADVERSE AND COMMON SIDE EFFECTS: Pain on injection has been noted in snakes and in tortoises. Skin rashes have developed after administration to desert tortoises.

DRUG INTERACTIONS: Carbenicillin is used primarily in combination with aminoglycosides to reduce the rate of development of bacterial resistance. Carbenicillin may have a deactivating effect on aminoglycoside antibiotics; therefore, the two drugs should not be mixed in vitro. Treatment with carbenicillin is sometimes delayed until 48 hours after the initiation of aminoglycoside administration.

CEFOTAXIME

INDICATIONS: Cefotaxime (Claforan ✤ ★) is a third-generation cephalosporin used in the treatment of bacterial infections, including those by *Pseudomonas aeruginosa*. For more information, see **CEFOTAXIME** in the Small Animal section.

CEFTAZIDIME

INDICATIONS: Ceftazidime (Fortaz ✚ ★) is a third-generation broad-spectrum cephalosporin with activity against gram-negative bacteria, similar to cefotaxime, but with greater activity against *Pseudomonas aeruginosa*. It is used as an alternative to the aminoglycosides. For more information, see **CEFTAZIDIME** in the Small Animal section.

In an experimental study in snakes held at 30°C, ceftazidime administered IM at 20 mg/kg reached peak blood levels in 1 to 8 hours; therapeutic levels (defined as > 8 µg/mL) persisted for at least 96 hours. Dosing every 72 hours was recommended. The snakes used in this work were clinically ill patients; pharmacokinetic studies have not been carried out in healthy animals.

ADVERSE AND COMMON SIDE EFFECTS: Ceftazidime is less nephrotoxic than other cephalosporins; however, renal damage can occur at high dose levels. The drug is poorly absorbed orally. Some variability in half-life was seen in the above study, but it could not be determined whether this was due to variability in dosing technique or species response.

CEFUROXIME

INDICATIONS: Cefuroxime (Ceftin ✚ ★, Zinacef ✚ ★, Kefurox ✚ ★, Cefuroxime★) is a broad-spectrum cephalosporin antibiotic used for treatment of gram-positive and gram-negative infections. Cefuroxime axetil is intended for oral use and cefuroxime sodium for parenteral administration. For more general information, see **CEPH-ALOSPORIN ANTIBIOTICS** in the Small Animal section.

ADVERSE AND COMMON SIDE EFFECTS: The concomitant administration of aminoglycosides and some cephalosporins has resulted in nephrotoxicity in humans. In humans, pseudomembranous colitis has been reported in association with treatment with cefuroxime.

DRUG INTERACTIONS: Cefuroxime has been used for the treatment of gram-negative infections in snakes, at a dosage of 100 mg/kg daily for 10 days, in combination with gentamicin.

SUPPLIED AS: HUMAN PRODUCTS
For oral medication tablets containing 125★, 250, and 500 mg [Ceftin ✚ ★]
Oral suspension containing 125 mg/5 mL [Ceftin ✚ ★] and 250 mg/5 mL [Ceftin ✚]
For injection containing 750 and 1,500 mg/vial [Cefuroxime★, Zinacef ✚ ★, and Kefurox ✚ ★]

CEPHALOTHIN SODIUM

INDICATIONS: Cephalothin (Keflin ✚ ★) is a broad-spectrum cephalosporin antibiotic used for the treatment of bacterial infections. For more information, see **CEPHALOSPORIN ANTIBIOTICS** in the Small Animal section.

CHLORAMPHENICOL

INDICATIONS: Chloramphenicol (Azramycine ✚, Chlor Palm ✚, Chlor Tablets ✚, Chloromycetin ✚ ★, Karomycin Palmitate ✚, Viceton ★, and many others) is a bacteriostatic antibiotic used for the treatment of superficial and systemic bacterial diseases, including septicemic cutaneous ulcerative disease in aquatic turtles. For more information, see **CHLORAMPHENICOL** in the Small Animal section.

In experimental work with gopher snakes, oral chloramphenicol at a dosage of 12 mg/kg was slowly absorbed and resulted in blood levels of only 10 µg/mL (therapeutic blood levels were defined as blood concentrations > 20–40 µg/mL). Clinical recommendations range from 50 to 100 mg/kg once daily PO.

The pharmacokinetics of parenteral chloramphenicol have also been studied in snakes. In one study involving 16 different species, erratic absorption after SC injection, a wide variation in the rate of elimination among the various species, wide standard deviations within species, and a difference in mean plasma concentrations between two commercial preparations were found. To maintain plasma concentrations of 5 µg/mL, IM injection of 50 mg/kg at the following hours was recommended: gray rat snake—7.7; indigo snake—9.8; boa constrictor—27.6; Burmese python— 29.6; hog-nose snake—30.7; copperhead—36.5; cotton mouth—39.1; Indian rock python—49; eastern diamond back rattlesnake—51; timber rattlesnake—53.4; red-bellied watersnake—61.3; Midland water snake—69.2. All animals were held at 26°C. In another study in gopher snakes kept at 29°C, SC injection of 40 mg/kg resulted in peak blood levels of 26 µg/mL in just over 3 hours, and a half-life of 5.25 hours. The authors suggested dosage once daily.

ADVERSE AND COMMON SIDE EFFECTS: Although mammalian side effects such as blood dyscrasias have not been reported in reptiles, one snake in a pharmacokinetic study became anemic and had green discolored plasma. Chloramphenicol in propylene glycol and benzyl alcohol base may cause focal indurated lesions at sites of injection.

DRUG INTERACTIONS: Lizards and tortoises have been reported cleared of enteric *Salmonella* spp by oral treatment with a combination of 250 mg chloramphenicol and 75 mg ampicillin daily for 10 days.

CHLORHEXIDINE

INDICATIONS: Chlorhexidine (Nolvasan ★, Hibitane ♣) is a chemical used for disinfection and as a base for a variety of antiseptic products. Diluted chlorhexidine solution has been used topically, in combination with systemic antibiotics, for the treatment of mouth rot in snakes and shell infections in chelonians. Clinically, it appears effective against *Pseudomonas*. For more information, see **CHLORHEXIDINE** in the Small Animal section.

ADVERSE AND COMMON SIDE EFFECTS: Two red-bellied short-necked turtles developed flaccid paralysis and corneal opacity after 45 minutes of immersion in 0.024% chlorhexidine (12 mL of 2% solution/L of water) at a temperature of 30°C. Both died. On necropsy, keratitis, tracheitis, pharyngitis, and myocardial necrosis were described.

SUPPLIED AS: VETERINARY PRODUCTS
0.5% solution [Hibitane Teat Dip ♣]
1.6% solution [Della-Prep ♣, Sani-Wash ♣, Hibitane Udder Wash ♣]
2% solution [Nolvasan solution ★, Nolvasan-S ★, Hibitane ♣]
4% solution [Nolvasan Udder Wash Concentrate ★, Nolvasan Teat Dip ★]
5% solution [Nolvasan 5% Teat Dip ★]
1% cream [Hibitane Veterinary Ointment ♣, Nolvasan Antiseptic Ointment ★]

CHLORTETRACYCLINE

INDICATIONS: Chlortetracycline (Aureomycin and others) is a broad-spectrum bacteriostatic antibiotic with activity against gram-positive and gram-negative organisms, chlamydiae, rickettsiae, mycoplasmas, and many anaerobes. For more information, see **TETRACYCLINE ANTIBIOTICS** in the Small Animal section.

DRUG INTERACTIONS: Oral absorption is inhibited by calcium, magnesium, and iron-containing substances.

SUPPLIED AS: VETERINARY PRODUCTS
Water-soluble powder containing, 55 mg/g [Aureomycin ♣], 25.6 g/6.4 oz, or 102.4 g/25.6 oz [Fermycin Soluble ★]
Tablets containing 25 mg [Aureomycin Tablets ★]
Many agricultural feed additives

CIPROFLOXACIN

INDICATIONS: Ciprofloxacin (Cipro ♣ ★) is a fluoroquinolone antibiotic with activity against *Escherichia coli*, *Klebsiella*, *Proteus*, *Pseudomonas*,

Staphylococcus, Salmonella, Shigella, Yersinia, Campylobacter, and *Vibrio* spp. Ciprofloxacin is also produced in vivo as a metabolite after the administration of enrofloxacin. It has been used primarily as an oral medication in reptiles. Although recommendations exist in the literature for formulation of an oral suspension using ciprofloxacin tablets, the duration of activity of the drug is very short when compounded in this manner. This suspension is probably appropriate for only immediate administration. For more information, see **CIPROFLOX-ACIN** and **FLUOROQUINOLONE ANTIBIOTICS** in the Small Animal section.

CLINDAMYCIN

INDICATIONS: Clindamycin (Antirobe ♣ ★, Cleocin ★) is a lincosamide antibiotic with activity against a wide range of gram-positive, gram-negative, and anaerobic bacteria, and some sporozoan organisms. Oral dosage of reptiles with clindamycin has been described. For more information, see **CLINDAMYCIN** in the Small Animal section.

DEXAMETHASONE

INDICATIONS: Dexamethasone (Azium ♣ ★, Azium SP ♣ ★, Dex-5 ♣) is a glucocorticoid that has been used in the treatment of septic shock and acute head trauma. In one report, dexamethasone appeared to stimulate appetite in a Ridley's sea turtle. For more information, see **DEXAMETHASONE** in the Small Animal section.

ADVERSE AND COMMON SIDE EFFECTS: The routine use of glucocorticoids in reptiles is not recommended because of immunosuppressive effects.

DICHLORVOS

INDICATIONS: Dichlorvos (Task ★) is a cholinesterase-inhibitor anthelmintic used for the elimination of nematodes. For more information, see **DICHLORVOS** in the Small Animal section.

DICHLORVOS IMPREGNATED RESIN STRIPS

INDICATIONS: Dichlorvos (Vapona No Pest Strip and others) impregnated resin strips are used for the treatment of ectoparasites including mites, ticks, and fleas. Sections of strip should be placed inside the cage within a ventilated container, such as a perforated plastic vial, to prevent direct contact or ingestion. The dose or length of strip used is empirical. For more information, see **DICHLORVOS** and **ORGANOPHOSPHATE ANTHELMINTICS** in the Small Animal section.

ADVERSE AND COMMON SIDE EFFECTS: This product may be hazardous for humans; headache and nausea may occur after breathing Vapona-laden air. Wear gloves while handling and allow strips to breathe outside for several hours before use. Some lizards, including anoles, may develop hind leg paralysis on exposure to this chemical.

SUPPLIED AS: COMMERCIAL PRODUCTS
Impregnated resin strips containing 20% dichlorvos [Vapona No Pest Strip, Black Flag Insect Strip, and many others]

DIETHYLCARBAMAZINE CITRATE

INDICATIONS: Diethylcarbamazine [DEC] (Carbam ★, Filaribits ✦ ★) is used for treatment of ascarids and microfilaria. For more information, see **DIETHYLCARBAMAZINE** in the Small Animal section.

DIHYDROSTREPTOMYCIN

INDICATIONS: Dihydrostreptomycin (Ethamycin ✦) is an aminoglycoside antibiotic used parenterally for the treatment of bacterial infections and topically for the treatment of abscesses and necrotic stomatitis in snakes. For more information, see **DIHYDROSTREPTOMYCIN** and **AMINOGLYCOSIDE ANTIBIOTICS** in the Small Animal section.

ADVERSE AND COMMON SIDE EFFECTS: During treatment, it is essential to maintain hydration by ensuring the availability of fresh water or by administration of oral, intraperitoneal, or SC isotonic fluids. For prolonged therapy, monitoring of plasma or serum uric acid levels may be appropriate. Streptomycin should not be used in the presence of impaired renal function or dehydration.

DILOXANIDE

INDICATIONS: Diloxanide furoate is an anti-infective agent that has been used for the treatment of amebiasis.

SUPPLIED AS: Diloxanide furoate is available in the United States by special request from the Centers for Disease Control and Prevention [Furamide★].

DIMETRIDAZOLE

INDICATIONS: Dimetridazole (Emtryl ✦) is a water-soluble antiprotozoal agent used for the treatment of amebiasis and trichomoniasis in snakes.

ADVERSE AND COMMON SIDE EFFECTS: Several species of snakes are considered sensitive to the use of metronidazole and dimetridazole as deaths have occurred after treatment with doses greater than 100 mg/kg. These include tricolor king snakes, milk snakes, indigo snakes, and Uracoan rattlesnakes. A lower dose of 40 mg/kg is recommended in these animals. Other species of snakes may react similarly.

SUPPLIED AS: VETERINARY PRODUCTS
Water-soluble powder with 40% W/W [Emtryl Soluble ✦]
Feed additives [Dimetridazole 30% Premix ✦, Emtryl Premix ✦]

DOXAPRAM

INDICATIONS: Doxapram (Dopram-V ✦ ★) has been recommended for use in reptiles to stimulate respiration in patients with postanesthetic respiratory depression or apnea. For more information, see **DOXAPRAM** in the Small Animal section.

DRUG INTERACTIONS: Halothane and enflurane may precipitate arrhythmias. It is recommended that doxapram use be delayed about 10 minutes after discontinuation of these anesthetic agents.

DOXYCYCLINE

INDICATIONS: Doxycycline (Vibramycin ✦ ★, Vibravet ✦) is a second-generation, long-acting, lipid-soluble tetracycline antibiotic used in the treatment of respiratory syndrome in desert tortoises. For more information, see **DOXYCYCLINE** in the Small Animal section.
Experimental pharmacokinetic work was carried out in spur-tailed tortoises held at 27°C in conjunction with investigations into the minimal inhibitory concentration values for bacteria isolated from reptiles. After IM injection of 25 and 50 mg/kg, therapeutic serum concentrations (defined as 8 µg/mL) were maintained for 36 and 70 hours, respectively. These dosages were considered appropriate for the treatment of infections by sensitive strains of *Klebsiella* and *Staphylococcus* spp, but not *Salmonella* spp. Secondary rises in blood doxycycline concentration, attributed to saturation of protein-binding capacity, and summation effects after repeated dosing were noted. The author suggested a dosage of 50 mg/kg would provide adequate blood concentrations for 8 days, after which a second dose of 25 mg/kg could be administered if necessary. Drug elimination half-lives were not noted.

ENROFLOXACIN

INDICATIONS: Enrofloxacin (Baytril ✦ ★) is a fluoroquinolone antibiotic used as a first-line drug for the treatment of bacterial infections in reptiles, including *Pseudomonas aeruginosa* infections and middle ear infections in box turtles. Parenteral administration, combined with nasal flushing, is the treatment of choice for upper respiratory tract disease in tortoises due to the drug's effectiveness against *Mycoplasma* spp and *Pasteurella testudinis*. A portion of the enrofloxacin dose is metabolized to ciprofloxacin in vivo. Both drugs are therefore involved in the therapeutic effect. The injectable formulation of enrofloxacin can be administered orally, and the oral tablets can be formulated into a suspension by a compounding pharmacy. For general information, see **ENROFLOXACIN** in the Small Animal section.

Pharmacokinetic studies have been carried out in juvenile Burmese pythons held at 26°C. Single and multiple dose trials using 5 mg/kg IM resulted in peak blood levels of 1.66 and 2.78 µg/mL, respectively. Half-lives were also different between the two trials: 6.37 and from 12.4 to 31.9 hours. Administration of 5 mg/kg every 48 hours was considered adequate to provide blood concentrations of enrofloxacin greater than the minimal inhibitory concentration for relatively susceptible gram-negative organisms, such as *Escherichia coli*, *Klebsiella*, and *Proteus*, but for *Pseudomonas* 10 mg/kg was recommended.

Experimental work has also been carried out in gopher, Indian star, and spur-tailed tortoises using single and multiple dosing of 5 mg/kg and single doses of 10 mg/kg, all administered IM. In gopher tortoises held at 30°C, plasma concentrations remained above 0.75 µg/mL for 24 hours and above 0.32 µg/mL for 48 hours. Dosage of 5 mg/kg every 24 to 48 hours was recommended for the treatment of respiratory pasteurellosis and other bacterial infections. In Indian star tortoises held at 26° to 30°C and given a single injection of 5 mg/kg, plasma levels remained above 0.2 µg/mL for at least 12 hours in most tortoises. The suggested dosage regime was 5 mg/kg every 24 hours for susceptible species, or every 12 hours for *Pseudomonas* and *Citrobacter* spp. Single-dose pharmacokinetics of dosages of 5 and 10 mg/kg were evaluated in spur-tailed tortoises held at 30°C. Twelve hours after the administration of 5 mg/kg serum levels of enrofloxacin were undetectable. After a dose of 10 mg/kg therapeutic concentrations, defined as 3.5 µg/mL, were maintained for 12 hours. When a second injection of 10 mg/kg was administered 24 hours after the first, therapeutic blood levels were maintained for 16 hours.

ADVERSE AND COMMON SIDE EFFECTS: Enrofloxacin may cause discoloration of the skin or tissue necrosis in some animals if given by the SC route. Muscular necrosis after injection has been described in many species and probably also occurs in reptiles. The largest available and appropriate muscle mass should be used for injection. Local pain or inappetence may be noted after administration.

Long-term usage in desert tortoises, boas and pythons, and green iguanas has been associated with increased uric acid levels. Maintenance of normal hydration through ensuring the availability of fresh water or the administration of oral, intracoelomic, or SC isotonic fluids as required is suggested. Monitoring of serum or plasma uric acid levels may also be appropriate.

FEBANTEL + PRAZIQUANTEL

See **PRAZIQUANTEL**

FENBENDAZOLE

INDICATIONS: Fenbendazole (Panacur ✦ ★) is an anthelmintic recommended for the treatment of nematodes including ascarid, strongyle, and strongyloides infections in snakes, lizards, and tortoises. Tortoises may require 2 to 3 weeks to expel the worms. For more information, see **FENBENDAZOLE** in the Small Animal section.

In an efficacy study in ball pythons positive for nematode ova on fecal examination, fenbendazole was administered at 10, 25, 50, and 100 mg/kg orally every 14 days. All snakes were cleared of infection after four treatments; 95.6% after three. All doses were equally effective. Efficacy of treatment at each weekly evaluation was slightly greater than for ivermectin, administered orally at 200 µg/kg every 14 days, for the first through third treatments. All animals were cleared by both compounds after the fourth treatment.

Fenbendazole was used via cloacal administration in Greek, Kleinmann's, and Indian star tortoises to treat oxyurid infestations. Treatment resulted in immediate expulsion of adult worms, and fecal flotations were negative for parasite ova 2 and 4 weeks later. Efficacy was greater than had been previously experienced using the oral route. This was attributed to the achievement of higher levels of fenbendazole within the lower intestine, the actual location of the worms.

GENTAMICIN SULFATE

INDICATIONS: Gentamicin (Gentocin ✦ ★) is an aminoglycoside antibiotic that was one of the most commonly used drugs for treating gram-negative infections in reptiles, especially in snakes. However, the nephrotoxicity of gentamicin and the development of newer antibiotics have decreased the popularity of this drug. Amikacin is now the most commonly used aminoglycoside in reptile medicine. For more general information, see **GENTAMICIN** in the Small Animal section.

Pharmacokinetic and toxicity studies have been performed in several species of snakes and turtles and in juvenile American alligators. Despite this, specific doses and dosage intervals are difficult to state conclusively. These studies have demonstrated significant variation in drug distribution and excretion relating to individual variation, species, dosage amount, and ambient/body temperature. For example, in Florida broad-banded water snakes administered 4 mg/kg of gentamicin IM, the clearance of the drug at 30°C was twice that at 15°C. At a dosage of 16 mg/kg, clearance was three times faster at the higher temperature. In juvenile American alligators, the gentamicin clearance half-life was significantly shorter for a dose of 1.25 as compared to 1.75 mg/kg. Route of administration did not appear to affect pharmacokinetic parameters when IM injections were administered into the fore or hind legs of Eastern box tortoises. This variation makes overdosage, leading to accumulation of serum gentamicin and nephrotoxicity, or underdosage, resulting in prolonged periods of subtherapeutic blood levels, quite possible.

In gopher snakes at 15°C, dosage with 2.5 mg/kg every 72 hours maintained adequate therapeutic levels (defined as 8–12 µg/mL) without reaching toxic concentrations (defined as > 15 µg/mL). However, a half-life of approximately 80 hours and the fact that blood levels did not drop below the recommended trough of 2 µg/mL between injections suggests that the dosing interval was too short. In blood pythons (temperature not stated), the recommended treatment regime was initially for 2.5 or 3 mg/kg (depending on the minimal inhibitory concentration desired), then 1.5 mg/ kg every 96 hours, based on a half-life of 2 to 3 days.

ADVERSE AND COMMON SIDE EFFECTS: Gentamicin is nephrotoxic in reptiles and has a low margin of safety. Due to interspecies variations in drug absorption and clearance, a dosage safe in one species may be toxic in another. In 2 boid snakes, gentamicin administered at 4.4 mg/kg twice daily for 2 days, then once daily for 5 days, resulted in nephrotoxicity and death. Nephrotoxicity, with a range of morphologic changes ranging from cloudy swelling to frank tubular necrosis, has been created in gopher snakes and banded water snakes with doses as low as 5 mg/kg once daily. Toxicity increased with increased dosage and decreased frequency of administration and was greater in banded water snakes held at 30°C as compared to 15°C. Toxicity may not be evident until after therapy has concluded.

Administration of supplemental isotonic fluids orally, SC, or intracoelomically is recommended during the course of treatment and for several days afterward. Plasma or serum uric acid levels should be monitored during treatment and for 2 weeks afterward. Fasting, to lower the protein load on the kidneys, may reduce the occurrence of renal damage. Determination of blood gentamicin levels would be valuable where possible.

Ototoxicity has been described in lizards that received more than 100 mg/kg for up to 3 weeks.

DRUG INTERACTIONS: Gentamicin is often used in combination with penicillins and cephalosporins for treatment of severe gram-negative infections. Cefuroxime has been given at 100 mg/kg once daily, in combination with gentamicin, for 10 days to treat *Proteus* infections in snakes. Gentamicin loses antimicrobial action in the presence of carbenicillin and cephalothin; therefore, these drugs should not be combined before administration. In mammals with decreased renal function in vivo inactivation may also occur. Because of this, some authors have suggested delaying carbenicillin administration until 48 hours after initial treatment with gentamicin. If renal function is unaltered, this precaution is probably unnecessary.

GLUCOSE

INDICATIONS: Glucose is used for oral treatment of fasting- and stress-induced hypoglycemia in crocodilians; D-glucose, or dextrose, is an equivalent product.

SUPPLIED AS: VETERINARY PRODUCT
Parenteral solutions containing 50% dextrose ✦ ★

GLYCOPYRROLATE

INDICATIONS: Glycopyrrolate (Robinul-V ★, Robinul ✦ ★) is an anticholinergic agent used as an alternative to atropine in preanesthetic regimens to prevent bradycardia and reduce oral and upper respiratory secretions and to reduce oral mucus in conjunction with systemic antibacterial therapy in snakes with necrotic stomatitis or respiratory tract infections. For more information, see **GLYCO-PYRROLATE** in the Small Animal section.

ITRACONAZOLE

INDICATIONS: Itraconazole (Sporanox ✦ ★) is a triazole antifungal drug active against many fungal pathogens. Itraconazole is best absorbed when given with a fatty meal. For general information, see **ITRACONAZOLE** in the Small Animal section.

The pharmacokinetics of itraconazole were studied in spiny lizards held at ambient temperature (not specifically stated) with a basking lamp. The animals were dosed orally with 23.5 mg/kg once daily for 3 days. Sporanox capsules were opened and the individual beads counted for each animal. The drug was well absorbed; potentially therapeutic plasma levels were obtained within 24 hours. It was predicted that steady-state blood concentrations would be reached within 10 days. The drug was present in high levels in liver within approximately 90 hours; muscle levels were minimal. Blood levels persisted within reported minimal inhibitory concentrations of common fungal pathogens for 6 days after peak concentration was reached and had an elimination half-life of 48 hours. A specific dosing interval was not recommended.

ADVERSE AND COMMON SIDE EFFECTS: The capsular formulation of itraconazole makes accurate dosing, especially of small patients, very difficult.

IVERMECTIN

INDICATIONS: Ivermectin (Heartgard ♣ ★, Ivomec ♣ ★, Eqvalan ♣ ★) is used for the treatment of infestations by nematodes and arthropod ectoparasites, especially skin mites in snakes. The drug may have some effect against pentastomes and subcutaneous dracunculosis. For more information, see **IVERMECTIN** in the Small Animal section.

Ivermectin has been widely recommended for the elimination of enteric nematode parasites in reptiles; however, several case reports describe poor results and/or suggest that the efficacy of fenbendazole or febantel/praziquantel is greater. In a study comparing the efficacy of fenbendazole (various doses) and ivermectin (200 µg/kg; PO) in ball pythons positive for nematode ova on fecal examination, the two drugs were administered every 14 days and fecal egg counts performed. The efficacy of fenbendazole was greater until the fourth treatment, at which point all animals ceased to shed eggs.

Ivermectin has been highly successful for the treatment of cutaneous mites in snakes, either by systemic administration or as a topical spray. Environmental clean-up is also required.

Two reports describe the oral use of ivermectin, administered once or twice at a 14 to 16 day interval, at a dose of 1,000 µg/kg in Tokay and Standing's day geckos. All animals treated ceased to shed pentastome eggs. Necropsies were not performed to determine whether all adult worms were in fact killed.

ADVERSE AND COMMON SIDE EFFECTS: Flaccid paresis, paralysis, and death have resulted from administration of ivermectin to chelonians. After IM administration of 400 µg/kg resulted in the death of 4 of 5 red-footed tortoises, an experimental trial was conducted in red-footed, leopard, and box tortoises and red-eared slider turtles. Neurologic signs were seen in leopard tortoises given 25 µg/kg, in some eastern box tortoises given 100 µg/kg, in some red-footed tortoises given 50 µg/kg, and in red-eared sliders given 150 µg/kg. Cumulative toxicosis was also noted after two red-footed tortoises were given a second dose 72 hours after the first. A separate study also described toxicity and death in red-eared slider turtles given 200 µg/kg orally. In red-footed tortoises a dosage of 50 µg/kg at 7-day intervals was found to be safe; however, elimination of parasites was not complete. Two spurred tortoises given 220 and 190 µg/kg SC did not show clinical signs of toxicity.

Neurologic signs have also been reported in ball pythons and a rough-necked monitor. Transitory and mild, but significant, tremors and stupor were noted in 6 of 98 ball pythons that had received 200 µg/kg orally. Seizure-like activity was described in the rough-necked monitor. One author has also described aggressive behaviors in king snakes after ivermectin therapy. In chameleons, skin discoloration may result at the site of injection.

DRUG INTERACTIONS: Concurrent administration of diazepam may potentiate the toxic effects of ivermectin as both act on the γ-aminobutyric acid–benzodiazepine receptor complex.

SUPPLIED AS: For oral medication the stock solution is diluted 1:10 or 1:100 in propylene glycol.

KANAMYCIN

INDICATIONS: Kanamycin (Kantrim ★) is an aminoglycoside antibiotic used for the treatment of gram-negative bacterial infections, especially *Pseudomonas* spp. For more information, see **KANAMYCIN** in the Small Animal section.

ADVERSE AND COMMON SIDE EFFECTS: Published dosages are empirical; no pharmacokinetic work has been done with this drug. Kanamycin is potentially nephrotoxic and should not be used in the presence of impaired renal function or dehydration. During treatment, it is essential to maintain hydration by ensuring the availability of fresh water or by administration of oral, intracolemic, or SC isotonic fluids. For prolonged therapy, monitoring of plasma or serum uric acid levels may be appropriate.

KETOCONAZOLE

INDICATIONS: Ketoconazole (Nizoral ✦ ★) is an antifungal agent used for the treatment of deep fungal and yeast infections, including dermatitis, shell rot, and pneumonia. For more information, see **KETOCONAZOLE** in the Small Animal section.

Single-dose and multidose pharmacokinetic studies in gopher tortoises have indicated that ketoconazole is absorbed orally and that therapeutic levels of the drug can be obtained and maintained in blood and tissue without evidence of toxicity. At an ambient temperature of 27°C, a dose of 15 mg/kg PO once daily was recommended to maintain plasma levels of ketoconazole above 1 µg/mL.

Much higher empirical doses are described in the literature without reports of toxicity.

DRUG INTERACTIONS: Ketoconazole has been used in combination with thiabendazole, each at 50 mg/kg PO once daily, in juvenile green turtles with mycotic pneumonia.

LEVAMISOLE

INDICATIONS: Levamisole (Levasole ♣ ★, Ripercol ♣, Tramisol ♣ ★) is an anthelmintic used for the treatment of infestations by nematodes, acanthocephalans, and pentastomes, and for pulmonary rhabdiasis in snakes. For more information, see **LEVAMISOLE** in the Small Animal section.

ADVERSE AND COMMON SIDE EFFECTS: Do not use in debilitated animals. The margin of safety may be narrow.

LINCOMYCIN

INDICATIONS: Lincomycin (Lincocin ♣ ★) is a lincosamide antibiotic used for the treatment of bacterial infections, including peptostreptococcal wound infections in snakes. For more information, see **LINCOMYCIN** in the Small Animal section.

ADVERSE AND COMMON SIDE EFFECTS: Lincomycin should not be used in the presence of impaired renal or hepatic function or dehydration.

MEBENDAZOLE

INDICATIONS: Mebendazole (Telmin ♣) is an anthelmintic used for the treatment of gastrointestinal nematode infections. A broad range of dosages exists in the literature. For more information, see **MEBENDAZOLE** in the Small Animal section.

MEPERIDINE

INDICATIONS: Meperidine (Demerol ♣ ★) is a short-acting narcotic analgesic used for the relief of moderate to severe pain and as a preanesthetic. For more information, see **MEPERIDINE** in the Small Animal section.

A controlled study of the responsiveness of juvenile Nile crocodiles to a hot plate indicated that the intraperitoneal administration of meperidine increased the latency of the response, with a plateau effect reached at doses of 2 to 4 mg/kg. This work suggests that crocodiles are very sensitive to the antinociceptor effects of this drug.

METRONIDAZOLE

INDICATIONS: Metronidazole (Flagyl ✤ ★) is a synthetic antibacterial, antiprotozoal agent that has been used in the treatment of amebiasis, trichomoniasis, and infection by other flagellates. In a study of the antimicrobial sensitivities of bacteria isolated from clinically affected reptiles, 19 of 19 anaerobic organisms cultured were sensitive to metronidazole. For more information, see **METRONIDAZOLE** in the Small Animal section.

Reported dosage regimens vary considerably, with the most common being 40 to 100 mg/kg PO once, then repeated in 2 weeks. Dosage with 75 to 275 mg/kg has been recommended for single day, once daily for up to 3, or according to one report, 10 days, or weekly administration. There have been no pharmacokinetic studies on metronidazole administration in reptiles.

The IV 5 mg/mL metronidazole preparation has been used in small chelonians (< 1 kg in weight) at a dosage of 60 to 80 mg/kg once daily for three treatments. Administration was SC in the axial area.

ADVERSE AND COMMON SIDE EFFECTS: Several species of snake are considered sensitive to the drug as deaths have occurred after treatment with doses greater than 100 mg/kg. These include tricolor king snakes, milk snakes, indigo snakes, and Uracoan rattlesnakes. A lower dose of 40 mg/kg is recommended in these animals. Other species of snakes may react similarly.

Metronidazole was inadvertently administered once daily, orally, at a dose of 142 mg/kg, for 8 days to a loggerhead musk turtle. From days 10 to 12 after the initiation of treatment the turtle became progressively weaker and anorectic; partial paralysis was noted. Supportive care was initiated and clinical signs gradually resolved over a period of 8 weeks. Anecdotal reports of snakes developing neurologic signs after administration also exist. Treatment with metronidazole may result in faunal imbalance in herbivorous species.

OTHER USES: Metronidazole has been used to stimulate the appetite of anorectic snakes. The mechanism of this effect is unclear.

MIDAZOLAM

INDICATIONS: Midazolam (Versed ✤ ★) is a short-acting parenteral benzodiazepine central nervous system depressant, with sedative-hypnotic, anxiolytic, muscle-relaxing, and anticonvulsant properties. The drug is two to three times more potent than diazepam and has a shorter half-life. For more information, see **MIDAZOLAM** in the Small Animal section.

The sedative effects of midazolam, alone and in conjunction with ketamine, have been studied in red-eared slider, painted, and snapping turtles. In snapping turtles at 21°C, mild sedation inadequate for manipulation was achieved using midazolam alone at 2 mg/kg. This dose combined with 20 or 40 mg/kg of ketamine resulted in sedation and chemical restraint adequate for extensive manipulation. Onset of effect was within 5 minutes, duration of sedation was 5 to 20 minutes, and all animals completely recovered within 210 minutes. In red-eared slider turtles held at 24° to 27°C, a dose of 1.5 mg/kg IM resulted in sedation with an onset of 4 to 28 minutes, a duration of 3 to 114 minutes, and a recovery of 20 to 60 minutes. Wide individual variation was noted, and one animal died. In painted turtles doses ranging from 2 to 20 mg/kg IM did not result in sedation.

ADVERSE AND COMMON SIDE EFFECTS: Myositis and edema developed at the thoracic inlet near the injection sites into the forelimbs in 3 of 12 red-eared slider turtles. Two of the 3 gradually recovered, but the third died. The study in which these turtles were involved included repeated doses of midazolam; volume of injection may have been high in these animals.

MILBEMYCIN

INDICATIONS: Milbemycin oxime (Interceptor ✦ ★) is an anthelmintic, insecticidal, and acaricidal compound. For more general information, see **MILBEMYCIN** in the Small Animal section.

Milbemycin was administered to red-eared slider turtles at dosages of 0.2, 0.5, and 1.0 mg/kg orally, and to the same species and Gulf coast box and ornate box turtles at a dose of 0.5 mg/kg SC with no adverse reactions. Milbemycin was effective in eliminating shedding of nematode eggs at a dose of 0.25 mg/kg SC once or twice at an 8-day interval. The drug was not effective against acanthocephalan parasites.

ADVERSE AND COMMON SIDE EFFECTS: Milbemycin has a mode of action and potential toxicity similar to that of ivermectin. The safety of milbemycin has been evaluated in only a small number of animals in a limited number of species.

NEOMYCIN

INDICATIONS: Neomycin (Biosol-M ✦, Mycifradin ✦ ★) is an aminoglycoside antibiotic used topically and, less commonly, orally for treatment of bacterial enteritis. For more information, see **NEOMYCIN** in the Small Animal section.

ADVERSE AND COMMON SIDE EFFECTS: Neomycin is generally less effective than amikacin and gentamicin, and when used systemically, is the most toxic aminoglycoside.

DRUG INTERACTIONS: Oral neomycin has been used in combination with systemic gentamicin and oral administration of live lactobacillus for treatment of severe enteritis and septicemia.

NYSTATIN

INDICATIONS: Nystatin (Mycostatin ✦ ★, Nilstat ✦ ★) is an antifungal agent used for the treatment of gastrointestinal yeast infections, including oral candidiasis. Although published recommendations are for once daily treatment, the activity of nystatin is based on topical contact and, therefore, more frequent administration may be more efficacious. For more information, see **NYSTATIN** in the Small Animal section.

OXYTETRACYCLINE

INDICATIONS: Oxytetracycline (Liquamycin ✦ ★, Terramycin ✦ ★) is a short-acting, water-soluble tetracycline used for the treatment of bacterial infections, including *Aeromonas* spp, septicemia in alligators, and ulcerative stomatitis in turtles and tortoises. For more information, see **OXYTETRACYCLINE** and **TETRACYCLINE ANTIBIOTICS** in the Small Animal section.

ADVERSE AND COMMON SIDE EFFECTS: Oxytetracycline may cause inflammation at sites of injection.

OXYTOCIN

INDICATIONS: Oxytocin (Pitocin★, Syntocinon ✦ ★) is used for the treatment of dystocia resulting from uterine inertia, most commonly in chelonians. For more information, see **OXYTOCIN** in the Small Animal section.

Oxytocin is not the hormone primarily responsible for oviposition in reptiles, which probably explains the variable results obtained with its use. It is not known whether estrogens are required to sensitize the reptilian uterus before oxytocin administration. Concurrent or prior treatment with calcium is usually recommended. Oviductal contractions usually occur in 30 to 60 minutes, although not all animals respond. Provision of environmental conditions conducive to oviposition, such as the correct nesting area and ambient temperature, are essential. Promising results have been obtained using vasotocin, a more appropriate but not readily available compound.

ADVERSE AND COMMON SIDE EFFECTS: Uterine rupture may occur if underlying uterine pathology prevents egg passage. Mortality has been reported after treatment with oxytocin, although the significance of the drug in directly causing death is unknown. Some animals will pass only a portion of the egg clutch after oxytocin administration.

PAROMOMYCIN

INDICATIONS: Paromomycin (Humatin ★) is an aminoglycoside antibiotic with a broad spectrum of activity against bacteria, protozoa, and cestodes. The drug has been used in the treatment of amebiasis in snakes. It acts primarily in the intestinal lumen, against trophozoite and encysted forms. Doses are empirical.

ADVERSE AND COMMON SIDE EFFECTS: Paromomycin is poorly absorbed from the intestinal tract. The drug is potentially nephrotoxic and ototoxic and may have neuromuscular blocking effects. Other adverse effects in humans include gastrointestinal upset.

SUPPLIED AS: HUMAN PRODUCT
Oral capsules containing 250 mg [Humatin★]

PENICILLIN G
PENICILLIN, BENZATHINE
PENICILLIN, PROCAINE

INDICATIONS: Penicillin compounds are used for the treatment of bacterial infections. Penicillin G is also used to lavage open wounds. For more information, see **PENICILLIN ANTIBIOTICS** in the Small Animal section.

PIPERACILLIN

INDICATIONS: Piperacillin (Pipracil ✲ ★) is a third-generation, broad-spectrum, semisynthetic penicillin with activity against most aerobic gram-negative bacteria and some gram-positive and anaerobic organisms. It is used to treat bacterial infections, including those caused by *Pseudomonas aeruginosa*. For more information, see **PENICILLIN ANTIBIOTICS** in the Small Animal section.

The pharmacokinetics of piperacillin were studied in five blood pythons held at 28° to 30°C. IM doses of 100 mg/kg and 200 mg/kg, followed by 100 mg/kg after 24 hours, were evaluated. Peak blood concentrations were achieved within 4 hours of injection, and blood piperacillin concentrations well above the minimal inhibitory concentration for a series of bacteria isolated from the glottises of snakes (0.25–4 μg/mL) were reached. The elimination half-life was approximately 12 to 17 hours. A dose of 100 mg/kg IM every 48 hours was recommended in this species. There was no elevation of serum uric acid levels in the one animal in which renal function was assessed.

ADVERSE AND COMMON SIDE EFFECTS: Thrombophlebitis and pain on injection have been noted in human patients. No such response was noted in the study described above.

DRUG INTERACTIONS: Piperacillin has been used in combination with amikacin or tobramycin for septic patients. Under these circumstances the low end of the dosage range has been recommended. Administer piperacillin and aminoglycosides separately because inactivation can occur if the drugs are mixed in vitro.

SUPPLIED AS: HUMAN PRODUCT
For injection, vials containing 2, 3, and 4 g [Pipracil ✚ ★]

PIPERAZINE

INDICATIONS: Piperazine (Hartz Once a Month ★, Once a Month Roundworm Treatment ✚, Pipa-Tabs ★, Purina Liquid Wormer ★) is an anthelmintic used for the treatment of gastrointestinal nematodes. For more information, see **PIPERAZINE** in the Small Animal section.

ADVERSE AND COMMON SIDE EFFECTS: Piperazine may be toxic in debilitated reptiles.

SUPPLIED AS: VETERINARY PRODUCT
See Small Animal section

POLYMYXIN B

INDICATIONS: Polymyxin B (Aerosporin ✚ ★) is used in the treatment of bacterial, especially gram-negative infections. For more information, see **POLYMYXIN B** in the Small Animal section.

PRAZIQUANTEL

INDICATIONS: Praziquantel (Droncit ✚ ★) is the anthelmintic drug of choice for treating trematode and cestode infections, especially extraintestinal forms. It has been used successfully for spirorchid infections in green turtles. For more information, see **PRAZIQUANTEL** in the Small Animal section.

DRUG INTERACTIONS: Oral praziquantel plus febantel (Vercom★) has been used successfully to clear nematode eggs from the feces of prehensile-tailed skinks. Efficacy was felt to be better than that of ivermectin.

SUPPLIED AS: VETERINARY PRODUCTS
Praziquantel: See Small Animal section
Praziquantel plus febantel:
Paste containing 3.4 mg praziquantel and 34 mg febantel/g [Vercom★]
Tablets containing 18.2 mg praziquantel and 72.6 mg febantel [Drontal Plus ❦]

PREDNISOLONE

INDICATIONS: Prednisolone (Delta-Cortef ★, Solu-Delta-Cortef ❦ ★, and others) is an intermediate-acting glucocorticoid agent. For more information, see **PREDNISOLONE** and **GLUCOCORTICOID AGENTS** in the Small Animal section.

ADVERSE AND COMMON SIDE EFFECTS: Routine use of glucocorticoids in reptiles is not recommended because of immunosuppressive effects.

PROPRANOLOL

INDICATIONS: Propranolol (Inderal ❦ ★) is a nonselective β_1- and β_2-blocking agent whose use in veterinary medicine is primarily in the management of cardiac disease. In reptiles, propranolol has been used to induce oviposition. For more information, see **PROPRANOLOL** in the Small Animal section and **VASOTOCIN** in this section.

DRUG INTERACTIONS: The plateau lizard was used as an experimental subject to investigate the hypothesis that adrenergic inhibition of uterine muscular activity exists in reptiles. Single doses of 1 mg/kg of propranolol used as an adrenergic blocking agent, 0.5 mg/kg arginine vasotocin, and 25 µg/kg prostaglandin $F_{2\alpha}$ resulted in oviposition in 4 of 8 animals (2 of the clutches were partial), 2 of 3 (1 partial) and 0 of 4 lizards, respectively. When animals were pretreated with propranolol, administration of arginine vasotocin or prostaglandin $F_{2\alpha}$ resulted in oviposition in 3 of 3 and 6 of 7 (1 partial clutch) lizards. Only animals that had received prostaglandin exhibited nesting or nest guarding behavior. Tunnelling and nest building were also seen in a green iguana that received 7.5 mg/kg of propranolol followed by 18.5 µg/kg of prostaglandin $F_{2\alpha}$. This animal did not pass eggs; this may have been due to the much lower dose of propranolol or to prior treatment with oxytocin and passage of a portion of the clutch.

PROSTAGLANDIN F$_{2\alpha}$, E$_2$

INDICATIONS: Prostaglandin $F_{2\alpha}$ (Lutalyse ❦ ★) is used for the management of reproductive conditions in mammals; the drug causes contraction of the myometrium and relaxation of the cervix.

Prostaglandin $F_{2\alpha}$ has been used to induce oviposition in some species of viviparous lizards. The drug also appears to stimulate nesting behavior in some species of lizards. A case report also describes the treatment of a spotted python that retained two eggs after oviposition. Dinoprostone gel (prostaglandin E_2) was applied intracloacally near the cervix, and 20 minutes later an IM injection of 0.6 mg/kg prostaglandin $F_{2\alpha}$ was administered. The snake passed the remaining two eggs within 8 hours. For more information, see **PROSTAGLANDIN $F_{2\alpha}$** in the Small Animal section and **PROPRANOLOL** in this section.

SUPPLIED AS: VETERINARY PRODUCT
Prostaglandin $F_{2\alpha}$: See Small and Large Animal sections

HUMAN PRODUCTS
Prostaglandin E (Dinoprostone)
Gel formulation containing 0.5 mg/3 mL [Prepidil ♣] and 1 and 2 mg/3 g [Prostin E_2 ♣]
Suppository containing 20 mg [Prostin E_2 ★]

PYRETHRIN-CONTAINING PRODUCTS

INDICATIONS: Pyrethrin-containing products (Sectrol ♣ ★, Ovitrol ♣ ★, and many others) are naturally occurring insecticides derived from the plant *Chrysanthemum cinerariae-folium*. Insect mortality is enhanced when these products are combined with piperonyl butoxide. These topical insecticides, in either dip or shampoo formulations, are used most frequently for the treatment of ectoparasites in lizards and snakes. For more information see **PYRETHRIN-CONTAINING PRODUCTS** in the Small Animal section.

ADVERSE AND COMMON SIDE EFFECTS: Avoid contact of the chemical with the eyes and mouths of animals. Pyrethrin products may be too toxic for neonatal reptiles. Pyrethrins act rapidly; therefore, animals can be blotted to remove excess product and/or rinsed thoroughly within a few minutes of application. Do not use with other cholinesterase inhibitors; toxicity was reported in a green tree python after being sprayed with permethrin, a synthetic pyrethroid. The animal had been treated with an organophosphate 10 days earlier.

SUPPLIED AS: VETERINARY PRODUCTS
Powder, spray, and shampoo formulations containing varying percentages of pyrethrin and piperonyl butoxide. Some products also contain carbaryl and other insecticidal compounds.

SELENIUM

See **VITAMIN E**

SILVER SULFADIAZINE

INDICATIONS Silver sulfadiazine (Flamazine ✤, Silvadene ★, SSD ★, Thermazene ★) is a water-miscible cream with bactericidal activity against a broad range of gram-positive and gram-negative bacteria, including *Pseudomonas* and *Aeromonas* spp, and some yeasts. It has been used most commonly for topical treatment of mouth rot and burns but is also effective for other cutaneous injuries and bacterial infections.

SUPPLIED AS: HUMAN PRODUCTS
1% topical cream [Flamazine ✤, Silvadene ★, SSD ★, Thermazene ★, Silver sulfadiazine cream ★]

STREPTOMYCIN

See **DIHYDROSTREPTOMYCIN**

SULFONAMIDE DRUGS

INDICATIONS: The sulfonamides are antibacterial, antiprotozoal drugs that have been used for the treatment of intestinal and biliary coccidiosis. They are not effective against gastric cryptosporidiosis. For more information, see **SULFONAMIDE ANTIBIOTICS** and **SULFADIMETHOXINE** in the Small Animal section, or **SULFON-AMIDES** in the Large Animal section.

ADVERSE AND COMMON SIDE EFFECTS: Sulfonamide drugs should not be used in the presence of dehydration or renal disease.

SUPPLIED AS: VETERINARY PRODUCTS
Sulfadiazine: See **TRIMETHOPRIM-SULFADIAZINE**
Sulfadimethoxine:
Various formulations for oral use in drinking water [Albon, Di-Methox, and others ★]
Oral suspension containing 250 mg/5 mL [Albon Oral Suspension-5% ★]
Tablets containing 125 [S-125 ✤, Albon ★] and 250 mg [S-250 ✤, Albon ★]
For injection containing 400 mg/mL [Albon Injection-40% ★]
Sulfamethazine:
Various formulations for oral use in drinking water [Sulmet ✤ ★, Sulfamethazine★, and others]
Sulfaquinoxyline:
Various liquid and powder formulations for oral use in drinking water [Sulfaquinoxaline 19.2% concentrate ✤, Purina Sulfa-Nox Liquid ★, and others]

TETRACYCLINE

INDICATIONS: Tetracycline (Panmycin Aquadrops ♣ ★, numerous formulations for drinking water) has been used for the treatment of bacterial infections, including *Aeromonas* spp septicemia in crocodilians and osteomyelitis in snakes. For more information, see **TETRACYCLINE ANTIBIOTICS** in the Small Animal section.

ADVERSE AND COMMON SIDE EFFECTS: Tissue damage may occur at the site of IM injection.

SUPPLIED AS: VETERINARY PRODUCTS
For oral administration containing 100 mg/mL [Panmycin Aquadrops Liquid ♣ ★]
For injection containing 100 [Tetroxy ♣] and 200 mg/mL [Tetraject ♣]
Numerous liquid and powder formulations for use in drinking water ♣ ★

THIABENDAZOLE

INDICATIONS: Thiabendazole (Equizole ★, Mintezol ★, Thibenzole ★) is an antiparasitic drug used for the elimination of gastrointestinal nematodes, including strongyloides. The drug is reported to be more effective against ascarids in tortoises than mebendazole or diethylcarbamazine citrate, although it may only reduce the worm burden. For more information, see **THIABENDAZOLE** in the Small Animal section.

DRUG INTERACTIONS: Thiabendazole has been used in combination with ketoconazole for the treatment of mycotic pneumonia in juvenile green turtles.

TILETAMINE ZOLAZEPAM

INDICATIONS: Tiletamine zolazepam (Telazol ★) is an injectable dissociative anesthetic/tranquilizer that has been used in reptiles for sedation and restraint, anesthetic induction, and anesthesia of short duration. Higher doses may result in prolonged recoveries. For more information, see **TILETAMINE ZOLAZEPAM** in the Small Animal section.

DRUG INTERACTIONS: Premedication with atropine or glycopyrrolate has been recommended.

TOBRAMYCIN

INDICATIONS: Tobramycin (Nebcin ♣ ★) is an aminoglycoside antibiotic used for the treatment of bacterial infections, especially those caused by *Pseudomonas* spp, against which it has better activity than gentamicin. For more information, see **TOBRAMYCIN** in the Small Animal section.

ADVERSE AND COMMON SIDE EFFECTS: Tobramycin is less nephrotoxic than gentamicin but may be more nephrotoxic than amikacin.

DRUG INTERACTIONS: Tobramycin is potentiated by β-lactam antibiotics.

TOLNAFTATE

INDICATIONS: Tolnaftate (Tinavet ★, Tinasol ★, Tinactin ♣, and others) is a topical fungicidal agent used for the treatment of superficial fungal infections. Tolnaftate has been described for the topical treatment of mycotic dermatitis in snakes, after the affected areas were soaked in dilute organic iodine, and for chronic dermatitis in Solo-mon Island prehensile-tailed skinks.

SUPPLIED AS: VETERINARY PRODUCTS
Cream containing 10 mg/g tolnaftate [Tinavet ★]
Solution containing 10 mg/mL tolnaftate [Tinasol ★]
HUMAN PRODUCTS
Cream and liquid containing 10 mg/g tolnaftate [Pitrex ♣, Tinactin ♣, Zeasorb ♣]

TRIMETHOPRIM SULFADIAZINE
TRIMETHOPRIM SULFADOXINE

INDICATIONS: Trimethoprim plus sulphadiazine (or sulfadiazine), sulfadoxine, and sulfamethoxazole (Tribrissen ♣ ★, Trivetrin ♣, Septra ♣ ★, Bactrim ♣ ★, and others), are bactericidal antibiotic combinations commonly used for the treatment of bacterial infections in reptiles, including pneumonia, osteomyelitis in snakes, and middle ear infections in box turtles, and as anticoccidial agents. These drugs have been used safely for long-term therapy, i.e., 90 days or more, for the treatment of chronic infections. It has been reported that long-term therapy may help reduce shedding and eliminate gastric cryptosporidiosis in snakes when combined with appropriate husbandry and supportive measures. A regimen of 30 mg/kg PO once daily for 4 weeks, then 60 mg/kg PO once daily for 2 months has been described. Despite the frequency of use of these drugs, and perhaps because of their safety, no pharmacokinetic evaluations have been performed. For more information, see **TRIMETHOPRIM-SULFADIAZINE** in the Small Animal section.

SUPPLIED AS: VETERINARY PRODUCTS
For injection containing 40 mg/mL trimethoprim and 200 mg/mL sulfadiazine [Tribrissen 24% ✤]
For injection containing 40 mg/mL trimethoprim and 200 mg/mL sulfadoxine [Bimotrin ✤, Borgal ✤, Trimidox ✤, Trivetrin ✤]
For injection containing 80 mg/mL trimethoprim and 400 mg/mL sulfadiazine [Tribrissen 48% ✤]
Tablets containing trimethoprim plus sulfadiazine in the following combinations: 5 + 25, 20 + 100, 80 + 400 [DiTrim★, Tribrissen ✤ ★]
Oral suspension containing 9.1 mg trimethoprim and 45.5 mg sulfadiazine/mL [Tribrissen ✤]

HUMAN PRODUCTS
Oral suspensions containing 40 mg trimethoprim and 200 mg sulfamethoxazole/5 mL [Bactrim ✤ ★, Septra ✤ ★, and many others]
Oral suspensions containing 45 mg trimethoprim and 205 mg sulfadiazine /5 mL [Coptin ✤]

TYLOSIN

INDICATIONS: Tylosin (Tylan ✤ ★, Tylocine ✤, Tylosin ★) is a macro-lide antibiotic that has been used for the treatment of bacterial infections, especially pneumonia in snakes and chelonians. Treatment with tylosin may help to alleviate the clinical signs of respiratory syndrome of desert tortoises. For more information, see **TYLOSIN** in the Small Animal section.

VASOTOCIN

INDICATIONS: Arginine vasotocin has been used experimentally and in small numbers of clinical reports to stimulate oviposition in reptiles. Experimental work on three species of lizards showed vasotocin to be 10 times more potent for this purpose than oxytocin. Another report describes a success rate of over 70% in inducing oviposition in a variety of snakes, lizards, and chelonians as compared to only 19% with oxytocin. A response is expected within 10 minutes to 24 hours after intracoelomic or IV injection. Repeat dosage may be necessary. Pretreatment with calcium is recommended by some authors.

ADVERSE AND COMMON SIDE EFFECTS: Precautions are similar to those for oxytocin; underlying uterine pathology may result in failure to pass eggs or in uterine rupture. Arginine vasotocin is poorly stable; small aliquots should be frozen after reconstitution from powder. No adverse responses were seen in a few individuals given up to 50 µg/kg.

DRUG INTERACTIONS: The plateau lizard was used as an experimental subject to investigate the hypothesis that adrenergic inhibition of uterine muscular activity exists in reptiles. Single doses of 1 mg/kg of propranolol, a β-blocking agent, 0.5 mg/kg arginine vasotocin, and 25 µg/kg prostaglandin $F_{2\alpha}$ resulted in oviposition in 4 of 8 animals (2 of the clutches were partial), 2 of 3 (1 partial) and 0 of 4 lizards, respectively. When animals were pretreated with propranolol, administration of arginine vasotocin or prostaglandin $F_{2\alpha}$ resulted in oviposition in 3 of 3 and 6 of 7 (1 partial clutch) lizards. Only animals that had received prostaglandin exhibited nesting or nest guarding behavior. Tunneling and nest building were also seen in a green iguana that received 7.5 mg/kg of propranolol followed by 18.5 µg/kg of prostaglandin $F_{2\alpha}$. This animal did not pass eggs; this may have been due to the much lower dose of propranolol or to prior treatment with oxytocin and passage of a portion of the clutch.

SUPPLIED AS: CHEMICAL PRODUCT
Arginine vasotocin (Sigma Chemicals)

VITAMIN A

INDICATIONS: Vitamin A (Aquasol A ★) is used as a supplement for sick reptiles and for the treatment of vitamin A deficiency, especially in pet turtles and tortoises. Published dosages include single, daily, and weekly treatment with 1,000 to 50,000 IU/kg per animal. Oral administration is recommended by some authors to decrease the risk of overdosage, whereas others prefer the parenteral route of administration.

ADVERSE AND COMMON SIDE EFFECTS: Overdose in terrestrial chelonians may result in subacute xeroderma followed by severe necrotizing dermatitis, epidermal lifting, and ulceration. These lesions were seen in 3 box turtles administered 5,000 IU/kg/week for 2 to 3 weeks, but have not been experimentally re-created. An anecdotal report describes similar and extremely severe sloughing of the skin in a snake that had received extensive supplementation with injectable vitamin A. Herbivorous species often receive adequate vitamin A in their diet and should not be treated before dietary evaluation.

SUPPLIED AS: HUMAN PRODUCTS
Capsules containing 10,000, 25,000, or 50,000 IU [Aquasol A ★]
Solution containing 50,000 IU/mL [Aquasol A ★]
For injection containing 50,000 USP U/mL [Aquasol A Parenteral ★]

VITAMIN B COMPLEX

INDICATIONS: Vitamin B ✦ ★ complex injections are used as a nutritional supplement for sick reptiles and to stimulate appetite, especially in chelonians and lizards.

SUPPLIED AS: VETERINARY PRODUCTS
For injection containing various vitamin level combinations [Vitamin B Complex ✦ ★, Vita-Jec B Complex Fortified ★, Vita-Jec B Complex ★, Compound 150 ✦, Hi-Po B Complex ★, Vitamin B Complex Forte ★, Vitamin B Complex Fortified ★, Vitamin B Complex Fortified injection ★, Vitamin B Complex injection ★]
Oral syrup [V.A.L. Syrup ★]

VITAMIN B₁ (THIAMINE)

INDICATIONS: Thiamine (various products ✦ ★) is used for the treatment of thiamine deficiency and as a dietary supplement, especially in fish-eating animals. For more information, see **THIAMINE** in the Small Animal section.

VITAMIN B₁₂ (CYANOCOBALAMIN)

INDICATIONS: Cyanocobalamin is used in the treatment of general nutritional debility.

SUPPLIED AS: VETERINARY PRODUCTS
For injection containing:
1,000 and 5,000 µg/mL [Vitamin B-12 ✦]
1,000, 3,000, and 5,000 µg/mL [Cyanocobalamin ★]
1,000 and 3,000 µg/mL [Vita-Jec B-12 ★]

VITAMIN C

See **ASCORBIC ACID**

VITAMIN D₃

INDICATIONS: Vitamin D₃ is used as a general oral supplement to ensure proper absorption and utilization of calcium and phosphorus, and parenterally for the treatment of nutritional secondary hyperparathyroidism and metabolic bone disease. Suggested dosages in the literature vary 10-fold, but at least weekly administration is generally recommended. Vitamin D therapy should occur in conjunction with calcium supplementation and, in some cases, administration of calcitonin. Parenteral treatment is generally discontinued when serum calcium/phosphorus ratios return to normal and dietary corrections are instituted.

ADVERSE AND COMMON SIDE EFFECTS: Excess vitamin D administration may result in vascular and/or renal calcification.

DRUG INTERACTIONS: Vitamin D is more commonly supplied in combination with vitamins A and E, or for oral use with calcium and phosphorus.

SUPPLIED AS: VETERINARY PRODUCTS
For injection containing:
80,000 IU/mL [Hydro-Vit D$_3$ ♣, Solu-Vit D$_3$ ♣]
1,000,000 IU/mL [Poten-D ♣, Downer-D ♣]

HUMAN PRODUCT
For injection containing 1 or 2 µg/mL of calcitriol [Calcijex ♣]

VITAMIN E + SELENIUM

INDICATIONS: A single case report describes a green iguana with muscular weakness, limb contractions, and fasciculations that apparently disappeared after treatment with vitamin E and selenium. The clinical presentation resembled hypocalcemia. Vitamin E is also used for treatment of steatitis in aquatic turtles and crocodilians. One unit of vitamin E equals the biologic activity of 1 mg of DL-α-tocopherol acetate, and of 735 µg of D-α-tocopheryl acetate. For more information, see **VITAMIN E** in the Small Animal section, and **SELENIUM** in the Large Animal section.

DRUG INTERACTIONS: Vitamin E is commonly used in combination with selenium.

SUPPLIED AS: VETERINARY PRODUCTS
For injection containing vitamin E:
200, 300, and 500 IU/mL [Vitamin E ★]
For injection containing vitamin E + selenium:
1 mg selenium and 50 mg vitamin E/mL [BO-SE ★, Seletoc ★]
2.5 mg selenium and 50 mg vitamin E/mL [E-SE ♣ ★]
3 mg selenium and 136 mg vitamin E/mL [Dystosel ♣, E-SEL ♣, Selon-E ♣]
5 mg selenium and 50 mg vitamin E/mL [MU-SE ★]
6.8 mg selenium and 136 mg vitamin E/mL [Dystosel DS ♣]

VITAMIN K

INDICATIONS: Vitamin K$_1$ or phytonadione (Aqua-Mephyton★, Mephyton★, Konakion★, Veta-K1♣★) is used for the treatment of vitamin K deficiency in crocodilians and as a supplement in debilitated animals to assist in the formation of coagulation factors. For more information, see **VITAMIN K** in the Small Animal section.

Handbook of Veterinary Drugs, Second Edition, edited by Dana Allen,
Lippincott–Raven Publishers, Philadelphia. © 1998

Section 17

The Use of Chemotherapeutic Agents in Avian Medicine

CHOICE OF MEDICATION

The majority of drug dosage and safety recommendations for pet birds are still empirical and based on clinical experience, although increasing numbers of pharmacokinetic and controlled studies are being undertaken. Most published informaton relates to the common caged bird species, raptors, and domestic poultry. Extrapolation from these reports, and from mammalian dosage regimes, is common practice. Unfortunately for the practitioner, there are considerable differences in drug uptake, distribution, and metabolism among the various species of birds. This is not surprising given the diversity in body size, physiology, and habits present in the class Aves. Metabolic scaling has been used to help tailor drug dosages to varied body size; however, it does not consider variations in drug metabolism or idiosyncratic reactions that may occur in certain species.

Few drugs are specifically licensed for use in avian species; therefore, most treatments are "extralabel" and require the experience and discretion of the veterinarian. It is important that medical therapy be tailored to the response of the patient. The compounds listed in this text are those described in the literature and currently marketed in Canada or the United States. Dosages that are based on pharmacokinetic or controlled efficacy trials are noted with an asterisk in the table.

ROUTES OF ADMINISTRATION

Drugs are usually administered to avian patients via the standard routes: PO, IM, SC, and IV. Often treatment is initiated using a parenteral route, and then continued orally. Liquid oral medications can be administered directly into the oral cavity or, more commonly, into the esophagus or crop with a metal or rubber tube. Few avian patients can be "pilled"; however, a small number of tablet formulations are marketed for use in pigeons. Many antibiotics are available in flavored syrups that are palatable to birds and can be placed in or on a favorite food item, thus avoiding stressful capture at frequent intervals. Medications can easily be mixed into formulas used to hand-raise baby birds.

Although medication of drinking water is common practice in the poultry industry, it is difficult to make standard recommendations in other species. Maintenance of adequate and consistent dosage depends on total water consumption, drinking patterns, palatability, bioavailability, absorption, and stability in solution of a given drug. Water consumption patterns vary widely among different types of birds; illness may result in increased or decreased water consumption, thereby affecting the dose of medication ingested. Taste preferences and sensitivities also vary; sweeteners such as aspartame or fruit drink crystals can be used to mask the taste of unpleasant or bitter compounds. Most medications must be changed on at least a daily basis. Most pet avian species will not drink adequate amounts of water to self-medicate when they are ill. Despite these drawbacks, medication of drinking water is sometimes the most practical way to treat birds in aviary or quarantine situations.

Medication-impregnated feeds are used primarily in aviary situations, and for the treatment of chlamydiosis. Millet and pellets containing chlortetracycline are commercially available. Other combinations, such as medicated mash diets, can be specially formulated for the treatment of individuals or groups of birds. The amount of medication consumed depends on its concentration in the feed, the amount of feed eaten, and the bioavailability of the drug. The amount of feed eaten depends on the palatability and energy content of the diet. Not all birds will readily accept an abrupt change in diet, especially when it consists of a switch from seed mix to pelleted diet. Ill birds often have reduced food intakes.

Intramuscular injection is the most common form of parenteral administration. The pectoral muscles are generally the best developed and most easily accessed. When treating young birds, it is important not to penetrate the poorly developed pectoral muscle and thin sternum to avoid making intrathoracic injections. Ratites do not have adequate pectoral musculature and the legs or epaxial muscles must be used for injection. Because birds have a renal portal system, injection into the hind legs is not recommended when drugs are nephrotoxic or excreted or metabolized by the kidneys. Experimental studies have not proven whether these precautions are necessary. Repeated IM injections may result in myonecrosis, especially if irritating solutions or large volumes are used.

Subcutaneous injections are less frequently recommended; drugs or fluids may be poorly absorbed because of the paucity of blood vessels in the thin avian dermis. Injections should not be made in the cervical area because penetration into the subcutaneous air sac extensions is possible. The shoulder, inguinal, or cranial thigh regions are most frequently used.

Intravenous injections are most commonly used for initiation of treatment in seriously ill birds. Continued IV therapy is not practical, especially in small species, because of difficulties in obtaining repeat venipuncture in small and often uncooperative patients. The frequency of hematoma formation often precludes making multiple injections into the same vein. Intraosseous injection is an alternative route for the administration of sterile, nonirritating compounds. Continued infusion or repeated injections are possible in this manner. Little information is available on the rate of absorption of medications administered by this technique; however, it is assumed to be rapid.

Nebulization and direct intratracheal or air sac administration of drugs have been used to treat respiratory disease. Higher local drug levels may be reached by these methods than by standard parenteral or oral routes. Concurrent parenteral therapy is advised.

Handbook of Veterinary Drugs, Second Edition, edited by Dana Allen,
Lippincott–Raven Publishers, Philadelphia. © 1998

Section 18

Common Dosages in Avian Medicine

Drug	Dosage	Indication/Species
Acetylcysteine 10%	2 to 5 drops in sterile saline per treatment	for nebulization or intranasal flushing
ACTH (corticotropin)	*15 to 25 U/bird; IM	various psittacines
ACTH (cosyntropin)	*0.125 mg/bird; IM	ACTH stimulation test, various psittacines, bald eagle, Andean condor
Acyclovir	*80 mg/kg tid; PO	Pacheco's disease, monk parakeets
	*40 mg/kg tid; IM	
	333 mg/kg; PO	
	200 mg/90 mL drinking water	during an outbreak of Pacheco's disease
	423 mg/L drinking water for 7 to 10 days	
	24 mg/bird bid; PO in food	large psittacines
	6 mg/bird bid; PO in food	small psittacines
	*400 mg capsular drug/2 qt parrot seed plus 1 mg (IV form)/mL drinking water	Quaker parakeets

Drug	Dosage	Indication/Species
Allopurinol	10 mg/kg tid to qid; PO initially. Reduce frequency to bid or once daily as required.	psittacines
	10 mg/30 mL drinking water. Change solution several times per day.	budgerigars
Amikacin	10 to 20 mg/kg bid–tid; SC, IM, IV	general recommendations in the literature
	*10 to 20 mg/kg bid–tid; IM, IV	African gray parrots
	*15 to 20 mg/kg bid–tid; IM	cockatiels
	*20 mg/kg tid; IM	chickens
	*7.6 mg/kg tid; IM	ostriches
Aminopentamide hydrogen sulfide	0.05 mg/kg bid–tid for 1 day, then reduce frequency of dosage for 2 additional days; SC, IM	to control acute vomiting in psittacines
Amoxicillin	*150 mg/kg q 4 hr; IM	pigeons
	*150 mg/kg qid; PO	pigeons
	150 to 175 mg/kg once to twice daily; PO	general recommendations in the literature
Amoxicillin/ clavulanate	14 mg/kg bid; PO	blue-fronted Amazon parrots
	*125 mg/kg once daily; PO	pigeons
Amphotericin B	*1.5 mg/kg tid; IV	turkeys, great horned owls, red-tailed hawks
	1.5 mg/kg 1 to 3 times daily; IV	raptors, psittacines; recommendations from 3 to 14 days of treatment
	1 mg/kg once, 2 or 3 times daily for up to 1 month; intratracheally	dilute with sterile water or saline, combined with flucytosine
	1 to 7 mg/mL; nebulize bid for 15 min	diluted with sterile water or saline
	once daily to bid; topically	oral candidiasis

Drug	Dosage	Indication/Species
Ampicillin	*15 to 20 mg/kg bid; IM	emus, cranes
	*15 mg/kg bid; IM	hawks
	*25 mg/kg tid; IM	gallinules, pigeons
	*25 to 120 mg/kg once or twice daily; PO (capsule form)	pigeons
	*100 mg/kg bid; IM	pigeons, sensitive organisms
	*50 mg/kg tid–qid; IM	Amazon and blue-naped parrots, localized infections
	*100 mg/kg q 4 hr; IM	Amazon and blue-naped parrots, systemic disease
Amprolium	0.5 mL of 9.6% solution/L drinking water for minimum 5 days	enteric coccidiosis
	30 mg/kg once daily for 6 days; PO	enteric coccidiosis in falcons
Ascorbic acid	20 to 40 mg/kg once daily to once weekly; IM	general supportive care
Atipamezole	equivalent volume to dosage of Domitor	reversal agent for medetomidine
Atropine	0.1 to 0.5 mg/kg q 3 to 4 hr as needed; ¼ dose can be given IV, the remainder IM or SC	organophosphate
	0.02 to 0.1 mg/kg once; SC, IM	preanesthetic
Azithromycin	50 to 80 mg/kg once daily for 3 consecutive days in each week; PO	for chlamydia (6-wk treatment) and mycoplasma (3-wk treatment)
BAL (dimercaprol)	25 to 35 mg/kg bid 5 days/wk for 3 to 5 wk; PO	lead poisoning
Biosol-M	1 to 4 drops/oz drinking water	enteric infections
Bismuth subsalicylate (Pepto-Bismol)	2 mL/kg bid; PO	gastrointestinal irritation

Drug	Dosage	Indication/Species
Butorphanol	1 to 3 mg/kg; SC, IM	postoperative analgesia
Calcium borogluconate/ glubionate	1 mL/30 mL drinking water (115 mg Ca/5 mL) 1 mL/kg once daily; PO (115 mg Ca/5 mL)	calcium supplementation
Calcium EDTA	20 to 50 mg/kg 1, 2, or 3 times daily; SC, IM, IV, PO	lead or zinc poisoning
Calcium gluconate	50 to 100 mg/kg slowly to effect; IV, IM if diluted	hypocalcemic tetany, convulsions
Calcium gluconate/ calcium lactate	5 to 10 mg/kg once or twice daily; SC, IM; can be repeated weekly for longer term therapy	calcium deficiency
Carbaryl (5% powder)	topical application, as needed	arthropod ectoparasites
Carbenicillin	100 to 200 mg/kg bid, tid, or qid; IM, IV	psittacines
	100 to 200 mg/kg once or twice daily; PO	psittacines, ground tablets mixed in food
	100 mg/kg once to twice daily; intratracheally	pneumonia in psittacines; in combination with parenteral aminoglycosides
	200 mg/10 mL saline for nebulization	
Carnidazole	*10 mg single dose; PO	trichomoniasis in pigeons
	*5 mg single dose; PO	newly weaned pigeons
Cefazolin	50 to 100 mg/kg bid; IM	raptors
Cefotaxime	50 to 100 mg/kg tid–qid; IM	
Ceftriaxone	*100 mg/kg; IV	blue-fronted Amazon parrots
	75 to 100 mg/kg tid, qid or q 4 hr; IM, IV	
Cephalexin	*35 to 50 mg/kg q 2 to 3 hr; PO	bobwhite quail, hybrid rosybill ducks
	*35 to 50 mg/kg qid; PO	pigeons, cranes, emus

Drug	Dosage	Indication/Species
Cephalothin	*100 mg/kg q 2 to 3 hr; IM, IV	bobwhite quail, hybrid rosybill ducks
	*100 mg/kg qid; IM, IV	pigeons, cranes, emus
Cephradine	as for cephalexin	
Chloramphenicol	*102 mg/kg qid; IM, IV	Chinese spot-billed ducks
	*50 mg/kg qid; IM	macaws, conures
	*50 mg/kg bid; IM	budgies, turkeys, chickens, Egyptian geese, buteo hawks, barred owls
	*50 mg/kg once daily; IM	peafowl, bald eagles
	200 mg/15 mL saline	for nebulization
	80 mg/kg bid–tid; IM	commonly recommended dosage
	50 mg/kg tid–qid; IV	
Chloramphenicol palmitate	75 to 100 mg/kg bid, tid, or qid; PO	psittacines
	50 mg/kg qid; PO	chickens, turkeys
Chlorhexidine	10 to 30 mL of 2% solution/gallon drinking water	oral candidiasis, during therapy for chlamydia
Chloroquine phosphate	10 mg/kg loading dose, then 5 mg/kg at 6, 18, and 24 hr; PO	Plasmodium spp, malaria in penguins; in combination with primaquine phosphate
	10 mg/kg of chloroquine plus 1 mg/kg primaquine, 1 day weekly; PO in drinking water	to prevent seasonal malaria in budgies, canaries, and finches
Chlortetracycline	*0.5% impregnated millet for 30 days	budgies, canaries, finches, parakeets (Keet Life)
	*1% impregnated pellets or mash for 45 days	other psittacines
	*95 mg/kg qid **OR** 190 mg/kg tid; PO	pigeons with calcium in diet
	*30 mg/kg qid **OR** 95 mg/kg tid; PO	pigeons with no calcium in diet
Cimetidine	5 mg/kg tid; PO, IM, IV	gastric ulceration and gastritis in psittacines

Drug	Dosage	Indication/Species
Ciprofloxacin	*50 mg/kg bid; PO 20 to 40 mg/kg bid; PO 793 mg/L drinking water, for 7 days	red-tailed hawks psittacines, including pediatrics
Clazuril	*2.5 mg single dose; PO	coccidiosis in pigeons
Clindamycin	100 mg/kg once daily; PO 50 to 100 mg/kg bid; PO	pigeons psittacines
Clomipramine	0.5 to 1.0 mg/kg once daily to bid; PO (adjust dosage as required)	psittacines for psychological feather picking
Deferoxamine	100 mg/kg once daily; SC	hepatic hemochromatosis in a channel-billed toucan
Dexamethasone	1 to 4 mg/kg as needed; IM, IV	shock, head trauma, anti-inflammatory
Diazepam	0.1 to 2 mg/kg bid–tid; IM, IV 2.5 to 4 mg/kg as needed; PO	sedation, for convulsions psittacines
Diclazuril	0.0001% in medicated feed	coccidiosis prevention in broiler chickens
Diethylstilboestrol	0.025 to 0.083 mg/kg once; IM 1 drop of 0.25 mg/mL solution/30 mL drinking water	
Digoxin	*0.02 mg/kg once daily; PO *0.05 mg/kg once daily; PO *0.019 mg/kg bid; IV *0.0035 mg/kg once daily; IV *0.0049 mg/kg bid; IV *0.01 mg/kg once daily; PO	budgies, sparrows Quaker parakeets male Pekin ducks male turkeys roosters Indian hill mynah, secretary bird
Dimetridazole	*0.02% to 0.04% in drinking water, 5 days treatment, 5 days rest, 5 days treatment 1.5 mg/30 g, 3 treatments 12 hr apart; PO	giardiasis in budgies giardiasis in budgies

Drug	Dosage	Indication/Species
Dimetridazole (continued)	50 mg/kg once daily for 5 days; PO	trichomoniasis in pigeons and doves
	1 tsp/gal drinking water (182 g/6.42 oz powder) for 5 days	most species (see comments in text)
	0.5 tsp/gal drinking water (182 g/6.42 oz powder) for 5 days	mynahs and lories
Diphenhydramine	2 to 4 mg/kg bid; PO, deep IM	treatment of feather picking in psittacines
	0.013 to 0.065 mg/mL drinking water. This equals 0.06 to 0.1 mL of pediatric Benadryl per 10 mL of drinking water	
DMSA	30 mg/kg bid; PO	lead and zinc toxicosis
Doxapram	5 to 10 mg/kg once; IM, IV	respiratory stimulant
Doxycycline (oral)	*40 to 50 mg/kg once daily for 45 days; PO	cockatiels, Senegal parrots, blue-fronted and orange-winged Amazon parrots
	*25 mg/kg once daily for 45 days; PO	African gray parrots, Goffin's cockatoos, blue and gold and green-winged macaws
	*25 mg/kg once daily OR 7.5 mg/kg bid; PO	pigeons with no calcium in diet
	*150 mg/kg once daily OR 25 mg/kg bid; PO	pigeons with calcium in diet
	25 to 30 mg/kg once daily for 45 days; PO	cockatoos and macaws
	25 to 50 mg/kg once daily for 45 days; PO	other psittacine species
Doxycycline (injectable)	75 to 100 mg/kg q 5 to 7 days for 4 wk, then every 5 days for the remainder of a 45-day treatment; IM	psittacines (Vibravenos or specially compounded formulations only)
	*80 mg/kg at intervals of 7, 7, 7, 6, 6, 6, 5 days; SC, IM	Houbara bustards

Drug	Dosage	Indication/Species
Doxycycline (injectable) (continued)	10 to 50 mg/kg once or twice; IV	initial aggressive therapy (vibramycin hyclate)
Doxycycline (in feed)	300 to 440 mg/kg food for 45 days *100 g of corn diet medicated with 0.1% fed bid for 45 days	blue and gold and scarlet macaws
Enilconazole	6 mg/kg bid; PO	eclectus parrot with glossal candidiasis
	200 mg/L drinking water	canary with cutaneous dermatophytosis
Enrofloxacin	*15 mg/kg bid; PO, IM *7.5 to 30 mg/kg bid; IM 5 to 20 mg/kg bid; PO, SC, IM	African gray parrots African gray parrots commonly recommended dosage
Enrofloxacin (in drinking water)	*100 to 200 ppm in drinking water for 7 days	pigeons
	*190 to 750 mg/L drinking water	African gray parrots
	*50 mg/L drinking water for 5 days	Mycoplasma iowae in turkey poults
Enrofloxacin (in food)	250 to 1,000 ppm	psittacines
Epinephrine	0.1 mg/kg; IV, intracardiac, intratracheal, intraosseous	for nonanesthetic-related cardiac arrest
	0.01 to 0.02 mg/kg; IV, intracardiac, intratracheal, intraosseous	for anesthetic-related cardiac arrest; use lower dosage for halothane than isoflurane
Ergonovine maleate	0.07 mg/kg once; IM	to stimulate egg expulsion
Erythromycin	10 to 20 mg/kg bid; PO 44 to 88 mg/kg bid; PO for 5 to 7 days 500 mg/gal drinking water, 10 days on, 5 days off, 10 days on 200 mg in 10 mL saline, nebulize for 15 min tid	psittacines psittacines

Drug	Dosage	Indication/Species
Fenbendazole	5 to 15 mg/kg once daily for 5 days; PO	anseriformes
	20 to 50 mg/kg once, repeat in 10 days; PO	ascarids
	20 to 50 mg/kg once daily for 5 to 7 days; PO	capillariasis
	20 to 50 mg/kg once daily for 3 days; PO	microfilaria, trematodes
	20 to 100 ppm in seed	note toxicity in some species of finch
Fluconazole	2 to 10 mg/kg once daily; PO	*Candida* spp infection of the digestive system
Flucytosine	*75 to 120 mg/kg qid; PO	turkeys, great horned owls, red-tailed hawks
	250 mg/kg bid; PO	psittacines
	18 to 40 mg/kg qid; PO	raptors
	50 mg/kg bid for 2 to 4 wk; PO	prophylactic treatment, swans
	100 to 200 mg/kg bid; PO	various species
Flunixin	1 to 10 mg/kg as needed; IM	analgesic
Furosemide	0.15 to 2.2 mg/kg once daily or bid; PO, IM	diuretic
Gentamicin	*2.5 mg/kg tid; IM	red-tailed hawks, great horned owls, golden eagles
	*3 mg/kg bid; IM	turkeys
	*5 mg/kg tid; IM	pheasants, cranes
	*10 mg/kg qid; IM	quail
	*5 to 10 mg/kg bid; IM	cockatiels
	10 mg/kg bid; IM	blue and gold macaws
	10 mg/kg tid; IM	African gray parrots
	2 to 5 mg/kg bid–tid; IM	see note re: toxicity
	40 mg/kg 1, 2, or 3 times daily for 2 to 3 days; PO	enteric infections
	50 mg/10 mL saline tid; nebulize for 15 min	sinusitis, air sacculitis
	5 to 10 mg/kg once daily; intratracheally	pneumonia, combined with IM carbenicillin or tylosin
Haloperidol	0.2 mg/kg bid; PO	feather picking, psittacines < 1 kg

Drug	Dosage	Indication/Species
Haloperidol (continued)	0.08 to 0.15 mg/kg once daily to bid; PO	psittacines > 1 kg
	1 to 2 mg/kg q 2 to 3 wk; IM	psittacines
Hydroxyzine	2.2 mg/kg tid; PO	red-lored Amazon parrot for feather picking
Injacom 100	0.3 to 0.7 mL/kg; IM. Can double dose first treatment, then treat once weekly as required.	vitamin deficiency, supportive care
Interferon	1,500 IU/kg once daily; PO	psittacines
	1 IU/mL 4,000 IU/gal drinking water for 14 to 28 days	pigeons for circoviral infection
Iodine	1 drop of stock solution per 30 to 250 mL drinking water. Stock solution contains 2 mL Lugol's (Strong) iodine in 30 mL water.	iodine deficiency goiter in budgies. Daily for treatment, 2 to 3 times weekly for prevention
	20% sodium iodine in saline for injection; 0.01 mL/ budgie once; IM	for initiation of therapy
	122 mg/kg of diatrizoate sodium (37% iodine); IM	
Iron dextran	10 mg/kg once, repeat in 7 to 10 days if needed; IM	iron deficiency anemia, after hemorrhage
Isoniazid	15 mg/kg bid; PO	mycobacteriosis
Itraconazole	*6 mg/kg bid; PO	pigeons
	*5 to 10 mg/kg once daily; PO	blue-fronted Amazon parrots
	5 to 10 mg/kg once daily; PO	raptors, psittacines, waterfowl; aspergillosis or systemic candidiasis
Ivermectin	0.2 mg/kg once, repeat in 10 to 14 days if necessary; PO, IM	nematode and arthropod parasites including *Knemidokoptes* and air sac mites
	0.4 mg/kg once monthly; SC	spirurid nematodes of the proventriculus in African jacanas
	0.05 mg once; topically in the eye	ocular oxyspirurids in crested wood partridges and chickens

Drug	Dosage	Indication/Species
Ivermectin (continued)	10 mg/5 gal drinking water	aviary treatment
Kanamycin	50 to 250 mg/gal drinking water for 3 to 5 days	enteric infections
Kaolin and pectin	2 mL/kg bid, tid, or qid; PO	antidiarrheal agent
Ketamine	5 to 75 mg/kg; IM	common range of dosage
Ketamine + diazepam	5 to 30 mg/kg + 0.5 to 2 mg/kg; IM	common range of dosage
	2.5 to 5 mg/kg + 0.5 to 2 mg/kg; IV	common range of dosage
Ketamine + xylazine	5 to 30 mg/kg; IM + 1 to 4 mg/kg; IM	common range of dosage
	2.5 to 5 mg/kg; IV + 0.25 to 0.5 mg/kg; IV	common range of dosage
Ketoconazole	20 to 50 mg/kg bid; PO	mycotic infections
	30 mg/kg bid; PO	Amazon parrots— cutaneous aspergillosis
	200 mg/L drinking water for 7 to 14 days	
Lactulose	0.1 mL of 667 mg/mL suspension per kg bid; PO	hepatic dysfunction in Amazon parrots
	0.3 mL of 667 mg/mL suspension per kg once daily; PO	hepatic dysfunction
Levamisole	*20 mg/bird single dose; PO	anthelmintic dose for pigeons (Spartrix)
	15 mg/kg once, repeat in 10 days; PO	anthelmintic dose, Australian parakeets
	20 to 50 mg/kg once, repeat in 10 days; PO	anthelmintic dose, waterfowl
	4 to 8 mg/kg once, repeat in 10 to 14 days; IM, SC	anthelmintic dose, general use
	5 to 15 mL of 13.65% injectable solution/gal drinking water for 1 to 3 days, repeat in 10 days	anthelmintic dose
	2 mg/kg 3 times at 14-day intervals; IM, SC	as an immunostimulant
	0.3 mL of 13.65% injectable solution/gal drinking water for several weeks	as an immunostimulant

Drug	Dosage	Indication/Species
Levothyroxine	15 to 20 μg/kg once daily to bid; PO	
	0.1 mg tablet/30 mL drinking water daily	budgies, birds who drink little water
	0.1 mg tablet dissolved in 100 to 300 mL drinking water	other species
	for both doses, stir water, offer for 15 min, then remove	
Lincomycin	1 drop of 50 mg/mL suspension bid for 7 to 14 days; PO	budgies
	75 to 85 mg/kg bid for 7 to 14 days; PO	Amazon parrots
	167 mg/kg once daily for 7 to 14 days; PO	Amazon parrots
	100 g/kg once daily; PO	raptors
	*16.9 mg/L drinking water for 7 days	necrotic enteritis in chickens
Lincomycin/ spectinomycin	2.5 mg lincomycin + 5 mg spectinomycin per chick; SC	day-old poultry chicks to reduce early mortality
	1 part lincomycin + 2 to 3 parts spectinomycin in drinking water at 2 g/gal for 10 days	mycoplasmosis in turkeys
	1/8 to 1/4 tsp LS-50 powder per pint of drinking water for 10 to 14 days	chronic respiratory disease
Magnesium sulfate	0.5 to 1.0 g/kg once daily; PO	oral cathartic and chelating agent
Mebendazole	25 mg/kg bid for 5 days; PO	raptors and psittacines
	5 to 15 mg/kg once daily for 2 days; PO	waterfowl
Medetomidine + ketamine	100 μg/kg medetomidine + 25 mg/kg ketamine; IM	psittacines, chickens, pigeons
	75 to 100 μg/kg medetomidine + 3 to 7 mg/kg ketamine; IM	psittacines

Drug	Dosage	Indication/Species
Medetomidine + Ketamine (continued)	50 to 100 µg/kg medetomidine + 2 to 5 mg/kg ketamine; IV	psittacines
	50 to 100 µg/kg medetomidine + 3 to 5 mg/kg ketamine; IM	raptors
	25 to 75 µg/kg medetomidine + 2 to 4 mg/kg ketamine; IV	raptors
	100 to 200 µg/kg medetomidine + 5 to 10 mg/kg ketamine; IM, IV	geese
Medroxy-progesterone	18 to 50 mg/kg (according to size) once q 4 to 12 wk; IM, SC 150 g = 50 mg/kg 150 to 300 g = 40 mg/kg 300 to 700 g = 30 mg/kg 700 g = 25 mg/kg umbrella cockatoo = 18 mg/kg	to suppress ovulation, possibly to reduce feather picking
	0.1% in feed	to suppress ovulation in pigeons
Meperidine	1 to 3 mg/kg as needed; IM	analgesia
Methylprednisolone	0.5 to 1 mg/kg; IM Stock solution of 1.4 mL of 40 mg/mL product in 7.5 mL lactulose; 1 drop per wk in problem mo, 1 drop per mo for remainder of year	anti-inflammatory to prevent seasonal recurrence of "Amazon foot necrosis" syndrome
Metoclopramide	0.5 mg/kg once daily to tid; IM, SC	promote gastric motility
Metronidazole	10 to 30 mg/kg bid for 10 days; PO	anaerobic bacterial infections, psittacines
	10 mg/kg once daily for 2 days; IM	psittacines

Drug	Dosage	Indication/Species
Metronidazole (continued)	50 mg/kg once daily for 5 days; PO	trichomoniasis in pigeons and doves
	200 to 400 ppm in drinking water for 5 days	giardiasis in budgie nestlings
Mibolerone	10 µg/kg once; PO	to stop oviposition
Miconazole	10 mg/kg once daily for 6 to 12 days; IM	aspergillosis in raptors
	20 mg/kg tid; IV (slowly)	systemic mycotic infections in psittacines
	topically bid to tid	cutaneous mycotic infections
	2 mg IV formulation in 300 mL of acetylcysteine; via nebulization	red-lored Amazon parrot
Midazolam	2 mg/kg; IM	psittacines, swans
	2 to 4 mg/kg; IM	geese
Minocycline	0.5% impregnated millet	chlamydiosis in small psittacines, canaries
Monensin	90 g/ton feed	poultry, quail; disseminated visceral coccidiosis in crane chicks
Neomycin	1 to 8 drops of the 50 mg/mL preparation per 28 mL of drinking water	
	5 g/gal of drinking water	
Nortriptyline	2 mg/110 mL drinking water	feather picking in psittacine birds
Nystatin	300,000 U/kg 1, 2, or 3 times daily for 7 to 14 days; PO	candidiasis of the oral cavity and gastro-intestinal system
Oxytetracycline	*43 mg/kg once daily; IM	ring-necked pheasants
	*16 mg/kg once daily; IM	great horned owls
	*58 mg/kg once daily; IM	Amazon parrots
	50 mg/kg bid; IM	psittacines
	50 to 100 mg/kg q 48 to 72 hr; SC, IM (long-acting formulation)	cockatoos
	152 mg/kg q 72 hr; SC (long-acting formulation)	*Pasteurella multocida* infection in turkeys

Drug	Dosage	Indication/Species
Oxytetracycline (continued)	*50 to 100 mg/kg q 2 to 3 days for 30 to 45 days; SC	Goffin's cockatoos, blue-fronted and orange-winged Amazon parrots, blue and gold macaws; for chlamydiosis
Oxytocin	0.2 to 2.0 U/bird once; IM	egg binding, uterine hemorrhage
Paramomycin	100 mg/kg PO for 5 days; in food	cryptosporidiosis in Lady Gouldian finches
Penicillamine	50 mg/kg bid; PO	lead poisoning
Penicillin G	*50 mg/kg bid–tid; IM (potassium penicillin G)	turkeys
	*100 mg procaine and 100 mg benzathine penicillin/kg once daily or every second day; IM	turkeys
Phenobarbital	1 to 5 mg/kg bid; PO	seizure control
Phenylbutazone	3.5 to 7 mg/kg bid–tid; PO	psittacines
	20 mg/kg tid; PO	raptors
Piperacillin	*50 mg/kg tid; IV	blue-fronted Amazon parrots
	*100 mg/kg tid; IM	blue-fronted Amazon parrots
	50 to 200 mg/kg bid–qid; IM	general range of recommendations
	4 mg/macaw egg, 2 mg/ smaller eggs, days 14, 18, and 22; into the air cell	to reduce embryo mortality
Piperazine	100 to 500 mg/kg once, repeat in 10 to 14 days; PO	ascarid nematodes in gallinaceous birds
	45 to 200 mg/kg once, repeat in 10 to 14 days; PO	ascarid nematodes in waterfowl
Polymixin B	333,000 IU (33.3 mg) in 5 mL saline, nebulize for 15 min; tid	pneumonia and air sacculitis
Polysulfated glycosamino-glycans	100 mg once weekly for 3 mo; IM	King vulture, frostbite and amputation of digits

Drug	Dosage	Indication/Species
Polysulfated glycosamino-glycans (continued)	12.5 to 25 mg once; intra-articularly	osteoarthritis in Palawan peacock pheasant, demoiselle crane
Pralidoxime chloride	10 to 30 mg/kg once, do not repeat; IM	organophosphate toxicity
Praziquantel	*10 mg/kg (tablet form) or 25 mg/kg (aqueous form); PO	*Raillietina tetragona* in chickens
	*8.5 mg/kg; IM or 11 mg/kg; SC	*R. tetragona* in chickens
	10 to 20 mg/kg once, repeat in 10 to 14 days; PO	cestodes
	5 to 9 mg/kg once, repeat in 10 to 14 days; IM	psittacines
	10 mg/kg once daily; IM for 3 days, then PO for 11 days	hepatic trematodes in a toucan
	0.06 mg/bird (0.05 mL of suspension of 23 mg tablet in 20 mL water); PO	enteric cestodes in Lady Gouldian finches
Prednisolone	6 to 7 mg/kg bid; PO	anti-inflammatory
	0.5 to 1 mg/kg once; IM	anti-inflammatory
	2 to 4 mg/kg; IM, IV	shock, trauma, endotoxemia (immunosuppressive)
Prednisolone sodium succinate	10 to 20 mg/kg q 15 min to effect; IV, IM	shock; decrease dose by half in larger birds
Prednisone	6.7 mg/kg bid, then use decreasing dosage schedule	anti-inflammatory, antipruritic
Primaquine	0.03 mg/kg once daily for 3 days; PO	plasmodial malaria in penguins
	10 mg/kg of chloroquine plus 1 mg/kg primaquine, 1 day weekly; PO in drinking water	to prevent seasonal malaria in budgies, canaries, and finches

Drug	Dosage	Indication/Species
Prostaglandin E_2	0.2 mg/kg topically to the uterovaginal junction, once	to facilitate oviposition
Pyrantel pamoate	4.5 mg/kg once, repeat in 10 to 14 days; PO	intestinal nematodes
Pyrethrin products	topical, light mist as needed	ectoparasites, especially lice
Pyrimethamine	0.5 mg/kg bid for 30 days; PO	sarcocystosis, toxoplasmosis, plasmodial malaria
Rifampin	10 to 20 mg/kg bid; PO	mycobacteriosis
Selenium	see vitamin E/selenium	
Spectinomycin	11 to 22 mg/kg SC; q 5 days 20 mL/gal drinking water for 5 to 10 days 1 g powder (500 mg drug)/L drinking water 200 mg/15 mL saline for nebulization	*Pasteurella multocida* in turkeys gram-negative enteric infections mycoplasmosis in turkeys and chickens pneumonia and air sacculitis
Stanozolol	25 to 50 mg/kg once or twice weekly; IM 2 mg tablet/120 mL drinking water	anabolic steroid
Streptomycin	10 to 50 mg/kg bid–tid; IM	galliformes, pigeons, large birds; do not use in pet birds
Sucralfate	25 mg/kg tid; PO	gastric protectant, psittacines
Sulfa-chlorpyridazine	¼ to ½ tsp/L drinking water for 5 to 10 days	*Escherichia coli* and other enteric infections
Sulfadimethoxine	25 to 50 mg/kg once daily, 3 days on, 3 days off, 3 days on 200 mg/mL saline for nebulization	coccidiosis in raptors pneumonia and air sacculitis

Drug	Dosage	Indication/Species
Sulfamethazine	0.1% to 0.2% in drinking water for 5 days; or for 3 days on, 3 days off, 3 days on	coccidiosis in budgies
	0.5% in drinking water for 4 days	coccidiosis in pigeons
	30 mg/30 mL drinking water	small psittacines
Testosterone	8 mg/kg once, repeat weekly for anemia as needed; IM	increase male libido, anemia, feather problems, debilitation
	2.5 mg/kg weekly for 6 wk; IM	canaries
	stock solution of 2×10 mg tablets **OR** 100 mg of injectable formulation in 30 mL water; 5 drops of this/30 mL drinking water, provide daily for 6 wk. If no response is seen after 2 wk double the dose.	to induce male canaries to sing
Tetracycline	200 to 250 mg/kg once daily to bid; PO	initial therapy for chlamydiosis
	250 mg of syrup/cup of soft food	in conjuction with switching to medicated pelleted feed
	1 tsp powder (10 g/6.4 oz)/ gal drinking water for 5 to 10 days change water 2 to 3 times daily	
Thiabendazole	250 to 500 mg/kg once, repeat in 10 to 14 days; PO	ascarids
	100 mg/kg once daily for 7 to 10 days; PO	*Syngamus trachea*
Ticarcillin	150 to 200 mg/kg bid, tid, or qid; IM, IV	
Tiletamine + zolazepam	2 to 10 mg/kg; IM	sedation and anesthesia in ratites

Drug	Dosage	Indication/Species
Tiletamine + zolazepam (continued)	1 to 3 mg/kg; IV	sedation and anesthesia in ratites
Tobramycin	2.5 to 10 mg/kg bid; IM	pheasants, cranes, psittacines
Toltrazuril	75 mg/L of drinking water for 2 days each wk, 4-wk treatment	atoxoplasmosis in canaries
	10 mg/kg once daily for 4 days; PO	*Caryospora neofalconis* infection in raptors
Trimethoprim sulfadiazine	15 to 30 mg/kg IM; bid	
Trimethoprim sulfamethox-azole	10 to 30 mg/kg once daily, bid–tid; IM	psittacines
	10 to 50 mg/kg once daily; PO	pigeons
	25 mg/kg once daily for 5 days; PO	coccidiosis in mynahs and toucans
Tylosin	*15 mg/kg tid; IM	cranes
	*25 mg/kg qid; IM	bobwhite quail, pigeons
	*25 mg/kg tid; IM	emus
	10 to 40 mg/kg bid–tid; IM	general range of dosage
	*1 g in 50 mL DMSO, nebulize for 1 hr	bobwhite quail, pigeons
	250 g/8.8 oz powder; 1/4 tsp/8 oz, or 2 tsp/gal of drinking water; 10 days on, 5 days off; 10 days on	chronic respiratory disease
	1.0 mg/mL in drinking water for more than 21 days	*Mycoplasma gallisepticum* conjunctivitis in house finches
	0.5 mg/mL drinking water for 4 to 8 days	*Mycoplasma* spp in poultry
	up to 300 g/ton of feed	*Mycoplasma synoviae* in poultry
	250 g/8.8 oz powder; 1:10 in water as eye spray; bid–tid	conjunctivitis

Drug	Dosage	Indication/Species
Vitamin A	50,000 U/kg twice during the first wk, then weekly as needed; IM	vitamin A deficiency
Vitamin A, D$_3$, E	see **INJACOM 100**	
Vitamin B complex	dose by thiamine content, 10 to 30 mg/kg once per wk; IM	
Vitamin B$_1$ (thiamine)	1 to 2 mg/kg daily in food	raptors, penguins, cranes
Vitamin B$_{12}$	250 to 500 µg/kg once per wk; SC, IM	
Vitamin C	20 to 40 mg/kg once daily to once weekly; IM	
Vitamin D	See **INJACOM 100**	
Vitamin E	200 to 400 IU/day; PO	great blue heron
Vitamin E/ selenium	0.06 mg/kg selenium q 72 hr; IM	myopathy
	same dose every 3 to 14 days	neuropathy in cockatiels
	0.05 to 0.1 mg selenium/kg q 14 days; IM	
	0.1 mL/kg of preparation containing 1 mg selenium + 50 mg vitamin E/mL; IM	0.01 mL—cockatiel 0.03 mL—African gray 0.05 mL—eclectus parrot 0.1 mL—macaw
Vitamin K	0.2 to 5.0 mg/kg 1 to 3 times; IM	
	10 to 20 mg/kg bid; IM	psittacines
	10 to 12.5 mg/kg bid for 4 days; SC	coagulopathy in pelicans
Viokase-V	⅛ tsp/kg food	pancreatic insufficiency, maldigestion
Xylazine	see **KETAMINE**	anesthesia combined with ketamine
Yohimbine	0.1 to 1 mg/kg; IV, IM	reversal agent for xylazine

Handbook of Veterinary Drugs, Second Edition, edited by Dana Allen,
Lippincott–Raven Publishers, Philadelphia. © 1998

Section 19

Description of Drugs for Birds

ACETYLCYSTEINE

INDICATIONS: Acetylcysteine (Mucomyst ✦ ★) is a mucolytic agent used to help liquefy abnormal viscous or inspissated mucous secretions of the respiratory tract and eye. The drug has been used in birds by nebulization and direct nasal and sinus flushes. For more information, see **ACETYLCYSTEINE** in the Small Animal section.

ADVERSE AND COMMON SIDE EFFECTS: Dyspnea, lethargy, tachycardia, and edema of the eyelids have been described in neonatal birds after nebulization with acetylcysteine.

DRUG INTERACTIONS: Formation of a precipitate or a change in the color or clarity may occur when acetylcysteine is combined with tetracycline, oxytetracycline, chlortetracycline, or hydrogen peroxide, suggesting incompatability of these drugs.

ACTH

INDICATIONS: ACTH, or corticotropin, is a polypeptide secreted by the anterior pituitary. Cosyntropin is a synthetic analogue that is preferred for use in testing for adrenocortical insufficiency. Each 0.25 mg of cosyntropin is equivalent to 25 U (25 mg) of corticotropin. Cosyntropin is injected IM to stimulate a rise in serum corticosterone levels. In birds serum cortisol does not elevate in response to exogenous ACTH administration.

ADVERSE AND COMMON SIDE EFFECTS: Hypersensitivity reactions occur rarely in humans.

DRUG INTERACTIONS: Patients should not receive pretest doses of cortisone or hydrocortisone.

SUPPLIED AS: HUMAN PRODUCTS (Cosyntropin)
For injection containing 0.25 mg/vial [Cortrosyn ★]
0.25 mg/vial [Cortrosyn ♣]
1.0 mg/mL [Synacthen ♣]
HUMAN PRODUCTS (Corticotropin)
For injection containing 25 [Acthar ★] and 40 U in gel [ACTH ★, Acthar ★]
VETERINARY PRODUCTS (Corticotropin)
For injection containing 40 and 80 U ACTH in gel [ACTH ♣, ACTH gel ★]

ACYCLOVIR

INDICATIONS: Acyclovir (Avirax ♣, Zovirax ♣ ★) is an antiviral drug with activity against various herpes viruses and cytomegalovirus. In birds, the drug is used to reduce mortality during outbreaks of Pacheco's disease, a herpesviral infection. Treatment is most effective in birds that are not yet showing clinical disease. The oral form, available in capsules, is relatively insoluble in water. It is best administered by direct gavage, although in large aviaries treatment of drinking water and feed has been used. The water-soluble sodium salt intended for IV use has been given IM. Birds should be treated for a minimum of 7 days.

ADVERSE AND COMMON SIDE EFFECTS: An IM injection of the sodium salt can result in hemorrhage and muscle necrosis. Phlebitis commonly follows IV administration. The reconstituted solution is unstable and should be divided into aliquots and frozen for future treatments. The drug has not produced toxic effects even at 240 mg/kg administered three times daily. In humans, headaches, vomiting, and diarrhea are the most common adverse reactions reported. Nephrotoxicity and, rarely, neurologic signs can occur with parenteral administration. Because acyclovir is incompletely absorbed from the gastrointestinal system, oral overdosage and toxicity is unlikely.

DRUG INTERACTIONS: Amphotericin B and ketoconazole increase the effectiveness of acyclovir against some viral diseases in humans.

SUPPLIED AS: HUMAN PRODUCTS
Capsules containing 200 mg [Zovirax ★]

Tablets containing 200, 400, and 800 mg [Avirax ♣, Zovirax ♣ ★]
Suspension containing 200 mg/5 mL [Zovirax ♣ ★]
For injection containing 500 mg or 1 g of acyclovir sodium
[Zovirax ♣ ★)

ALLOPURINOL

INDICATIONS: Allopurinol (Zyloprim ♣ ★) inhibits the enzyme
xanthine oxidase and blocks the formation and urinary excretion of
uric acid. For more information, see **ALLOPURINOL** in the Small
Animal section.
   Allopurinol has been used in birds to reduce circulating uric acid
levels and treat articular gout. Improvement may be seen after 2 to 3
days of treatment; however, not all patients respond. The drug is
well absorbed after oral administration. Success has been described
using direct oral administration and medication of the drinking
water. Allopurinol tablets can be crushed and made into suspension
with sterile water or simple syrup.

ADVERSE AND COMMON SIDE EFFECTS: Allopurinol was administered to red-tailed hawks to prevent postprandial hyperuricemia; however, in three of six birds marked increases in serum
uric acid and visceral gout occurred. The other three birds showed
no effect of the drug. This suggests there may be considerable
species and individual variability.

DRUG INTERACTIONS: A number of significant drug interactions
exist. See **ALLOPURINOL** in the Small Animal section.

AMIKACIN

INDICATIONS: Amikacin (Amiglyde-V ♣ ★, Amikin ♣ ★) is an
aminoglycoside antibiotic indicated in the treatment of infections
caused by many gram-negative bacteria including susceptible
strains of *Escherichia coli*, *Klebsiella* spp, *Proteus* spp, and *Pseudomonas*
spp. For more information, see **AMIKACIN** and **AMINOGLYCO-
SIDE ANTIBIOTICS** in the Small Animal section.
   Amikacin is commonly used in pediatric avian medicine, where
it may be injected SC. In a pharmacokinetic study in African gray
parrots, amikacin given IM was rapidly absorbed with a peak serum
level reached by 45 minutes. The half-life was similar to that found
in other vertebrates. Almost all serum amikacin was eliminated by 8
hours after injection. Based on pharmacokinetic calculations, no accumulation was predicted at an IM or IV dosage of 10 to 20 mg/kg
every 8 to 12 hours. Similar pharmacokinetic data were recorded in
a study in cockatiels. At a dosage of 15 mg/kg IM twice daily, peak
and trough levels of 27.3 and 0.6 µg/mL, respectively, were reached.
Human guidelines for peak and trough amikacin levels are 15 to 30
µg/mL and 5 to 10 µg/mL, respectively. In ostriches given 2.12

mg/kg, SC injection resulted in lower blood levels than did injection into the muscles of the axial or thigh regions.

ADVERSE AND COMMON SIDE EFFECTS: In some species amikacin is less nephrotoxic than gentamicin; however, toxic effects have been described in birds. Although some sources recommend dosages up to 40 mg/kg, an Amazon parrot given 40 mg/kg twice daily IM developed polydipsia and polyuria on the second day of treatment. These signs continued until 3 weeks after treatment ended. Mild polyuria and polydipsia and elevated creatinine phosphokinase (CPK) and aspartate aminotransferase (AST) levels were also noted in orange-winged Amazon parrots given a dose of 13 mg/kg IM tid, or 20 mg/kg IM bid. Concurrent administration of balanced electrolyte fluids is recommended to reduce the chance of renal damage, especially in neonates. Measurement of blood antibiotic concentrations would help prevent toxicity. Pain on injection, transient lameness after injection, and elevated CPK levels have been described in ostriches. The toxicity of amikacin is enhanced under a number of conditions. See **AMINOGLYCOSIDE ANTIBIOTICS** in the Small Animal section for information on specific drug interactions.

DRUG INTERACTIONS: Amikacin is often used in combination with penicillins such as carbenicillin and piperacillin.

AMINOPENTAMIDE HYDROGEN SULFATE

INDICATIONS: Aminopentamide hydrogen sulfate (Centrine ★) is an anticholinergic drug indicated for the treatment of acute abdominal visceral spasm, pylorospasm, and nausea, vomiting, and diarrhea in dogs and cats. The actions of this drug are similar to those of atropine, with lesser mydriatic and salivary effects.

Aminopentamide hydrogen sulfate has been used to control acute vomiting in psittacines.

ADVERSE AND COMMON SIDE EFFECTS: Aminopentamide hydrogen sulfate delays gastric emptying and should not be used in cases of pyloric obstruction. Use of this drug may mask clinical signs indicative of gastrointestinal blockage.

SUPPLIED AS: VETERINARY PRODUCTS
For injection containing 0.5 mg/mL [Centrine ★]
Tablets containing 0.2 mg [Centrine ★]

AMOXICILLIN

INDICATIONS: Amoxicillin (Amoxi-Tabs ★, Amoxi-Drop ★, Amoxi-Inject ★, Amoxil ♣ ★, Moxilean ♣, Robamox-V ★) is indicated for the treatment of superficial and systemic bacterial infections. For more information, see **AMOXICILLIN** in the Small Animal section.

Pharmacokinetic studies have been carried out in a number of species of birds, including pigeons, chickens, and ducks. Parenteral use provided higher and more predictable antibiotic levels than did oral administration. Oily parenteral formulations resulted in a lower peak plasma level, but were more slowly excreted and, therefore, longer lasting as compared to the sodium salt. Tissue levels were greater than those in extravascular fluids. In these studies, amoxicillin had a greater bioavailability than similar dosages of ampicillin. In pigeons the use of oral tablets did not produce reliable antibiotic levels. General recommendations in the literature often recommend doses much lower than those suggested by pharmacokinetic studies.

AMOXICILLIN + CLAVULANATE

INDICATIONS: Amoxicillin combined with clavulanate (Clavamox ✦ ★), a β-lactamase inhibitor, extends the bactericidal spectrum of amoxicillin to include many β-lactamase-producing organisms. The combination diffuses readily into most body tissues, with the exception of brain and spinal fluid. For more information, see **CLAVAMOX** and **PENICILLIN ANTIBIOTICS** in the Small Animal section.

An experimental trial evaluated the safety and efficacy of amoxicillin + clavulanate in pigeons. Ten birds were given a 125 mg tablet PO once daily for 7 days. The only clinical abnormalities noted were 9 episodes of regurgitation and pink or red-brown discoloration of the feces. After 7 days of treatment, no bacteria were isolated from the feces of 4/10 birds, in comparison with control birds from which *Escherichia coli* and *Streptococcus faecalis* were ientified. Treatment did not seem to affect the development of lesions resulting from the inoculation of *Staphylococcus aureus* into the foot pad of 5 birds receiving antibiotics. Pharmacokinetic parameters for the drug were not evaluated.

AMPHOTERICIN B

INDICATIONS: Amphotericin B (Fungizone ✦ ★) is an effective fungicidal agent that has been the traditional first-line treatment for various systemic mycotic infections. For more information, see **AMPHOTERICIN B** in the Small Animal section.

Amphotericin B has been used for the treatment of aspergillosis in many species of birds, especially raptors, penguins, and psittacines. The drug can be administered IV, intratracheally, or by nebulization. The SC and intraosseous routes have been suggested when venous access is not available; however, their efficacy has not been proven. When used via nebulization, amphotericin B is poorly absorbed by the respiratory epithelium and has a primarily topical effect. It has been suggested that fluconazole and clotrimazole may be more effective than amphotericin B for nebulization. Amphotericin B can also be used topically for oral candidiasis that is refractory to nystatin.

In a pharmacokinetic study in turkeys, great horned owls, and red-tailed hawks given IV amphotericin B, plasma levels above the minimal inhibitory concentration for *Aspergillus fumigatus* were reached; however, clearance of the drug from the bloodstream was extremely rapid. Intratracheal injection of 1.5 mg/kg did not produce measurable plasma levels.

Once reconstituted, amphotericin B has a shelf life of only a few hours at room temperature and approximately 1 week if refrigerated. The drug can be reconstituted with sterile water and frozen in aliquots, then diluted in 5% dextrose or water as necessary for IV use or nebulization, respectively.

ADVERSE AND COMMON SIDE EFFECTS: Amphotericin B may be nephrotoxic and may induce bone marrow suppression. In turkeys given a single dose of the drug IV at 1.5 mg/kg, or 1 mg/kg once daily for 3 days, and great horned owls and red-tailed hawks given three injections of 1.5 mg/kg at 2-hour intervals, no evidence of renal toxicity was seen. Rapid IV injection of doses above 1.0 mg/kg resulted in transitory incoordination and mild convulsions. The use of amphotericin B as a nasal flush for 14 days in an African gray parrot resulted in severe inflammation and necrosis in the sinuses and adjacent muscle and led to the bird's death. Concern was also raised that the drug may have been absorbed through inflamed tissue, creating a risk for systemic (i.e., renal) toxicity.

DRUG INTERACTIONS: Amphotericin B can be used in combination with other antifungal agents such as ketoconazole or flucytosine.

AMPICILLIN

INDICATIONS: Ampicillin (Omnipen ★, Penbriton ♣, Polyflex ♣ ★) is indicated in the treatment of bacterial diseases, including some *Pasteurella* spp infections. For more information, see **AMPICILLIN** in the Small Animal section.

Pharmacokinetic studies have been carried out in pigeons, Amazon parrots, blue-naped parrots, emus, and chickens. Oral administration of ampicillin results in low and erratic blood levels, possibly due to excretion in the bile and intestinal wall immediately after absorption. Pharmacokinetic parameters vary among species. Sodium ampicillin injected IM resulted in a lower peak plasma level in pigeons than in parrots. In pigeons, the use of oily suspensions resulted in lower peak plasma concentrations, but slower excretion and longer duration than did the sodium salt. Administration of the same dosage of amoxicillin resulted in higher antibiotic levels. Although dosages for oral administration of ampicillin are commonly found, poor absorption makes oral use of this drug suitable only for the treatment of extremely susceptible organisms or for intestinal disease. Ampicillin was found to be more effective than erythromycin, enrofloxacin, or trimethoprim (all drugs administered in the drinking water) in preventing morbidity in pigeons experimentally infected with *Streptococcus bovis*.

AMPROLIUM

INDICATIONS: Amprolium (Amprol ♣, Corid ★) is an antiprotozoal agent and coccidiostat. For more information, see **AMPROLIUM** in the Small or Large Animal sections.

In birds, amprolium is used for the treatment of enteric coccidiosis. Some strains of parasites found in mynahs and toucans may be resistant to this drug; however, resistance has been described in several groups of birds after repeated use.

ADVERSE AND COMMON SIDE EFFECTS: Thiamine-responsive seizures were reported in a juvenile merlin with enteric *Caryospora neofalconis*, which was treated with amprolium for 16 days.

ASCORBIC ACID

INDICATIONS: Ascorbic acid or vitamin C (Apo-C ♣, Redoxon ♣) is essential for the synthesis and maintenance of collagen and intercellular ground substance of body tissues, blood vessels, bone, cartilage, tendons, and teeth. It is also important in wound healing and resistance to infection. It may influence the immune response. For more information, see **ASCORBIC ACID** in the Small Animal section.

Ascorbic acid has been used in the general supportive care of debilitated avian patients.

SUPPLIED AS: VETERINARY PRODUCT
For injection containing 250 mg/mL [Vitamin C ♣ ★]
HUMAN PRODUCT
Tablets containing 100, 250, 500, or 1,000 mg

ATROPINE

INDICATIONS: Atropine ♣ ★ is an anticholinergic, antispasmodic, and mydriatic drug also used to treat organophosphate toxicity. For more information, see **ATROPINE** in the Small Animal section.

In birds, atropine can be used as a preanesthetic agent to prevent bradycardia, although it may cause thickening of tracheal secretions and therefore predispose to blockage of an endotracheal tube. Atropine is used for the treatment of organophosphate and carbamate toxicity, to control vomiting, and as an antispasmodic. Atropine is not effective for inducing mydriasis in birds as the iris is composed of striated rather than smooth muscle.

ADVERSE AND COMMON SIDE EFFECTS: Thickening of tracheal secretions during anesthesia may result in the development of mucous plugs within the endotracheal tube. Gastrointestinal paralysis or stasis may become worse after treatment with atropine.

AZITHROMYCIN

INDICATIONS: Azithromycin (Zithromax ✚ ★) is a semisynthetic macrolide antibiotic with a narrow spectrum of activity that includes chlamydia, mycoplasma, and some streptococci and staphylococci. The drug accumulates in tissue and has a prolonged half-life. In human medicine, a single dose of azithromycin is used to treat uncomplicated venereal chlamydiosis.

No pharmacokinetic or efficacy studies have been carried out in birds, but the drug has been used orally to treat chlamydial and mycoplasmal infections. Lactulose and water have been used as the base for compounded oral suspensions.

ADVERSE AND COMMON SIDE EFFECTS: In humans, the presence of food in the stomach decreases the rate and extent of gastrointestinal absorption. Azithromycin is eliminated principally via the liver; therefore, caution is recommended in treating humans with hepatic disease.

SUPPLIED AS: HUMAN PRODUCTS
Capsules containing 250 mg [Zithromax ✚ ★]
Tablets containing 250 mg [Zithromax ✚]
Powder (suspension base) containing 300, 600, and 900 mg [Zithromax ✚ ★]

BAL (DIMERCAPROL)

INDICATIONS: BAL ✚ ★, or dimercaprol, is a sulfhydryl-containing compound that chelates arsenic. It is principally used for the treatment of arsenic toxicity and occasionally for toxicity caused by lead, mercury, and gold. BAL is not very effective in advanced cases. It is, therefore, best to administer the drug shortly after exposure. For more information, see **BAL-DIMERCAPROL** in the Small Animal section.

Dimercaprol has been used to treat lead toxicosis in birds. The drug can be given orally. It may be more effective than calcium EDTA in removing lead from the central nervous system and in rapidly decreasing blood lead levels.

ADVERSE AND COMMON SIDE EFFECTS: See **BAL-DIMERCAPROL** in the Small Animal section. IM injection is painful.

BIOSOL-M

See **NEOMYCIN**

BISMUTH SUBSALICYLATE

INDICATIONS: Bismuth subsalicylate (Pepto-Bismol ✤ ★) is used in the treatment of gastritis and diarrhea. It inhibits the synthesis of prostaglandins responsible for gastrointestinal tract hypermotility and inflammation. The drug may also have antibacterial and antisecretory properties. Bismuth subsalicylate relieves indigestion by forming insoluble complexes with offending noxious agents and by forming a protective coating.

ADVERSE AND COMMON SIDE EFFECTS: See BISMUTH SUBSALICYLATE and ASPIRIN in the Small Animal section.

DRUG INTERACTIONS: The antimicrobial action of tetracyclines may be reduced if these drugs are used concurrently. It is advised that tetracycline be given at least 2 hours before or after bismuth administration.

BUTORPHANOL

INDICATIONS: Butorphanol (Torbugesic ✤ ★, Torbutrol ✤ ★) is a narcotic agonist/antagonist analgesic with potent antitussive activity in some species. For more information, see BUTORPHANOL in the Small Animal section.

In birds butorphanol is most commonly used as a postoperative analgesic.

ADVERSE AND COMMON SIDE EFFECTS: In experimental trials in budgies given 0.1 mg (approximately 3–4 mg/kg), half of the birds showed motor deficits and were unable to perch tightly for 2 to 4 hours. The birds remained alert and had stable heart and respiratory rates.

CALCIUM BOROGLUCONATE
CALCIUM GLUCONATE
CALCIUM GLUCONATE/CALCIUM LACTATE

INDICATIONS: Calcium products are used for the treatment of hypocalcemia and for calcium supplementation. Calcium borogluconate, glubionate (Neo-Calglucon ★), gluconate (Calcet ✤ ★) and lactate ✤ ★ can be administered orally. Calcium glubionate should be given before feeding to enhance calcium absorption. Calcium gluconate and calcium glycerophosphate/lactate combinations are administered IV, or, if venous access is unavailable, IM or SC in a diluted form. Calcium gluconate/lactate combinations are used for IM injection. For more information, see **CALCIUM GLUCONATE** or **CALCIUM LACTATE** in the Small Animal section.

In birds, calcium products are used for the treatment of clinical calcium deficiency including hypocalcemic tetany and egg binding, for the pretreatment of uterine inertia and egg binding before the administration of oxytocin, and for supplementation of birds with mineral deficiency. Initial administration is usually by the parenteral route; oral supplementation is used for long-term therapy.

DRUG INTERACTIONS: Oral calcium supplements should not be given to birds being treated with tetracycline-medicated feed because uptake of the medication is significantly reduced. Injectable supplementation is recommended.

SUPPLIED AS: HUMAN PRODUCTS
Calcium glubionate: oral solution containing 115 mg elemental calcium/5 mL [Neo-Calglucon Syrup ★], 110 mg elemental calcium/5 mL, Calcium Sandoz ✦]
Calcium glycerophosphate powder
Calcium glycerophosphate/lactate: parenteral solution containing 5 mg of each element/mL [Calphosan ★]

VETERINARY PRODUCTS
Calcium glycerophosphate/lactate: solution containing 5 mg/mL of each element for IM and SC use [Calphosan Solution ★], and IM, SC, and IV use [Cal-pho-sol solution SA ★]
Calcium gluconate or borogluconate: numerous solutions for IV, SC, IP use (see individual product information for recommended route of administration) containing 230 mg/mL [23% solution ✦ ★] and 257.5 mg/mL [25.7% solution ✦ ★]

CALCIUM DISODIUM EDETATE (EDTA)

INDICATIONS: Calcium disodium EDTA (Calcium Disodium Versenate ✦ ★) is the most common chelating agent used for the treatment of lead toxicity. Before administration, calcium EDTA is diluted to a 1% solution using 5% dextrose in water. For more information, see **CALCIUM EDTA** in the Small Animal section.

In birds, calcium EDTA is used in the treatment of heavy metal poisoning, particularly lead and zinc. The drug also chelates, but to a much lesser extent, cadmium, copper, iron, and manganese. Calcium disodium EDTA chelates lead in the bone and plasma, creating insoluble complexes that are excreted by the kidneys. There is less risk of blood calcium chelation with disodium EDTA than with EDTA-acid or sodium EDTA. Oral administration will result in chelation of lead and zinc in the gastrointestinal tract. Other drugs used in the treatment of lead poisoning in birds include dimercaprol, DMSA, and penicillamine.

Calcium EDTA has been used IM or IV for the complete treatment period, or for initial therapy followed by oral treatment. Some authors recommend DMSA as an alternative for long-term oral therapy. Treatment should continue for 5 to 7 days, until no lead is visible radiographically, or until clinical signs abate. Patients should be watched carefully for the reappearance of clinical signs because lead in tissues continues to leach into the circulation.

ADVERSE AND COMMON SIDE EFFECTS: Calcium EDTA is nephrotoxic in mammals and should be used with caution in patients with impaired renal function or dehydration. Concurrent fluid therapy may be appropriate. In dogs, vomiting, diarrhea, and depression have also been described. Polydipsia has been reported in psittacines. Although birds are commonly treated PO, some sources indicate that this may increase absorption of lead from the gastrointestinal tract. Because IM injection of the drug is painful, diluting with sterile water and combining with an equal volume of 1% procaine hydrochloride have been recommended. Despite successful chelation therapy, clinical signs referable to peripheral neuropathy may not completely resolve, and birds may die of persistent gizzard impaction and stasis. Long-term treatment (i.e., several weeks) may result in chelation and depletion of normal blood cations.

DRUG INTERACTIONS: Do not use calcium EDTA in combination with nephrotoxic drugs. Renal toxicity may be enhanced by concurrent administration of glucocorticoids. Oral administration of fiber laxatives or peanut butter may assist in passage of lead particles from the gastrointestinal tract.

SUPPLIED AS: HUMAN PRODUCT
Calcium Disodium Versonate ✤ ★ 200 mg/mL

VETERINARY PRODUCT
6.6 % solution for injection [Leadidate ✤]

CARBARYL

INDICATIONS: Carbaryl (Sevin ✤, Zodiac Flea and Tick Powder ✤, and many others), a carbamate insecticide and cholinesterase inhibitor, is used for the eradication of arthropod ectoparasites. For more information, see **CARBAMATE INSECTICIDES** in the Small Animal section.

In birds, 5% carbaryl dust is used either by direct application to the bird or by addition to nest box litter. Approximately 1 teaspoon is required for a cockatiel nest, 2 tablespoons for a large macaw nestbox. Carbaryl may also be used to reduce ant infestations of the cage or nestbox.

SUPPLIED AS: VETERINARY PRODUCTS
Numerous dusting powders containing 5% carbaryl ♣ ★

CARBENICILLIN

INDICATIONS: Carbenicillin (Geopen ♣ ★, Pyopen ♣ ★) is an extended- spectrum, penicillinase-sensitive, semisynthetic penicillin used for the treatment of a variety of bacterial infections. It is effective against *Pseudomonas* and *Aeromonas* spp and in abscesses. For more information, see **CARBENICILLIN** and **PENICILLIN ANTIBIOTICS** in the Small Animal section.

In birds, carbenicillin is used IM, IV, and orally. Ground carbenicillin tablets can be mixed in food and given orally. Although the drug has been placed in drinking water, the ground tablets are not water soluble and form a suspension with uneven distribution. Respiratory disease can be treated by nebulization or by direct intratracheal injection.

ADVERSE AND COMMON SIDE EFFECTS: Carbenicillin is unstable once reconstituted. Some authors have suggested freezing the reconstituted drug in aliquots for subsequent treatments; however, subsequent stability has not been investigated. Ground tablets have an objectionable taste and odor that must be camouflaged with sweeteners or flavored compounds for use in drinking water.

DRUG INTERACTIONS: Carbenicillin is frequently used in combination with aminoglycosides, including gentamicin and amikacin. Separate syringes should be used to avoid in vitro inactivation of the aminoglycoside. Amikacin is more resistant to this inactivation than gentamicin. Intratracheal administration of carbenicillin has been used in combination with parenteral gentamicin for the treatment of *Pseudomonas* spp pneumonia.

CARNIDAZOLE

INDICATIONS: Carnidazole (Carnidazole ♣ ★) is an antiprotozoal drug licensed for the treatment of trichomoniasis in nonfood pigeons. It is also effective against hexamitiasis and histomoniasis. The drug is administered as a single oral dose in tablet form. Newly weaned birds are given half the adult dose. The drug was previously marketed under the trade name of Spartrix.

ADVERSE AND COMMON SIDE EFFECTS: Carnidazole was administered to pigeons in single doses of 40, 160, 320, and 640 mg/kg and at 40 mg/kg once daily for 7 days without adverse effects.

SUPPLIED AS: Tablets containing 10 mg [Carnidazole ♣ ★]

CEFAZOLIN

INDICATIONS: Cefazolin (Ancef ♣ ★, Kefzol ♣ ★) is a rapidly acting, first-generation cephalosporin. Of the cephalosporins, it achieves the greatest serum concentrations and has the longest half-life, and is the most active against *Escherichia coli*, *Klebsiella*, and *Enterobacter*. For additional information, see **CEFAZOLIN** and **CEPHALOSPORIN ANTIBIOTICS** in the Small Animal section.

Cefazolin has been recommended for the treatment of osteomyelitis, especially in raptors.

ADVERSE AND COMMON SIDE EFFECTS: Administration of cefazolin IM to great horned owls, red-tailed hawks, brown pelicans, and great blue herons has resulted in extensive hemorrhage in the pectoral muscles at the site of injection. One great horned owl had a hematocrit of 10% after treatment. In humans, thrombocytopenia is a recognized adverse effect; it is possible that this also occurs in birds.

CEFOTAXIME

INDICATIONS: Cefotaxime (Claforan ♣ ★) is a third-generation, broad-spectrum cephalosporin used in the treatment of bacterial infections, especially by gram-negative organisms. For more information, see **CEFOTAXIME** and **CEPHALOSPORIN ANTIBIOTICS** in the Small Animal section.

In a single dose pharmacokinetic study in blue-fronted Amazon parrots given 50 mg/kg IV or 100 mg/kg IM, cefotaxime was rapidly absorbed with a terminal half-life of less than 45 minutes. Dosage at least three times daily was recommended.

Reconstituted cefotaxime is stable for 10 days under refrigeration or can be frozen in aliquots for up to 6 months. Greater dilution of the drug is necessary for IV, as compared to IM, administration.

ADVERSE AND COMMON SIDE EFFECTS: Treatment with cefotaxime may result in an elevation in aspartate aminotransferase (AST) in some birds.

DRUG INTERACTIONS: Cefotaxime potentiates the antibacterial effects of aminoglycosides.

CEFOXITIN

INDICATIONS: Cefoxitin (Mefoxin ♣ ★) is a semisynthetic broad-spectrum, second-generation cephalosporin antibiotic. Cefoxitin has some activity against gram-positive cocci, good activity against many strains of *Escherichia coli* and *Klebsiella* and *Proteus* organisms, and is highly effective against many anaerobic infections. For more

information, see **CEFOXITIN** and **CEPHALOSPORIN ANTIBI-
OTICS** in the Small Animal section.

Reconstituted cefoxitin is stable for 10 days under refrigeration
or can be frozen in aliquots for up to 6 months. Greater dilution of
the drug is necessary for IV, as compared to IM, administration.

DRUG INTERACTIONS: Synergistic effects are seen against some
organisms when cefoxitin is used in conjunction with the penicillins
or chloramphenicol. Cefoxitin should not be administered with
aminoglycoside antibiotics because of possible incompatibility.
Nephrotoxicity is of concern in mammals when cefoxitin is used in
conjunction with aminoglycosides, vancomycin, polymyxin B, or diuretics. Pain may occur on IM injection.

CEFTRIAXONE

INDICATIONS: Ceftriaxone (Rocephin ✥ ★) is a semisynthetic
third-generation cephalosporin antibiotic with expanded activity
against gram-negative organisms. The drug's spectrum of activity is
similar to those of cefotaxime, ceftazidime, and ceftizoxime. For
more general information, see **CEPHALOSPORIN ANTIBIOTICS**
in the Small Animal section.

In a single dose pharmacokinetic study in blue-fronted Amazon
parrots given 100 mg/kg IV, ceftriaxone was rapidly absorbed and
had a terminal half-life of less than 45 minutes. Dosage at least three
times daily was recommended.

A second study was conducted in chickens. After a single IM injection of 100 mg/kg, serum antibiotic levels had peaked by 30 minutes after injection (18.03 μg/mL), and were undetectable by 4 to 6
hours. Peak blood concentrations were above the minimal inhibitory
concentration values for *Escherichia coli*, enterobacteria, and *Salmonella* spp isolated from psittacine cloacal swabs, but not for *Proteus,
Pseudomonas,* or *Klebsiella* spp. Birds were also nebulized with 40
mg/mL in sterile water, and with 40 and 200 mg/mL in sterile water
and DMSO. Ceftriaxone was detectable in the serum of only one bird
immediately after the cessation of nebulization. Level of drug in the
respiratory tissues was not assessed.

Reconstituted ceftriaxone is stable for 10 days under refrigeration
or can be frozen in aliquots for up to 6 months. Greater dilution of
the drug is necessary for IV, as compared to IM, administration.

ADVERSE AND COMMON SIDE EFFECTS: Adverse effects reported for ceftriaxone in humans are similar to those of other
cephalosporins.

DRUG INTERACTIONS: The antibacterial action of ceftriaxone and
the aminoglycosides, amikacin, gentamicin, and tobramycin, may be
additive or synergistic against some strains of Enterobacteriaceae

and *Pseudomonas aeruginosa*. In vitro inactivation has occurred with these combinations; separate syringes should therefore be used for administration.

SUPPLIED AS: HUMAN PRODUCTS
For injection containing 0.25, 1, and 2 g/vial [Rocephin ✦]; 0.25, 0.5, 1 and 2 g/vial [Rocephin ★] 20 and 40 mg/mL (frozen) [Rocephin ★]

CEPHALEXIN

INDICATIONS: Cephalexin (Keflex ✦ ★) is a broad-spectrum, first-generation cephalosporin. For more information, see **CEPHALEXIN** and **CEPHALOSPORIN ANTIBIOTICS** in the Small Animal section.

In a pharmacokinetic study involving pigeons, bobwhite quail, hybrid rosy-bill ducks, emus, and greater sandhill cranes given oral cephalexin, the biologic half-life was 36 to 126 minutes and varied directly with body weight. No difference in pharmacokinetic parameters was seen in fasted as compared to nonfasted quail.

CEPHALOTHIN

INDICATIONS: Cephalothin (Keflin ✦ ★) is a broad-spectrum, first-generation cephalosporin antibiotic. For more information, see **CEPHALOTHIN** and **CEPHALOSPORIN ANTIBIOTICS** in the Small Animal section.

In a pharmacokinetic study involving pigeons, bobwhite quail, hybrid rosy-bill ducks, emus, and greater sandhill cranes given cephalothin IM, the biologic half-life ranged from 16 to 54 minutes and varied directly with body weight in all species except the ducks. The frequency of dosing was such that use of this drug is impractical in many situations.

ADVERSE AND COMMON SIDE EFFECTS: Cephalothin is potentially nephrotoxic. The parenteral form is acid sensitive and should not be given orally.

CEPHRADINE

INDICATIONS: Cephradine (Velosef ★) is a first-generation cephalosporin with a spectrum of activity similar to that of cephalexin. The drug is available in oral as well as an injectable formulation. For further information, see **CEPHRADINE** and **CEPHALOSPORIN ANTIBIOTICS** in the Small Animal section.

No pharmacokinetic work has been carried out in birds; however, it is assumed that treatment should parallel that with cephalexin.

CHLORAMPHENICOL

INDICATIONS: Chloramphenicol (Azramycine ♣, Chlor Palm ♣, Chlor Tablets ♣, Chloromycetin ♣ ★, Karomycin Palmitate ♣, Viceton ★, and many others) is a bacteriostatic antibiotic with activity against a number of pathogens including gram-positive and gram-negative bacteria, chlamydiae, rickettsiae, coxiella, mycoplasmas, and some protozoa. For more information, see **CHLORAMPHENICOL** in the Small Animal section.

In pharmacokinetic studies using various doses of chloramphenicol in 18 species of birds, half-lives ranging from 26 minutes in the pigeon to 288 minutes in the bald eagle were found. Oral administration resulted in lower blood chloramphenicol levels than did IM injection. In chickens, oral use resulted in minimally effective blood levels. In pigeons, elimination was so rapid that frequency of administration was impractical. IV or IM injection of the succinate ester resulted in plasma concentrations 1.5 times less than those produced by the ethanol, benzyl alcohol, or propylene glycol formulations.

In Chinese spot-billed ducks, oral absorption was also variable. Blood levels resulting from 55 mg/kg did not reach therapeutic levels. Peak blood levels were reached within an hour of IV or IM injection of 22 mg/kg. It was suggested that, due to the high volume of distribution, tissue levels may be greater than those in plasma.

In chickens, therapeutic blood levels could be reached by oral administration of 50 mg/kg; however, there was considerable individual variation. Increasing the dose to 200 mg/kg PO increased the half-life, but not the peak serum level.

Despite its erratic absorption, chloramphenicol palmitate is a frequently used medication. It is palatable and is commonly added to food, including mixtures for hand-fed neonates. Parenteral administration should be used for serious infections. Chloramphenicol succinate has been used for the treatment of respiratory disease by nebulization. Chloramphenicol powder from capsules has been mixed with seed or mash diets to medicate entire flocks, especially for infections by *Salmonella* spp. The drug does not remain in solution in drinking water.

ADVERSE AND COMMON SIDE EFFECTS: Reversible, dose-dependent anemia, anorexia, and depression have been described in chickens, turkeys, and ducks. Vomiting and diarrhea may also occur. Temporary infertility has been described in male pigeons. Owners of pet birds should be warned about the potential risks to humans from this drug.

CHLORHEXIDINE

INDICATIONS: Chlorhexidine (Hibitane ♣, Nolvadent ♣ ★, Nolvasan ★, Savlon ♣, and others) is a chemical used for disinfection and as a base for a variety of antiseptic products. Diluted chlorhexidine solutions are used topically and orally, and the compound is also formulated into a number of topical creams. For more information, see **CHLORHEXIDINE** in the Small Animal section.

Two percent chlorhexidine solution in drinking water is used to prevent and treat candidiasis, especially in birds receiving long-term therapy with chlortetracycline-impregnated feed. Chlorhexidine is not absorbed from the intestine.

ADVERSE AND COMMON SIDE EFFECTS: Chlorhexidine may not be palatable to canaries, especially in the drug's scented form. Reduced water consumption, possibly to a fatal degree, can result from offering treated drinking water.

SUPPLIED AS: VETERINARY PRODUCTS
0.5% solution [Hibitane Teat Dip ✪]
1.6% solution [Della-Prep ✪, Sani-Wash ✪, Hibitane Udder Wash ✪]
2% solution [Nolvasan solution ★, Nolvasan-S ★, Hibitane ✪]
4% solution [Nolvasan Udder Wash Concentrate ★, Nolvasan Teat Dip ✪]
5% solution [Nolvasan 5% Teat Dip ★]
1% cream [Hibitane Veterinary Ointment ✪, Nolvasan Antiseptic Ointment★]

CHLOROQUINE PHOSPHATE

INDICATIONS: Chloroquine (Aralen✪★) is a synthetic antimalarial agent available for oral administration as the phosphate salt. It is effective against the circulating forms of many strains of *Plasmodium* spp and as a tissue amebicide, and has anti-inflammatory actions. Preerythrocytic and exoerythrocytic forms are not affected by the drug.

Chloroquine combined with primaquine has been used for the initial therapy of *Plasmodium* spp malaria in penguins, and prophylactically, in drinking water, to prevent seasonal malaria in outdoor budgies, canaries, and finches. The tablets can be dissolved in water (up to a concentration of 1 g/15 mL) and dosage based on estimated water intake.

ADVERSE AND COMMON SIDE EFFECTS: The bioavailability of chloroquine phosphate is greater, and adverse gastrointestinal effects lesser, in humans when the drug is administered with food. A number of significant side effects have been described in humans. Overdosage may lead rapidly to cardiovascular collapse.

DRUG INTERACTIONS: Therapy should be combined with primaquine phosphate.

SUPPLIED AS: HUMAN PRODUCTS
Tablets containing 150 ♣ and 300 ★ mg [Aralen phosphate]
Tablets containing 300 mg chloroquine + 45 mg primaquine phosphate [Aralen phosphate with primaquine phosphate★]

CHLORTETRACYCLINE

INDICATIONS: Chlortetracycline (Aureomycin ♣ ★, Fermycin Soluble ★ and others) is a broad-spectrum bacteriostatic antibiotic with activity against gram-positive and gram-negative organisms, chlamydiae, rickettsiae, mycoplasmas, and many anaerobes. For more information, see **TETRACYCLINE ANTIBIOTICS** in the Small Animal section.

Chlortetracycline-impregnated feed has historically been the most common compound used to treat birds infected with *Chlamydia psittaci*, especially in aviaries and quarantine facilities. Birds are provided with only treated feed for 30 to 45 days to maintain blood chlortetracycline levels greater than 1 μg/mL. Blood levels drop rapidly if consumption of medicated feed is interrupted. Medication of water does not provide consistent blood levels. Doxycycline and enrofloxacin are now preferred by many for the treatment of individual patients.

Commercially available millet impregnated with 0.5% chlortetracycline is fed to budgies, canaries, and finches. Therapeutic blood levels are reached within 24 hours.

In North America, the recommended level of chlortetracycline for mash or pelleted diets is 1%. In Europe, 5% is the general recommendation; however, 2.0% to 2.5% is used for some psittacines including large macaws, lovebirds, rosellas, and parakeets. Impregnated pellets are available from a number of commercial suppliers. As compared to specially formulated mash diets, pellets have a longer shelf life, are easier to feed, and have more consistent nutritional and therapeutic values. Mash diets must be made fresh daily.

Nectar solutions for nectar-feeding birds should contain 0.5% chlortetracycline.

Oral, as compared to IV, administration of chlortetracycline to chickens and turkeys results in much lower bioavailability. This may be due to filtering by the liver and excretion into the bile immediately after intestinal absorption.

ADVERSE AND COMMON SIDE EFFECTS: Many birds are reluctant to eat new foods; therefore, pelleted diets must be introduced carefully to ensure adequate food intake. Direct medication with oxytetracycline or doxycycline may need to be carried out during the transition period. Long-term chlortetracycline therapy may predispose birds to fungal and yeast overgrowth, especially oral and gastrointestinal candidiasis, and to gastrointestinal upset due to disruption of normal flora. Tetracyclines, especially chlortetracycline, inhibit protein synthesis and are immunosuppressive.

DRUG INTERACTIONS: Dietary calcium reduces absorption of chlortetracycline and, therefore, reduces therapeutic effect. Diets should contain no more than 0.7% calcium. A decrease in dietary calcium from 1% to 0.5% increased chlortetracycline absorption by 2.5 times in one study. In pigeons the half-life of oral chlortetracycline doubled when no grit was provided.

SUPPLIED AS: VETERINARY PRODUCTS
Water-soluble powder containing
55 mg/g [Aureomycin ✦]
25.6 g/6.4 oz, 102.4 g/25.6 oz [Fermycin Soluble ★]
Tablets containing 25 mg [Aureomycin Tablets ★]
Many agricultural feed additives
Millet impregnated with 0.5% chlortetracycline [Keet Life ★] Pellets impregnated with 1.0% chlortetracycline [Lafeber, Zeigler Brothers, Bird Life, Wings of Life, and others]

CIMETIDINE

INDICATIONS: Cimetidine (Tagamet ✦ ★), a histamine (H_2)-blocking agent, reduces gastric acid secretion and is used in the management of gastric and duodenal ulceration that does not result from the administration of nonsteroidal anti-inflammatory drugs. Cimetidine also increases caudal esophageal sphincter tone and promotes gastric emptying in mammals. The drug is available for oral use and for injection. For further information, see **CIMETIDINE** in the Small Animal section.

DRUG INTERACTIONS: By interfering with hepatic microenzyme systems, cimetidine affects the metabolism of many drugs. For further information, see **CIMETIDINE** in the Small Animal section.

CIPROFLOXACIN

INDICATIONS: Ciprofloxacin (Cipro ✦ ★) is a fluoroquinolone antibiotic available for oral, IV, and ophthalmic use. For more information, see **CIPROFLOXACIN** and **FLUOROQUINOLONE ANTIBIOTICS** in the Small Animal section.
   Ciprofloxacin has been recommended for oral gavage in individual birds or for use in drinking water for the treatment of flocks. Tablets dissolve well in water once the protective outer coating is removed; however, the duration of activity once in suspension may be very short.
   A pharmacokinetic trial using a single oral dose of 50 mg/kg was carried out in fasted red-tailed hawks. The drug was rapidly absorbed from the gastrointestinal tract. Mean peak serum concentration was 3.64 µg/mL; dosage with 50 mg/kg every 12 hours was recommended to maintain blood levels above 1.38 µg/mL, the minimal inhibitory concentration for many susceptible bacteria.

A series of wild house finches infected with *Mycoplasma gallisepticum* were treated with ciprofloxacin ophthalmic ointment for 5 to 7 days, in combination with tylosin in the drinking water for at least 21 days at a dose of approximately 1 mg/mL. This therapy was highly effective in eliminating clinical signs and preventing relapses, but the presence of a continued carrier state could not be ruled out. Birds treated with ciprofloxacin ophthalmic drops alone had a high rate of recurrence of conjunctivitis.

ADVERSE AND COMMON SIDE EFFECTS: Ciprofloxacin in water has a salty, bitter taste that should be masked by a sweetener or flavored compound. There is one report of a lilac-crowned mealy Amazon that became aggressive while being treated. Similar behavior has been reported in birds treated with enrofloxacin.

CLAZURIL

INDICATIONS: Clazuril (Appertex) is an anticoccidial drug licensed for use in nonfood pigeons in Europe against *Eimeria labbeana* and *E. columbarum*. The drug was previously marketed in North America. For information on similar compounds, see **TOLTRAZURIL** and **DICLAZURIL** in this section.

ADVERSE AND COMMON SIDE EFFECTS: At 125 times the recommended dose, pigeons developed mild, transient vomiting and watery diarrhea. Clazuril is safe to use during the breeding season. No adverse effects were noted in cranes given five times the recommended dose. Clazuril was suggested as a treatment for *Caryospora neofalconis* in juvenile merlins instead of sulfadimidine or amprolium.

SUPPLIED AS: VETERINARY PRODUCT
Tablets containing 2.5 mg [Appertex]

CLINDAMYCIN

INDICATIONS: Clindamycin (Antirobe ♣ ★, Cleocin ★) is a lincosamide antibiotic with activity against a wide range of infectious organisms. The drug is widely distributed in most body tissues and may penetrate the cerebrospinal fluid and ocular tissue if inflammation is present. For more information, see **CLINDAMYCIN** in the Small Animal section.
    Clindamycin has been recommended for the treatment of conditions such as osteomyelitis where long-term therapy is required. Treatment with clindamycin stopped the passage of clostridial spores and improved fecal character in a Catalina macaw with voluminous malodorous feces.

ADVERSE AND COMMON SIDE EFFECTS: Renal and hepatic function should be monitored during long-term use. Overgrowth of gastrointestinal yeasts may also occur.

CLOMIPRAMINE

INDICATIONS: Clomipramine (Anafranil ✦) is tricyclic antidepressant and antiobsessional human medication that has been used in psittacine birds to try and control psychological feather picking and self-mutilation. The drug has been effective in some birds in some case reports; however, the response of each patient is as yet completely unpredictable. Birds should be started on a low dose, which can be adjusted over several days according to response.

ADVERSE AND COMMON SIDE EFFECTS: Adverse effects described in psittacine birds include drowsiness, occasional regurgitation, and an episode of ataxia in a cockatoo. A variety of anticholinergic, psychiatric, neurologic, and cardiovascular adverse effects are described in humans. The effects of long-term treatment have not been systematically evaluated.

DRUG INTERACTIONS: In humans clomipramine should not be given with or within 14 days of treatment with an MAO inhibitor, e.g., possibly Amitraz, as this combination may predispose to hypertension. Clomipramine may potentiate the cardiovascular effects of sympathomimetic drugs, e.g., epinephrine.

SUPPLIED AS: HUMAN PRODUCTS
Tablets containing 10, 25, and 50 mg [Anafranil ✦, Apo-Clomipramine ✦, Gen-Clomipramine ✦, Novo-Clomipramine ✦]

CLOTRIMAZOLE

INDICATIONS: Clotrimazole (Canesten ✦, Lotrimin ★, Mycelex ★) is a topical imidazole antifungal agent useful in the treatment of localized dermatophytosis, candidal stomatitis, and nasal aspergillosis in dogs. For more information, see **CLOTRIMAZOLE** in the Small Animal section.

Clotrimazole has been used via nebulization for the successful treatment of confirmed respiratory aspergillosis in five birds (psittacines and raptors). Treatment was initiated with systemic therapeutic agents, including amphotericin B, flucytosine, or itraconazole, and nebulization begun once the birds were out of respiratory distress. The clotrimazole was solubilized in polyethylene glycol with a resulting pH of 6 to 6.5, and nebulized at a particle size of 0.5 to 5 microns. Clinical improvement was seen within a week in several cases. Treatment was continued for 2 to 4 months and could be carried out by the owners at home. Birds were monitored closely during treatment and showed no evidence of renal or hepatic dysfunction.

ADVERSE AND COMMON SIDE EFFECTS: Two of the three psittacines showed mild discomfort during nebulization, perhaps because of the dense fog produced. Once Amazon parrot regurgitated during the first few minutes of a treatment. A white film developed in the nares of one bird after 3 months of treatment; this was manually removed without difficulty. Ophthalmic lubricant should be used to reduce ocular irritation. Hepatic function should be monitored during therapy.

DEFEROXAMINE

INDICATIONS: Deferoxamine is a chelating agent that complexes primarily with trivalent iron and aluminum ions. It is used in humans to treat acute or chronic iron intoxication. The drug forms complexes with free iron or iron-binding proteins such as ferritin and hemosiderin. The resulting complex, ferrioxamine, is excreted in the urine and feces. Deferoxamine is poorly absorbed orally but well absorbed after IM or SC injection.

Deferoxamine was used effectively in a channel-billed toucan with iron storage disease. The bird's condition was monitored closely while under treatment; chemical and image analyses for iron levels were carried out on monthly liver biopsies. The bird improved clinically, but died 4 months later of cardiac fibrosis. Liver iron levels were unremarkable at that point.

ADVERSE AND COMMON SIDE EFFECTS: A variety of adverse effects are described in humans, including gastrointestinal upset; disturbances of hearing and vision; decreased blood sugar, serum calcium, and sodium; and increased coagulability.

DRUG INTERACTIONS: In humans with ascorbic acid deficiency, supplementation with vitamin C enhances the excretion of iron complexes. Patients receiving high amounts of vitamin C may, however, be predisposed to cardiac impairment as a result of toxic levels of labile iron within tissues. Vitamin C supplements should not be given to patients with cardiac disease.

SUPPLIED AS: HUMAN PRODUCT
For injection containing 500 mg/vial ♣ ★ and 2 g/vial ♣ [Desferal]

DEXAMETHASONE

INDICATIONS: Dexamethasone (Azium ♣ ★, Azium SP ♣ ★, Dex-5 ♣) is a glucocorticoid anti-inflammatory agent. For more information, see **DEXAMETHASONE** in the Small Animal section.

In birds, dexamethasone is used for the treatment of acute head trauma, shock, and at a lower dose as an anti-inflammatory agent. It may be helpful in reducing the inflammation associated with egg yolk peritonitis, and in the treatment of goiter in budgies, in combination with iodine. For long-term therapy, a decreasing dose schedule is recommended. Dexamethasone has been used in combination with antibiotics for the treatment of the "Amazon foot necrosis" syndrome.

ADVERSE AND COMMON SIDE EFFECTS: Concern is frequently expressed regarding the high sensitivity of birds to the immuno-suppressive effects of glucocorticoids. This has been supported by experimental work in pigeons, which showed that the hypothalamic–pituitary–adrenal system is more sensitive to suppression by gluco-corticoids than that of mammals, and that suppression is dose depen-dent. The minimum intravenous dose required to suppress plasma corticosterone levels was 50 μg/kg. Administration of 1 mg/kg IM once daily for 6 weeks resulted in complete suppression of the pitu-itary–adrenal system. When administration of dexamethasone was stopped, 6–7 weeks were required for basal plasma corticosterone lev-els to return to normal ranges. The duration of suppression by dex-amethasone was greater than that of prednisolone, which was also evaluated in these studies. In another study, dexamethasone was ad-ministered orally at 50 μg/kg, topically to bare skin at approximately 10 μg/kg, topically in combination with DMSO to bare skin at doses of 50 to 0.05 μg/kg, and ophthalmically at approximately 8 μg/kg. Suppression of corticosterone levels for up to 28 hours occurred in the groups given oral, ophthalmic, and topical dexamethasone with DMSO at 50 μg/kg. An oral dose of 3 drops of Azium (2 or 4 mg/mL, strength not stated) per gallon drinking water was found to be im-munosuppressive in another study. Elevations in liver enzymes, poly-dipsia, polyuria, and diarrhea can occur secondary to treatment.

DIAZEPAM

INDICATIONS: Diazepam (Valium ✤ ★, Valrelease ★) is a benzodi-azepine used as an anticonvulsant for the control of seizures, as a preanesthetic, in combination with anesthetic agents such as keta-mine, and for sedation. For more information, see **DIAZEPAM** in the Small Animal section.

DICLAZURIL

INDICATIONS: Diclazuril (Clinicox ✤) is licensed for the preven-tion of coccidiosis in broiler chickens. A related drug, clazuril, was previously available in tablet formulation for use in pigeons.

SUPPLIED AS: VETERINARY PRODUCT
Premix for medicated feed, containing 0.5% diclazuril [Clinicox ✤]

DIETHYLSTILBOESTROL

INDICATIONS: Diethylstilboestrol or DES (Stilboestrol ✤) is a non-steroidal estrogen used in the management of estrogen-responsive reproductive problems in females and plumage problems in both sexes. Tablets are insoluble (diethylstilboestrol) or sparingly soluble (diethylstilboestrol diphosphate) in water, but soluble in alcohol. For more information, see **DIETHYLSTILBOESTROL** in the Small Ani-mal section.

ADVERSE AND COMMON SIDE EFFECTS: Overdose may result in anemia.

SUPPLIED AS: VETERINARY PRODUCT
Tablets containing 1 mg DES [Stilboestrol ♣]

HUMAN PRODUCTS
Tablets containing 0.1, 0.5, and 1 mg DES [Stilbestrol ♣]; 1 and 5 mg [diethylstilbestrol ★], 50 mg [Stilphostrol ★], and 100 mg [Honvol ♣]
For injection containing 250 mg/5 mL Honvol ♣] and 50 mg/mL [Stilphostrol ★]

DIGOXIN

INDICATIONS: Digoxin (Lanoxin ★, Cardoxin ♣ ★) is a positive inotropic and negative chronotropic agent used in the treatment of congestive heart failure. For more information, see **DIGOXIN** in the Small Animal section.

The pharmacokinetic properties of digoxin have been studied in a number of avian species, including chickens, turkeys, ducks, Quaker parakeets, sparrows, and budgies. Digoxin elixir is rapidly absorbed after oral administration. The elimination half-life varied among the species tested, from a low of 6.67 hours in roosters to 25.9 hours in Quaker parakeets. In turkeys, pharmacokinetic variables changed with age of the bird and disposition with dosage levels. In budgies 0.02 mg/kg (approximately 0.0005 mg) produced blood levels in the therapeutic range for mammals. The digoxin elixir was diluted 1:4 to draw a measurable dose. A dosage of 0.05 mg/kg per day was recommended as a safe initial dose in Quaker parakeets.

Digoxin has been used clinically to treat birds in congestive heart failure, but little investigative work has been done on the efficacy of digoxin in avian species. In a trial involving chickens, a dose of 0.1 mg/kg daily reduced the incidence of ascites. When possible, measurement of blood plasma levels should be undertaken. In an Indian hill mynah with congestive heart failure, digoxin administered at 0.01 mg/kg once daily improved cardiac function; trough digoxin levels were 1.6 ng/mL. Dosage of 0.01 mg/kg once daily to a secretary bird with dilative cardiomegaly resulted in a trough level of 1.4 ng/mL. The bird improved clinically for a short period, but was eventually euthanized.

ADVERSE AND COMMON SIDE EFFECTS: In chickens, roosters, turkeys, and ducks, no toxic effects were seen at high plasma levels. In the Indian hill mynah described above, dosage with 0.02 mg/kg resulted in second-degree heart block. Trough levels were 2.4 ng/mL, above the therapeutic range in cats of 1 to 2 ng/mL. Dosage with 0.1 mg/kg in pigeons induced cardiac arrhythmias.

DIHYDROSTREPTOMYCIN

See **STREPTOMYCIN**

DIMETRIDAZOLE

INDICATIONS: Dimetridazole (Emtryl ♣) is an antimicrobial agent effective against anaerobic bacteria and protozoa.

In birds, dimetridazole has been used orally or in the drinking water to treat trichomoniasis in pigeons, doves, cockatiels, and budgies; giardiasis in budgie nestlings; and histomoniasis and hexamitiasis. In homing pigeons medicated water containing 400 mg/L had to be provided for at least 3 days to suppress infection by *Trichomonas gallinae*. Treatment once daily for 2 days using 20 mg tablets was ineffective in fasted and fed pigeons. The bioavailability of the tablet formation was 83.8%; however, this was decreased by 20% if the drug was administered with food.

Dimetridazole has also been suggested for the treatment of infections by anaerobic bacteria.

ADVERSE AND COMMON SIDE EFFECTS: In situations where water intake is increased, birds may ingest toxic quantities of dimetridazole. These include periods of hot weather, when parents are feeding young, and during the breeding season when males increase their activity level. Extended therapy with dimetridazole may result in toxicity or overgrowth of *Candida*. Cockatiels, budgerigars, and pigeons have been reported to have developed incoordination and acute seizures and to have died after receiving 1 teaspoon (182 g dimetridazole/6.42 oz product) per gallon of drinking water. Dimetridazole is toxic or lethal in Pekin robins, and possibly in other passerine birds. Acute hepatitis has been reported in cockatiel chicks. B vitamins may help resolve clinical signs.

SUPPLIED AS: VETERINARY PRODUCTS
Water-soluble powder with 40% W/W [Emtryl Soluble ♣]
Feed additives [Dimetridazole 30% Premix ♣, Emtryl Premix ♣]

DIPHENHYDRAMINE

INDICATIONS: Diphenhydramine (Benadryl ♣ ★) is an antihistamine also used as an antiemetic. For more information, see **DIPHENHYDRAMINE** and **ANTIHISTAMINES** in the Small Animal section.

Diphenhydramine is used in psittacine birds to try and control feather picking or as a mild sedative. Results are extremely variable.

ADVERSE AND COMMON SIDE EFFECTS: Birds become sleepy if the dosage is too high; tailoring treatment to each individual patient is necessary. Caution must be taken when with dosage recommendations are phrased simply as a volume (i.e., mL, tsp). The adult Benadryl elixir contains twice the concentration of the pediatric product that is commonly used (12.5 versus 6.25 mg/mL) and is formulated in an alcohol base. Veterinarians must ensure that clients are clear about which preparation they should use.

DMSA (2,3 DIMERCAPTOSUCCINIC ACID)

INDICATIONS: DMSA, or Succimer (Chemet ★), is an oral chelating agent with a high affinity for lead that is used in the treatment of lead poisoning in children. Children with blood lead levels greater than 70 µg/mL, or with clinical signs of encephalopathy, should receive initial or concurrent therapy with parenteral calcium EDTA and dimercaprol. In humans the initial dosage is 10 mg/kg tid for 5 days, then bid for an additional 14 days. Repeated treatment courses at a minimum of 14-day intervals may be appropriate.

DMSA has been used orally for the treatment of lead and zinc poisoning in birds. The drug forms water-soluble chelates that are excreted in the urine. Rational therapy would be to use calcium EDTA for initial parenteral therapy, then switch to oral medication with DMSA once lead levels have decreased and clinical signs have begun to resolve.

ADVERSE AND COMMON SIDE EFFECTS: Toxic side effects have not been described in birds.

SUPPLIED AS: HUMAN PRODUCT
Capsules containing 100 mg [Chemet ★]

DOXAPRAM

INDICATIONS: Doxapram (Dopram-V ♣ ★) is used to stimulate respiration in patients with postanesthetic respiratory depression or apnea and to encourage the return of laryngopharyngeal reflexes in patients with mild to moderate respiratory and central nervous system depression due to anesthetic overdose. For more information, see **DOXAPRAM** in the Small Animal section.

DOXYCYCLINE

INDICATIONS: Doxycycline (Vibramycin ♣ ★, Vibravet ♣, and others) is a second-generation, long-acting, lipid-soluble tetracycline antibiotic used in the treatment of bacterial, rickettsial, chlamydial, and mycoplasmal infections. As compared to other tetracyclines, doxycycline and minocycline are rapidly and almost completely absorbed by the gastrointestinal system and have greater activity against anaerobes and facultative intracellular bacteria. The half-life of doxycycline is almost three times that of chlortetracycline. For more information, see **DOXYCYCLINE** and **TETRACYCLINE ANTIBIOTICS** in the Small Animal section.

Doxycycline is currently the treatment of choice for chlamydiosis, especially in individual birds. Doxycycline can be administered by the IV, IM, and oral routes. IV injection has been recommended for the initial treatment of severely ill birds. The IM route is practical; however, to avoid severe necrosis of muscle at the site of injection only neutral pH solutions can be injected. Vibramycin hyclate, reconstituted according to the manufacturer's instructions, cannot be used in this way. Because Vibravenos, the formulation recommended for IM use, has not been available in the United States and has recently become unavailable in Canada, veterinarians have had compounding pharmacists create neutral sodium phosphate-buffered solutions of doxycycline for IM injection. Severe muscle damage in two caiques was reported after use of such a product, although no problems were seen in other psittacine species given the same formulation. A switch to oral therapy, either directly or through medication of the food, is often made once clinical signs begin to resolve. Treatment should continue for a period of 45 days, regardless of the method of administration. Pharmacokinetic studies have been performed in a variety of avian species, with minimum inhibitory concentrations of greater than 1 µg/mL in plasma being the objective.

In psittacine birds, IM doses of 80 to 100 mg/kg provide adequate blood levels for 5 to 6 days; however, the rate of elimination of the drug increases over time. A reducing time interval is therefore recommended for injection. Two recommended treatment schedules are: eight injections given at intervals of 7, 7, 7, 7, 6, 5, and 5 days; and six injections at 5-day intervals followed by four injections at 4-day intervals. Effective blood levels are reached within a few hours; shedding of chlamydia stops within 24 hours. Species such as the large macaws; lovebirds (*Agapornis*); eastern, western, and pale-headed rosellas; Bourke's, red-winged, turquoise, and mulga parrots; and red-fronted, canary-winged, and gray-cheeked parakeets, which require lower amounts of chlortetracycline for treatment, can be treated with doxycycline at 75 mg/kg on the same schedule. Half-lives of doxycycline in psittacines are species specific, ranging from 10 to over 20 hours.

Houbara bustards injected IM or SC with 100 mg/kg of Vibravenos seven times over a 38-day period maintained plasma levels greater than 1 µg/mL. With SC injection, absorption was slightly slower and elimination more rapid. This route was preferred to deliver the large volume of the drug. Mild irritation was noted at the sites of injection. Over 250 birds were treated based on the results of this study.

Once daily administration of 25 to 50 mg/kg in seven psittacine species produced therapeutic blood levels. In chickens given 10 mg/kg once daily orally, blood concentrations peaked at over 50 µg/mL and remained above 1 µg/mL for at least 12 hours. Oral absorption of doxycycline was erratic in growing chickens fed a liquid diet; this may have relevance for administration in the hand-feeding formula to psittacine chicks.

Doxycycline can be formulated into pelleted or mash diets; because of its greater bioavailability the dosage required is probably less than that for chlortetracycline. This may improve diet palatability. Seeds impregnated with 0.24% doxycycline fed to budgies and grass parakeets resulted in therapeutic blood levels; levels in birds fed mash diets containing 0.1%, 0.2%, and 0.4% for 6 weeks varied among birds and in individual birds from day to day. In one study, blue and gold and scarlet macaws were fed 100 g of a corn diet medicated with 0.1% doxycycline hyclate daily for 45 days. Blood levels greater than 1 µg/mL were obtained by day 3 and maintained through the period of treatment. Although absorption of oral doxycycline is less affected by calcium levels than is chlortetracycline, dietary calcium levels should probably be kept below 0.7%. Chickens medicated with 0.02 g/L in the drinking water did not attain serum levels of 1 µg/mL; however, levels in kidney and lung were greater than in serum.

ADVERSE AND COMMON SIDE EFFECTS: The IM administration of most IV preparations results in severe muscle damage due to the acid pH of these solutions. Vibravenos or specially compounded formulations must be used for this route. The oral LD_{50} in week-old chickens was 2,500 mg/kg. In Goffin's cockatoos treated with doxycycline in a mash diet, aspartate aminotransferase (AST) increased during treatment.

Vomiting has been reported in blue and gold macaws after both IM and oral administration of the drug. Reducing the dosage in this species has been suggested, as has dividing the dose for twice daily administration. Because of its more complete absorption and enteric secretion as an inactive conjugate, doxycycline has less disruptive effects on gastrointestinal flora than does chlortetracycline. Birds should, nevertheless, be monitored for the overgrowth of gastrointestinal yeasts such as *Candida* spp. Treatment with doxycycline may halt oviposition in hens and has been associated with bone deformities in toucans, especially in young birds. One report describes hemorrhages and delays in blood coagulation associated with repeated doxycycline injections. Vitamin K administered at the same time appeared to partially protect against this. Red discoloration of the feces may occur in treated birds.

As with all tetracyclines, doxycycline should be protected from light to prevent formation of toxic oxidation by-products.

DRUG INTERACTIONS: The effect of dietary calcium on oral absorption of doxycycline is less pronounced than with chlortetracycline. In pigeons without calcium in the diet the half-life was 6.25 hours; the presence of calcium decreased it to 3.81 hours. Calcium and zinc in the intestinal tract may bind to excreted doxycycline and block enterohepatic cycling, thus decreasing the drug's half-life. Dietary iron decreases absorption by 80% to 90%, whereas the presence of organic acids such as citric acid increases absorption by two to five times. The absorption of oral doxycycline was reduced by the presence of grit in the diet of pigeons.

SUPPLIED AS: VETERINARY PRODUCTS
Avian product: for injection containing 20 mg/mL [Vibravenos]
Water-soluble powder containing 50 mg/g [Vibravet 5% ♣]
Oral suspension containing 5 mg/mL after reconstitution [Vibravet ♣]
HUMAN PRODUCTS
Oral suspension containing 50 mg/5 mL [Vibramycin calcium syrup ★]
Capsules containing 50 and 100 mg [numerous products ♣ ★]
Tablets containing 100 mg [Apo-Doxy-Tabs ♣, Doxycin ♣, Nu-doxy-cycline ♣, Rho-doxycycline ♣]
For IV injection in vials of 100 and 200 mg [Doxy 100 ★, Doxy 200 ★, Vibramycin hyclate ★, doxycycline hyclate ★, Vibramycin-IV ♣]

ENILCONAZOLE

INDICATIONS: Enilconazole (Imaverol ♣) is an imidazole antifungal agent that has activity against *Penicillium* and the dermatophytes. For more information, see **ENILCONAZOLE** in the Small Animal section.

   In birds, enilconazole has been used in the drinking water to prevent and treat pulmonary aspergillosis in chicks. Enilconazole has also been used successfully against oral candidiasis and topical dermatophyte infections.

ADVERSE AND COMMON SIDE EFFECTS: Some birds reduce consumption of drinking water medicated with enilconazole. In some reported cases alternate day therapy was efficacious. An elevation in aspartate aminotransferase (AST) was seen in an eclectus parrot treated orally with 6 mg/kg twice daily for 7 days.

ENROFLOXACIN

INDICATIONS: Enrofloxacin (Baytril ♣ ★) is a fluoroquinolone antibiotic with activity against a range of gram-positive and gram-negative bacteria, mycoplasmas, chlamydiae, rickettsia, and atypical mycobacteria. Enrofloxacin has limited activity against anaerobes. For more information, see **ENROFLOXACIN** and **FLUORO-QUINOLONE ANTIBIOTICS** in the Small Animal section.

   Enrofloxacin is one of the most commonly used antibiotics in avian medicine; hence, some bacterial resistance is developing. Oral suspensions formulated from the injectable product are commonly used as an alternative to long-term therapy by injection. Enrofloxacin is effective against *Chlamydia psittaci*, but insufficient research is available to supplant doxycycline as the recommended therapeutic agent. Enrofloxacin is partially metabolized to ciprofloxacin, also an effective antibacterial agent.

Several pharmacokinetic studies have been carried out in African gray parrots. In a single-dose trial, enrofloxacin was administered at 15 mg/kg IM and 3, 15, and 30 mg/kg orally. Peak plasma concentrations were reached 2 to 4 hours after oral administration, and 1 hour after IM injection. The bioavailability of the oral medication was 51% of that of the IM dose. IM injection resulted in a higher peak plasma concentration than the oral dose; however, 2 hours after administration there was no difference between the two.

In a multidose trial, birds were given 30 mg/kg orally twice daily for 10 days. The disposition of enrofloxacin changed over this period, suggesting that an increase in dosage might be necessary for prolonged treatment.

In an additional study in African gray parrots, enrofloxacin in the drinking water produced lower plasma levels than the previous two routes. Birds given 0.09, 0.19, 0.38, and 0.75 mg/mL drinking water had similar serum levels of enrofloxacin and showed no significant differences in mean daily water consumption or weight loss as compared to control birds. Birds administered 1.5 and 3.0 mg/mL became depressed and exhibited polyuria and polydipsia, although no biochemical abnormalities were detected. Adverse signs resolved within 3 days of ending treatment. Birds had poor acceptance of water containing more than 0.75 mg/mL. The African gray parrots had lower blood levels than broilers or turkeys given enrofloxacin at a dosage of 0.1 mg/mL, suggesting that interspecies generalizations may not be accurate.

Protection trials were performed in Muscovy ducks challenged with intratracheal *Escherichia coli* and in canaries challenged with *Yersinia pseudotuberculosis*. Birds were experimentally infected then treated with enrofloxacin in the drinking water. Good therapeutic efficacy was described in ducks who had access to water containing 12.5 or 25 ppm for 4 hours daily for 5 days and in the canaries who were treated with 150 mg/L. Enrofloxacin provided in drinking water at 150 mg/L is recommended for the treatment of enteric *Campylobacter* spp infections in Lady Gouldian finches.

ADVERSE AND COMMON SIDE EFFECTS: Myonecrosis at injection sites can be severe. In a study in which 102 birds were given 100 or 200 ppm enrofloxacin in drinking water or 10 mg/kg IM once daily for 10 days, 22 birds developed polyuria and polydipsia that resolved after the trial ended, 19 had reduced food intake, and 8 had infections due to mycotic overgrowth. Depression, polyuria, and polydipsia were also seen in African gray parrots given enrofloxacin in the drinking water at concentrations of 1.5 and 3.0 mg/mL. Renal damage was identified in a Senegal parrot treated for 10 days with enrofloxacin and ketoconazole. Vomiting and inappetance have also been described in birds receiving enrofloxacin. Agitation and aggression have been recorded in a yellow-naped and a red-headed Amazon parrot being treated with enrofloxacin.

In an experimental trial in racing pigeons given 200, 400, or 800 ppm in drinking water over a long term, no abnormalities were noted in the birds themselves; however, there was a dose-related increasing embryo mortality in eggs from treated parents. Chicks raised by parents given 800 ppm had a slightly delayed increase in body weight and growth of long feathers, and in some birds joint lesions occurred. There was no long-term effect on growth or fertility of the chicks. It has been suggested that treatment with enrofloxacin may cause joint problems in some young psittacines and pigeons; however, the drug is widely used in pediatric patients.

EPINEPHRINE

INDICATIONS: Epinephrine ♣ ★ is indicated in cardiac arrest associated with ventricular asystole. It accelerates atrial and ventricular rates. It has been suggested that the avian heart is more sensitive to norepinephrine. For more information, see **EPINEPHRINE** in the Small Animal section.

ERGONOVINE MALEATE

INDICATIONS: Ergonovine maleate is an oxytocin principle of ergot used in conjunction with calcium and vitamin A injections to aid in egg expulsion. The drug should be diluted for use in small birds.

ADVERSE AND COMMON SIDE EFFECTS: The use of ergonovine is contraindicated where there is physical obstruction to the passage of an egg. In humans, hypertension may follow IV administration; overdose results in a variety of clinical signs including gangrene and seizures. Ergonovine is not used in patients with cardiovascular disease.

SUPPLIED AS: HUMAN PRODUCTS
For injection containing 0.2 mg/mL [Ergotrate Maleate ★] and 0.25 mg/mL [Ergonovine Maleate ♣]
Tablets containing 0.2 mg [Ergotrate Maleate ♣ ★]

ERYTHROMYCIN

INDICATIONS: Erythromycin (Erythro-100★, Gallimycin ♣ ★) is a macrolide antibiotic with primary activity against gram-positive bacteria. The drug also has activity against *Campylobacter fetus*, mycoplasmas, chlamydiae, rickettsiae, spirochetes, and some atypical mycobacteria, leptospires, and amebae. For more information, see **ERYTHROMYCIN** in the Small Animal section.

In birds, erythromycin is primarily used by oral administration or by nebulization with the injectable formulation for the treatment of chronic respiratory disease, especially air sacculitis and sinusitis, when mycoplasmas are suspected. Most psittacine gram-negative infections are resistant to the drug. The drug has been used in the drinking water at a concentration of 300 mg/L for the treatment of enteric *Campylobacter* spp infections in Lady Gouldian finches.

ADVERSE AND COMMON SIDE EFFECTS: The injectable solution given IM may result in severe muscle necrosis.

FENBENDAZOLE

INDICATIONS: Fenbendazole (Panacur ♣ ★) is an anthelmintic recommended for the elimination of nematodes and some tapeworms. It is also effective against giardia and some trematodes and microfilaria. For more information, see **FENBENDAZOLE** in the Small Animal section.

In birds, fenbendazole is used for the treatment of nematode infections, including capillariasis and *Syngamus* spp infection. It is not effective against gizzard worms in finches. The drug has been used by direct oral administration or mixed in feed. In a pharmacokinetic study in white Pekin ducks given 5 mg/kg orally or IV, no significant abnormalities were noted in complete blood cell counts, serum biochemistry, corticosterone levels, or thyroid function. Fenbendazole was not effective against hepatic trematodes in cockatoos at doses up to 100 mg/kg three times daily for three days.

ADVERSE AND COMMON SIDE EFFECTS: In one report a preparation of 200 mg fenbendazole impregnated into 1 kg of finch seed and fed for 6 to 7 days was toxic to long-tailed, blue-faced parrot and diamond fir-tail finches, and chestnut-breasted mannikins. Toxicity was not seen in parrots, pigeons, or doves. Deaths have been reported 3 to 5 days after administration of 1,000 mg/L in drinking water. Ataxia, mydriasis, and depression have also been described in canaries at this dose. Fenbendazole should not be used during molting because it may stunt feather growth, or during nesting.

SUPPLIED AS: VETERINARY PRODUCTS
Granules (222 mg fenbendazole/gram) to be mixed with food [Panacur ♣ ★]
Oral paste containing 10% fenbendazole [Panacur ♣ ★, Safe-Guard ★]
Oral suspension containing 10% fenbendazole [Panacur ♣ ★, Safe-Guard ♣ ★]

FLUCONAZOLE

INDICATIONS: Fluconazole (Diflucan ✚ ★) is a synthetic azole derivative antimycotic agent. Fluconazole has greater water solubility, better oral bioavailability, higher plasma and extravascular levels, and a longer plasma half-life than ketoconazole. Fluconazole is only recommended if topical treatment (e.g., enilconazole) is not feasible. Fluconazole penetrates well into the brain, cerebrospinal fluid, and eyes. For more information, see **FLUCONAZOLE** in the Small Animal section.

In birds, fluconazole has been used primarily to treat mucosal and systemic infections with *Candida* spp. Absorption of the drug is not affected by gastric pH, a feature useful in the treatment of pediatric patients whose gastric pH is relatively high. Fluconazole has been successfully used to reduce the number of candidial organisms in oral and fecal smears from psittacines at doses of 2, 5, and 10 mg/kg per day for 2 to 4 days. Umbrella cockatoos and blue-fronted Amazon parrots required 5 mg/kg to reduce numbers of organisms in feces to normal within 48 hours. Tablets were dissolved in water and the resulting suspension administered orally.

Fluconazole has also been used in the treatment of *Aspergillus* spp infections. Outbreaks of mycotic respiratory disease, caused by *Aspergillus* spp and *Alternaria* spp, in hummingbird colonies were successfully controlled by providing the birds with a 9% protein-supplemented nectar containing 25 mg/L of fluconazole for up to 2 weeks.

ADVERSE AND COMMON SIDE EFFECTS: Transient regurgitation has been reported after treatment with fluconazole, especially in cockatoos and cockatiels. Increases in aspartate aminotransferase (AST) and lactic dehydrogenase (LDH) were seen during treatment; however, by 2 weeks after treatment, enzyme levels had returned to normal.

FLUCYTOSINE (5-FLUOROCYTOSINE)

INDICATIONS: Flucytosine (Ancobon ★, Ancotil ✚) is a fluorinated pyrimidine antifungal agent often used in combination with amphotericin B, with which it is synergistic. For more information, see **FLUCYTOSINE** in the Small Animal section.

In birds, flucytosine has been used for the treatment of severe candidiasis in the digestive system and systemic candidial infections, and for the prevention and treatment of respiratory aspergillosis. Some work has shown, however, that in vitro, significant numbers of these organisms are resistant to the drug. Preventive treatment has been especially recommended for high-risk patients such as immunosuppressed birds, birds with severe chlamydia infections, and stressed raptors, particularly accipiter hawks new to captivity.

In a pharmacokinetic study involving turkeys, great horned owls, and red-tailed hawks, oral administration of flucytosine at doses of 75 to 120 mg/kg was recommended at 6-hour intervals to maintain plasma levels above the minimum inhibitory concentration for *Aspergillus fumigatus*.

ADVERSE AND COMMON SIDE EFFECTS: Gastrointestinal irritation has been described in some birds. Because of potential bone marrow toxicity, hematologic parameters should be monitored in birds on long-term therapy.

DRUG INTERACTIONS: Flucytosine can be used in combination with amphotericin B.

FLUNIXIN MEGLUMINE

INDICATIONS: Flunixin meglumine (Banamine ♣ ★) is a potent nonsteroidal antiprostaglandin agent with anti-inflammatory and antipyretic properties that make it useful in the treatment of inflammation and pain associated with musculoskeletal disease. For more information, see **FLUNIXIN** in the Small Animal section.

Flunixin has been recommended for use in pediatric patients with intestinal pain and anorexia and for birds in shock or with traumatic injuries.

ADVERSE AND COMMON SIDE EFFECTS: In an experimental trial in budgies given 10 mg/kg, five of seven birds vomited between 2 and 5 minutes after administration, but appeared normal after that. Diarrhea has also been reported.

FUROSEMIDE

INDICATIONS: Furosemide (Lasix ♣ ★) is a potent loop diuretic that is effective in reducing edema of cardiac origin and promoting diuresis. For more information, see **FUROSEMIDE** in the Small Animal section.

ADVERSE AND COMMON SIDE EFFECTS: Overdosage may result in dehydration and electrolyte abnormalities. Neurologic signs and death have also been reported. Some species, such as lories, are very sensitive to furosemide and are easily overdosed. The therapeutic index in birds appears to be low.

GENTAMICIN

INDICATIONS: Gentamicin (Gentocin ♣ ★) is an aminoglycoside antibiotic used in the treatment of bacterial infections, especially those caused by gram-negative organisms. For more information, see **GENTAMICIN** and **AMINOGLYCOSIDE ANTIBIOTICS** in the Small Animal section.

Gentamicin has been used widely in avian medicine, but nephrotoxicity is a real concern. Pharmacokinetic parameters vary widely among avian species; therefore, direct application of dosage recommendations from one species to another may be inappropriate. In recent years, amikacin has been a less toxic alternative when an aminoglycoside antibiotic is desired.

In pharmacokinetic studies carried out in bobwhite quail, pheasants, and greater sandhill cranes given from 5 to 20 mg/kg IM, peak plasma concentrations varied with increasing drug dose. The mean half-life ranged from approximately 40 minutes in quail to 165 minutes in cranes. In another study involving red-tailed hawks, great horned owls, and golden eagles given 10 mg/kg IV, significant differences in serum half-life and total body clearance were seen among the different species. This dose resulted in peak and trough levels greater than those associated with nephro- and ototoxicity in humans.

In a study in quail, cranes, and ducks, levels of gentamicin in lung and leg muscle parallelled those in plasma; levels in liver and kidney were greater. Movement and elimination of the drug differed among the species examined. Similar findings were described for hawks, owls, chickens, and turkeys. Gentamicin was present in renal tissue for 3 to 4 weeks after cessation of treatment in chickens and turkeys.

A pharmacokinetic study in cockatiels concluded that a dosage of 5 to 10 mg/kg IM two to three times daily was appropriate. A half-life of 71 minutes was calculated in this species based on an IM dose of 5 mg/kg twice daily. The mean peak and trough levels were 4.6 μg/mL and 0.2 μg/mL, respectively. In human medicine, the desired peak and trough levels of gentamicin are 8–10 μg/mL and less than 2 μg/mL.

Gentamicin has been used to treat sinusitis and air sacculitis by nebulization, where it has a primarily topical effect due to poor absorption from the respiratory epithelium. Sinusitis can also be treated by direct intranasal administration of gentamicin ophthalmic solution. Direct intratracheal injection has also been suggested for the treatment of respiratory disease.

Gentamicin is not absorbed through intact intestinal mucosa; therefore, oral therapy is limited to treatment of infections confined to the gut.

ADVERSE AND COMMON SIDE EFFECTS: Gentamicin is nephrotoxic, especially in birds that are dehydrated or suffering from pre-existing renal disease. Concurrent administration of balanced electrolyte solutions may help reduce renal damage. Measurement of blood antibiotic concentrations should be carried out whenever possible.

Renal toxicity has been described in a wide variety of avian species, including psittacines, given gentamicin at a total dose of 10 mg/kg per day and greater. Polyuria and polydipsia were commonly seen; however, neither clinical signs nor serum biochemical parameters were considered good indicators of the degree of renal damage. Renal function did not return to normal for up to several weeks after cessation of treatment. Recent work suggests that less frequent administration of aminoglycoside antibiotics (allowing trough levels to drop to 1 µg/mL) reduces the likelihood of toxicity. Deaths occurred frequently in birds given daily doses of 20 mg/kg or greater. Lories may be particularly susceptible to the toxic effects. Weakness, apnea, and sudden death attributed to neuromuscular blockade has been described in hawks and great horned owls. Some birds also showed ataxia, which was presumed to result from vestibular damage.

DRUG INTERACTIONS: Gentamicin is inactivated in vitro if mixed with carbenicillin or ticarcillin. In vivo inactivation may occur in the presence of these drugs and renal disease. Some cephalosporins potentiate the effect of gentamicin.

HALOPERIDOL

INDICATIONS: Haloperidol (Haldol ✦ ★, Peridol ✦, and others) is an antipsychotic drug, similar in structure to droperidol, which is used to treat human psychiatric disorders. An oral and a long-acting (decanoate) IM formulation are available.

In birds, haloperidol has been used for the treatment of feather picking and self-mutilation. There is tremendous variability in response, and the dosage must be carefully adjusted for each individual patient. The greatest success appears to have been obtained in cockatoos. Attention to environmental and other factors is an important component of therapy.

ADVERSE AND COMMON SIDE EFFECTS: In humans, there is a narrow range between the effective therapeutic dose and that causing extrapyramidal neurologic symptoms. Adverse effects related to other body systems are also described. In birds, African gray parrots and Quaker parakeets have shown disorientation or abnormal behaviors when on treatment. Quaker parakeets and Moluccan and umbrella cockatoos may require a lower dose than other psittacine species.

DRUG INTERACTIONS: Haloperidol may be additive with or potentiate the effects of central nervous system depressants, including opiates and other analgesics, and anesthetics.

SUPPLIED AS: HUMAN PRODUCTS
Tablets containing 0.5, 1, 2, 5, 10, and 20 mg [Apo-peridol ✦, Novo-peridol ✦, Peridol ✦, Haldol ✦ ★]

Oral suspension containing 2 mg/mL [Haldol Concentrate ★, Haloperidol Intensol ★, PMS-Haloperidol ✦]
For injection containing 5 mg/mL [Haldol ★, Haloperidol Injection ★]

HYDROXYZINE

INDICATIONS: Hydroxyzine [Atarax ✦ ★, Vistaril ★, and others] is a piperazine derivative antihistamine agent with sedative and tranquilizing effects. The drug is used in humans primarily for the symptomatic management of anxiety and the management of pruritus caused by allergy.

In birds, hydroxyzine has been used to treat feather picking. There is tremendous variability in response, and the dosage must be carefully adjusted for each individual patient. Attention to environmental and other factors is also an essential component of therapy.

ADVERSE AND COMMON SIDE EFFECTS: The most common adverse effects in humans are drowsiness and dry mouth. A variety of other reactions are described.

DRUG INTERACTIONS: Hydroxyzine may be additive with or potentiate the effects of central nervous system depressants including opiates and other analgesics, anesthetics, and anticholinergic agents.

SUPPLIED AS: HUMAN PRODUCTS
Tablets containing 10, 25, and 50 mg [Atarax ✦ ★, Anxanil ★]
Capsules containing 25 and 50 mg [Hy-Pam ★, Vistaril ★, Apo-Hydroxyzine ✦]
Oral syrup containing 2 mg/mL [PMS-Hydroxyzine ✦]
Oral solution containing 10 mg/5 mL [Atarax ✦ ★]
Oral suspension containing 25 mg/5 mL [Vistaril ★]
For injection containing 50 mg/mL [numerous products ★]

INJACOM 100

INDICATIONS: Injacom 100 ★ is an aqueous multivitamin solution for IM use in the treatment of vitamin deficiencies and as a general supportive measure. Because it contains vitamin D_3, the product may help in the treatment of soft bones, soft eggs and egg binding, and bone repair.

ADVERSE AND COMMON SIDE EFFECTS: African gray parrots should be treated once only to avoid problems with calcium metabolism. Vitamin D toxicity is a potential hazard of repeated injection; however, it has not been described in practice. Injacom, the large animal formulation, is oil based and contains excess vitamin D.

SUPPLIED AS: VETERINARY PRODUCTS
Injacom 100 ★ containing 100,000 IU vitamin A, 10,000 IU vitamin D₃,
and 20 IU vitamin E
No Canadian product contains the same proportions
Vitamin A-D ♣ containing 500,000 IU vitamin A, 75,000 IU vitamin
D₃, and 50 IU vitamin E
Numerous veterinary and human oral preparations with similar
composition

INTERFERON

INDICATIONS: Interferon (Roferon A ♣ ★) has immunomodulating
and antiproliferative capabilities and antiviral activity. It has been
used in birds infected or exposed to the virus that causes psittacine
proventricular dilation disease (PDD). Results are still preliminary;
however, the drug appeared to halt the spread of PDD virus through
a psittacine breeding nursery when administered once daily for 6
weeks and may have some effect on slowing the progress of disease
in infected birds. Interferon has also been suggested for the treatment of pigeons with circoviral infection. For more information, see
INTERFERON in the Small Animal section.

IODINE

INDICATIONS: Iodine is used for the treatment and prevention of
iodine deficiency, or goiter, in budgies. The drug is usually provided
in a dilute form in the drinking water; however, in birds that are
vomiting, injectable use of sodium iodide is possible.

DRUG INTERACTIONS: Iodine products oxidize when exposed to
light and should be stored in dark bottles. Medicated drinking water
should be replaced daily.

SUPPLIED AS: Lugol's iodine ♣ ★

IRON DEXTRAN

INDICATIONS: Iron dextran is used for the treatment of iron deficiency anemia and after hemorrhage. In mammals, 90% of the drug
is absorbed after 1 to 3 weeks. For more information, see **IRON
DEXTRAN** in the Small Animal section.

ADVERSE AND COMMON SIDE EFFECTS: Iron dextran should
be used with caution in avian species that are predisposed to he-
mochromatosis.

DRUG INTERACTIONS: Iron dextran is reported to be incompatible with chlortetracycline and sulfadiazine sodium.

ISONIAZID

INDICATIONS: Isoniazid [Isoniazid ✦ ★, Isotamine ✦] is an antimicrobial agent active only against organisms of the genus *Mycobacterium*. The drug is bacteriostatic or bactericidal depending on concentrations in tissue and the susceptibility of the organism. It is only active against replicating organisms. Humans are treated with the drug for a minimum of 6 months. Isoniazid is also used prophylactically in high-risk situations.

Isoniazid has been used to treat birds infected with mycobacterial organisms. Veterinarians differ in their willingness to treat avian mycobacteriosis based on concerns over poor success rate of treatment and the potential for spread of the disease to humans under certain conditions.

ADVERSE AND COMMON SIDE EFFECTS: In humans, administration with food reduces absorption and peak plasma concentrations. A variety of adverse effects are reported, including hepatic dysfunction, hypersensitivity, and peripheral neuritis.

DRUG INTERACTIONS: In humans, isoniazid is used alone or in combination with rifampin or rifampin and pyrazinamide.

SUPPLIED AS: HUMAN PRODUCTS
Syrup containing 10 mg/5 mL [Isotamine ✦] and 50 mg/5 mL [Isotamine ✦, Isoniazid syrup ★]
Tablets containing 50 [Isoniazid ✦], 100 [Isoniazid ✦ ★] and 300 mg [Isoniazid ✦ ★, Isotamine ✦]

ITRACONAZOLE

INDICATIONS: Itraconazole (Sporanox ✦ ★) is a triazole antifungal agent active against histoplasmosis, blastomycosis, aspergillosis, cryptococcosis, dermatophytosis, and candidiasis. Unlike ketoconazole, itraconazole reaches adequate levels in the central nervous system at therapeutic doses. The drug is used orally and is best absorbed with a fatty meal. Itraconazole is partially converted by hepatic biotransformation to hydroxyitraconazole, which is also fungicidal. In humans, treatment from 6 months to a year is recommended.

A 10 mg/mL liquid formulation of itraconazole has recently become available for the treatment of oral and esophageal candidiasis in humans. The human absorption profile of this and the capsular format differ; Sporanox liquid should not be taken with food. The two drugs are not considered interchangeable in humans. In humans, the relative bioavailability is as follows: empty stomach 0.5, capsules with food 1.0, liquid with food 1.25, liquid empty stomach 1.6. Sporanox capsules contain lactose granules coated with itraconazole. In the past, dosage was determined by the laborious process of counting the number of granules in a capsule and then dividing the total milligrams of drug in the capsule by this number, or by solubilizing the contents of a capsule in 0.1 N HCl (50 mg/mL) by sonication, and then diluting it in orange juice to a final concentration of 5 mg/mL. The new oral formulation eliminates the need to solubilize Sporonox capsules; however, it may still be more convenient to use individual granules for treatment in food.

There has been considerable interest in the use of itraconazole to treat respiratory aspergillosis in birds, and some pharmacokinetic studies, using the capsular formulation, have been carried out. Maximum blood and tissue concentrations were reached in pigeons 4 hours after a single oral dose of 10 mg/kg. After 12 treatments at 6-hour intervals, steady-state plasma concentrations of 3.6 µg/mL and a half-life of 13.3 hours were recorded. A dosage of 6 mg/kg twice daily was recommended to maintain plasma fungicidal concentrations and reduce fluctuations in the concentration of the drug. Levels of itraconazole in pulmonary parenchyma were much lower than in plasma. It was suggested that a dosage as high as 26 mg/kg bid might be necessary to maintain a minimal inhibitory concentration (MIC) of greater than 1 µg/mL in the lung; however, concern was expressed that this dose might be toxic.

In a second study in pigeons, itraconazole was administered orally at a dose of 5 mg/kg either once or once daily for 14 days. Birds received the drug as is from the capsules or solubilized in acid. Plasma and tissue levels were measured. By day 14 of treatment, the group receiving the acid formulation had higher plasma levels. This was attributed to better absorption, which perhaps saturated the elimination pathways. Concentrations of itraconazole and hydroxy-itraconazole were measured in tissue; their concentrations increased in the lungs and air sacs over the 14 days of treatment, and, combined, were above the MIC for most strains of *Aspergillus*.

Blue-fronted Amazon parrots were treated with 5 or 10 mg/kg orally once daily for 14 days. The itraconazole was dissolved in acid and diluted in orange juice before administration. Plasma concentrations were up to 10 times greater in these parrots than in the pigeons in the previous study. It is not known whether this relates to a species difference or if there is a greater bioavailability of the acid formulation used in the parrot study. The half-life after 14 days of treatment was 6 to 7 hours, shorter than that of the pigeons. Bioaccumulation of itraconazole was noted at the 10 mg/kg dose. A dose of 5 mg/kg once daily was expected to be effective in most cases of aspergillosis; 10 mg/kg was recommended for *Candida* spp and when there was not good clinical response at the lower dose. Amazon parrots have been treated for up to 3 months at the higher dose without adverse effects.

The pharmacokinetics of itraconazole were looked at in two gentoo penguins that received 10 and 20 mg/kg once daily for 6 days. Trough serum itraconazole levels were 2.5 times greater at day 6 than on day 3, but were not substantially different between the two doses.

Case reports describe the use of itraconazole in a range of species, including psittacines, raptors, and penguins, against *Candida* and *Aspergillus* spp. Doses of 8 to 10 mg/kg once daily resulted in serum trough levels above the MIC for the organism cultured in several of these cases in which measurements were taken. Itraconazole is also widely used for the prevention and treatment of aspergillosis in waterfowl.

ADVERSE AND COMMON SIDE EFFECTS: Anorexia and depression have been reported in two African gray parrots given 8 and 10 mg/kg once daily. One bird died. Amazon parrots have been treated at 10 mg/kg without evidence of toxicity, although in one report an Amazon parrot became lethargic and anorectic after 1 year of treatment. The bird returned to normal demeanor once treatment was withheld. Concerns have also been noted relating to unexplained deaths in African gray parrots being treated with itraconazole.

In one case report, half the penguins that received itraconazole at 20 mg/kg showed moderately reduced appetites. Aspartate aminotransferase elevations were noted while on the drug; changes in uric acid levels were not consistent.

IVERMECTIN

INDICATIONS: Ivermectin (Heartgard ♣ ★, Ivomec ♣ ★, Eqvalan ♣ ★) is used for the eradication of endo- and ectoparasites. For more information, see **IVERMECTIN** in the Small Animal section.

In birds, ivermectin is the treatment of choice for cutaneous *Knemidokoptes* spp and tracheal mites. The commercial bovine 10 mg/mL product is diluted 1:4 in propylene glycol for more accurate dosing. Although the equine injectable product is sometimes described as water soluble, propylene glycol remains the best diluent. Ivermectin can be administered PO, in the drinking water for aviary situations, or IM. In very small species, ivermectin has been used topically over the right jugular vein at the calculated dose or using a concentration of approximately 0.5 mg/mL (10 mg/mL solution diluted by 1:20) and a dose of 1 drop per bird. In a study of the efficacy of ivermectin against ocular oxyspirurids in crested wood partridges and chickens, doses from 0.005 to 0.05 mg placed in the conjunctival sac eliminated the parasites, whereas 0.01 mg given orally or parenterally did not. No ocular toxicity was noted in chickens treated with up to 1 mg ocularly once daily for 10 days. Systemic treatment with ivermectin, at the standard dosage, is useful in eradicating maggots from wounds.

ADVERSE AND COMMON SIDE EFFECTS: In aviaries treated for tracheal mites, mortalities of 3% to 12% have been reported. This is attributed to tracheal occlusion with dead mites and inflammatory debris and exudate. The propylene glycol base may cause adverse effects when administered IM, especially in small birds. Toxicity has been reported in bullfinches and goldfinches that received a dose of 0.4 mg/kg topically. Deaths have occurred in budgerigars and finches after IM administration of the equine product at the standard dose of 0.2 mg/kg. Particular concern should be taken when administering ivermectin by the droplet technique to avoid accidental overdosage.

KANAMYCIN

INDICATIONS: Kanamycin (Kantrim ★) is an aminoglycoside antibiotic used for the treatment of gram-negative bacterial infections, especially *Pseudomonas* spp. For more information, see **KANAMYCIN** and **AMINOGLYCOSIDE ANTIBIOTICS** in the Small Animal section.

Kanamycin has been recommended for use in drinking water to control enteric infections and as a preventive measure in stressed birds, especially finches.

KAOLIN-PECTIN

INDICATIONS: Kaolin-pectin (Kaopectate ✦ ★, others) is a gastrointestinal protectant used in the management of diarrhea. For more information, see **KAOLIN-PECTIN** in the Small Animal section.

KETOCONAZOLE

INDICATIONS: Ketoconazole (Nizoral ✦ ★) is an antifungal agent used for the treatment of deep fungal and yeast infections. Ketoconazole is fungistatic at low concentrations, and fungicidal at higher levels. Absorption of ketoconazole is enhanced in an acid environment and with a high fat meal. High levels of dietary carbohydrate reduce absorption in humans. For more information, see **KETOCONAZOLE** in the Small Animal section.

In birds, ketoconazole is used orally in the treatment of yeast infections, particularly candidiasis that is refractory to nystatin therapy. Ketoconazole is used less frequently to treat pulmonary aspergillosis. Ketoconazole tablets are not soluble in water, but ground tablets have been suspended in methyl cellulose mixed 50:50 with cherry-based syrup by a compounding pharmacist. This suspension was stable for 6 months. One-fourth of a 200 mg tablet can also be dissolved in 0.2 mL 1 N HCl and 0.8 mL water. The liquid turns pink when the drug is dissolved.

Minimal pharmacokinetic information is available on the use of ketoconazole in birds. Pigeons given a single oral dose of 30 mg/kg attained peak serum levels in 0.5 to 4 hours; the elimination half-life was 2.3 hours. In Moluccan cockatoos given the same dose, the half-life was 3.8 hours.

Ketoconazole has also been suggested as a treatment for gastric megabacteriosis.

ADVERSE AND COMMON SIDE EFFECTS: Regurgitation has been described in psittacines receiving ketoconazole. No adverse effects were noted in pigeons given 30 mg/kg bid orally for 30 days. Serum alanine aminotransferase, aspartate aminotransferase, and uric acid were monitored as well as behavioral parameters. Because hepatotoxicity is described in mammals, caution should be used in prescribing ketoconazole to birds with hepatic dysfunction. Changes in adrenal or hormonal steroid production have not been noted in birds; however, the drug has not been studied in any detail in avian species.

DRUG INTERACTIONS: Ketoconazole has been used in birds in combination with amphotericin B.

LACTULOSE

INDICATIONS: Lactulose (Cephulac ♣ ★, Chronulac ♣ ★) is a synthetic nonabsorbable disaccharide. It acts as a mild osmotic laxative, increases the rate of passage of ingesta, and leads to the reduction of bacterial production of ammonia making it useful in the management of hepatic encephalopathy. For more information, see **LACTULOSE** in the Small Animal section.

In birds, lactulose may also be effective as an appetite stimulant and to help re-establish natural enteric flora.

ADVERSE AND COMMON SIDE EFFECTS: Reduce dosage if diarrhea occurs.

LEVAMISOLE

INDICATIONS: Levamisole (Levasole ♣ ★, Ripercol ♣, Tramisol ♣ ★) is an anthelmintic used for the treatment of infestations by nematodes. Levamisole may help restore immune function by increasing the number and function of T lymphocytes and macrophages. It has also been reported to stimulate antibody production, increase phagocytosis by macrophages, inhibit tumor growth, and stimulate suppressor cell activity. For more information, see **LEVAMISOLE** in the Small Animal section.

Tablets containing 20 mg levamisole (Spartakon) were previously available in North America for the treatment of *Ascaridia columbae* and *Capillaria obsignata* in nonfood pigeons. It was recommended that birds be fasted for 24 hours before and 3 hours after treatment.

Levamisole is also effective against tetrameriasis. The injectable form of the drug can be administered by IM or SC injection, orally in the drinking water, or by gavage.

Levamisole has also been used to stimulate the immune system in immunosuppressed birds. Experimental work in chickens suggested that doses of 1.25 to 2.5 mg/kg orally or SC were effective for this purpose.

ADVERSE AND COMMON SIDE EFFECTS: Levamisole has a low therapeutic index in birds and should be used with caution, especially by the IM route. It should not be used in debilitated birds or lories. Doses of two to four times the recommended dosage may result in depression. Vomiting, neurologic signs including mydriasis and ataxia, and death may occur. These clinical problems have been described in cockatoos, budgies, and mynah birds at a dose of 40 mg/kg injected IM or SC. Hepatotoxicity in budgies has been associated with a dose of 25 mg/kg IM. Swelling at sites of injection has also been noted. Vomiting has been reported in pigeons treated with the tablet formulation. Lethal doses have included 35 mg/kg IM in pigeons, 66 mg/kg IM in peach-faced lovebirds, and 22 mg/kg IM in white ibis.

SUPPLIED AS: VETERINARY PRODUCT
Avian product: Tablets containing 20 mg [Spartakon]
See also Small and Large Animal sections

LEVOTHYROXINE

INDICATIONS: Levothyroxine (Eltroxin ✤ ★, Synthroid ✤ ★) is a synthetic form of T_4 used in the treatment of hypothyroid disease. For more information, see **LEVOTHYROXINE** in the Small Animal section.

Levothyroxine has been used for the treatment of birds with thyroid insufficiency, for goiter in budgies, for thyroid-responsive syndromes including obesity, delayed molting and poor feathering, and to shrink subcutaneous lipomas. Response to therapy is extremely variable; therefore, caution should be taken to monitor treated birds carefully. Measurement of T_4 levels may be helpful. Published dosages vary widely; all are empirical.

ADVERSE AND COMMON SIDE EFFECTS: Overdose may result in hyperthyroidism manifested by tachycardia, polyuria, polydipsia, hyperesthesia, vomiting, weight loss, and death.

LINCOMYCIN

INDICATIONS: Lincomycin (Lincocin ✤ ★, Lincomix Powder ✤ ★) is a lincosamide antibiotic primarily active against gram-positive cocci, particularly *Staphylococcus* and *Streptococcus* spp. It can also be used to treat infections by *Clostridium tetani* and *C. perfringens*, and *Mycoplasma* spp. For more information, see **LINCOMYCIN** in the Small Animal section.

Lincomycin alone has poor activity against most infections in psittacines, which are usually caused by gram-negative organisms. It has been used for the treatment of necrotic enteritis caused by *C. perfringens* in chickens.

ADVERSE AND COMMON SIDE EFFECTS: Deaths have occurred after IV injection. Secondary yeast infections can occur after prolonged treatment.

DRUG INTERACTIONS: Lincomycin is used in combination with spectinomycin, especially for mycoplasmal infections. The minimal inhibitory concentration for the combination of these two drugs is lower than that of either used alone.

SUPPLIED AS: VETERINARY PRODUCTS
See also Small and Large Animal sections.
Water-soluble powder containing 16 g/40 g packet [Lincomix Powder ♣ ★]
Containing Lincomycin and Spectinomycin
Water-soluble powder containing 16.7 g lincomycin and 33.3 g spectinomycin/75 g packet [L-S 50 Water Soluble ★]
Water-soluble powder containing 33.3 g lincomycin and 66.6 g spectinomycin/150 g packet [L-S 100 Water Soluble Powder ♣, Linco-Spectin 100 soluble powder ♣]
For injection containing 50 mg lincomycin and 100 mg spectinomycin/mL [Linco-Spectin Sterile solution ♣ ★]

MAGNESIUM SULFATE

INDICATIONS: Magnesium is essential for electrolyte balance across all membranes. Magnesium sulfate (Epsom salts) has been used in birds with heavy metal poisoning as an oral chelating agent and osmotic cathartic. Concurrent therapy with calcium EDTA is required.

ADVERSE AND COMMON SIDE EFFECTS: Magnesium sulfate must be diluted to prevent damage to the epithelium of the intestinal tract.

SUPPLIED AS: CHEMICAL SUPPLY
As salts containing 98% to 100% magnesium sulfate (Epsom salts)

MEBENDAZOLE

INDICATIONS: Mebendazole (Telmin ♣) is an anthelmintic useful for the elimination of a variety of nematode parasites, including *Capillaria* spp. For more information, see **MEBENDAZOLE** in the Small Animal section.

Mebendazole has been used in a variety of avian species, but toxicity has been reported in a number of these. Mebendazole is commonly used in food to treat waterfowl.

ADVERSE AND COMMON SIDE EFFECTS: Acute toxic hepatitis has been reported in raptors. A dose of 12 mg/kg has been reported to have caused death in *Columbiformes*. Toxicity is also described in cormorants and pelicans. Deaths secondary to intestinal obstruction with dead nematodes have been reported in heavily parasitized finches and psittacine birds.

MEDETOMIDINE

INDICATIONS: Medetomidine (Domitor ✢ ★) is an α_2-agonist pre-anesthetic agent with sedative and analgesic properties. The drug should not be used alone. For more information, see **MEDETOMIDINE** in the Small Animal section.

Medetomidine has been used as an anesthetic agent in birds in combination with ketamine. Twenty-three psittacine species, chickens, and pigeons were given 100 µg/kg medetomidine plus 25 mg/kg ketamine IM, with rapid induction and maintenance of a surgical plane of anesthesia for 30 minutes. Anesthesia in one bird was reversed with atipamezole due to the presence of hypopnea and bradycardia. Recovery was rapid. A volume of atipamezole equal to the volume of Domitor was administered. A second study in psittacines, raptors, and geese used IM doses of medetomidine, from 50 to 200 µg/kg, and much lower doses of ketamine, from 3 to 10 mg/kg. Doses for IV use in raptors and psittacines were slightly lower.

DRUG INTERACTIONS: In mammals, atropine and glycopyrrolate given at the same time as or after medetomidine may induce bradycardia, heart block, premature ventricular contraction, and sinus tachycardia.

MEDROXYPROGESTERONE

INDICATIONS: Medroxyprogesterone (Depo-Provera ✢ ★, Provera ✢ ★) is a synthetic prolonged-action progestational compound that suppresses secretion of follicle-stimulating hormone (FSH) and luteinizing hormone (LH), thus arresting the development of graafian follicles and corpora lutea within the ovary. For more information, see **MEDROXYPROGESTERONE ACETATE** in the Small Animal section.

In birds, medroxyprogesterone has been used to stop egg laying in chronic layers. A single dose may be effective for up to 6 months in some birds. The drug has been used, with variable success, to reduce feather picking and self-mutilation.

ADVERSE AND COMMON SIDE EFFECTS: Treatment may result in obesity, polyuria, polydipsia, lethargy, and fatty liver syndrome. Cockatoos and Quaker parakeets should receive a lower dose than is generally recommended. Necrosis can occur at the site of IM injection.

MEPERIDINE

INDICATIONS: Meperidine (Demerol ♣ ★) is a short-acting narcotic analgesic used for the relief of moderate to severe pain or as a pre-anesthetic. It has minimal sedative effects. For more information, see **MEPERIDINE** in the Small Animal section.

In birds, meperidine is used by the parenteral route. No information is available on blood levels or duration of activity; however, it appears that a single dose of the drug may have longer lasting effects than would be expected based on the half-life in mammals.

METHYLPREDNISOLONE

INDICATIONS: Methylprednisolone (Medrol ♣ ★, Depo-Medrol ♣ ★) is an intermediate-acting glucocorticoid used in mammals for its anti-inflammatory properties to control autoimmune skin diseases, as adjunctive therapy in spinal cord trauma, and in the treatment of shock. For more information, see **METHYLPREDNISOLONE** and **GLUCOCORTICOIDS** in the Small Animal section.

In birds, methylprednisolone has also been used to prevent the seasonal recurrence of "Amazon foot necrosis" syndrome in Amazon parrots.

METOCLOPRAMIDE

INDICATIONS: Metoclopramide (Maxeran♣, Reglan♣★) is an antiemetic agent with central (chemoreceptor trigger zone) and peripheral activity. It contributes to lower esophageal sphincter competence and promotes gastric emptying. It is useful in the management of vomiting, gastroesophageal reflux, and gastric motility disorders. For more information, see **METOCLOPRAMIDE** in the Small Animal section.

In birds, metoclopramide has been used to stimulate motility of the crop, proventriculus and ventriculus, and intestines, particularly in pediatric medicine and for birds with delayed gastrointestinal motility as a result of proventricular dilation disease.

ADVERSE AND COMMON SIDE EFFECTS: Hyperactivity was reported in a baby blue and gold macaw treated with metoclopramide. Metoclopramide should not be used when there is mechanical blockage to the flow of ingesta or when there is gastrointestinal bleeding or perforation.

METRONIDAZOLE

INDICATIONS: Metronidazole (Flagyl ♣ ★) is a synthetic antibacterial, antiprotozoal agent with activity against anaerobic bacteria, *Giardia*, trichomonads, amebae, balantidiae, and trypanosomes. The drug may also have immunosuppressive or immunostimulatory properties. For more information, see **METRONIDAZOLE** in the Small Animal section.

In birds, metronidazole is used orally by gavage or in the drinking water to treat protozoal infections such as trichomoniasis and giardiasis, or anaerobic bacterial infections.

ADVERSE AND COMMON SIDE EFFECTS: Metronidazole was not effective in clearing budgie aviaries of *Giardia* at 200 ppm in one report but, in a second, treatment with 200 to 400 ppm was successful. The use of metronidazole is contraindicated in finches. The IV product causes myonecrosis if used IM.

MIBOLERONE

INDICATIONS: Mibolerone (Cheque Drops ★) is an androgenic, anabolic, antigonadotropic agent. For more information, see **MIBOLERONE** in the Small Animal section.

Mibolerone has been used experimentally in birds to stop oviposition.

MICONAZOLE

INDICATIONS: Miconazole (Monistat ♣ ★, Micatin ♣) is a synthetic imidazole-derived antifungal agent active against most pathogenic fungi, gram-positive bacteria, and some *Acanthamoeba* spp.

Miconazole has been used topically for the treatment of dermatophytosis and cutaneous candidiasis and for nebulization of psittacine birds. For nebulization, the drug has been either compounded as an aqueous solution or combined with acetylcysteine. IM administration of the IV formulation was used successfully for the treatment of aspergillosis in raptors in one report; however, the same regimen was not effective in two psittacine species.

ADVERSE AND COMMON SIDE EFFECTS: No safety or efficacy trials have been performed in birds. In humans, miconazole is less toxic than amphotericin B. Phlebitis, hepatitis, and pruritus have been recorded after IV injection, possibly due to the castor oil diluent. Gastrointestinal upset, transient anemia, thrombocytopenia, and hyperlipidemia are some of the reported adverse effects in people.

DRUG INTERACTIONS: Miconazole enhances the activity of coumarin anticoagulants. Antagonism may exist between amphotericin B and miconazole.

SUPPLIED AS: HUMAN PRODUCTS
For injection containing 10 mg/mL [Monistat i.v. ★]
Several topical gynecologic preparations [Micatin ♣, Monistat ♣]

VETERINARY PRODUCTS
Cream containing 20 mg/g [Conofite ♣ ★]
Lotion and spray containing 1% [Conofite ★]
Shampoo containing 2% [Dermaxzole ★]

MIDAZOLAM

INDICATIONS: Midazolam (Versed ♣ ★) is a short-acting parenteral benzodiazepine central nervous system depressant with sedative-hypnotic, anxiolytic, muscle relaxant, and anticonvulsant properties. The drug is two to three times more potent than diazepam and has a shorter half-life. For more information, see **MIDAZOLAM** in the Small Animal section.

In birds, midazolam is used to provide sedation for diagnostic and nonpainful procedures, and as a preanesthetic. In a controlled trial in Canada geese given 2 mg/kg IM, maximum sedation was seen 15 to 20 minutes after injection. Minimal cardiovascular or respiratory changes occurred.

ADVERSE AND COMMON SIDE EFFECTS: Ducks are poorly sedated by midazolam at doses up to 8 to 10 mg/kg IM.

MINOCYCLINE

INDICATIONS: Minocycline (Minocin ♣ ★) is a second-generation, long-acting, lipid-soluble tetracycline. It is more active against anaerobes and several facultative intracellular bacteria than are other tetracyclines, with the exception of doxycycline. Minocycline is also more active against *Nocardia* spp and staphylococci than other tetracyclines. For more information, see **MINOCYCLINE** and **TETRACYCLINE ANTIBIOTICS** in the Small Animal section.

In avian medicine, minocycline has been used primarily in the treatment of chlamydiosis. A dosage of 100 mg/kg minocycline produces slightly higher, but of shorter duration, blood levels than does the same dose of doxycycline. Millet impregnated with 0.5% minocycline was fed to yellow-naped, orange-cheeked, and blue-crowned parakeets. Blood levels greater than 5 µg/mL were achieved; levels greater than 1 µg/mL persisted for 48 hours after medicated feed was withdrawn. The authors commented that a lower concentration of drug would probably be adequate to maintain therapeutic blood levels greater than 1 µg/mL.

MONENSIN

INDICATIONS: Monensin (Coban ♣ ★, Rumensin ♣ ★) is an ionophore antibiotic used commonly as a feed additive in the poultry and livestock industries for control of coccidiosis. Coban 60 is also licensed for use in quail in the United States. For more information, see **MON-ENSIN** in the Large Animal section.

Monensin has been used to control coccidiosis in galliform birds and pigeons, and may be more effective than amprolium or clazuril. Monensin was a candidate drug for the control of visceral coccidiosis in whooping cranes; thus, a safety trial was conducted in sandhill cranes. Monensin was safe when fed at one, two, and five times the recommended poultry dose of 99 ppm (90 g/ton). Some reduction in appetite was noted in birds fed the highest concentration of medicated feed, but no abnormalities were noted on careful clinical and necropsy evaluations. An efficacy trial was not conducted, but coccidia were not noted in the feces or viscera of treated birds, in contrast to control birds.

ADVERSE AND COMMON SIDE EFFECTS: Toxicity most frequently results from errors in mixing of the feed. Clinical signs of anorexia, dyspnea, ataxia, depression, recumbency, and death and pathologic lesions of skeletal and cardiac myodegeneration have been reported in a variety of species, including guinea fowl, chickens, and turkeys. The drug may be lethal to adult turkeys or guinea fowl. No toxicity was seen in crane chicks given five times the recommended poultry dose.

SUPPLIED AS: VETERINARY PRODUCTS
As a feed additive containing 132.2 g/kg (60 g/lb) [Coban 60 ✦ ★, Rumensin 60 ✦ ★]

NEOMYCIN

INDICATIONS: Neomycin (Biosol-M ✦, Mycifradin ✦ ★), an aminoglycoside antibiotic, can be used topically or orally. It is not absorbed from the gastrointestinal tract and is, therefore, active only against enteric bacteria. Neomycin is generally less effective than amikacin or gentamicin. The drug is extremely toxic if administered systemically.

Neomycin has been administered by direct oral gavage or in the drinking water.

ADVERSE AND COMMON SIDE EFFECTS: Biosol M, which also contains methscopolamine bromide, can be toxic in birds.

NORTRIPTYLINE

INDICATIONS: Nortriptyline (Aventyl ✦ ★, Nortriptyline HCl ★, Pameloc ★) is an oral tricyclic antidepressant drug used in humans.

Nortriptyline has been used, with very limited success, to treat feather picking in psittacine birds. In humans, it is suggested that dosage should be low initially and gradually adjusted for each individual. Maximal antidepressant effects may require 2 weeks or more of therapy. Once symptoms are controlled the dose is gradually reduced to the lowest effect level.

ADVERSE AND COMMON SIDE EFFECTS: Hyperactivity has been reported in treated birds. If this occurs, the dosage should be reduced or, if the bird does not return to normal activity patterns, treatment with nortriptyline halted. Withdrawal symptoms are seen in humans after abrupt withdrawal of the drug.

SUPPLIED AS: HUMAN PRODUCTS
Capsules containing 10 and 25 mg [Aventyl ♣ ★, Nortriptyline HCl ★] and 50 and 75 mg [Nortriptyline HCl ★, Pameloc ★]
Oral solution containing 10 mg/5 mL [Aventyl ★, Pameloc ★]

NYSTATIN

INDICATIONS: Nystatin (Mycostatin ♣ ★, Nilstat ♣ ★) is an antifungal agent used for the treatment of gastrointestinal yeast infections, including oral candidiasis. For more information, see **NYSTATIN** in the Small Animal section.

In birds, nystatin is used for the prevention and treatment of oral and gastrointestinal candidiasis, especially in hand-fed neonates and birds on long-term antibiotic therapy. The drug is effective topically and is not systemically absorbed across intact epithelium. Oral lesions must be treated by direct contact with the medication. When treating hand-fed neonates, it is probably better to administer nystatin separately from formula to maximize nystatin's concentration and epithelial contact time. Doses are empirical and vary widely in the literature.

ADVERSE AND COMMON SIDE EFFECTS: Regurgitation is seen infrequently.

OXYTETRACYCLINE

INDICATIONS: Oxytetracycline (Liquamycin ♣ ★, Terramycin ♣ ★) is a short-acting, water-soluble tetracycline with activity against a broad range of gram-positive and gram-negative organisms as well as chlamydiae, rickettsiae, and mycoplasmas. For more information, see **OXYTETRACYCLINE** and **TETRACYCLINE ANTIBIOTICS** in the Small Animal section.

In birds, oxytetracycline is used IM or SC in the treatment of bacterial infections and chlamydiosis. Oxytetracycline is eliminated through the bile and the kidneys. In chickens given oxytetracycline IM, the highest tissue levels were found in liver, then in gluteal muscle, heart, kidney, and pectoral muscle. In a pharmacokinetic study involving ring-necked pheasants, great horned owls, and several species of Amazon parrots, no correlation of half-life with body weight was noted. In another study involving Goffin's cockatoos given single doses of 50, 75, and 100 mg/kg IM and SC, increased dosage resulted in increased blood levels, but there were significant differences between the two routes of administration at only one time-dose point. There was no accumulation of drug in the plasma of birds given 100 mg/kg SC every 72 hours for 30 days. No adverse effects, other than those attributed to damage at the sites of injections, were noted. The half-life of oxytetracycline in these cockatoos was shorter than that in the three species previously mentioned and in turkeys.

In turkeys given the long-acting oxytetracycline formulation at 152 mg/kg SC, the half-life of the drug was 12 hours and blood concentrations remained greater than 1 µg/mL (the target point for *Chlamydia psittaci* and *Pasteurella multocida*) for 72 hours. In a separate study using the standard formulation of oxytetracycline, 12-week-old turkeys received 200 mg/bird SC. Blood levels had dropped below 1 µg/mL by day 2 after injection.

In Pekin ducks infected with *Salmonella* spp, oral oxytetracycline fed at 50 and 200 mg/kg feed decreased the duration of shedding of oxytetracycline-sensitive bacterial strains but increased the duration of shedding of resistant strains.

ADVERSE AND COMMON SIDE EFFECTS: Irritation and necrosis occur at the sites of both SC and IM injections. In cockatoos, damage was dose related, was more severe at IM sites, and increased in severity after multiple injections. Concurrent elevations in aspartate aminotransferase, creatinine kinase, and lactic dehydrogenase were noted.

OXYTOCIN

INDICATIONS: Oxytocin (Pitocin ★, Syntocinon ✦ ★) is a hormone of the posterior pituitary gland. For more information, see **OXYTOCIN** in the Small Animal section.

In avian medicine, oxytocin is used to stimulate uterine contractions in egg-bound birds. Concurrent administration of injectable calcium and vitamin A have been recommended. The drug has also been used to control uterine hemorrhage. Oxytocin is preferable to prostaglandin $F_{2\alpha}$, which may cause systemic reactions when used parenterally. Oxytocin receptors are located only in the uterus.

ADVERSE AND COMMON SIDE EFFECTS: Because oxytocin does not relax the uterovaginal sphincter, shell rupture can occur. Oxytocin is contraindicated where physical reasons prevent passage of the egg. Oxytocin may not be effective in hypocalcemic birds.

DRUG INTERACTIONS: Topical application of prostaglandin E_2 relaxes the uterovaginal sphincter, allowing easier passage of the egg.

PAROMOMYCIN

INDICATIONS: Paromomycin (Humatin ★) is an aminoglycoside antibiotic with a broad spectrum of activity against bacteria, protozoa, and cestodes. A case report describes the use of paromomycin to reduce morbidity and mortality in a flock of Lady Gouldian finches with cryptosporidiosis. The dose of the drug was calculated for the flock weight of all birds and administered in food. The amount of treated food provided was doubled for wastage.

ADVERSE AND COMMON SIDE EFFECTS: Paromomycin is poorly absorbed from the intestinal tract. The drug is potentially nephrotoxic and ototoxic and may have neuromuscular blocking effects. Other adverse effects in humans include gastrointestinal upset.

SUPPLIED AS: HUMAN PRODUCT
Oral capsules containing 250 mg [Humatin ★]

PENICILLAMINE

INDICATIONS: Penicillamine (Cuprimine ✤ ★, Depen ✤ ★) is a thiol compound that chelates cystine, lead, and copper and promotes their excretion in the urine. For more information, see **PENICILLAMINE** in the Small Animal section.

Penicillamine has been used orally in birds to treat lead poisoning.

ADVERSE AND COMMON SIDE EFFECTS: Regurgitation has been recorded in birds. The therapeutic index in mammals is low. For more information, see **PENICILLAMINE** in the Small Animal section.

PENICILLIN G

INDICATIONS: For more information, see **PENICILLIN ANTIBIOTICS** in the Small Animal section.

In a pharmacokinetic study in turkeys, a combination of procaine and benzathine penicillins was better absorbed than the potassium salt or either drug alone. In chickens, aqueous penicillin was absorbed more rapidly than procaine penicillin after IM administration; however, serum concentrations were undetectable 4 hours after injection of 6 to 50 mg/kg. Oral penicillin was poorly absorbed, resulting in low serum levels. Procaine penicillin may maintain therapeutic blood levels for up to 48 hours in some species. The drug is most commonly used in gallinaceous birds and waterfowl that are difficult to treat on a daily basis.

Equivalency of milligram and United States Pharmacopeia units:

Penicillin G sodium—1 mg = 1,500 to 1,750 USP units
Penicillin G sodium powder—1 mg = 1420 to 1,667 USP units
Penicillin G procaine—1 mg = 900 to 1,050 USP units
Penicillin G benzathine—1 mg = 1,090 to 1,272 USP units

ADVERSE AND COMMON SIDE EFFECTS: Adverse reactions to the injection of the procaine/benzathine combination have been reported in small birds even at doses of 1 mg/kg, probably due to procaine toxicity. Other reactions include vomiting and acute collapse in a South American black-collared hawk and regurgitation and trembling in pigeons given 500 mg/kg (833,500 IU/kg). No reactions were seen in pigeons given 100 or 200 mg/kg, or in chickens and turkeys given 100 mg/kg.

PHENOBARBITAL

INDICATIONS: Phenobarbital ✤ ★ is the drug of choice for the control of seizure activity in small animals and has been used for this purpose in psittacine birds. Monitoring of serum levels is important in determining optimum dosage. For more information, see **PHENOBARBITAL** and **BARBITURATES** in the Small Animal section.

PHENYLBUTAZONE

INDICATIONS: Phenylbutazone (Butazone ✤, Butazolidin ✤, Bute ✤, Phenylbutazone ✤ ★) has analgesic, antipyretic, and anti-inflammatory properties that make it useful in the treatment of osteoarthritis, rheumatism, and inflammation of the skin and soft tissue. For more information, see **PHENYLBUTAZONE** in the Small Animal section.

Phenylbutazone has been used orally in psittacines and raptorial birds for its anti-inflammatory properties.

PIPERACILLIN

INDICATIONS: Piperacillin (Pipracil ✤ ★) is a broad-spectrum, semisynthetic penicillin with activity against most aerobic gram-negative bacteria and some gram-positive and anaerobic organisms. It is used to treat bacterial infections, including those caused by *Pseudomonas aeruginosa*. For more information, see **PENICILLIN ANTIBIOTICS** in the Small Animal section.

A single-dose pharmacokinetic study of piperacillin has been carried out in blue-fronted Amazon parrots. The drug has been also been used to increase egg hatchability by injection into the air cell of the egg.

ADVERSE AND COMMON SIDE EFFECTS: Piperacillin is unstable once reconstituted. Some authors have suggested freezing the reconstituted drug in aliquots for subsequent treatments; however, subsequent stability has not been investigated. Adverse effects are similar to those of other extended-spectrum penicillins.

DRUG INTERACTIONS: Piperacillin can be used in combination with the aminoglycosides.

SUPPLIED AS: HUMAN PRODUCT
For injection in vials containing 2, 3, and 4 g [Pipracil ❦ ★]

PIPERAZINE

INDICATIONS: Piperazine (Hartz Once a Month ★, Once a Month Roundworm Treatment ❦, Pipa-Tabs ★, Purina Liquid Wormer ★) is an anthelmintic used for the eradication of roundworms. For more information, see **PIPERAZINE** in the Small Animal section.

Piperazine has been used for the treatment of ascarid nematodes in gallinaceous birds but has not proved effective for psittacines or finches.

POLYMYXIN B

INDICATIONS: Polymyxin B (Aerosporin ❦ ★) is used in the treatment of gram-negative infections, especially those resistant to aminoglycosides. The drug is used frequently as a topical preparation. For more information, see **POLYMYXIN B** in the Small Animal section.

Polymyxin has been used by nebulization for the treatment of pneumonia and air sacculitis in birds. The drug is poorly absorbed by the respiratory epithelium and has primarily a topical effect.

ADVERSE AND COMMON SIDE EFFECTS: Weakness, incoordination, vomiting, and death have been reported in Amazon parrots receiving parenteral doses of 5 to 10 mg/kg.

POLYSULFATED GLYCOSAMINOGLYCANS

INDICATIONS: Polysulfated glycosaminoglycans (Adequan IM ❦ ★) may be beneficial in the treatment of osteoarthritis through a variety of mechanisms. To maximize therapeutic benefit, treatment should begin soon after the inciting traumatic event. For more information, see **POLYSULFATED GLYCOSAMINOGLYCANS** in the Small Animal section.

Polysulfated glycosaminoglycans have been used IM in a king vulture, and intra-articularly in a demoiselle crane and a Palawan peacock pheasant to treat arthritic lesions.

PRALIDOXIME CHLORIDE

INDICATIONS: Pralidoxime chloride ❦ ★, or 2-PAM chloride, is a cholinesterase reactivator used to treat organophosphate toxicity. The drug is most effective when given within 24 hours of exposure and is usually not of value after 36 to 48 hours have passed. In humans, administration by slow IV injection is suggested; the IM and SC routes are alternates when venous access is not possible. The use of pralidoxime in the treatment of carbamate toxicity is controversial and generally not recommended.

ADVERSE AND COMMON SIDE EFFECTS: IM administration of pralidoxime may result in pain at the site of injection. There is an anecdotal report of death in a bald eagle after treatment.

DRUG INTERACTIONS: Pralidoxime has little effect on muscarinic activity; animals should be pretreated with atropine. Pralidoxime is contraindicated in cases of carbaryl exposure because toxicity appears to increase.

SUPPLIED AS: HUMAN PRODUCT
For injection containing 1 g/vial [Protopam chloride ✦ ★]

PRAZIQUANTEL

INDICATIONS: Praziquantel (Droncit ✦ ★) is an anthelmintic used for the elimination of cestodes and some trematodes. For more information, see **PRAZIQUANTEL** in the Small Animal section
   In birds, praziquantel is used parenterally and orally for the elimination of cestodes. The injectable formulation can also be used for oral administration. Several reports describe the drug's use against hepatic trematodes. An IM dose of 10 mg/kg once daily for 3 days, then once daily for 11 days PO in toucans halted the shedding of trematode eggs. In a Moluccan cockatoo given 10 mg/kg once daily for 3 days SC, there was a sharp decrease in shedding of eggs, but at autospy adult flukes of abnormal appearance were still present in the liver.

ADVERSE AND COMMON SIDE EFFECTS: The injectable form of the drug is toxic to finches. There is an anecdotal report of weakness, disorientation, and even deaths in baby and juvenile African gray parrots that were treated with 9 mg/kg IM in quarantine stations. Adults of the same species showed no adverse effects. Depression and death have been described in birds receiving doses of 100 to 250 mg/kg IM.

PREDNISOLONE
PREDNISOLONE SODIUM SUCCINATE
PREDNISONE

INDICATIONS: Prednisolone (Delta-Cortef ★) and Prednisone (Deltasone ✦ ★) are intermediate-acting glucocorticoid agents. Prednisone is converted by the liver to prednisolone. Except for cases of liver failure, the drugs can essentially be used interchangeably. For more information, see **PREDNISOLONE** and **GLUCOCORTI-COID AGENTS** in the Small Animal section.

These drugs are used by parenteral administration for the treatment of shock, trauma, and endotoxemia, and PO as anti-inflammatory agents. Tablets can be suspended in water to make a solution of appropriate concentration. A decreasing dosage schedule should be used for long-term therapy. Prednisone has been used in the supportive care of birds with acute head trauma and after treatment of canaries for respiratory mites.

ADVERSE AND COMMON SIDE EFFECTS: Concern is frequently expressed regarding the high sensitivity of birds to the immunosuppressive effects of glucocorticoids. This has been supported by experimental work in pigeons, which showed that the hypothalamic–pituitary–adrenal system is more sensitive to suppression by glucocorticoids than that of mammals, and that suppression is dose dependent. The minimum intravenous dose of prednisolone required to suppress plasma corticosterone levels was 0.7 µg/kg. The duration of suppression by prednisolone was shorter than that of dexamethasone, which was also evaluated in these studies. In another study, prednisolone was administered orally at 350 µg/kg, topically to bare skin at approximately 500 µg/kg, topically in combination with DMSO to bare skin at doses of 350 µg/kg, and ophthalmically at approximately 70 µg/kg. Suppression of corticosterone levels occurred in all groups except those treated topically without DMSO.

PRIMAQUINE

INDICATIONS: Primaquine ✤ ★ is a synthetic antimalarial agent used in combination with chloroquine for the therapy of malaria caused by *Plasmodium* spp, especially in penguins. The combination can also be used prophylactically, in drinking water, to prevent seasonal malaria in outdoor budgies, canaries, and finches. The tablets can be dissolved in water (up to a concentration of 1 g/15 mL) and dosage based on estimated water intake. A suitable medicated water formulation for these species can be made by dissolving one 500 mg chloroquine/75 mg primaquine tablet in 15 mL of water as a stock solution and placing 1 mL of stock solution in 480 mL of drinking water as treatment.

DRUG INTERACTIONS: Because primaquine is not active against asexual erythrocytic plasmodial forms, concurrent treatment with an agent active against the schizont form, such as chloroquine, should be carried out.

SUPPLIED AS: HUMAN PRODUCT
Tablets containing 15 mg ★ or 26.3 mg primaquine phosphate ✤

PROSTAGLANDIN E₂

INDICATIONS: Prostaglandin E_2 gel is applied to the uterovaginal junction of dystocic birds to stimulate relaxation of this region and aid in passage of the egg. The egg will often pass within 5 to 10 minutes of application. Low doses of oxytocin may increase the strength of the contractions in the shell gland, which are responsible for expulsion of the egg.

ADVERSE AND COMMON SIDE EFFECTS: Excessive doses of prostaglandin E_2 may result in smooth muscle relaxation. Caution must be taken to ensure that there are no mechanical obstructions to passage of the egg.

SUPPLIED AS: VETERINARY PRODUCT
Prostaglandin $F_{2\alpha}$: See Small and Large Animal sections

HUMAN PRODUCTS
Prostaglandin E (Dinoprostone)
Gel formulation containing 0.5 mg/3 mL [Prepidil ♣] and 1 and 2 mg/3 g [Prostin E2 ♣]
Suppository containing 20 mg [Prostin E2 ★]

PYRANTEL PAMOATE

INDICATIONS: Pyrantel pamoate (Pyr-A-Pam ♣, Pyran ♣, Nemex ★) is an anthelmintic used for the eradication of intestinal nematodes. The drug has a high therapeutic index. For more information, see **PYRANTEL PAMOATE** in the Small Animal section.

PYRETHRIN-CONTAINING PRODUCTS

INDICATIONS: Pyrethrin-containing products (Sectrol ♣ ★, Ovitrol ♣ ★, and many others) are naturally occurring insecticides derived from the plant *Chrysanthemum cinerariae-folium*. These drugs are γ-aminobutyric acid (GABA) agonists, which stimulate the insect's central nervous system causing muscular excitation, convulsions, and paralysis. Insect mortality is enhanced when these products are combined with piperonyl butoxide, which inhibits pyrethrin metabolism. For more information, see **PYRETHRIN-CONTAINING PRODUCTS** in the Small Animal section.
  In birds, pyrethrin products are used topically as a spray for the treatment of external arthropod parasites, especially lice. Care should be taken to spray the axillary area with the wings of the bird extended to contact all the parasites.

ADVERSE AND COMMON SIDE EFFECTS: Avoid contact of the chemical with the eyes and oral cavity.

PYRIMETHAMINE

INDICATIONS: Pyrimethamine (Daraprim ✤ ★) is an antiparasitic drug that is highly selective against plasmodium and is used in combination with the sulfonamides (e.g., sulfadiazine) in the treatment of infections with *Toxoplasma gondii*. For more information, see **PYRIMETHAMINE** in the Small Animal section.

Pyrimethamine has also been used successfully in the treatment of *Sarcocystis* spp infection in two Amazon and one eclectus parrots. Trimethoprim-sulfadiazine (30 mg/kg bid; IM) was administered concurrently for the first 7 days of the 30-day treatment. Pyrimethamine was made into an oral solution by suspending a 25 mg tablet in 21 mL of water, and adding 4 mL of a water-soluble lubricating jelly to create a 1 mg/mL suspension.

RIFAMPIN

INDICATIONS: Rifampin (Rifadin ✤ ★, Rimactane ✤ ★) is an antibiotic used alone or in combination with other agents in the treatment of actinomycosis, *Coxiella burnetii* (Q fever), feline leprosy, listeriosis, Rocky Mountain spotted fever, and tuberculosis. It is active against staphylococcus and other intracellular organisms (e.g., *Chlamydia*). The drug may also be useful in the treatment of chronic staphylococcal infection, such as severe pyoderma and chronic osteomyelitis, but it should always be used with another antibiotic because resistance develops rapidly. For more information, see **RIFAMPIN** in the Small Animal section.

In birds, rifampin has been used most frequently in combinations with isoniazid to treat mycobacterial infections. Veterinarians vary in their willingness to treat avian mycobacteriosis; concerns include poor success rate of treatment in many cases and the potential for spread of the disease to humans.

SELENIUM

See **VITAMIN E + SELENIUM** in this section.

SPECTINOMYCIN

INDICATIONS: Spectinomycin (Spectam ✤ ★) is an aminocyclitol broad-spectrum antibiotic effective against gram-negative bacteria including *Escherichia coli*, *Klebsiella*, *Salmonella*, *Proteus*, and *Enterobacter* spp as well as gram-positive bacteria, including streptococci, and staphylococci. Spectinomycin is related structurally to the aminoglycosides and it shares many similar properties. For more information, see **SPECTINOMYCIN** in the Small Animal section.

Spectinomycin is registered for SC use in turkeys to reduce mortality resulting from infection by sensitive strains of *Pasteurella multocida* and for use in the drinking water to control mycoplasmal infections in chickens and turkeys. The drug has been used by nebulization for the treatment of pneumonia and air sacculitis and in drinking water for the treatment of gram-negative enteric infections.

ADVERSE AND COMMON SIDE EFFECTS: Spectinomycin has a low degree of toxicity. SC injections of up to 50 mg/turkey poult caused no adverse effects. Transient ataxia and coma, of up to 4 hours' duration, resulted from administration of 90 mg/poult.

Some humans who handle spectinomycin develop serious cutaneous reactions.

DRUG INTERACTIONS: Spectinomycin is most frequently used in conjunction with lincomycin. See **LINCOMYCIN** in this section.

SUPPLIED AS: VETERINARY PRODUCTS
For injection containing 100 mg/mL [Spectam ✤ ★]
Oral solution containing 50 mg/mL [Spectam ✤ ★]
Water-soluble powder containing 500 mg/g [Spectam ✤ ★]

STANOZOLOL

INDICATIONS: Stanozolol (Winstrol-V ✤ ★) is an anabolic steroid with strong anabolic and weak androgenic activity. For more information, see **STANOZOLOL** and **ANABOLIC STEROIDS** in the Small Animal section.

Stanozolol has been used orally or by injection for anabolic therapy in birds that are debilitated, anemic, or anorectic to stimulate appetite and weight gain.

ADVERSE AND COMMON SIDE EFFECTS: Stanozolol should be used with caution in birds with hepatic or renal disease and in laying hens.

STREPTOMYCIN
DIHYDROSTREPTOMYCIN

INDICATIONS: Streptomycin and dihydrostreptomycin (Ethamycin ✤) are aminoglycoside antibiotics. For more information, see **DIHYDROSTREPTOMYCIN** and **AMINOGLYCOSIDE ANTIBIOTICS** in the Small Animal section.

Streptomycin is used most commonly in the poultry industry. In chickens, streptomycin is absorbed rapidly and is excreted slowly after IM injection. The drug has also been used in pigeons.

ADVERSE AND COMMON SIDE EFFECTS: Streptomycin should not be used in pet birds due to the risk of toxicity. Paralysis and death have been reported in some species.

SUCRALFATE

INDICATIONS: Sucralfate (Carafate ★, Sulcrate ✦) accelerates the healing of oral, esophageal, gastric, and duodenal ulcers through several mechanisms. For more information, see **SUCRALFATE** in the Small Animal section.

Sucralfate has been recommended for use in psittacine birds for the above-mentioned conditions. The tablets can be ground and mixed with water for administration.

SULFACHLORPYRIZIDINE
SULFADIMETHOXINE
SULFADIMIDINE
SULFAMETHAZINE

INDICATIONS: The sulfonamides are antibacterial, antiprotozoal drugs used for the treatment of bacterial diseases and intestinal and biliary coccidiosis. For more information, see **SULFONAMIDE ANTIBIOTICS** and **SULFADIMETHOXINE** in the Small Animal section.

Sulfamethazine is used primarily as a drinking water treatment for the control of enteric coccidia. Sulfadimethoxine has also been used for this purpose, and by nebulization to treat pneumonia and air sacculitis. Sulfachlorpyridazine is used in the drinking water to treat enteric infections, including those caused by *Escherichia coli*.

Sulfadimidine has been used to treat enteric *Caryospora neofalconis* infections in juvenile merlins in a breeding facility. Based on a recommended dose of 50 to 100 mg/kg once daily for 5 to 7 days, birds were treated with 50 mg/kg orally or IM for up to 10 days. The parenteral route was preferred because of concurrent vomiting. One bird received 25 mg/kg bid orally for 6 weeks without adverse effects. Clinical response was variable. Oocyst production declined after treatment, but in some birds increased again within 7 to 10 days. The authors concluded that the drug was effective, but that clazuril or toltrazuril might be better choices. Sulfadimidine has also been suggested as a treatment for clostridial enteritis in psittacines.

SUPPLIED AS: VETERINARY PRODUCTS
Sulfadimethoxine:
Various formulations for oral use in drinking water [Albon, Di-Methox, and others ★]
Oral suspension containing 250 mg/5 mL [Albon Oral Suspension-5% ★]
Tablets containing 125 [S-125 ✦, Albon ★] and 250 mg [S-250 ✦, Albon ★]
For injection containing 400 mg/mL [Albon Injection-40% ★]
Sulfamethazine:
Various formulations for oral use in drinking water [Sulmet ✦ ★, Sulfamethazine ★, and others]

Sulfachlorpyridazine:
For injection containing 200 mg/mL [Vetisulid ★]
Oral powder containing 50 g/bottle [Vetisulid ★]

TESTOSTERONE

INDICATIONS: Testosterone is an androgenic steroid. For more information, see **TESTOSTERONE** and **ANABOLIC STEROIDS** in the Small Animal section.

In birds, testosterone has been used by injection or PO in the drinking water to increase male libido, for anemia, debilitation, and feather loss, and to stimulate male canaries to sing. The use of testosterone in birds that have stopped singing may discourage owners from investigating underlying health problems. Testosterone has also been used to break the cycle of hens in persistent lay.

ADVERSE AND COMMON SIDE EFFECTS: Long-term testosterone therapy will interfere with the normal hormonal feedback systems. Testosterone therapy is contraindicated in birds with hepatic or renal disease.

SUPPLIED AS: VETERINARY PRODUCTS
Tablets containing 10 mg methyltestosterone ♣
Injectable products: see **TESTOSTERONE** in the Small Animal section

TETRACYCLINE

INDICATIONS: Tetracycline (Panmycin Aquadrops Liquid ♣ ★) is a bacteriostatic antibiotic effective against many aerobic and anaerobic gram-positive and gram-negative bacteria, spirochetes, mycoplasmas, and rickettsial organisms. It is used to medicate drinking water or for direct oral administration. For more information, see **TETRACYCLINE ANTIBIOTICS** in the Small or Large Animal section.

The primary use of tetracycline in avian medicine has been as an initial treatment for chlamydiosis while birds acclimate to medicated diets. It is unsuitable for long-term therapy. Syrup formulations are palatable to birds and can be added to soft food mixes. Birds may not consume adequate amounts of medicated water to ensure therapeutic blood levels of the drug. Doxycycline is now preferred by most veterinarians for the direct oral treatment of birds with chlamydiosis.

ADVERSE AND COMMON SIDE EFFECTS: Calcium, magnesium, and iron chelate tetracycline resulting in formation of insoluble complexes. Long-term use may predispose to yeast infections; therefore, antifungal agents are often administered concurrently. Disruption of the enteric flora resulting in vitamin K deficiency is also of concern. Tetracycline is potentially nephrotoxic and may be immunosuppressive. Bone deformities may develop in toucans, especially young birds, after the use of tetracyclines.

SUPPLIED AS: VETERINARY PRODUCTS
For oral administration containing 100 mg/mL [Panmycin Aquadrops Liquid ✦ ★]
Various water-soluble powder formulations that can also be mixed in feed

THIABENDAZOLE

INDICATIONS: Thiabendazole (Equizole ★, Mintezol ★, Thibenzole ★) is a broad-spectrum anthelmintic drug that also has antipyretic and anti-inflammatory effects and fungicidal activity. For more information, see **THIABENDAZOLE** in the Small Animal section.

In birds, thiabendazole has been used orally for the treatment of nematode parasites, including ascarids and *Syngamus trachea*. A pharmacokinetic study was conducted in turkeys, red-tailed hawks, broad-winged hawks, and great horned owls to evaluate the potential for use of thiabendazole in the treatment of pulmonary aspergillosis. Serum from birds that received oral doses of 20, 60, and 120 mg/kg did not inhibit the growth of *Aspergillus* spp isolates in vitro. The drug was not recommended for this purpose.

ADVERSE AND COMMON SIDE EFFECTS: Thiabendazole may be toxic in ostriches, diving ducks, and cranes.

TICARCILLIN

INDICATIONS: Ticarcillin (Ticar ✦ ★) is an extended-spectrum parenteral penicillin antibiotic with activity similar to, but more potent than, carbenicillin. Ticarcillin is especially useful for the treatment of resistant gram-negative infections, including those by *Pseudomonas* spp. For more information, see **TICARCILLIN** and **PENICILLIN ANTIBIOTICS** in the Small Animal section.

ADVERSE AND COMMON SIDE EFFECTS: Once reconstituted, ticarcillin is stable for only 72 hours. Some authors have suggested freezing the reconstituted drug in aliquots for subsequent treatments; however, stability has not been investigated. Hepatoxicity was described in a rose-breasted cockatoo treated with the combination of ticarcillin and tobramycin.

DRUG INTERACTIONS: Ticarcillin is synergistic with aminoglycosides but may inactivate them in vitro so solutions should not be mixed. Ticarcillin in combination with clavulanic acid (Timentin ✦ ★) is effective against many penicillinase-producing strains of bacteria.

TILETAMINE ZOLAZEPAM

INDICATIONS: Tiletamine plus zolazepam (Telazol ★) is an injectable dissociative anesthetic/tranquilizer combination useful for sedation and restraint and anesthetic induction or anesthesia of short duration (30 minutes) requiring mild to moderate analgesia. For more information, see **TILETAMINE ZOLAZEPAM** in the Small Animal section.

Telazol has been used IM and IV in ratites to induce anesthesia or for short, relatively nonpainful procedures such as radiography.

ADVERSE AND COMMON SIDE EFFECTS: Some reports describe violent recoveries from anesthesia with Telazol.

DRUG INTERACTIONS: Because the half-life of tiletamine is shorter than that of zolazepam, one should administer ketamine rather than additional Telazol as a top-up to prolong sedation or anesthesia. Flumazenil, a reversal agent for benzodiazepine tranquilizers, will help reverse the effects of zolazepam.

TOBRAMYCIN

INDICATIONS: Tobramycin (Nebcin ♣ ★) is an aminoglycoside antibiotic used for the treatment of bacterial infections, especially those caused by *Pseudomonas* spp., against which it has better activity than gentamicin. For more information, see **TOBRAMYCIN** and **AMINOGLYCOSIDE ANTIBIOTICS** in the Small Animal section.

ADVERSE AND COMMON SIDE EFFECTS: Tobramycin is less nephrotoxic than gentamicin, with 40% to 65% less accumulation in the kidneys of red-tailed hawks, great horned owls, and barred owls. Hepatoxicity was described in a rose-breasted cockatoo treated with the combination of ticarcillin and tobramycin.

DRUG INTERACTIONS: Tobramycin is potentiated by penicillins and cefotaxime; a lower dose should be used when in combination.

TOLTRAZURIL

INDICATIONS: Toltrazuril (Baycox) is licensed for the prevention of coccidiosis in broiler chickens and is available in Canada by Emergency Drug Release. A related drug, clazuril, was previously available in tablet formulation for use in pigeons.

Toltrazuril has been administered in the drinking water to treat atoxoplasmosis in canaries and has been recommended for the treatment of *Caryospora neofalconis* in raptors.

SUPPLIED AS: VETERINARY PRODUCT
For use in the drinking water [Baycox]

TRIMETHOPRIM SULFADIAZINE
TRIMETHOPRIM SULFADOXINE
TRIMETHOPRIM SULFAMETHOXAZOLE

INDICATIONS: Trimethoprim sulfadiazine, trimethoprim sulfadoxine and trimethoprim sulfamethoxazole (Tribrissen ✦ ★, Trivetrin ✦, Borgal ✦) are bactericidal antibiotic combinations. For more
information, see **TRIMETHOPRIM SULFADIAZINE** in the Small
Animal section or **SULFONAMIDES; POTENTIATED** in the Large
Animal section.

Trimethoprim-sulfonamide combinations are widely used in
avian medicine, especially for respiratory and enteric infections and
for the treatment of hand-fed baby psittacines. The drug combination is effective against some protozoa, including coccidia of toucans
and mynahs. A dose of 50 mg/kg twice daily IM for 9 days resulted
in the clinical recovery of a cassowary with presumptive toxoplasmosis. Because the half-life of trimethoprim is short, 2.5 hours in
geese, it is combined with short-acting sulfonamide drugs. Oral
bioavailability is excellent in birds.

ADVERSE AND COMMON SIDE EFFECTS: Regurgitation has
been reported after oral administration of trimethoprim-sulfonamide drugs to raptors and psittacines, especially macaws. Facial
flushing and gastrointestinal stasis have also been reported in some
species, again particularly in macaws. Pigeons tolerate oral medication well. Decreased food and water consumption and anemia have
been described in 6-week broiler chickens given up to 4.4 times the
recommended dose.

DRUG INTERACTIONS: Trimethoprim sulfadiazine has been used
in combination with pyrimethamine for the treatment of sarcocystosis in one eclectus and two Amazon parrots.

SUPPLIED AS: VETERINARY PRODUCTS
For injection containing 40 mg/mL trimethoprim and 200 mg/mL
sulfadiazine [Tribrissen 24% ✦]
For injection containing 40 mg/mL trimethoprim and 200 mg/mL
sulfadoxine [Bimotrin ✦, Borgal ✦, Trimidox ✦, Trivetrin ✦]
For injection containing 80 mg/mL trimethoprim and 400 mg/mL
sulfadiazine [Tribrissen 48% ✦]
Tablets containing trimethoprim plus sulfadiazine in the following
combinations: 5 + 25, 20 + 100, 80 + 400 [DiTrim ★, Tribrissen ✦ ★]
Oral suspension containing 9.1 mg trimethoprim and 45.5 mg sulfa-
diazine/mL [Tribrissen ★]

HUMAN PRODUCTS
Oral suspensions containing 40 mg trimethoprim and 200 mg sulfamethoxazole/5 mL [Bactrim ✚ ★, Septra ✚ ★, and many others]
Oral suspensions containing 45 mg trimethoprim and 205 mg sulfadiazine /5 mL [Coptin ✚]

TYLOSIN

INDICATIONS: Tylosin (Tylan ✚ ★, Tylocine ✚, Tylosin ★) is a macrolide antibiotic. It has activity against some gram-negative and gram-positive bacteria, spirochetes, chlamydiae, and mycoplasmas. For more information, see **TYLOSIN** in the Small Animal section.

In avian medicine, tylosin is used primarily for the treatment of mycoplasmal infections, especially of the respiratory tract, and conjunctivitis. In pharmacokinetic studies in chickens, bobwhite quail, pigeons, sandhill cranes, and emus, a positive correlation was found between half-life and body weight. Tylosin was rapidly absorbed, attaining peak plasma levels within 30 to 90 minutes, and penetrated rapidly into tissues. Tissue levels, especially kidney and liver, were higher than those of plasma. Six hours after administration, tylosin levels in lung, liver, and kidney were greater than 1 µg/mL, the minimal inhibitory concentration for many susceptible microorganisms, even though plasma levels were barely detectable. Nebulization for 1 hour resulted in effective antibiotic levels in the lungs and air sacs of pigeons and quail; however, in quail tissue levels were negligible by 1 and 3 hours, respectively, after nebulization was completed. Systemic absorption was minimal.

Tylosin was used successfully to treat *Mycoplasma gallisepticum* conjunctivitis in house finches. The drug was placed in the drinking water at a concentration of 1 mg/mL for 21 to 77 days. The recommended dose in poultry is 0.5 mg/mL for 4 to 8 days. The birds were also treated ophthalmically with ciprofloxacin for 5 to 7 days. At the end of the treatment period, conjunctival cultures on all birds were negative; however 2 of 18 birds were positive on polymerase chain reaction. The carrier status could not be ruled out based on this research, but *M. gallisepticum* could not be isolated from necropsied birds.

Rheas with respiratory and ocular disease, from whose tracheal swabs *Mycoplasma synoviae* and *Escherichia coli* were isolated, responded rapidly to a single shot of long-acting doxycycline, medication of the drinking water with 1.1 g/mL tylosin for 4 weeks, and direct ophthalmic therapy with tylosin powder diluted 1:10 in sterile water.

ADVERSE AND COMMON SIDE EFFECTS: Drinking water containing tylosin powder has a bitter taste that may need to be masked for adequate water consumption.

DRUG INTERACTIONS: In an experimental study, DMSO added to tylosin for nebulization resulted in a greater level and longer duration of antibiotic concentration in the lung and air sacs.

SUPPLIED AS: VETERINARY PRODUCTS
See **TYLOSIN** in the Small Animal section for injectable and tablet formulations, and in the Large Animal section for products intended for the drinking water.

VIOKASE-V

INDICATIONS: Viokase ✦ ★ is a mixture containing standardized activities of the pancreatic enzymes lipase, amylase, and protease used for the management of pancreatic exocrine insufficiency.

In birds, Viokase is used for the treatment of pancreatic insufficiency, delayed crop emptying, and maldigestion. The compound is mixed with moistened food or given by gavage. Food should be incubated for 15 minutes before feeding. Other commercial products are also available.

SUPPLIED AS: VETERINARY PRODUCT
Powder or tablets containing lipase, protease, and amylase [Viokase-V ★]
HUMAN PRODUCT
Powder or tablets containing lipase, protease, and amylase [Viokase ✦ ★]

VITAMIN A

INDICATIONS: Vitamin A [Aquasol A ★] is used in the treatment of hypovitaminosis A and during the therapy of avian pox virus infections, chronic sinusitis, and ophthalmic disorders. Long-term therapy may be required to replenish liver stores.

SUPPLIED AS: HUMAN PRODUCTS
Capsules containing 10,000, 25,000 or 50,000 IU [Aquasol A ★]
Solution containing 50,000 IU/mL [Aquasol A ★]
For injection containing 50,000 USP U/mL [Aquasol A Parenteral ★]

VITAMIN B₁ (THIAMINE)

INDICATIONS: Thiamine is used orally as a nutritional supplement in birds on fish diets that may be deficient in thiamine due to dietary thiaminase. Thiamine powder or capsules can be added to the food. Thiamine may also be helpful in the treatment of heavy metal toxicosis in some species. For more information, see **THIAMINE** in the Small Animal section.

DRUG INTERACTIONS: Injectable thiamine is also available in multiple B complex.

VITAMIN B COMPLEX

INDICATIONS: Vitamin B complex ♣ ★ is administered as a supportive therapy in the treatment of diseases characterized by debility, anemia, peripheral neuropathy, muscular weakness; to stimulate appetite; and following long-term antibiotic therapy.

ADVERSE AND COMMON SIDE EFFECTS: Overdose may result in anaphylaxis. Dose by thiamine content.

SUPPLIED AS: VETERINARY PRODUCTS
For injection containing various vitamin level combinations [Vitamin B Complex ♣ ★, Vita-Jec B Complex Fortified ★, Vita-Jec B Complex ★, Compound 150 ♣, Hi-Po B Complex ★, Vitamin B Complex Forte ★, Vitamin B Complex Fortified ★, Vitamin B Complex Fortified injection ★, Vitamin B Complex injection ★]
Oral syrup [V.A.L. Syrup ★]

VITAMIN B₁₂ (CYANOCOBALAMIN)

INDICATIONS: Vitamin B_{12} is used for the treatment of anemia.

ADVERSE AND COMMON SIDE EFFECTS: Pink droppings may result.

SUPPLIED AS: VETERINARY PRODUCTS
For injection containing
1,000 and 5,000 µg/mL [Vitamin B-12 ♣]
1,000, 3,000, and 5,000 µg/mL [Cyanocabalamin ★]
1,000 and 3,000 µg/mL [Vita-Jec B-12 ★]

VITAMIN C

See **ASCORBIC ACID**

VITAMIN D₃

INDICATIONS: Vitamin D_3 is used as a supplement for birds with calcium deficiency, and, in combination with vitamins A and E, as a general nutritional supplement. See **INJACOM 100** in this section.

ADVERSE AND COMMON SIDE EFFECTS: Particular caution should be taken in treating young psittacine birds on heavily fortified diets. Clinical hypervitaminosis D was described in a nursery containing macaw chicks.

SUPPLIED AS: VETERINARY PRODUCTS
For injection containing
80,000 IU/mL [Hydro-Vit D$_3$ ✚, Solu-Vit D$_3$ ✚]
1,000,000 IU/mL [Poten-D ✚, Downer-D ✚]

HUMAN PRODUCT
For injection containing 1 or 2 µg/mL of calcitriol [Calcijex ✚]

VITAMIN E + SELENIUM

INDICATIONS: Vitamin E has been used in the treatment of steatitis. Vitamin E and selenium are used in combination for the treatment of myopathies and muscular weakness. A syndrome of paralysis in cockatiels is vitamin E + selenium responsive. Supplementation may assist in the treatment of limb dysfunction in chicks. One report describes a positive clinical response to vitamin E + selenium therapy in mockingbirds that developed ascending paralysis while on a diet of cat food. Vitamin E + selenium is often administered to large birds after severe muscular exertion to prevent the occurrence of or reduce the severity of capture myopathy.

ADVERSE AND COMMON SIDE EFFECTS: Overdosage can result in selenium toxicity.

SUPPLIED AS: VETERINARY PRODUCTS
For injection containing Vitamin E
200, 300, 500 IU/mL [Vitamin E ★]
For injection containing Vitamin E + selenium
1 mg selenium and 50 mg vitamin E/mL [BO-SE ★, Seletoc ★]
2.5 mg selenium and 50 mg vitamin E/mL [E-SE ✚ ★]
3 mg selenium and 136 mg vitamin E/mL [Dystosel ✚, E-SEL ✚, Selon-E ✚]
5 mg selenium and 50 mg vitamin E/mL [MU-SE ★]
6.8 mg selenium and 136 mg vitamin E/mL [Dystosel DS ✚]

VITAMIN K$_1$

INDICATIONS: Vitamin K$_1$ or phytonadione, (Aqua-Mephyton ★, Mephyton ★, Konakion ★, Veta-K1 ✚ ★) is used to treat coagulopathies due to fat-soluble vitamin malabsorption such as occurs with long-term use of antibacterial agents, and vitamin K antagonism caused by salicylates, coumarins, and indanediones, including warfarin poisoning. For more information, see **VITAMIN K** in the Small Animal section.

In birds, vitamin K is used in the treatment of hemorrhagic disorders and as a preventive measure during long-term medication with amprolium or sulfonamide drugs. Decreased coagulability and hemorrhages have been seen in psittacine birds receiving the injectable doxycycline product Vibravenos. Concurrent treatment with vitamin K was partially protective.

XYLAZINE

INDICATIONS: Xylazine (Anased ♣ ★, Rompun ♣ ★) is an anesthetic agent characterized by a rapid onset, good to excellent sedation, excellent analgesia, and a smooth recovery. Its sedative effects last longer. For more information, see **XYLAZINE** in the Small Animal section.

In birds, xylazine is used in combination with ketamine for injectable anesthesia. This combination is not recommended for pet birds; the safety of inhalant agents such as isoflurane is considerably greater.

YOHIMBINE

INDICATIONS: Yohimbine (Yobine ♣ ★, Antagonil ♣ ★) is a competitive α_2-adrenergic blocking agent used to reverse the effects of xylazine and speed anesthetic recovery in a wide variety of avian species. Yohimbine is generally thought to have little effect on the cardiovascular system. For more information, see **XYLAZINE** in the Small Animal section.

ADVERSE AND COMMON SIDE EFFECTS: Excitement and mortality have been described in mammals receiving doses of more than 1 mg/kg.

DRUG INTERACTIONS: Administration of yohimbine should be delayed for approximately 20 to 30 minutes if ketamine has been used in combination with xylazine. Otherwise, reversal of the xylazine will leave an animal under the influence of ketamine alone, and recovery from anesthesia may not be smooth.

SUPPLIED AS: VETERINARY PRODUCTS
For injection containing 2 [Yobine ♣ ★] and 5 [Antagonil ♣ ★] mg/mL

INDEX

Numbers followed by a "t" indicate tabular material.